Advanced Image Processing and Computer Vision

Advanced Image Processing and Computer Vision

Guest Editors

Selene Tomassini
M. Ali Akber Dewan

MDPI

Basel • Beijing • Wuhan • Barcelona • Belgrade • Novi Sad • Cluj • Manchester

Guest Editors
Selene Tomassini
Department of Information Engineering and Computer Science
University of Trento
Trento
Italy

M. Ali Akber Dewan
School of Computing and Information Systems
Athabasca University
Athabasca, AB
Canada

Editorial Office
MDPI AG
Grosspeteranlage 5
4052 Basel, Switzerland

This is a reprint of the Special Issue, published open access by the journal *Computers* (ISSN 2073-431X), freely accessible at: http://www.mdpi.com.

For citation purposes, cite each article independently as indicated on the article page online and as indicated below:

Lastname, A.A.; Lastname, B.B. Article Title. *Journal Name* **Year**, *Volume Number*, Page Range.

ISBN 978-3-7258-5783-8 (Hbk)
ISBN 978-3-7258-5784-5 (PDF)
https://doi.org/10.3390/books978-3-7258-5784-5

Contents

Preface . . . . **vii**

Wejdan Alarefah, Salma Kammoun Jarraya and Nihal Abuzinadah
Transformer-Based Student Engagement Recognition Using Few-Shot Learning
Reprinted from: *Computers* **2025**, *14*, 109, https://doi.org/10.3390/computers14030109 . . . . . . **1**

Praveen Kumar Sekharamantry, Farid Melgani, Jonni Malacarne, Riccardo Ricci, Rodrigo de Almeida Silva and Jose Marcato Junior
A Seamless Deep Learning Approach for Apple Detection, Depth Estimation, and Tracking Using YOLO Models Enhanced by Multi-Head Attention Mechanism
Reprinted from: *Computers* **2025**, *13*, 83, https://doi.org/10.3390/computers13030083 . . . . . . **16**

Atsuki Matsui, Ryuto Ishibashi and Lin Meng
Optimizing Loss Functions for You Only Look Once Models: Improving Object Detection in Agricultural Datasets
Reprinted from: *Computers* **2025**, *14*, 44, https://doi.org/10.3390/computers14020044 . . . . . . **41**

Artyom M. Grigoryan and Alexis A. Gomez
Commutative Quaternion Algebra with Quaternion Fourier Transform-Based Alpha-Rooting Color Image Enhancement †
Reprinted from: *Computers* **2025**, *14*, 37, https://doi.org/10.3390/computers14020037 . . . . . . **58**

Christopher Henshaw, Jacob Dennis, Jonathan Nadzam and Alan J. Michaels
Number Recognition Through Color Distortion Using Convolutional Neural Networks
Reprinted from: *Computers* **2025**, *14*, 34, https://doi.org/10.3390/computers14020034 . . . . . . **84**

Ningning Xu and Jidong J. Yang
Leveraging Scene Geometry and Depth Information for Robust Image Deraining
Reprinted from: *Computers* **2025**, *14*, 11, https://doi.org/10.3390/computers14010011 . . . . . . **115**

Hina Kotani, Atsushi Teramoto, Tomoyuki Ohno, Yoshihiro Sobue, Eiichi Watanabe and Hiroshi Fujita
Atrial Fibrillation Type Classification by a Convolutional Neural Network Using Contrast-Enhanced Computed Tomography Images
Reprinted from: *Computers* **2024**, *13*, 309, https://doi.org/10.3390/computers13120309 . . . . . . **128**

Osmar Antonio Espinosa-Bernal, Jesús Carlos Pedraza-Ortega, Marco Antonio Aceves-Fernandez, Juan Manuel Ramos-Arreguín, Saul Tovar-Arriaga and Efrén Gorrostieta-Hurtado
Modified Multiresolution Convolutional Neural Network for Quasi-Periodic Noise Reduction in Phase Shifting Profilometry for 3D Reconstruction
Reprinted from: *Computers* **2024**, *13*, 290, https://doi.org/10.3390/computers14030109 . . . . . . **145**

R. S. Abdul Ameer, M. A. Ahmed, Z. T. Al-Qaysi, M. M. Salih and Moceheb Lazam Shuwandy
Empowering Communication: A Deep Learning Framework for Arabic Sign Language Recognition with an Attention Mechanism
Reprinted from: *Computers* **2024**, *13*, 153, https://doi.org/10.3390/computers13060153 . . . . . . **164**

Abdelaziz Daoudi and Saïd Mahmoudi
Enhancing Brain Segmentation in MRI through Integration of Hidden Markov Random Field Model and Whale Optimization Algorithm
Reprinted from: *Computers* **2024**, *13*, 124, https://doi.org/10.3390/computers13050124 . . . . . . **188**

Ihar Volkau, Sergei Krasovskii, Abdul Mujeeb and Helen Balinsky
Computer Vision Approach in Monitoring for Illicit and Copyrighted Objects in Digital Manufacturing
Reprinted from: *Computers* **2024**, *13*, 90, https://doi.org/10.3390/computers13040090 . . . . . . **210**

Momina Liaqat Ali and Zhou Zhang
The YOLO Framework: A Comprehensive Review of Evolution, Applications, and Benchmarks in Object Detection
Reprinted from: *Computers* **2024**, *13*, 336, https://doi.org/10.3390/computers13120336 . . . . . . **223**

Pushkar Kadam, Gu Fang and Ju Jia Zou
Object Tracking Using Computer Vision: A Review
Reprinted from: *Computers* **2024**, *13*, 136, https://doi.org/10.3390/computers13060136 . . . . . . **260**

Sowmik Kanti Deb and W. David Pan
Quantum Image Compression: Fundamentals, Algorithms, and Advances
Reprinted from: *Computers* **2024**, *13*, 185, https://doi.org/10.3390/computers13080185 . . . . . . **304**

Preface

This Reprint explores the rapidly evolving domain of AI-driven image processing and analysis, become central to modern technological innovation.

The scope of this Reprint spans fundamental research, algorithmic development, and applied methodologies, highlighting how AI has transformed the way visual information is interpreted, analyzed, and used across diverse scenarios. Particular attention is given to innovative AI-based algorithms that operate effectively under real-world constraints such as limited data availability, heterogeneous data quality, and the need for robust, adaptive solutions.

The motivation for compiling this Reprint arises from the growing demand for intelligent, human-centric technologies that are reliable. By bringing together contributions from leading experts and emerging researchers, this Reprint reflects both the maturity of established methods and the creativity of novel approaches.

This Reprint is intended for a broad audience, including academic researchers, graduate students, health/industry professionals, and policymakers interested in the current state and future directions of AI-driven image processing and analysis in order to inspire further research and foster interdisciplinary collaboration in fields such as medicine, agriculture, environmental monitoring, and beyond.

Selene Tomassini and M. Ali Akber Dewan
Guest Editors

computers

MDPI

Article

Transformer-Based Student Engagement Recognition Using Few-Shot Learning

Wejdan Alarefah *, Salma Kammoun Jarraya * and Nihal Abuzinadah

Computer Science Department, Faculty of Computing and Information Technology, King Abdulaziz University (KAU), Jeddah 21589, Saudi Arabia; nabuznadah@kau.edu.sa
* Correspondence: wabdullahalghamdi0002@stu.kau.edu.sa (W.A.); smohamad1@kau.edu.sa (S.K.J.)

Abstract: Improving the recognition of online learning engagement is a critical issue in educational information technology, due to the complexities of student behavior and varying assessment standards. Additionally, the scarcity of publicly available datasets for engagement recognition exacerbates this challenge. The majority of existing methods for detecting student engagement necessitate significant amounts of annotated data to capture variations in behaviors and interaction patterns. To address these limitations, we investigate few-shot learning (FSL) techniques to reduce the dependency on extensive training data. Transformer-based models have shown comprehensive results for video-based facial recognition tasks, thus paving new ground for understanding complicated patterns. In this research, we propose an innovative FSL model that employs a prototypical network with the vision transformer (ViT) model pre-trained on a face recognition dataset (e.g., MS1MV2) for spatial feature extraction, followed by an LSTM layer for temporal feature extraction. This approach effectively addresses the challenges of limited labeled data in engagement recognition. Our proposed approach achieves state-of-the-art performance on the EngageNet dataset, demonstrating its efficacy and potential in advancing engagement recognition research.

Keywords: few-shot learning; vision transformer; student engagement recognition

1. Introduction

The use of online learning has become mainstream, and it has recently played a key role in the educational field. Online learning helps students by taking advantage of computer techniques, allowing teachers to provide lessons to students efficiently [1].

However, the recognition of e-learning engagement is a critical issue in educational technology. Traditional methodologies are insufficient to assess engagement in all situations, and student performance in online learning environments often suffers due to the limited interaction between teachers and students [1]. In addition, due to the complexities of student participation, as well as the influence of diverse definitions and standards, its evaluation and measurement are also challenging. As a result, teachers are unable to assess the level of student engagement; thus, methods for the efficient and automatic recognition of students' learning engagement are required.

Typical approaches for identifying and assessing engagement include (a) self-reporting, (b) observational checklists and rating scales, and (c) automated measures that use technical tools to detect students' engagement, such as facial expression recognition [2] [3,4], body gesture recognition [5], and head pose and eye gaze tracking [6].

The automated measurements are more objective than the other two methods [3]. Most of these measurements come from computer vision-based tools which have been

https://doi.org/10.3390/computers14030109

shown to be effective in detecting e-learners' degrees of engagement [5]. Computer vision methodologies have demonstrated greater appropriateness for online learning due to their reduced distractibility for users, alongside the widespread availability and affordability of the requisite equipment and software for data recording and evaluation [7]. One of the biggest challenges in this field is the extremely limited number of datasets relating to student engagement. The majority of existing methods for detecting student engagement necessitate significant amounts of annotated data to capture variations in behaviors and interaction patterns, which can be expensive at times [8]. Moreover, traditional supervised learning methods demonstrated limited performance in the student engagement recognition task. However, few-shot learning techniques can be implemented in order to reduce the amount of data used/required in training. Although few-shot learning approaches have significantly advanced computer vision, to the best of our knowledge, they have not yet been explored in the context of student engagement recognition in online learning.

In this research, we aim to investigate the appropriateness of few-shot learning for student engagement recognition using the dataset produced by [5] and the EngageNet dataset [9].

Few-shot learning (FSL) is a meta-learning problem in which models are evaluated through an N-way, K-shot classification problem [10], in which the model learns k samples from N classes. The few-shot learning technique can identify novel classes using only a few samples once it has been deployed [8]. The objective of FSL is to overcome the obstacles faced by deep learning techniques, which include the rarity of samples, the high effort required for collecting data, and the high cost of the computational process [8]. FSL is a step on the way to mimicking human-like learning. Hence, FSL has been used in a wide range of real-world applications, including computer vision, robotics, acoustic signal processing, and natural language processing [8].

Vision Transformers (ViTs), as proposed in [11], have become a powerful feature representation model and were recently used widely, including the following research works: [11–13]. Vision Transformers provide comparable performance for understanding video-based facial recognition context.

In this research, we propose an FSL model that employs a prototypical network with the vision transformer (ViT) model pre-trained on a face recognition dataset (e.g., MS1MV2) for spatial feature extraction, followed by an LSTM layer for temporal feature extraction. We investigated the suitability of few-shot learning for recognition of student engagement level and explored the accuracy achieved through utilizing the specific architecture on the dataset collected in [5]. The novelty of our approach lies in the combination of Vision Transformers and Few-Shot Learning to handle the challenges of limited labeled data in engagement recognition, unlike traditional ML methods which rely hugely on the amount of training data.

The rest of this paper is organized as follows: Section 2 reviews the related work on student engagement recognition, few-shot learning, and Vision Transformers. Section 3 details the proposed methodology. Section 4 presents the experimental setup and results, including the dataset and model architecture, and Section 5 concludes with a discussion and future directions.

2. Literature Review

2.1. Student Engagement Recognition

In the context of online learning, many uncontrollable factors affect student engagement, such as the learning environment and information interruption; therefore, teachers must use a system that can recognize student engagement during online learning [1]. Various studies have explored student engagement recognition in online learning, ranging from single-model to multi-model approaches [14]. Visual cues are used in computer vision-based approaches, such as facial expressions [2–4], body gestures [5], and eye gaze [6].

Zhang et al. [3] used mouse movements from students' facial expressions to improve labeling accuracy. Later on, adaptive weighted Local Gray Code Patterns and quick sparse representation techniques were employed for feature extraction and classification. Altuwairqi et al. [2] carried out a number of investigations into the recognition of students' engagement levels depending on their emotions; they linked each level of engagement with specific emotions by computing the Matching-Score (MS) and Mis-Matching Score (MisMS) for both matched and unmatched emotions at each engagement level.

The usability of convolutional neural networks (CNNs) has been investigated in this field. Nezami et al. [4] proposed a CNN model that was adapted from the VGG-B framework, and then they pre-trained the model on the FER-2013 dataset and fine-tuned it using their engagement recognition dataset (ER). Khenkar et al. [5] investigated a deep three-dimensional CNN model for the recognition of e-learners' engagements based on spatio-temporal features of micro-body gestures. The authors also used a transfer learning approach to the 3D CNN model trained on the Sports-1M dataset. The resulting accuracy shows the efficiency of using body gestures for engagement recognition. Another work [7] used multiple CNN architectures, including All-Convolutional-Network (ALL-CNN), Network-in Network (NiN-CNN), and Very-Deep-Convolutional-Network (VD-CNN). In addition, motivated by these models, the authors proposed a model that achieved higher accuracy for the students' engagement classification. Kaur et al. [6] used a Multi-Instance Learning (MIL) deep network for the prediction and localization of the learners' eye gaze movements and head pose characteristics, then passed these features through the LSTM-based network and flattened the output. The resulting vector passed through three dense layers and average pooling, producing a single regressed engagement value.

While Hasnine et al. [14] associated student emotions with engagement levels, their approach lacked validation with diverse datasets, which we address using few-shot learning techniques. The developed model consists of four phases conducted in the following order: the first phase involves face recognition using the OpenCV Library, emotion detection using CNN, eye detection, and engagement recognition using the Concentration index. The model was tested using videos captured from a web camera available on YouTube, including eleven students; therefore, the validation of the model did not use an appropriate dataset. While numerous machine learning and deep learning methodologies have been explored for the recognition of student engagement, few-shot learning techniques have not been thoroughly investigated for this purpose, to the best of our knowledge.

2.2. Few-Shot Learning Technique

Most deep learning methods are unable to learn from a few examples in real-world scenarios where data are scarce, and they tend to overfit. Therefore, there is a large volume of published studies describing the role of using only a few samples. A novel paradigm shift known as few-shot learning allows for the development of models that can rapidly learn a new category from a small number of training examples. Supervised machine learning models, on the other hand, need a significant volume of data to be more accurate. In few-shot learning, the model is trained using numerous training tasks (also called episodes) [8]. Each task contains its own support set and query set that include N classes and K samples (known as N-way, K-shot), as shown in Figure 1, and few-shot learning is called "one-shot learning" when there is only one sample per class. In each task, the model is trained on the support set and verified using the query set, after which the model is evaluated using a test task that contains its own support and query sets that are not included in the training [15]. In other words, once the few-shot learning model has been trained, it will be able to classify new classes using previously acquired information and with the help of additional information (the support set) [16].

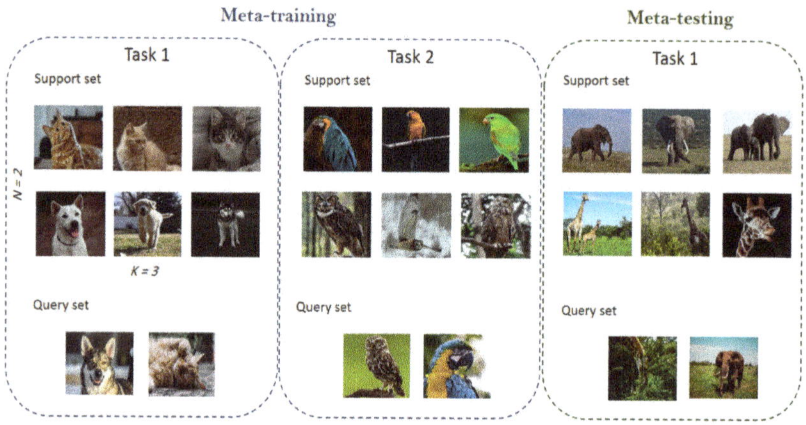

Figure 1. An example of a 2-way 3-shots classification task for few-shot learning.

According to Liu et al. [10], few-shot learning approaches based on meta-learning can be categorized into metric-, optimization-, and model-based learning.

Metric-based learning mainly consists of three phases, as follows. The initial step is to derive a metric space from a set of training samples using a network in which samples from the same class are near together and samples from other classes are far apart [17]. After the network has been trained, it can be regarded as an embedding function. The second phase is to extract features from all the testing data set samples. The final phase involves classifying the testing samples using similarity function (Euclidean or Cosine distance) [18].

Maddula et al. [17] introduced a Meta-Learning Approach to Recognize Emotions (MLARE), utilizing a Siamese network alongside a binary cross-entropy loss mechanism (BCE) combined with sigmoid activation as the loss function in order to improve accuracy. The Prototypical Network [15] is another metric-based learning approach that uses a non-linear neural network which maps the input into an embedding space and defines the prototype of each class as the average of its support set within the embedding space. The classification of an embedded query point is subsequently executed by locating the closest class prototype.

Sung et al. [19] proposed Relation Network, a flexible metric-based model comprised of two modules; first, the used embedding module concatenates the resulting feature vector of each sample in the support set with the feature vector of the query sample, then feeds them into the relation module, which calculates the relation score between the query sample and each sample in the support set.

2.3. Vision Transformer

Transformers' uncomplicated architecture enables the processing of a variety of modalities (e.g., images, videos, text, and audio) with comparable processing blocks. Additionally, it has the capability to efficiently replace the CNN models in deep neural networks since the pioneering development of the Vision Transformer (ViT) [11], which introduced the use of transformers for image classification tasks with minimal changes by dividing each image into patches, embedding them, and concatenating the embeddings with positional encodings before passing them to the transformer block. As illustrated in Figure 2, the transformer block comprises a multi-head attention layer and a multi-layer perceptron (MLP) layer, each preceded by normalization layers. Dosovitskiy et al. [11] trained the transformers on very large dataset, revealing that data-hungry models. Then, Touvron et al. [20] produced the Data-efficient Image Transformer (DeiT) to demonstrate that transformers can be trained with mid-size datasets (e.g., ImageNet-1k) by leveraging several data augmentation methods and novel distillation techniques. The research [12] explored that the ViT can perform well on smaller datasets in the field of face recognition through employing patch-level data augmentation techniques.

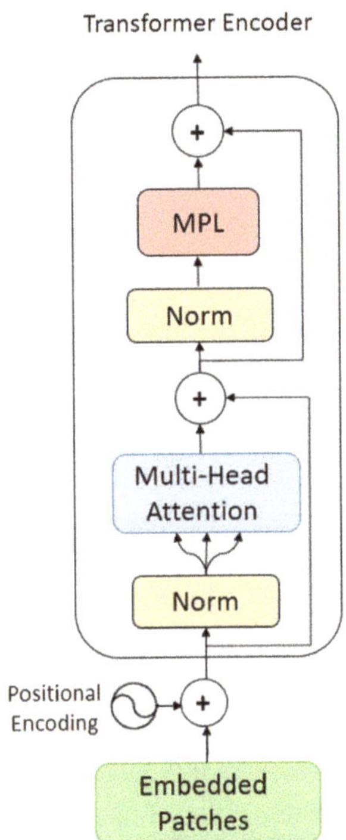

Figure 2. The architecture of the Vision Transformer Encoder.

Some studies have investigated the use of transformers for recognizing student engagement [13,16,21]. However, as previously stated, a major challenge in this field is the extremely limited availability of data for recognizing student engagement levels.

Therefore, this research investigates the efficiency of applying few-shot learning techniques to improve online learning methods. To the best of our knowledge, combining Vision Transformers (ViTs) with LSTM layers in few-shot learning scenarios remains a relatively unexplored area of research.

3. Proposed Architecture

The proposed few-shot learning model (see Figure 3) integrates a Vision Transformer (ViT) with a Long Short-Term Memory (LSTM) network to extract spatio-temporal features for engagement recognition in videos of students learning online. Additionally, it leverages the episodic training approach with prototypical loss to improve the generalization capability when using limited labeled data. The first stage involves preprocessing videos by extracting 16 frames from each, followed by normalization and resizing to 112 $\times$ 112 pixels. The second stage involves the feature extraction model, and the last stage includes computing the prototypes and the losses.

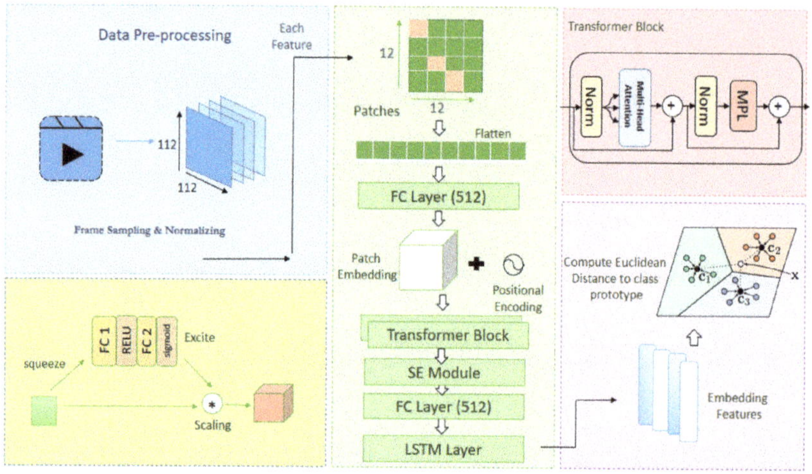

Figure 3. The overall architecture of our approach. We utilized the vision transformer model with the SE module to enhance the extracted features, followed by a dimensionality reduction layer and LSTM layer for temporal feature extraction; then, the prototypes were computed for classification.

Vision Transformer Backbone

We selected the TransFace ViT model [12] pre-trained on the MS1MV2 dataset, due to its proven performance in facial recognition tasks, which are critical for detecting engagement cues. Figure 3 shows how we integrate the TransFace model with the LSTM layer.

The Vision Transformer (ViT) processes each frame independently to extract spatial features. We follow the typical Transformer formulation. Key operations in this module include patch embedding, positional encoding, and transformer-based feature extraction. Each frame is divided into P × P non-overlapping patches; then, each patch is flattened and projected into an embedding space of dimension D. To retain spatial information, a learnable positional encoding is added to the patch embeddings.

A stack of transformer blocks processes the token sequence. Each block consists of normalization layers, a multi-head self-attention mechanism and a feed-forward network (FFN).

$$H = A(Q,K,V) = softmax\left(\frac{QK^T}{\sqrt{d}}\right)V \tag{1}$$

The self-attention mechanism A enhances the dot-product attention operation by organizing three components: queries, keys, and values (q,k,v) into matrix structures (Q,K,V). The mechanism for self-attention utilizes a softmax function to determine the weights of attention for each value in V by calculating a dot product among all queries in Q and all keys in K.

The output of the ViT for each frame is a high-dimensional feature vector, which is flattened into a 1D representation for further processing. Next, each feature vector is scaled using the squeeze and excitation module which highly improve the accuracy. Then, to reduce the computational complexity and align the feature dimensions with the LSTM input requirements, a linear layer is applied. The LSTM network processes sequences of feature vectors to capture temporal dynamics.

The model is trained using prototypical loss in an episodic manner of training. For each class c, a prototype P_c is computed as the mean of the support embeddings. We use

Euclidean distance as a similarity function, and then the probability of the query be-longing to class c is given by the softmax over distances, as follows:

$$P(y = c|f_{query}) = \frac{exp\ (-d(f_{query}, P_c))}{\sum_{\acute{c}} exp\ (-d(f_{query}, P_{\acute{c}}))} \quad (2)$$

The prototypical loss minimizes the negative log-likelihood of the correct class:

$$L_{proto} = -\frac{1}{n_{query}} \sum_{i=1}^{n_{query}} log\ P(y_i = c_i | f_{query,i}) \quad (3)$$

4. Experimental Results

4.1. Dataset

To evaluate our approach, we employed two student engagement recognition datasets: the Khenkar Dataset [5] for training and the EngageNet dataset [9] for testing to follow the few-shot learning settings.

Khenkar Dataset [4]: The datasets in the field of student engagement recognition are very limited, and one of the most reliable available datasets is the Khenkar Dataset [5], which contains multi-class videos (High-, Medium-, Low-Engagement and Disengagement) annotated by experts using the emotion-based affective model [2]. Over 2476 video clips are included in the dataset. Each video clip ranges from 2 to 40 s long and was collected from 24 lectures involving five college students. The dataset was collected in an uncontrolled setting and captured using built-in webcams, representative of the natural environment of an e-learning student. We used the color jetter and horizontal flip augmentation techniques to balance the unbalanced classes in the dataset. The final class distribution is shown in Table 1. We then split the dataset as 70% for training and 30% for validation.

Table 1. The sample distribution on the Khenkar Dataset.

Engagement Level	# of Samples
High engagement	2936
Medium engagement	2199
Low engagement	1890
Disengagement	1090

EnagageNet dataset [9]: The EngageNet dataset was utilized in the meta-testing stage of our approach. Each clip contains 10 s of video at a frame rate of 30 frames per second and a size of 1280 × 720 pixels. Four levels of engagement have been assigned to the video records of the subjects: "Not Engaged", "Barely Engaged", "Engaged", and "Highly Engaged". A subject-independent data split method was used to divide the dataset into 7983 samples for training, 1071 samples for validation, and 2257 samples for testing [9]. However, the testing data are not available to the public, so we used the validation set to test our model. During the experiments, we observed a high overlap between classes from the EngageNet dataset. We used Maximum Mean Discrepancy (*MMD*) [22], which represents the distance between distributions as follows.

$$MMD^2 = \frac{\sum_{i \neq j} K(X_i, X_j)}{n(n-1)} + \frac{\sum_{i \neq j} K(Y_i, Y_j)}{m(m-1)} - 2 \cdot \frac{\sum_{i,j} K(X_i, Y_j)}{n \cdot m} \quad (4)$$

The results of computing the *MMD* between the highly engaged class with the en-gaged and barely engaged classes were 0.003 and 0.01, respectively. This indicates a very small difference between their distributions. Therefore, we combined these three labels

"Highly-engaged", "Engaged", "Barely-engaged", into a single label, "Engaged", while the latter label, "Not-Engaged", remained unchanged. This then yielded a binary classification task, as outlined in Table 2. The testing process was episodic, and we selected relatively equal samples from each class.

Table 2. Sample distribution among the combined classes in the EnagageNet dataset.

Before	After	# of Samples
Highly-Engaged Engaged Barely-Engaged	Engaged	130
Not-Engaged	Not-Engaged	130

4.2. Implementation Details

In this research, we incorporated the TransFace pre-trained model [12] in our framework as a spatial feature extractor with an LSTM network for temporal features. We first split the video clips into smaller clips ranging from 3 to 10 s in length, and the number of samples in each class is shown in Table 1. Then, we used uniform sampling for frame extraction, which involves selecting 16 frames at regular intervals from a video and then normalizing and resizing each frame to be 112 × 112, which is the expected shape for the ViT model. We trained our model for 100 epochs with 20 episodes. Adam was chosen as the optimizer with a learning rate of 0.0001 and 0.001 as a weight decay. To optimize the learning process and prevent overfitting during training, we employed the ReduceLROn-Plateau learning rate scheduler. This scheduler adaptively reduced the learning rate when validation loss plateaued, ensuring more efficient convergence.

The TransFace model was fine-tuned with 12 transformer blocks, each with eight attention heads; see Table 3.

Table 3. The details of the proposed model.

	Model
# of Frames/clip	16
Learning Rate	0.0001
Weight Decay	0.001
Epochs	100
Iterations/Episodes	20
Batch-Size	40
Transformer Blocks	12 each with 512 dim
Attention Heads	8
Optimizer	ReduceLROnPlateau
Loss	Prototypical Loss
Similarity Measure	Euclidean Distance

We trained the framework with four classes: high-engagement, medium-engagement, low-engagement, and disengagement classes. The proposed model achieved 97% training accuracy and 90% validation accuracy during the meta-training stage in a 4-way 5-shot scenario.

4.3. Evaluation Metrics

To assess our results we employed multiple performance measures including Accuracy, Precision, Recall, and F1-measure as follows:

$$\text{Accuracy} = \frac{True\ Positives + True\ Negatives}{Total\ Number\ of\ Samples} \times 100\% \tag{5}$$

$$\text{Precision} = \frac{True\ Positives}{True\ Positives + False\ Positives} \tag{6}$$

$$\text{Recall} = \frac{True\ Positives}{True\ Positives + False\ Negatives} \tag{7}$$

$$\text{F1-measure} = 2 \times \frac{Precision \times Recall}{Precision + Recall} \tag{8}$$

These metrics were selected to provide a comprehensive evaluation of our model's performance in different aspects.

4.4. Results on the Unseen: EngageNet

Table 4 and Figure 4 present the testing results on the EngageNet dataset. Our results are obtained over 10 runs, each consisting of 26 iterations, where each iteration includes 5 support samples and 5 query samples. The proposed model achieved an overall accuracy of 73.62% $\pm$ 2.66% in the binary classification task, indicating a 95% confidence interval (CI) between 70.96% and 76.28%. According to the confusion matrix shown in Figure 4, the model correctly classified 75% ($\pm$4.9%) of Engaged instances (true positive rate) and 76% ($\pm$4.7%) of Not-Engaged instances (true negative rate). However, 25% of Engaged instances were misclassified as Not-Engaged, while 24% of Not-Engaged instances were misclassified as Engaged, suggesting challenges in differentiating subtle engagement cues.

Table 4. The few-shot evaluation with EngageNet dataset.

Metric	2-Way 5-Shot					
	TransFace ViT			Swin ViT		
	Engaged	Not-Engaged	Avg.	Engaged	Not-Engaged	Avg.
Precision	0.7495 ± 0.1153	0.7597 ± 0.1244	0.7546	0.5758 ± 0.15033	0.57615 ± 0.1412	0.5759
Recall	0.7251 ± 0.1527	0.7348 ± 0.1467	0.7299	0.5552 ± 0.1743	0.5819 ± 0.1740	0.5686
F1-Measure	0.7158 ± 0.1094	0.7235 ± 0.1077	0.7197	0.5445 ± 0.1385	0.5560 ± 0.1350	0.5503
Accuracy	0.7362 ± 0.0266			0.5686 ± 0.0231		

The confusion matrix reveals higher misclassification rates for engaged students, which is likely due to subtle differences between the 'Engaged' and 'Not-Engaged' classes that the model struggles to differentiate. Additionally, due to the limited number of samples in the 'Not-Engaged' class, some samples were repeated as part of the support set, while the 'Engaged' class contained more diverse samples.

As illustrated in Table 4 and Figure 5, the Not-Engaged class has higher recall (0.76) and a better F1 score (0.72) compared to the Engaged class (recall 0.74, F1 0.71). This indicates that the model is better at detecting "Not-Engaged" examples.

Furthermore, we evaluated the inference speed to assess the model's feasibility for real-time applications. We utilized an end device equipped with an Intel Core(TM) i7-7500U CPU (2.70 GHz) and 8 GB RAM, running python 3.10 with Pytorch 1.13. The proposed approach achieves an average inference time of 36.5705 s per image with a 95% confidence interval of ±2.7354 s, indicating its potential for real-time engagement recognition in classrooms.

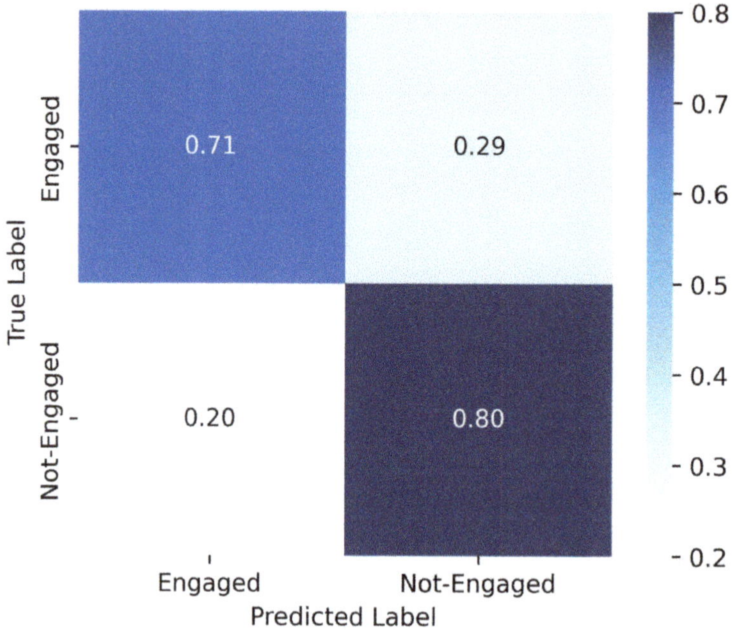

Figure 4. Confusion matrix of the proposed TransFace ViT + LSTM model on EngageNet dataset.

To evaluate our results, we explore our approach with the Swin ViT model [23], which is a benchmark backbone that demonstrated strong results in the field of image classification due to its robust hierarchical feature extraction capabilities, making it suitable for addressing challenges in engagement classification.

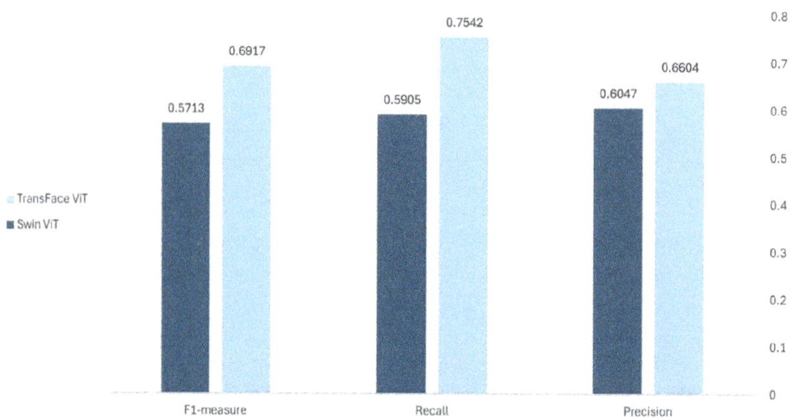

Figure 5. Comparison between the TransFace ViT model and the Swin ViT.

Under the same conditions, we combined the Swin ViT pre-trained model on the ImageNet-1K dataset with the LSTM layer. The model was fine-tuned alongside the remaining components using the same settings outlined in Table 2. The Swin ViT model achieved 98% training accuracy and 92% validation accuracy.

The TransFace ViT model outperforms the Swin ViT model with a significantly higher accuracy of 74% compared to 57%. This demonstrates the effectiveness of the TransFace ViT model in correctly classifying engagement levels. The results further confirm that the TransFace ViT model is better suited for binary classification tasks involving engagement recognition. While Swin ViT has shown success in image classification tasks, its performance in engagement recognition is comparatively weaker, particularly in terms of recall (0.57) compared to TransFace ViT's (0.74) and F1-measure (0.55) compared to TransFace ViT's (0.73). The overall performance of the proposed approach with the TransFace ViT model demonstrated consistent and promising results.

4.5. Comparison Performance

Table 5 compares various models that have been explored for student engagement recognition, utilizing diverse methods. The deep learning approaches, such as the EfficientNet B7 + LSTM model [24], and the transformer-based models, such as the Video Vision Transformer (ViViT) [25] and the Vision Transformer + Temporal Convolutional Network [16], have been implemented, and they, respectively, achieved 67.48%, 63.9%, and 65.58% improvements in temporal understanding. However, these methods face some challenges in distinguishing engagement levels. Another work employed the VGG16 fine-tuned model [26] and achieved 74.9% accuracy. However, traditional convolutional neural networks (CNNs) have been widely implemented but often require large amounts of labeled data. The Temporal Convolutional Network with Autoencoder (TCN-AE) [27] utilizes time-series data to capture behavioral and emotional cues, reporting an AUC ROC of 0.7489.

Table 5. Comparison of previous engagement measurement approaches with the proposed approach in this paper.

Ref	Feature Extraction	Method	Task Type	Accuracy
Mandia et al. [25]	Detect faces using the Multi-task Cascaded Convolutional Network (MTCNN)	Video Vision Transformer (ViViT) based architecture named Transformer Encoder with Low Complexity (TELC)	Multi-class	63.9%
Zhang et al. [16]	Facial features	Vision transformer + Temporal convolutional network	Multi-class	65.58
Selim et al. [24]	CNN	EfficientNet B7 + LSTM	Multi-class	67.48%
Abedi et al. [27]	Time-series data sequences extracted from both the behavioral feature and emotional states	Temporal convolutional network with autoencoder TCN-AE	Binary	(AUC ROC) 0.7489
Tieu et al. [26]	CNN	Fine-tune the VGG16	Binary	74.9%
(Proposed model)	Vision transformer	Proposed Model (ViT + LSTM + FSL)	Binary	74%

The proposed model (ViT + LSTM + few-shot learning) outperforms binary classification methods with 74% accuracy, demonstrating its effectiveness in student engagement recognition and addressing the challenges of limited labeled data. Integrating Vision Transformers for spatial feature extraction, LSTMs for temporal feature extraction, and few-shot learning to generalize from limited samples, the model enhances engagement recognition compared to traditional CNN- or LSTM-based methods. These findings suggest that leveraging transformer architectures with few-shot learning can significantly improve engagement recognition in real-world educational settings.

5. Discussion

As the proposed few-shot learning model, which integrates a Vision Transformer (ViT) with an LSTM layer, was trained on a limited set of video clips and generalizes to unseen data with 75% accuracy, teachers can implement it in real classroom settings to automatically assess student engagement levels from video recordings captured via a webcam. This approach automates engagement recognition and helps educators adapt their teaching strategies based on students' responsiveness.

Our model showed lower classification rates on the Engaged students due to the challenges regarding the engagement recognition of the data collected in a realistic setting with diverse conditions and different participants' ages. The participants were free to move around and sometimes become far from their devices with no restrictions on lighting or backgrounds. These factors contributed to increased variability, making engagement recognition more complex.

To further investigate the results proposed by our model, we have utilized the t-SNE (t-distributed Stochastic Neighbor Embedding) model to visualize the feature space learned during the training. However, as shown in Figure 6, the t-SNE plot indicates that data points from different engagement levels (i.e., "Engaged" vs. "Not-Engaged") cluster closely in the reduced dimensional space, suggesting substantial overlap in their underlying features. Moreover, engagement is frequently a subtle, continuous cue rather than a precisely defined category variable. Our t-SNE results highlight that certain "borderline" samples share characteristics of both classes.

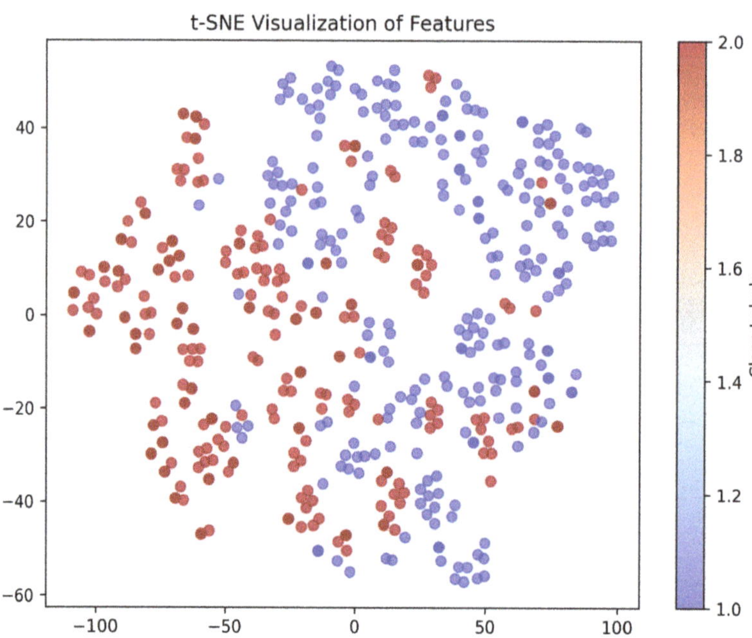

Figure 6. T-SNE visualization of extracted features from the EngageNet dataset.

Despite the model's promising performance, certain constraints about the utilized datasets must be noted. The Khenkar dataset, used for training, consists of only five students with video clips collected from their devices under varying lighting conditions and camera angles. While this introduces some diversity, the small sample size may limit the model's ability to generalize to broader student populations. The EngageNet dataset, with 127 participants aged 18 to 37 years, provides a wider range of engagement expressions and was annotated by three expert observers. Both datasets include computer-based and in-the-wild settings and were annotated using behavioral (facial and body cues) and cognitive (self-reports) dimensions. However, a notable imbalance exists in the engagement labels, with the 'not engaged' class being significantly smaller than the other categories, limiting the number of test clips to 130. To improve generalizability, future work should explore the model's performance on larger and more diverse datasets, including different educational settings, age groups, and cultural backgrounds.

6. Conclusions and Future Directions

We introduced a novel approach for recognizing student engagement in online learning environments, integrating few-shot learning with Vision Transformers (ViT) and Long Short-Term Memory (LSTM) networks. The proposed model was combined with a prototypical loss in an episodic training approach to address the challenge of limited labeled data. The experimental results indicate that the proposed model achieved highly promising results on the EngageNet dataset. The results highlight the importance of incorporating specialized models such as TransFace ViT for engagement classification tasks.

Future research directions involve investigating real-time deployment scenarios and integrating additional few-shot learning techniques, such as optimization-based methods, to enhance model performance. Moreover, to enhance the practicality of the proposed model, future work should focus on improving inference speed and computational efficiency for real-time classroom applications. We intend to benchmark latency, memory usage, and energy consumption against existing models, addressing the trade-offs between accuracy and resource constraints. Additionally, future research should incorporate multimodal data (audio features and physiological signals). Integrating these modalities with the vision cue data will significantly enhance the model's performance for recognizing subtle features of engagement.

Author Contributions: Conceptualization, W.A. and S.K.J.; data curation, W.A. and S.K.J.; formal analysis, W.A.; funding acquisition, W.A., S.K.J. and N.A.; investigation, W.A.; methodology, W.A. and S.K.J.; project administration, S.K.J.; resources, W.A.; software, W.A.; supervision, S.K.J. and N.A.; validation, S.K.J. and N.A.; visualization, W.A.; writing—original draft, W.A.; writing—review and editing, S.K.J. and N.A. All authors have read and agreed to the published version of the manuscript.

Funding: This research was funded by Deputyship for Research and Innovation, Ministry of Education in Saudi Arabia, through project number (IFPRC-054-612-2020) and King Abdulaziz University, DSR, Jeddah, Saudi Arabia.

Data Availability Statement: The dataset is not publicly available, due to privacy and institutional restrictions.

Conflicts of Interest: The authors declare no conflicts of interest.

References

1. Hu, M.; Li, H. Student engagement in online learning: A review. In Proceedings of the 2017 International Symposium on Educational Technology, ISET 2017, Hong Kong, China, 27–29 June 2017; Institute of Electrical and Electronics Engineers Inc.: Piscataway, NJ, USA, 2017; pp. 39–43. [CrossRef]
2. Altuwairqi, K.; Jarraya, S.K.; Allinjawi, A.; Hammami, M. A new emotion–based affective model to detect student's engagement. *J. King Saud Univ.-Comput. Inf. Sci.* **2021**, *33*, 99–109. [CrossRef]
3. Zhang, Z.; Li, Z.; Liu, H.; Cao, T.; Liu, S. Data-driven Online Learning Engagement Detection via Facial Expression and Mouse Behavior Recognition Technology. *J. Educ. Comput. Res.* **2020**, *58*, 63–86. [CrossRef]

4. Mohamad Nezami, O.; Dras, M.; Hamey, L.; Richards, D.; Wan, S.; Paris, C. Automatic Recognition of Student Engagement Using Deep Learning and Facial Expression. In *Lecture Notes in Computer Science (Including Subseries Lecture Notes in Artificial Intelligence and Lecture Notes in Bioinformatics)*; Springer: Berlin/Heidelberg, Germany, 2020; pp. 273–289. [CrossRef]
5. Khenkar, S.; Jarraya, S.K. Engagement detection based on analyzing micro body gestures using 3D CNN. *Comput. Mater. Contin.* **2022**, *70*, 2655–2677. [CrossRef]
6. Kaur, A.; Mustafa, A.; Mehta, L.; Dhall, A. Prediction and Localization of Student Engagement in the Wild. In Proceedings of the 2018 Digital Image Computing: Techniques and Applications (DICTA), Canberra, ACT, Australia, 10–13 December 2018. Available online: http://arxiv.org/abs/1804.00858 (accessed on 26 June 2018).
7. Murshed, M.; Dewan, M.A.A.; Lin, F.; Wen, D. Engagement Detection in e-Learning Environments using Convolutional Neural Networks. In Proceedings of the 2019 IEEE International Conference on Dependable, Autonomic and Secure Computing, International Conference on Pervasive Intelligence and Computing, International Conference on Cloud and Big Data Computing, International Conference on Cyber Science and Technology Congress (DASC/PiCom/CBDCom/CyberSciTech), Fukuoka, Japan, 5–8 August 2019; IEEE: Piscataway, NJ, USA, 2019; pp. 80–86. [CrossRef]
8. Wang, Y.; Yao, Q.; Kwok, J.T.; Ni, L.M. Generalizing from a Few Examples: A Survey on Few-shot Learning. *ACM Comput. Surv.* **2020**, *53*, 63. [CrossRef]
9. Singh, M.; Hoque, X.; Zeng, D.; Wang, Y.; Ikeda, K.; Dhall, A. Do I Have Your Attention: A Large Scale Engagement Prediction Dataset and Baselines. In Proceedings of the 25th International Conference on Multimodal Interaction, Paris, France, 9–13 October 2023; Association for Computing Machinery: New York, NY, USA, 2023; pp. 174–182. [CrossRef]
10. Liu, Y.; Zhang, H.; Zhang, W.; Lu, G.; Tian, Q.; Ling, N. Few-Shot Image Classification: Current Status and Research Trends. *Electronics* **2022**, *11*, 1752. [CrossRef]
11. Dosovitskiy, A.; Beyer, L.; Kolesnikov, A.; Weissenborn, D.; Zhai, X.; Unterthiner, T.; Dehghani, M.; Minderer, M.; Heigold, G.; Gelly, S.; et al. An Image is Worth 16x16 Words: Transformers for Image Recognition at Scale. *arXiv* **2020**, arXiv:2010.11929.
12. Dan, J.; Liu, Y.; Xie, H.; Deng, J.; Xie, H.; Xie, X.; Sun, B. TransFace: Calibrating Transformer Training for Face Recognition from a Data-Centric Perspective. In Proceedings of the IEEE/CVF International Conference on Computer Vision, Paris, France, 2–6 October 2023.
13. Mandia, S.; Singh, K.; Mitharwal, R. Vision Transformer for Automatic Student Engagement Estimation. In Proceedings of the 2022 IEEE 5th International Conference on Image Processing Applications and Systems (IPAS), Genova, Italy, 5–7 December 2022; IEEE: Piscataway, NJ, USA, 2022; pp. 1–6. [CrossRef]
14. Hasnine, M.N.; Bui, H.T.T.; Tran, T.T.T.; Nguyen, H.T.; Akçapõnar, G.; Ueda, H. Students' emotion extraction and visualization for engagement detection in online learning. In *Procedia Computer Science*; Elsevier B.V.: Amsterdam, The Netherlands, 2021; pp. 3423–3431. [CrossRef]
15. Snell, J.; Swersky, K.; Zemel, T.R. Prototypical Networks for Few-shot Learning. In Proceedings of the 31st Annual Conference on Neural Information Processing Systems (NIPS 2017), Long Beach, CA, USA, 4–9 December 2017.
16. Zhang, H.; Fu, Y.; Meng, J. Engagement Detection in Online Learning Based on Pre-trained Vision Transformer and Temporal Convolutional Network. In Proceedings of the 2024 36th Chinese Control and Decision Conference (CCDC), Xi'an, China, 25–27 May 2024; IEEE: Piscataway, NJ, USA, 2024; pp. 1310–1317. [CrossRef]
17. Maddula, N.V.S.S.; Nair, L.R.; Addepalli, H.; Palaniswamy, S. Emotion Recognition from Facial Expressions Using Siamese Network. In *Communications in Computer and Information Science*; Springer Science and Business Media Deutschland GmbH: Berlin/Heidelberg, Germany, 2021; pp. 63–72. [CrossRef]
18. Liu, B.; Yu, X.; Yu, A.; Zhang, P.; Wan, G.; Wang, R. Deep Few-Shot Learning for Hyperspectral Image Classification. *IEEE Trans. Geosci. Remote Sens.* **2019**, *57*, 2290–2304. [CrossRef]
19. Sung, F.; Yang, Y.; Zhang, L.; Xiang, T.; Torr, P.H.; Hospedales, T.M. Learning to Compare: Relation Network for Few-Shot Learning. In Proceedings of the IEEE Conference on Computer Vision and Pattern Recognition, Salt Lake City, UT, USA, 18–22 June 2018; pp. 1199–1208.
20. Touvron, H.; Cord, M.; Douze, M.; Massa, F.; Sablayrolles, A.; Jégou, H. Training data-efficient image transformers & distillation through attention. In Proceedings of the International Conference on Machine Learning, Online, 18–24 July 2021.
21. Su, R.; He, L.; Luo, M. Leveraging part-and-sensitive attention network and transformer for learner engagement detection. *Alex. Eng. J.* **2024**, *107*, 198–204. [CrossRef]
22. Gretton, A.; Borgwardt, K.M.; Rasch, M.; Schölkopf, B.; Smola, A.J. A Kernel Method for the Two-Sample-Problem. In *Advances in Neural Information Processing Systems*; Schölkopf, B., Platt, J., Hoffman, T., Eds.; MIT Press: Cambridge, MA, USA, 2006; Volume 19.
23. Liu, Z.; Lin, Y.; Cao, Y.; Hu, H.; Wei, Y.; Zhang, Z.; Lin, S.; Guo, B. Swin Transformer: Hierarchical Vision Transformer Using Shifted Windows. In Proceedings of the IEEE/CVF International Conference on Computer Vision, Montreal, QC, Canada, 11–17 October 2021.
24. Selim, T.; Elkabani, I.; Abdou, M.A. Students Engagement Level Detection in Online e-Learning Using Hybrid EfficientNetB7 Together With TCN, LSTM, and Bi-LSTM. *IEEE Access* **2022**, *10*, 99573–99583. [CrossRef]

5. Mandia, S.; Singh, K.; Mitharwal, R.; Mushtaq, F.; Janu, D. Transformer-Driven Modeling of Variable Frequency Features for Classifying Student Engagement in Online Learning. *arXiv* **2025**, arXiv:2502.10813.
6. Tieu, B.H.; Nguyen, T.T.; Nguyen, T.T. Detecting Student Engagement in Classrooms for Intelligent Tutoring Systems. In Proceedings of the 2019 6th NAFOSTED Conference on Information and Computer Science (NICS), Hanoi, Vietnam, 12–13 December 2019; pp. 145–149. [CrossRef]
7. Abedi, A.; Khan, S.S. Detecting Disengagement in Virtual Learning as an Anomaly using Temporal Convolutional Network Autoencoder. *Signal Image Video Process.* **2023**, *17*, 3535–3543. [CrossRef]

computers

MDPI

Article

A Seamless Deep Learning Approach for Apple Detection, Depth Estimation, and Tracking Using YOLO Models Enhanced by Multi-Head Attention Mechanism

Praveen Kumar Sekharamantry [1,2,*], Farid Melgani [1], Jonni Malacarne [1], Riccardo Ricci [1], Rodrigo de Almeida Silva [3] and Jose Marcato Junior [3]

[1] Department of Information Engineering and Computer Science, University of Trento, 38123 Trento, Italy; farid.melgani@unitn.it (F.M.); riccardo.ricci-1@unitn.it (R.R.)
[2] Department of Computer Science and Engineering, GITAM School of Technology, GITAM (Deemed to be University), Visakhapatnam 530045, India
[3] Faculty of Engineering, Architecture and Urbanism and Geography, Federal University of Mato Grosso do Sul, Campo Grande 79070-900, Brazil; rodrigo.a.silva@ufms.br (R.d.A.S.); jose.marcato@ufms.br (J.M.J.)
* Correspondence: pk.sekharamantry@unitn.it

Abstract: Considering precision agriculture, recent technological developments have sparked the emergence of several new tools that can help to automate the agricultural process. For instance, accurately detecting and counting apples in orchards is essential for maximizing harvests and ensuring effective resource management. However, there are several intrinsic difficulties with traditional techniques for identifying and counting apples in orchards. To identify, recognize, and detect apples, apple target detection algorithms, such as YOLOv7, have shown a great deal of reflection and accuracy. But occlusions, electrical wiring, branches, and overlapping pose severe issues for precisely detecting apples. Thus, to overcome these issues and accurately recognize apples and find the depth of apples from drone-based videos in complicated backdrops, our proposed model combines a multi-head attention system with the YOLOv7 object identification framework. Furthermore, we provide the ByteTrack method for apple counting in real time, which guarantees effective monitoring of apples. To verify the efficacy of our suggested model, a thorough comparison assessment is performed with several current apple detection and counting techniques. The outcomes adequately proved the effectiveness of our strategy, which continuously surpassed competing methods to achieve exceptional accuracies of 0.92, 0.96, and 0.95 with respect to precision, recall, and F1 score, and a low MAPE of 0.027, respectively.

Keywords: apple detection; depth estimation; multi-head attention mechanism; ByteTrack

1. Introduction

Apples are a major agricultural export across the world, contributing significantly to agricultural economic growth. Recently, computer vision-based systems have been employed in a wide range of applications, including biomedical [1,2], remote sensing, agricultural and farming monitoring, multimedia, and so on. The study's purpose is to develop a deep learning-based technology for agricultural automation. However, experienced farmers continue to be the driving force behind agricultural production. Manual labor wastes time and raises production costs, and workers with insufficient expertise and experience are prone to errors [3]. The advent of smart agriculture has fueled the integration of intelligence in orchards, which has emerged as a critical aspect in obtaining exact product information [4]. A visual system with automatic recognition based on support vector machine was proposed to identify fruit in orchards for autonomous growth evaluation, robotic harvesting, and yield calculation [5,6]. The vision system controlled the end result of the robot collecting apples from trees by identifying and localizing the apples.

As a result, detecting and tracking of apples is a critical challenge for these applications. Conversely, effectively recognizing fruits in natural situations poses substantial hurdles. Fruit detection can be inaccurate due to factors such as changing lighting conditions, overlapping shading, and similarities between distant little fruits and the backdrop. Many overlapping occlusions, leaf occlusions, branch occlusions, and other issues have also been identified, resulting in fruit target identification challenges that make fruits difficult to detect, recognize, and identify with high accuracy. The data collection of apples from farm fields is rather complex, as shown in Figure 1a–d.

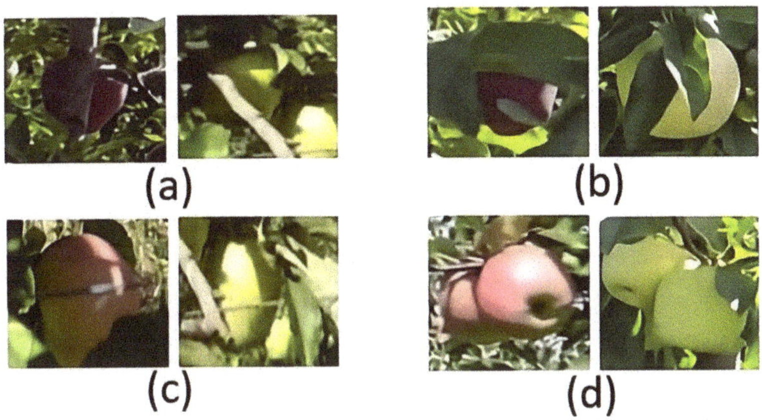

Figure 1. (**a**) Fruits concealed by branches; (**b**) Fruits obscured by leaves; (**c**) Fruits occluded by trellis wire; (**d**) Overlapping or bunched fruits.

In images, objects may overlap or be placed close together, with one object partially concealing the other. Obscured objects cannot be completely identified or annotated if occlusion is not handled correctly. Smaller or thinner objects, which have more of their surface area blocked, are more severely affected by occlusion. The concrete way of handling the problem would be to label the occlusion at the bounding box level to instruct the model as to which areas of an item are hidden. Thus, when producing a detection prediction, the model can then factor out the obscured characteristics. Also, image segmentation masks, bounding box overlays, and other techniques can be used to artificially occlude dataset objects. This demonstrates to the model how various items seem while partially obscured. The likelihood of missing or incorrectly packaging or labeling these difficult-to-see items is higher. Predicting the apple yield for a specific crop is a challenging task. For instance, an existing method for optimal thresholding for automatic recognition of apple fruits [7] claims that a low threshold of 0.2 has an extremely high recall. We face the possibility of obtaining too many false positives, which is the drawback. Similarly, according to Bin Yan et al. [8], a model will be extremely accurate with a threshold of 0.8, but the number of unrecognized apples will significantly increase. The most logical starting point would seem to be a threshold of 0.5 [9]. The detection of unidentified apples is much better with a confidence threshold of 0.5. The traditional methods are dedicated to the maturity of apples analyzed by the shape, size, and color of the apples [10,11] before detection and harvesting. Bulanon et al. [12] used threshold segmentation to improve the color difference of the red channel of the apple picture and extract the apple fruit target. The processing recognition rate reached 88.0%; however, it was only 18.0% in the backlight environment. Tian et al. [13] suggested a localization strategy based on depth information in pictures to determine the circular center, match the shape, and increase identification accuracy to 96.61%.

According to Lei Hu et al. [14], their proposed model offers an enhanced YOLOv5 algorithm for mature apple target detection in challenging situations. To improve accuracy and efficiency, it includes an adaptive scaling mechanism and a position focus loss function. To categorize and correlate the apple targets, the method uses the concept of feature information extraction and employs the position focal loss function. This helps to prevent feature information loss while also improving the algorithm's accuracy and efficiency. The new algorithm displays an 8.1% improvement in accuracy and 3.9 frames per second increase in pattern recognition speed through experimental examination of apple target feature data under varied conditions. The suggested method provides a solution for effectively detecting and locating ripe apples in complicated surroundings, which is useful for apple-picking robots and other applications. In spite of this, the study does not go into great depth about the adaptive scaling technique and position focus loss function employed in the enhanced YOLOv5 method. The report does not specify which complicated contexts were used to test and assess the new technique, nor does it compare the enhanced algorithm's performance to that of other current methods for detecting targets under challenging situations.

The work proposed by Jiuxin et al. [15] on apple-picking robots provides a quick technique for apple recognition and processing based on a modified version of the YOLOv5 algorithm. The enhanced model is easier to migrate and apply to hardware devices since it is smaller (57% smaller) and faster (27.6% faster) at processing data. The target association identification method increases efficiency by cutting the model selection process processing time by 89%. When compared to previous deep networks, the enhanced YOLOv5 model performs more quickly and accurately, making it a useful tool for apple recognition [16].

The lightweight MobileNetv2 network uses the inverted residual convolution module in place of the YOLOv5 backbone standard convolution module. The least-squares method is used to fix the model's inaccurate data output findings, making it better suited for distinguishing different apple forms. The approach of target association recognition is introduced when developing multi-target picking pathways according to the correlation among the confidence levels of the recognized targets. These methods are combined to enhance YOLOv5s, the model size is reduced, and the detection speed is increased, making it easy to migrate to and use in hardware devices. The suggested path planning method, which is based on the enhanced YOLOv5 model, lowers computation costs and successfully addresses the issues of processing massive volumes of information and repeating processing that arise throughout the apple picking activity. The target recognition information can be further utilized to provide suggestions for obstacle avoidance in the apple picking process.

An automated vision system was created employing stereo cameras synced to a customized LED strobe for on-tree measuring of apples in photos using excellent measurement precision [17]. Faster R-CNN and Mask R-CNN, two deep neural network models, were trained to find fruit candidates for size and extrapolate obscured fruit sections to enhance size estimation. The stereo cameras' spatial resolution and depth data were used to translate the segmented fruit shapes into metric specific surface areas and diameters. The camera system was used in monthly field tests from June to October to measure fruit size in the range of 22 to 82 mm and compare them to ground truth diameters. To determine the effect of fruit form on size estimation using images, a laboratory setting experiment was carried out. The 2D surface of an apple in an image, calculated in metric units that used the camera system, was used to describe fruit shape. In the experiment, altogether 100 apples (50 "Candy Crisp" and 50 "Rome") were imaged in various orientations to mimic field settings. In an analysis of the link between focal length, camera field-of-view, and size accuracy, it was discovered that increasing the distance from the tree reduced the pixel count and size accuracy. The imaging system delivered accurate measurements of fruit size and weight, as demonstrated by in-field comparisons of the readings with ground truth data. The study also included details on the dates and types of data acquired during the field experiment, including monthly image capture, ground truth size measurements, and fruit weight records. However, for fruit recognition and occlusion handling, the study used a specific pair of models of deep neural networks (Faster R-CNN and Mask R-CNN), and the effectiveness of other models or techniques was not examined, similar to the few traditional works on apple fields [18,19]. The use of stereo vision and machine learning in agricultural imagery may have drawbacks or difficulties, which include issues with illumination, image quality, and processing needs.

The YOLOv7-tiny-Apple model, which has been proposed as a lightweight small-target apple recognition and counting tool, can be used for autonomous orchard management, assisting in real-time apple detection and more efficient orchard management by identifying and counting apples [20]. The model provides theoretical support for developing apple identification and counting models by providing new insights on hardware installations and orchard yield estimation. It may be used in orchard management in real time to improve labor efficiency, product quality, and agricultural operational efficiency. The work makes use of the publicly available MinneApple dataset, which has been processed to create a collection of photos with diverse weather conditions, such as scenarios with fog and rain. The suggested detection algorithm is built on the updated YOLOv7-tiny model, which includes skip connections to shallower features, P2BiFPN for multi-scale feature fusion [21], and a lightweight ULSAM attention mechanism to minimize the loss of small target features. The suggested model, YOLOv7-tiny-Apple, demonstrated better detection accuracy with a mean average precision (mAP) of 80.4%, as well as a loss rate of 0.0316, which was 5.5% higher than the baseline model. The mean absolute error (MAE) was 2.737 and the root mean square error (RMSE) was 4.220 in terms of counts [22], which were 5.69% and 8.97% less than the original model, respectively. The amount of equipment needed was decreased by 15.81% due to the smaller size of the model. The suggested model showed improved generalization and resilience, making it appropriate for tiny target apple detection in a natural context with complicated backdrops and shifting weather conditions. The model needs to improve technological monitoring and management of smart orchards, lightweight optimization, greater detection accuracy, and mobile device deployment.

However, the efficacy of all of these systems is compromised due to backdrop complexity, motion blurriness, poor light, obstacle avoidance, and other factors. In this work, we propose a novel deep learning strategy based on the YOLOv7 model to address these concerns. In addition to this design, we have included a multi-head attention mechanism (MAM) technique to deal with size changes and predict the depth of apples in the orchard field. The following are the primary innovations and authors contributions of the proposed approach:

- To make our training dataset more effective, we included an attribute augmentation approach to offset the issue of contextual data loss and a feature improvement model that would enhance the representation of features and speed up inference.
- The YOLOv7 model is implemented on the augmented data for apple detection in live apple orchard fields.
- A multi-head attention mechanism is integrated with YOLOv7 to compute the depth of apples.
- The apples are tracked and counted using an enhanced ByteTrack technique.

The article is organized as follows: Section 2 deals with the proposed system in which data acquisition and data augmentation are applied on the dataset of apples to eliminate various factors of external sources that will affect the accuracy of the model. The detection of apples is dealt with by the improved YOLOv7 on the pre-processed data after data augmentation. A multi-head attention mechanism is applied to YOLOv7 to find the depth of apples along with the detection accuracy. Collaborating with these, the ByteTrack approach is finally used to track and count the number of apples. Section 3 presents the experimental results of the proposed methodology and a comparative analysis to demonstrate the robustness of the suggested method in comparison to standard object detection techniques. Section 4 clarifies the discussion of the methodologies and results obtained. Finally, Section 5 gives the conclusion and future potential of this seamless apple detecting and counting approach. By combining these elements, a complete system that can track and identify apples and comprehend the distance between apples and drones is obtained, opening up a valuable application.

2. Proposed Methodology

The recommended approach deals with a complete introspection of apple detection, finding the depth of apples and finally tracking and counting of the number of apples by the drone based on live apple orchard videos.

2.1. Data Acquisition and Pre-Processing

For the drone-cantered apple identification structure to be trained and evaluated, a refined custom dataset is required. The preparation process for data acquisition plays a vital role in the overall accuracy of the model. Reflex, stereo cameras, and a drone were used to gather the data on two distinct fields. The data collection was carried out in Val di Non in Trento, Italy, where the apple fields are situated, as shown in Figure 2a,b. The photos and videos were taken between the plants at a distance of 30 and 60 cm. The data were collected by the drone on a day in September with a variety of weather conditions, as shown in Figure 2c,d. There were no additional lights or artificial lighting used during the flight. The drone settings were processed via the rtmp protocol, which connects the camera to the drone's backend storage. It has an interference-free maximum transmission range of 80 m and height of 50 m.

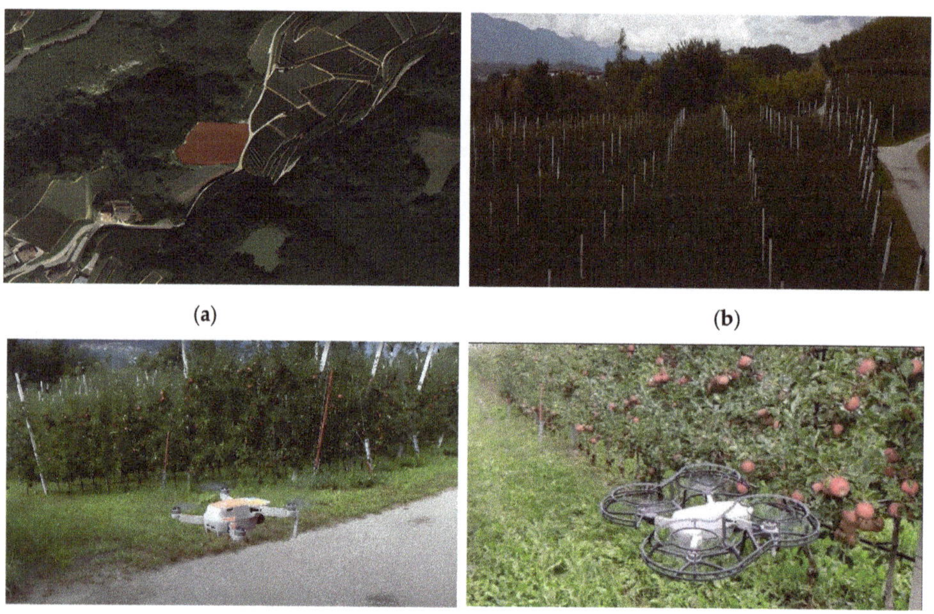

(a) (b) (c) (d)

Figure 2. (**a**) Geomap location of the apple orchard; (**b**) Drone camera view of the apple field; (**c**) Drone flying in the apple field; (**d**) Drone camera recording the apples.

A DJI Mavic mini 3 drone and a Stereo Labs ZED 2iw Polarizing Filter were used. It has a 249 g ultra-light option and 5-kilometre HD video transmission, and it can record high-resolution drone videos. The drone has GPS-precise hover and a vision sensor. With streamlined recording and editing, the three-axis Gimbal 2688 $\times$ 1520 resolution camera provides a detailed image. The camera's field of vision is 44° in the vertical and 81° in the depth. To confirm the robustness of the model, additional material included different lighting situations, angles, and orchard layouts.

(a) Annotations: A fraction of the image are captioned by labeling the apples for each frame of the 10 GB entire footage, which is divided into many frames. Each apple has a bounding box drawn around it, and the depth labels indicate how close it is to the drone. The dataset is particularly confined to apples that are ready to harvest, and the immature apples are curtailed during the first labeling effort. As a result, our trained method will be able to distinguish only mature apples under varied environmental conditions. The ground truth data from the annotations are used to train and test the model's accuracy.

(b) Dataset classification: A training dataset, a testing set, and a validation dataset are created from the full dataset. A considerable portion of the images are from the training set, while only 30% and 10% of the images are from the testing and validation sets, respectively. The testing set evaluates the trained model's performance.

2.2. Data Agumentations

In computer vision applications, data augmentation [23] is a critical part since many elements must be taken into account when the data collected are affected by external sources. We noticed that the distance between the camera and the trees fluctuated during the process since several apple images were relatively small while others were pretty large. There was a significant asymmetry in the original data. Also, applications that operate in real time suffered from this sort of input data uncertainty. Hence, training with this type of unbalanced data may result in over-fitting and reduce detection accuracy. In a similar way, the apple image data collection mechanism faces same issues during image capture. As a result, data augmentation becomes an essential duty in these sorts of tasks where object sizes differ often. Hence, the following augmentation approaches were taken into consideration:

Image radiance: In order to match the actual low light and bad illumination circumstances, the brightness is alternately increased and decreased. With the function "hsv2rgb", the image is first converted to HSV and then to RGB.

Flipping of Image: To help the image classifier recognize apples in various situations, the vertical as well as horizontal pixels are mirrored.

Rotating the image: When the capturing angle is constrained, the drone angle is not fixed. So the model needs to be trained to be capable of capturing and identifying the apple from a variety of perspectives.

Image blur: The drone moves at various speeds, and the video frequently records ambiguous information. The model can be trained using blurry images to help with accurate detection standards.

Noisy image: Images are subjected to a standard 0.02 of Gaussian variance [24,25]. High heat and electronic circuit noise may be produced by the drone. By utilizing Gaussian noise, this process would assist in creating a model of human motion with human qualities.

The cautiously improved dataset serves as the foundation for developing and testing the suggested drone-based apple recognition system. It consists of annotated drone-taken images of apples with corresponding depth labels.

2.3. YOLOv7 Architecture

The YOLOv7 model is a current-time object identification system for detecting apples in pictures or videos. YOLOv7 is an improved variation of the popular You Only Look Once (YOLO) approach, which estimates box boundaries and probabilities of classes for each object in a picture [26–28]. The YOLOv7 algorithm provides the best accuracy of any real-time object identification model while maintaining 30 frames per second or more. It uses far less hardware than conventional neural networks and therefore can be trained considerably more quickly on tiny datasets with no pre-learned weights. Researchers have presented many approaches for detecting apples utilizing the YOLOv7 model. One study, for example, developed a better method built on the YOLOv7 model to solve the poor performance of apple fruit detection due to the complex backdrop and occluded apple fruit. Other research employed an updated YOLOv7 framework and multi-object tracking algorithms to recognize and count apples in apple orchards [29,30]. The approach dealt with transformers to determine apple ripeness from digitized photos of several apple varieties.

In general, the YOLOv7 algorithm provides a robust tool for identifying apples in various contexts, and researchers are always looking for new ways to increase its precision as well as efficacy. The model design as well as the training method were optimized using YOLOv7. In model architecture, YOLOv7 provides an expanded, adequate layers aggregation network and scaling model skills. During the training phase, YOLOv7 replaces the original module with model re-parameterized skills and employs a dynamic label assignment technique to apply labels to distinct output layers. The standard YOLOv7 model's architecture for detection of apples involves basic components such as the inputs, backbone, neck, detection heads, and prediction output, as shown in Figure 3.

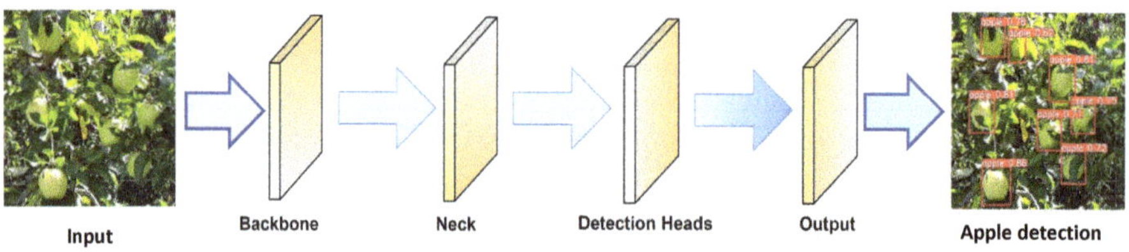

Figure 3. Basic description of YOLOv7 architecture.

The initial process in the procedure is to analyze the input image, which comprises different variants of apples images that need to be identified. The selection of a proper backbone network is essential for apple detection. The backbone network passes the input image through a number of convolutional layers. Specific filters are applied with the help of the convolution layer to the source images to capture varied features at diverse spatial resolutions. For object boundary detection, the network will first learn to recognize basic features like edges and colors in the first layers. The hierarchical feature learning is processed by the backbone network deeper layers by picking up on more complicated and abstract properties. At these deeper layers, features like texture, patterns, and object portions are learned, enabling the network to comprehend the fine details of apples. Higher-level semantic characteristics are extracted as the image is being processed through the backbone.

To identify apples from other items, these traits encode characteristics about object shape. One of the best features of the backbone is that it is made to be resistant to variations in scale and rotation. As a result, the network is able to recognize apples in the input image regardless of their dimension or orientation. The backbone network produces feature maps that spatially map the learned features on the image. Subsequent layers use these feature maps, which are packed with data about the input apple images, to detect objects. The network neck receives the feature maps that were retrieved from the backbone. The neck further enhances these features, frequently forming a feature pyramid that aids in the detection of objects of various sizes. The detection head processes the feature maps at the end and predicts the bounding box dimensions and class probabilities for the discovered apples.

The neck's role is to build a pyramid structure in which lower-resolution maps are obtained from higher-resolution ones (having finer information). As apples can exist in images in a variety of sizes, their pyramidal structure is crucial. The network can efficiently detect both large and small apples since it has features at many scales. Further feature fusion aids in capturing contextual data for apple detection. For instance, it enables the network to recognize how an apple interacts with its environment, facilitating precise detection. The neck also deals with the contextual information. Apples can be distinguished from other items and backgrounds using contextual information [31]. As an illustration, the existence of leaves, branches, or specific colors around an apple can serve as helpful detection cues. The neck network improves the semantic understanding by recognizing the whole shape of apple roundness and other unique structural properties. The enhanced and refined attributes from the neck are then handed to the head. These characteristics are used by the detection head to forecast apple-specific bounding box dimensions and class probabilities. The information from the neck is essential for the detection head to accurately estimate the location of the apples in the input image. Accuracy, real-time performance, good recognition efficiency, scalability, and effective hardware utilization are just a few benefits of using YOLOv7 to detect apples. Because of these benefits, YOLOv7 is a good choice for apple detection in a variety of applications, including monitoring systems and automated vehicles.

2.4. Improved YOLOv7 Architecture with Multi-Head Attention Mechanism

The improved YOLOv7 architecture in this section deals with the integration of the multi-head attention mechanism aimed at apple detection [32]. The modified framework accurately predicts the depth of apples and their confined features. The architecture diagram shown in Figure 4 depicts the addition of the multi-head attention mechanism within the framework of YOLOv7.

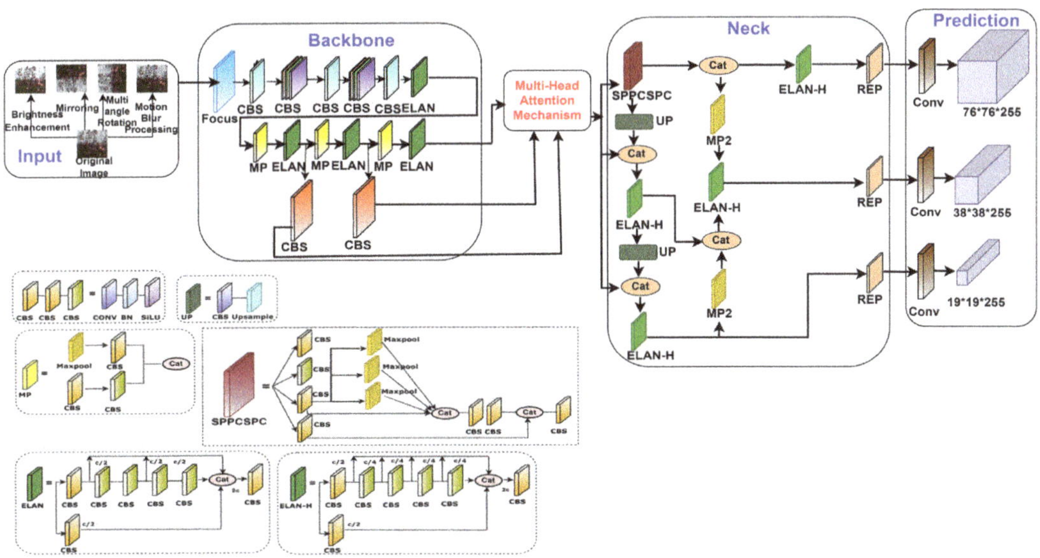

Figure 4. Architecture of YOLOv7 with multi-head attention mechanism.

In the architecture, the CBS layer performs the convolution, normalization of batches, and SiLU activation operations, which is the fundamental convolutional unit in the backbone. The feature map output of the ELAN (efficient layer aggregation network) layer is divided into three sections and is composed of several CBS structures. Here, the channel divides the feature map into two equal groups. The initial group then applies five convolution processes to produce the first component, the second group applies one convolution process to obtain the second one, and the third part is made up of the outputs of the first group's first convolution and third convolution. The feature map is divided into two groups by the MP (Max Pool) layer. Maximum pooling is used by the first group to extract more crucial information, and convolution is used by the second group to extract feature information. The outcome is finally obtained by joining two groups [33]. The CSPNet (convolutional spatial pyramid) including an SPP (spatial pyramid pooling) block makes up the SPPCSPC (spatial pyramid pooling and convolutional spatial pyramid pooling) layer. The CSPNet is a particular kind of network that incorporates data from several scales and resolutions to increase the detection precision. Spatial pyramid pooling, a technique used by the SPP block to gather more contextual data, involves combining characteristics at several measures. The REP layer is a revolutionary idea that uses structural re-parameterization to modify the framework in inference to enhance the model performance. The REP layer can obtain the output of the feature map in three sections during training. Convolution and batch normalization are implemented in the first and second phases and only batch normalization is implemented in the third phase Structural re-parameterization uses less computational power, and model performance is enhanced as REP inference only keeps the second portion of the structure.

Multi-Head Attention Mechanism

In the real-world scenario, tasks capturing long range dependencies and their respective contextual data often become crucial. So, integrating the YOLOv7 model, as shown in Figure 5, with the multi-head attention mechanism offers a great advantage to deal with such problems. Convolutional neural networks (CNNs) that have undergone prior training can extract feature maps from input images. As an attention mechanism is incapable of identifying the spatial relationships between pixels, positional encoding must be added to the feature maps to provide the details about the positions of the image core components. Techniques like 1×1 convolutions can be used to lower the dimensionality of the features.

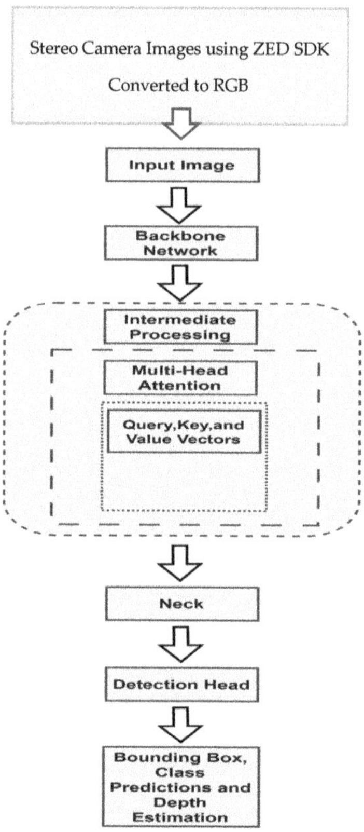

Figure 5. YOLOv7 architecture for apple detection and depth estimation.

The stereo cameras used in this work can capture high-resolution 3D video footage of apple orchards and determine depth by comparing the pixel displacement among the left and right pictures. Their two eyes are spaced 6 to 12 cm apart [34,35]. For every pixel (X, Y) in the picture, the ZED's depth maps record a distance value (Z). Measuring from the rear of the camera's left eye to the scene object, the distance is given in metric units (meters, for example). The ZED's default depth-detecting mode is called standard. The standard mode operates more quickly while maintaining distance metrics and shapes. We used the ValidMeasure function to determine valid depth data. Additionally, the ultra-depth mode provides computer vision-based techniques with the widest depth range and the best retained Z-accuracy across the sensing range. A feature called depth stabilization merges and filters the depth maps over many frames in a temporal manner. This makes it possible to reduce jitter and enhance the accuracy of depth on stationary objects like apples. By utilizing the ZED SDK's positional tracking feature, depth stabilization is still effective despite the fact that the camera is moving. To prevent merging the depth of dynamic regions, it may also identify moving objects. The depth resolution of a stereo camera varies across its range, and the formula $Dr = Z\hat{}2*\alpha$ describes how stereo vision employs triangulation to infer depth from a disparity image, where Dr is the depth resolution, Z is the distance, and α is a constant. The ZED SDK and accompanying tools are the only programs that can read the proprietary SVO file format. Together with metadata like timestamps and IMU (inertial measurement unit) data, it includes the camera's raw photos. Multiple file types can be created from SVO files for applications elsewhere. SVO may be exported into several formats using the sample ZED_SVO_Export SDK.

The source feature maps are linearly altered into several sets of queries, keys, and values. The input data maps are captured in a variety of ways by separately calculating the scaled dot-product attention scores. A residual connection is added from the input to the output of the multi-head attention. Also, a layer normalization is applied to make the training process more stable and efficient. After multi-head attention, the feature maps are trained over position-wise feed-forward neural networks. ReLU (rectified linear unit) activations and fully connected layers make up these networks. The network can more successfully capture the apples of different sizes because of multi-scale feature fusion. The detecting head predicts object class probability, bounding box coordinates, and other data required for object detection. Non-maximum suppression (NMS) is applied to exclude repetitive detections and choose the most certain predictions [36,37]. The model gains the ability to identify apples, forecast the bounding boxes, allocate class probabilities, and calculate their depths by minimizing the gap between estimated parameters as well as the ground truth labels.

The multi-head attention model is made up of the three components, query, key, and value, as shown in Figure 6. These components allow the model to concentrate on different input locations and collect relevant data. The concern is a representation of the area of interest that requires attention. A single feature or a collection of features describing an area in the feature maps connected to apples may be the query for apple detection. A query vector is created and then applied to every position in the input sequence. When compared to the key vectors, all query vectors are utilized to calculate the attention scores. Keys can represent either specific features that assist the model to recognize context, such as features from surrounding objects or regions, or features from the whole input image. To calculate the resemblance between queries and keys, key vectors are employed. If there is a lot of similarity, it means that the related portions of the data input need to be addressed.

The value, in accordance with the attention mechanism, refers to the properties that have been weighed and aggregated. The context of apple detection may benefit from the features that provide specific information about the recognized apples or their surroundings. Each attention head in the multi-head attention mechanism is in charge of mastering a different selective attention pattern or capturing a different aspect of the input material [38–40]. According to the calculated attention scores, value vectors are combined. Higher attention ratings indicate that the model places greater trust in the associated values when making predictions. Each attention head performs the computations for the query, key, and value separately. The weighted sum of the associated value vectors is computed using the attention results achieved from the SoftMax normalization. This weighted total, which reflects the focused information, is the result of each query attention mechanism. The model can determine which areas of the images are important for identifying apples by employing attention techniques. For instance, the attention mechanism could assist the model in focusing on the visible parts of an apple if the apple is partially obscured by another object, increasing detection accuracy. In contrast, queries, keys, and values work together to create a multi-head attention mechanism that allows the model to dynamically focus on different elements of the input data. This feature is especially useful for detecting apples in complex scenarios.

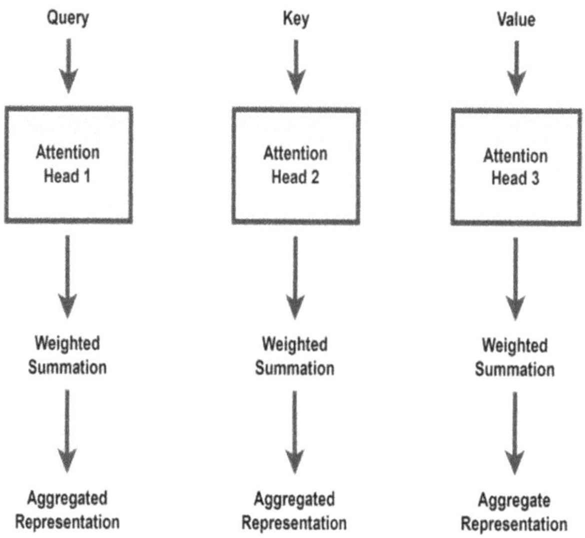

Figure 6. Components of multi-head model.

2.5. Box Prediction and Loss Function

The proposed YOLOv7 architecture neck module, which is defined above, is responsible of bounding box prediction. The ground truth of the bounding box is shown as W = (x_1, y_1, x_2, y_2). With these coordinates [41], Equation (1) is applied to determine W boundaries, as follows:

$$t_{x_1} = log\frac{(s_l(x+0.5)-x_1)}{r_l}, t_{y_1} = log\frac{(s_l(y+0.5)-y_1)}{r_l}, \quad t_{x_2} = log\frac{(x_2 - s_l(x+0.5))}{r_l}, t_{y_2} = log\frac{(y_2 - s_l(y+0.5))}{r_l} \quad (1)$$

The ground truth boxes and projection coordinates are taken into account to calculate the normalized offsets between the coordinates, where s_l is the scaling factor, r_l is the basic scale, and the coordinates of the image (x, y) are subsequently mapped to the original picture by applying down sampling. Using the log-space function at this point, we incorporate regularization. Later, the loss function is trained using the smooth L_1 loss function, and the bounding box prediction is performed using L_{reg}. Through iterative optimization, the loss function increases the accuracy of the target detection [42]. Classification and regression are the two primary components of the target loss detector loss function. The classification loss L_{cls} is among confidence, whereas the regression loss is in between the normalized border and regression target. The loss function is articulated as follows in Equation (2):

$$L(\{p_{sl}\},\{t_l\}) = L_{cls} + L_{reg} \frac{1}{N_{cls}} \sum_1 L_{cls}(p_{sl}, p_l) + \lambda \frac{1}{N_{reg}} \sum_1 p_l L_{reg}(t_i, t_l)$$
$$where = \begin{cases} p_i \, tf \, p_i = 1 \\ 1 - p_i \, otherwise \end{cases}, \alpha_s = \begin{cases} \alpha \, if \, p_i = 1 \\ 1 - otherwise \end{cases} \text{and } C = \begin{cases} 1 \left| t_{ij} - t_{ij} \right| < 1 \\ 0 \, otherwise \end{cases} \quad (2)$$

Here, α is utilized to correct the positive and negative sample imbalance that results from the target image having fewer samples than the overall image, i.e., there are fewer samples of apple images than there are of the complete images. As a result, the model obtains accurate bounding boxes, which improves accuracy. The proposed focal loss function aids in estimating the classification loss, and α function is utilized to balance the effects of the proposed positive and negative loss functions. Additionally, it prevents the samples from producing a dominant amount of classification loss. L_1 loss is used for estimating the regression loss in order to determine the bounding boxes, and β aids in choosing the L_1 or L_2 loss function depending on the range of the loss. Furthermore, N_{reg} and N_{cls} regularize these loss functions. In order to construct the final optimal model, the overall loss L is propagated backward in a gradient way. In the process of apple detection, YOLOv7 + MAM is trained to identify apples in pictures or videos. Bounding boxes and class labels surrounding the identified apples, together with an estimate of their depth, will be generated as output by the model.

2.6. ByteTrack

Multiple object tracking (MOT) is a vital computer vision task that involves recognizing how various apples move over time in a video clip acquired from a drone. The objective is to identify, locate, and track every apple in the video, even when they are partially or entirely occluded by other elements of the scene.

Typically, there are two processes involved in multiple object tracking, object detection and object association, as shown in Figure 7. With object detectors like Faster-RCNN or YOLO, object detection is the process of recognizing all possible objects of interest within the present frame. Object association is the method of connecting tracklets or objects found in the current frame with their corresponding tracklets from earlier frames. Despite significant advancements, MOT is still a difficult task. There are some crucial problems that have prevented high-quality performance and contributed as the foundation for current methods.

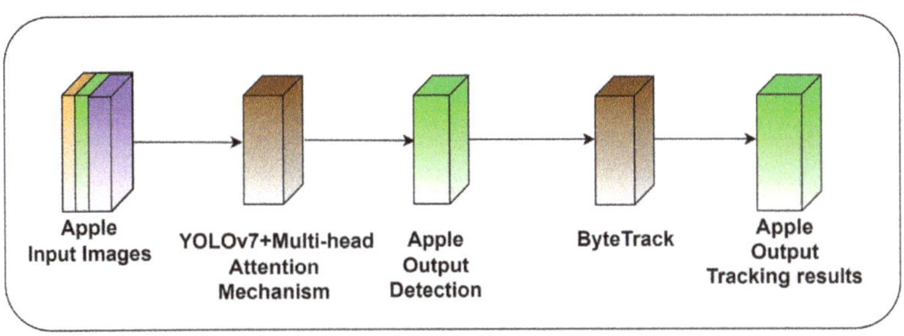

Figure 7. Proposed structure of multi-head detection and tracking of apples.

The visual input itself may cause complications. For instance, a single object motion and look can change significantly over the video sequence. Items in a scene can move in a variety of directions and at varying speeds. They can also alter in shape or size, as well as be completely or partially obscured by other objects. Several issues, such as object ID swapping or assigning numerous tracklets to the same item, lead to MOT tracking errors. Also, every apple object in the current frame must be consistently connected to its equivalent object in the previous frame, and the tracking system should be able to handle these deviations. A practical problem is the video inference speed while performing live video inference on apple orchards.

In our case, relying simply on a detection model makes counting unreliable because there is a significant chance the model may record numerous counts of identical apples if they occur in subsequent frames. Duplicate counts will lead to more false positive cases, which will reduce the model effectiveness and dependability for commercial application. The counting strategy should therefore be based on a method that is not only reliant on detections. So, a reliable method is to use an object tracking mechanism to follow each apple during the course of the video until the counter is incremented. According to the tracking-by-detection paradigm, a multi-object tracker (MOT) keeps track of numerous items of interest by detecting them in each time frame (t), connecting them to objects that were present in the previous frame ($t-1$), and predicting their position in the next frame, ($t+1$), thus tracking the items throughout time by repeating for each frame of the video sequence. The state of the object is predicted and updated using a Kalman filter in basic MOT methods like SORT [43], and the objects are associated using a Hungarian algorithm. The result of the MOT is bounding boxes with an ID produced specifically for each object to aid in object identification. However, these models may be prone to ID switching. As a result, the multi-object tracking accuracy (MOTA) is measured to assess the MOT's accuracy, as shown in Equation (3):

$$MOTA = 1 - \frac{\sum_t FN_t + FP_t + IDS_t}{\sum_t GT_t} \tag{3}$$

In this case, the terms FN, FP, IDS, and GT, respectively, refer to false negative, false positive, ID switch, and ground truth counts.

Building of ByteTrack

ByteTrack can resolve this issue by employing a motion model that controls a queue, called tracklets, to store the objects being tracked and conducts tracking and matching among bounding boxes having low confidence values. The main advancement of ByteTrack is the retention of non-background low confidence detection boxes, which are generally destroyed after the initial filtering of detections, and the use of these low-score boxes for a subsequent association phase [44,45]. Occluded detection boxes typically have confidence ratings that are below the threshold but still contain some information about the objects, giving them a better confidence score than background-only boxes. So, throughout the association phase, it is still important to maintain track of these low confidence boxes.

After the detection phase, the detected bounding boxes are filtered with preset upper and lower thresholds into high level of confidence boxes, low level of confidence boxes, and background boxes. After this procedure, background boxes are eliminated, but low- and high-confidence detection boxes are preserved for subsequent association stages. The detection accuracy boxes of present frames are matched with estimated boxes from previous frame tracklets (using Kalman filter) [46,47], which contain all active tracklets and lost tracklets from current frames, in a manner similar to normal association stages from other algorithms. The feature embeddings are matched using a simple IoU score or cosine similarity score (using feature extractors such as DeepSORT, QDTrack, etc.) using nearest neighbor distance and the Hungarian method or matching cascade [48,49]. Only if the similarity score exceeds a predetermined match threshold is the linear allocation among groups of bounding boxes confirmed. In the real implementation, mismatched high-score detection boxes are matched with tracklets that have updates from a single image before even being assigned to a new tracklet, as shown in Figure 8.

In the next step of association, the leftover unmatched predicted boxes of earlier frames are compared against low-score detection boxes. As it makes sense that obscured boxes should be less well linked to boxes from earlier frames, the matching method is the same as the first association step; however, the matching threshold is scaled lower.

Unmatched detecting boxes are deleted, whereas unmatched prediction boxes are given the label lost tracklets. Prior to Kalman filter prediction, the lost tracklets are stored for a certain time of frames and added to the active tracklets. This enables the trackers to retrieve certain tracklets that were lost as a result of objects briefly going completely missing for a limited number of frames. The basic detector in the present work is YOLOv7. Users can choose from a variety of matching measures among IoU and ReID, depending on the characteristics of the datasets. The initial phase identification of high-score detections can be performed using either IoU or ReID. ReID performs best on videos with low frame rates or videos with noticeable frame-to-frame motion, whereas IoU is more trustworthy in extreme occlusion situations when ReID characteristics are unreliable. Consequently, second phase association should always employ IoU as the matching criterion since we can expect that low-score detection boxes will contain occluded apples with ReID features that might not be accurate depictions of the objects.

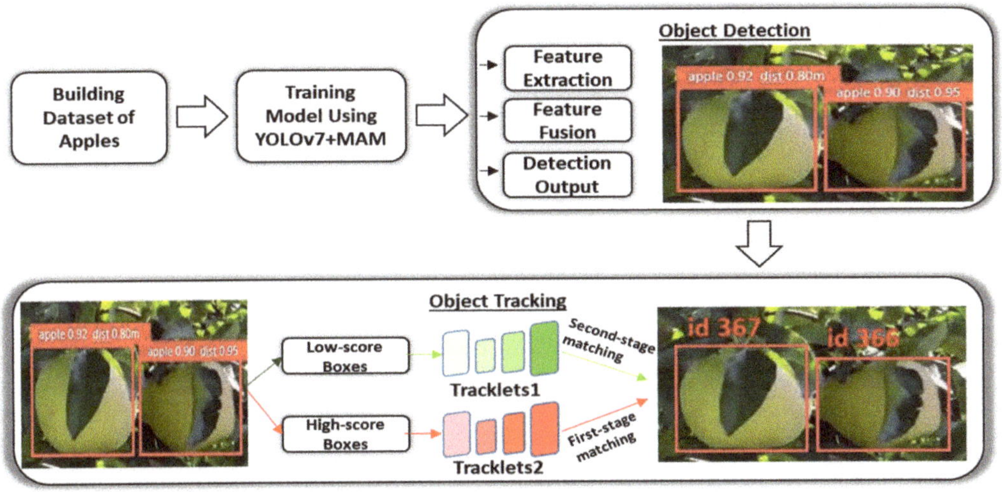

Figure 8. Proposed build of the model for detection and tracking of apples.

3. Results

The results of the suggested YOLOv7 + MAM architecture are shown in this section. Using real-time videos and images of apple orchards, this model was tested. The suggested method for apple tracking and detection was built with the Ubuntu 22.04 Linux operating system with the aid of the PyTorch deep learning framework. The operating system was installed with an Intel i7 processor, 24 GB of RAM, and an NVIDIA GeForce RTX 3090 linked to a 384-bit memory interface. The GPU operated at a rate of 1395 MHz. The Python programming language was used to develop the entire model. This model used YOLOv7, which was enhanced with a multi-head attention framework along with tracking using ByteTrack, and each model's performance was assessed with the aid of the CUDNN library and CUDA toolkit. The entire experiment was run with an IoU threshold set at 0.75.

The processing time examined in the current study is the duration the algorithm takes to analyze each frame of the drone-recorded input video stream. By contrast, memory usage is the amount of GPU-enabled system memory required for algorithm execution. The computational cost of our solution was calculated using a GPU-enabled computer system. We built the algorithm in Python and used the OpenCV package to process images. To determine the processing time, we measured the total execution time acquired by the algorithm on the video frames. Using the Python 'time' package, we recorded the start and end times of the processing pipeline and determined the average processing time per frame. Memory usage was analyzed using the 'memory_profiler' Python library, which allowed us to monitor the algorithm's memory consumption throughout execution. We measured peak memory consumption and averaged it across numerous iterations for a representative measure. Our computational cost evaluation revealed a 20 millisecond average processing time per frame and 2 millisecond standard deviation. Peak memory utilization during algorithm running was found to be around 300 MB.

3.1. Performance Assessment

The performance of the proposed approach was assessed using three indicators of accuracy: precision, recall, and F1 score. The following Equation (4) was applied to compute these parameters:

$$P_r = \frac{T_P}{F_P + T_P},\ Rec = \frac{T_P}{T_P + F_N},\ F1 - score = \frac{2P_r Rec}{P_r + Rec} \tag{4}$$

where T_P, F_P, and F_N represents the true positive, false positive, and false negative values.

3.2. Performance of Apple Detection

The results of the suggested approach to identify each apple in the picture are provided in this section. The performance that was attained was compared with that of the remaining models. To demonstrate the resilience of the suggested approach, we have considered several variables that impact system performance, like variations in illumination. We employed the PIL library in Python to account for changes in illumination, assigning a 0.5 factor for images with low brightness and 1.5 factor for pictures with high definition. The comparative study of the suggested method in terms of recall, precision, and F1 score for the original picture is shown in this section. The performance of the suggested approach was compared to that of several existing systems, including Faster RCNN, AlexNet With Faster RCNN, ResNet + FasterRCNN, YOLOv3, YOLOv5, YOLOv7, and finally with YOLOv7 + MAM. Table 1 displays the comparison outcomes for the detection performance.

Table 1. Performance comparison for the original images and under different lighting conditions.

	Original Images			Illumination Variations		
Detection Method	**Precision**	**Recall**	**F1 Score**	**Precision**	**Recall**	**F1 Score**
Faster RCNN	0.84	0.78	0.80	0.68	0.72	0.71
AlexNet + Faster RCNN	0.88	0.83	0.86	0.69	0.75	0.71
ResNet + FasterRCNN	0.87	0.64	0.74	0.72	0.75	0.72
YOLOv5	0.82	0.86	0.84	0.71	0.77	0.73
YOLOv7	0.83	0.91	0.86	0.82	0.85	0.84
YOLOv5 + MAM	0.88	0.94	0.92	0.85	0.91	0.87
YOLOv7 + MAM	0.92	0.96	0.95	0.87	0.93	0.89

Figure 9a illustrates a comparison bar chart of original images with the different available methods and Figure 9b illustrates a comparison bar chart of illuminated images with the different available methods. The performance of the proposed methodology in detecting apples in live orchards is depicted in Figure 10. Figure 10a illustrates a straightforward frame of apples from an input video that was shot by a drone. Figure 10b presents the results of the detection of apples with YOLOv5 along with the multi-head attention mechanism. Figure 10c demonstrates the outcome of the improved detection of apples using YOLOv7 with the multi-head attention mechanism.

In comparison between the YOLOv5 + MAM model and YOLOv7 + MAM model, as shown in Figure 10, the number of apples identified by the proposed model was enhanced by comparing the output images. A few apples were undetectable and unidentifiable by the previous models. This problem was completely resolved by the proposed YOLOv7 + MAM model. Every apple had its depth displayed, which made it easier for us to see how far apart the apples were from one another and from the drone's spatial configurations. Taking into account the depth, the basic three-dimensional image of the apple from a different perspective would offer an estimate of apple yield. Increasing the localization accuracy is feasible to deal with occlusions. The results of estimating depth and detecting every potential apple are presented in the outputs. A few ground truth problems, such as sunlight and shade, can be fixed by altering the confidence and non-maximum suppression threshold. The model's accuracy was tested under various illumination conditions, like low, normal, and high illumination, and the proposed model accuracy was optimal under all conditions, as shown in Figure 11. Each bar represents a distinct environmental condition and the rise of the bar signifies the model's improved accuracy under varied conditions. The obtained performance was compared with the other models' performances. The agility of the proposed architecture was demonstrated by evaluating a number of factors that affect system performance, including noise, light change, and blurry images. Using a kernel of (3 × 3), the Gaussian blur method was used in the blurriness stage.

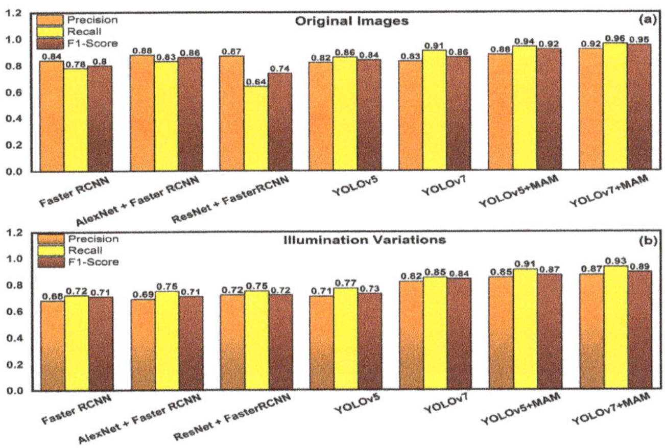

Figure 9. (**a**) Performance comparison bar graph of original images with existing models; (**b**) Performance comparison bar graph of illumination variation images with existing models.

3.3. *Performance of Apple Tracking*

To evaluate the effectiveness of the multi-object tracking methods, we considered the DeepSORT method and proposed the ByteTrack method for tracking and counting the apples [50,51]. Regarding multi-object tracking, the approach suggested in this study used deep learning. Therefore, it may be considered as an identical benchmark. In addition, the effectiveness of multi-object tracking was evaluated by directly using the trained YOLOv7 + MAM model for video detection. For the tracking and counting studies, three apple videos were chosen, and the following Equation (5) for mean absolute percent error (MAPE) was applied to compare the counting accuracy of the automated system with the manually recorded results:

$$\mathrm{MAPE} = \frac{1}{n}\sum_{i=1}^{n}\left|\frac{X_t^i - Y_t^i}{Y_t^i}\right| \tag{5}$$

where Y_t^i indicates the entire number of manually counted apples in the collected video sequence, X_t^i shows the results of the apples counting process utilizing two multi-objective tracking algorithms, n is the total number of videos that need to be recognized, and i represents the current initial video. The choice of this indicator makes it feasible to observe the general characteristics of the model visually. Table 2 presents the comparative results of apple tracking and counting results using the methods DeepSORT and ByteTrack. The three apple videos considered were apple video ID1, apple video ID2, and apple video ID3. The video lengths of live inference of apples were 2.51 min, 1.48 min, and 0.41 s, respectively. After video detection with the proposed model, the detected results were forwarded to tracking using the ByteTrack algorithm. We employed the ByteTrack implementation with the developed YOLOv7 + MAM detection model. In this proposed execution, a tracker class was initiated, and appropriate tracks of the tracker instances were updated for every image in the video stream using the detections. Two formats were available for entering the detection: [h1, g1, h2, g2, score] or [h1, g1, h2, g2, object_score, class_score, class_id]. A set of active tracklets with attributes such as track_id, present frame bounding box, and confidence score may be found in the output online targets. The performance comparison is illustrated in Figure 12a,b with respect to the apple counting applied by the DeepSORT and ByteTrack techniques.For unblemished transparency of the tracking count of apples, only the count of tracking ID for each apple was displayed in the output, as shown in Figure 13a–c. The output also displayed the count of the number of apples being tracked in the left top corner of the video stream considered for the experiments at different intervals of time.

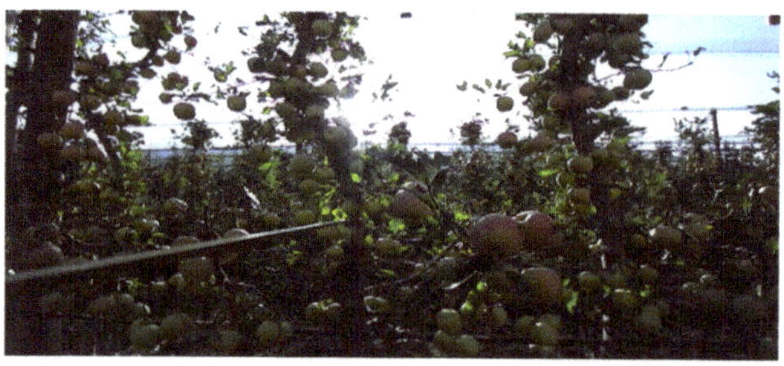

(a)

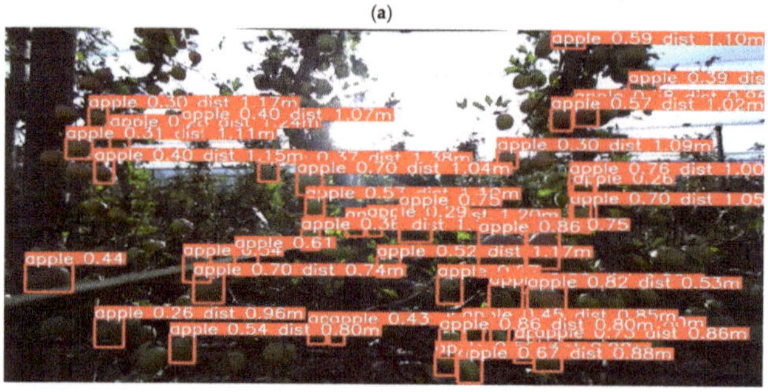

(b)

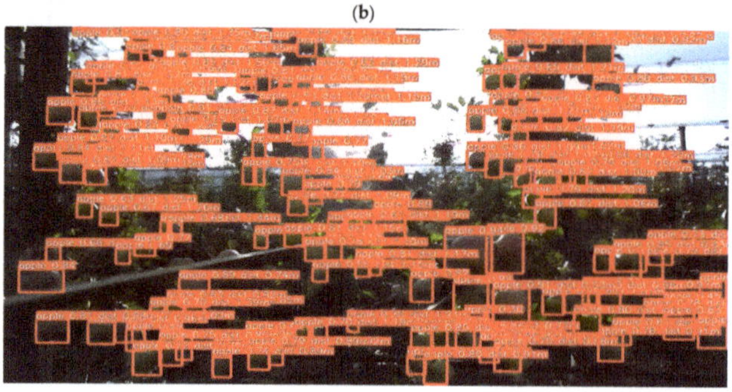

(c)

Figure 10. (**a**) Drone-centered image for apple detection in an apple orchard; (**b**) Inference of apple detection in an apple orchard using YOLOv5 + MAM; (**c**) Inference of apple detection in an orchard using proposed YOLOv7 + MAM.

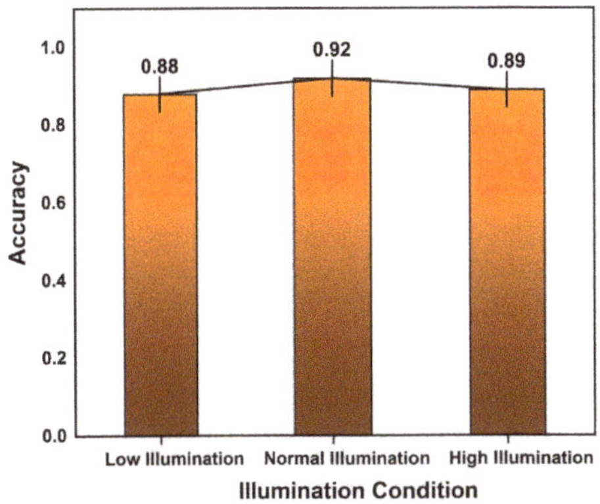

Figure 11. Model's accuracy under various lighting conditions.

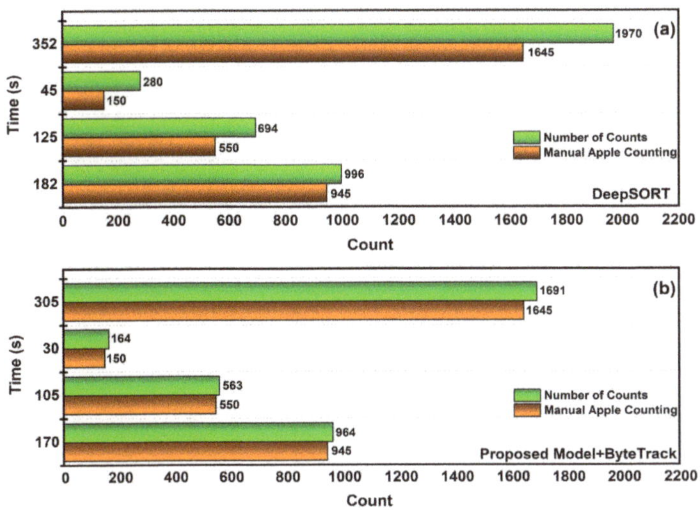

Figure 12. (**a**) Performance comparison graph of manual counting and DeepSORT tracking technique; (**b**) Performance comparison graph of manual counting and proposed tracking technique.

Table 2. Obtained experimental MAPE results of counting apples in live video inference.

Apple Video ID	Manual Apple Counting	Tracking Methods Employed after YOLOv7 + MAM	Count Time in Seconds	Number of Counts	MAPE
1	945	DeepSORT	182	996	0.053
		Proposed Model + ByteTrack	170	964	0.026
2	550	DeepSORT	125	694	0.261
		Proposed Model + ByteTrack	105	563	0.023
3	150	DeepSORT	45	280	0.866
		Proposed Model + ByteTrack	30	164	0.093
All	1645	DeepSORT	352	1970	0.197
		Proposed Model + ByteTrack	305	1691	0.027

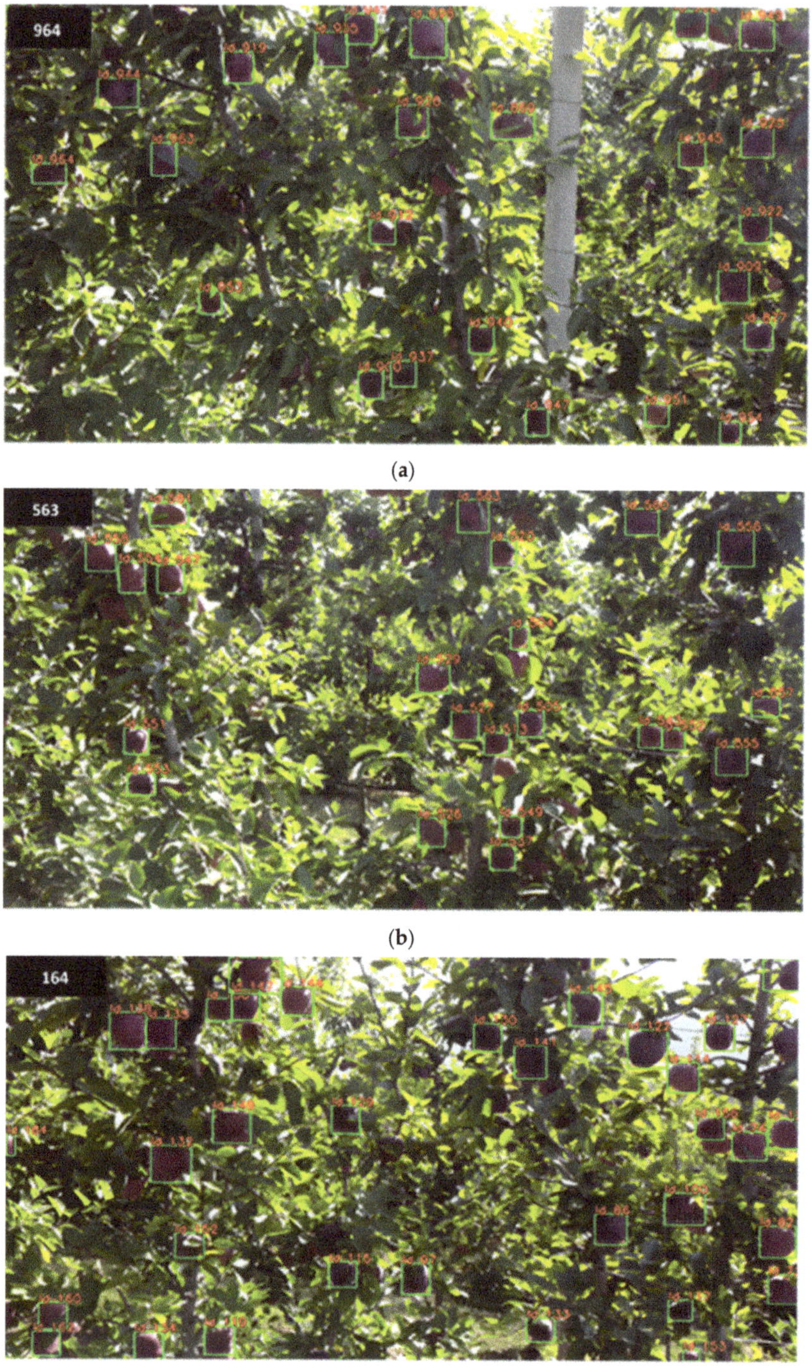

(a)

(b)

(c)

Figure 13. (**a**) The apple tracking results of Video ID1 after applyingYOLOv7 + MAM + ByteTrack; (**b**) The apple tracking results of Video ID2 after applying YOLOv7 + MAM + ByteTrack; (**c**) The apple tracking results of Video ID3 after applying YOLOv7 + MAM + ByteTrack.

4. Discussion

Based on the results mentioned in Table 1, we observed that YOLOv7+ MAM demonstrated a significant increase in overall performance along with enhancements in precision, recall, and F1 score. The results presented here imply that including an attention mechanism improves the capacity to recognize apples using YOLOv5 and YOLOv7. Interestingly, adding the multi-head attention mechanism did not significantly alter the model's size impact on running speed. YOLOv7, nevertheless, performed better overall compared to the YOLOv5 network. Deep neural networks can combine fruit graphs with various feature distributions to enhance overall generalization performance in light of migration learning. As a result, the prediction model may be built using several factors discovered by localized migration learning. This study revealed that the multi-head attention mechanism's inclusion had no appreciable impact on the model's size scale. This could be because the attention mechanism additional layer deepened the model's understanding of small objects while adding little to the overall complexity of the computation. As a result, the model's size remained relatively high. This could facilitate model deployment by allowing the compression to concentrate primarily on the optimization aspect of backbone network pruning rather than the structure's overall compression [52]. The primary benefit of this method is labeling the apple center and not the bounding box. This is quite beneficial in dense orchards. In addition to using cutting-edge technologies, YOLOv5 performed more accurately than previous models [53]. However, low light, motion blur, and complex backgrounds can affect how well these systems operate. We developed a novel deep learning mechanism based on YOLOv7 and a multi-head attention mechanism to address these issues. To address size changes, we implemented an attribute extension model operation on top of this architecture. In distinguishing between mature and immature apples, size is a critical aspect. Mature apples have larger diameters than immature ones. During training, the model learned to distinguish ripe apples based on the average size of their bounding boxes in the training sample. Therefore, the model implicitly learned a limit or range of permissible bounding box sizes for mature apples. When the model was applied for inference on live videos, it used the previously learned criteria to assess if a detected apple was likely to be a mature apple. If the bounding box associated with an object was inside the learned threshold for matured apples, the model considered it a valid detection. However, if the bounding box size was less than this criterion, signifying that the apple detected was most likely an immature apple, the model did not consider it a valid detection. Determining the three-dimensional location of every identified apple in the environment is essential for apple detection, and here is where depth estimation comes into play. This may be used to determine the distance between each apple and the camera. The YOLOv7 bounding boxes and depth information were linked to provide the three-dimensional location data (x, y, z) for every detected apple. ByteTrack used the identified apples' 3D coordinates as the starting point for tracking objects.

The counting results depicted that our suggested YOLOv7 + MAM + ByteTrack tracking approach outperformed the DeepSORT tracking method. Given that the suggested machine learning model produced the least amount of error, it was regarded as an efficient model and had the lowest MAPE [54,55]. The proposed model tracking experiment was performed on three different videos, and the consolidated MAPE applying DeepSORT was 0.197 and our proposed model attained a low MAPE of 0.027. The DeepSORT [56] technique also provided almost near results, but the duplication of apples and background apples that were not measured for the series of sequence counts made the model vulnerable. However, ByteTrack along with the recommended detection method categorized the apples in the foreground and background and included only the targeted apples in the count. When bounding boxes of apples were recognized, DeepSORT employed the ReID identifying model to link them across frames. If an apple could not be connected, SORT used the Kalman filter's predicted bounding box movements to link it between frames. It included only the bounding boxes with relatively high confidence. On the contrary, ByteTrack tracked the apples between frames solely by predicting their movements, using bounding boxes that were computed using the Kalman filter, eliminating the need for ReID. As a result, it shared technical similarities with DeepSort's Sort process. Nevertheless, dividing the processing into two stages, the first procedure aimed at the boundaries of the boxes having high confidence values and the second one with low confidence values, enhanced the performance.

To enhance the tracker performance, specific hyper parameters were utilized, such as MIN_THRESHOLD, which was set to 0.001 to retrieve nearly all detections. Bounding boxes, which were regarded as background boxes, were further filtered in the current model by a hard-coded background threshold set at 0.1. We could adjust MIN_THRESHOLD to values greater than 0.1 if we require more precision in our detection. However, this could exclude critical occluded object detection. To determine whether the threshold chosen offers the right quality, we should qualitatively review the situation.

It should also be emphasized that counting apples and recognizing their positions are two independent problems in the context of apple detection and tracking. The detection and tracking approaches also require different algorithms. The detection phase refers to the physical coordinates or bounding box of each apple within an image or video frame. This challenge requires recognizing the existence of apples and precisely determining their locations. From a technical aspect, detecting positions demands the creation of object identification algorithms capable of not only identifying objects but also providing precise spatial localization data. In terms of detecting apple positions, the algorithm's purpose is to provide bounding box coordinates for each discovered apple. These coordinates define the exact geographical location and size of each apple in the scene.

The counting refers to determining the total number of apples in a given scene or image. This assignment often entails identifying each apple and then adding it to the count of the total. The ID generated for each individual bounding box for each apple is not repeated. Each object is recognized with a unique ID in the live video captured by drone. The primary goal of the counting apples algorithm is to identify whether each observed apple object correlates precisely with the incremented ID number and the number of apples counted in the scene.

The comparative analysis illustrates that the proposed integrated approach achieved optimum performance even under different lightening conditions. Table 3 shows the time complexity for the YOLOv5 and YOLOv7 models combined with DeepSORT and ByteTrack at an mAP of 0.5 accuracy, including CPU and GPU time. The proposed approach resulted in the best accuracy, with low CPU and GPU time.

Table 3. Analyzing the performance of time complexity of tested models.

Models	Parameters (Million)	Accuracy (mAP 0.5)	CPU Time (ms)	GPU Time (ms)
YOLOv5 + MAM + DeepSORT	32.5	75.20	320	11.3
YOLOv7 + MAM + DeepSORT	24.6	79.32	220	9.1
YOLOv5 + MAM + ByteTrack	17.3	83.55	161	8.2
YOLOv7 + MAM + ByteTrack	11.5	92.35	71	6.4

To summarize the discussion, we found that the YOLOv7 + MAM detection head in conjunction with the ByteTrack tracking algorithm produced the best experimental results. The essential parameters for this approach are provided in Section 3. These findings suggest that a multi-head attention mechanism can enhance the detector's performance and that processing images with ByteTrack can improve its efficacy in multi-object tracking. These findings also provide a better framework for fruit counting research in the future. There are a few factors that should be considered, like deployment of GPU in different farm fields of apples that vary based on different geographical and growth environment conditions. The research is low cost and the proposed systems are scalable, allowing monitoring of orchards of all sizes, from small family farms to large commercial enterprises. Whether tracking acres or thousands of hectares, the proposed model offers a versatile and scalable alternative for apple detection, depth estimate, and agricultural monitoring. The client could obtain an exact count of the apples ready for harvest. Although color, shape, and size are minimal factors as limitations, the speed of the drone and the detection and tracking rate are major concerns that might affect the overall present fruit counting methodology. In the future, we plan to integrate different attention mechanisms with the latest lightweight models to attain a balance between speed and performance in fruit counting.

5. Conclusions

In this work, we proposed a YOLOv7 framework with a multi-head attention mechanism integrated with a ByteTrack multi-object tracking system to detect and count apple fruits in orchards. The results of our experiments demonstrated that the accuracy and robustness of apple identification were significantly improved by combining YOLOv7 with a multi-head attention mechanism. Even with difficult lighting circumstances and a variety of apple orientations, the model could successfully detect the apples along with the depth estimation of each apple, which enabled determination of the distance between each apple and the drone camera. Furthermore, ByteTrack for apple counting ensured our system's effectiveness. Apple counting was made simple and quick by seamlessly integrating ByteTrack for apple detection and tracking. ByteTrack ensured that tracking continued even if the apples moved, varied in appearance, or momentarily disappeared from the drone's vision. The method successfully dealt with occlusions and various sizes of apples in the orchard, which helped to provide precise and accurate counting outcomes. To verify the efficacy of our suggested model, we carried out comprehensive comparison tests with many current detection and counting techniques. The outcomes demonstrated how well the model performed in achieving the ideal balance between speed and precision, which makes it an invaluable tool for precision agriculture. We believe that our work paves the way for more developments in agricultural automation and establishes a solid basis for future research on object recognition and counting in complicated contexts.

Author Contributions: Conceptualization, P.K.S., F.M. and R.R.; methodology, P.K.S., F.M., R.R. and R.d.A.S.; software, R.R., R.d.A.S. and P.K.S.; formal analysis, P.K.S., F.M., J.M. and J.M.J.; resources, F.M., J.M.J. and J.M.; data curation, P.K.S. and R.R.; writing—original draft preparation, P.K.S. and F.M.; writing—review and editing, P.K.S., R.R., R.d.A.S. and F.M.; supervision, F.M., J.M.J. and J.M.; project administration, F.M., J.M.J. and J.M.; funding acquisition, F.M. and J.M. All authors have read and agreed to the published version of the manuscript.

Funding: This research was funded by the Fondazione Caritro (Trento, Italy) under the program 'Bando Post-doc 2021'. International collaboration is co-funded by the Italian Ministry of Foreign Affairs and International Cooperation and the Brazilian National Council of State Funding Agencies.

Institutional Review Board Statement: Not applicable.

Informed Consent Statement: Not applicable.

Data Availability Statement: Data are contained within the article.

Acknowledgments: This research was carried out within the framework of a project entitled 'System based on Artificial Intelligence and Drones for Apple Picking Automation in Trentino' funded by the Fondazione Caritro (Trento, Italy). International collaboration was possible thanks to the project entitled "Deep Learning for Precision Farming Mapping", co-founded by the Italian Ministry of Foreign Affairs and International Cooperation and the Brazilian National Council of State Funding Agencies. We would also like to acknowledge the use of Grammarly to improve the clarity and correctness of the English language in the manuscript.

Conflicts of Interest: The authors declare no conflicts of interest. The funders had no role in the design of the study; in the collection, analyses, or interpretation of data; in the writing of the manuscript; or in the decision to publish the results.

References

1. Zou, Z.; Chen, K.; Shi, Z.; Guo, Y.; Ye, J. Object detection in 20 years: A survey. *arXiv* **2019**, arXiv:1905.05055. [CrossRef]
2. Murala, S.; Vipparthi, S.K.; Akhtar, Z. Vision Based Computing Systems for Healthcare Applications. *J. Healthc. Eng.* **2019**, *2019*, 9581275. [CrossRef] [PubMed]
3. Tian, Y.; Yang, G.; Wang, Z.; Wang, H.; Li, E.; Liang, Z. Apple Detection during Different Growth Stages in Orchards Using the Improved YOLO-V3 Model. *Comput. Electron. Agric.* **2019**, *157*, 417–426. [CrossRef]
4. Zhao, C. Current situations and prospects of smart agriculture. *J. South China Agric. Univ.* **2021**, *42*, 1–7.
5. Cohen, O.; Linker, R.; Naor, A. Estimation of the number of apples in color images recorded in orchards. In Proceedings of the International Conference on Computer and Computing Technologies in Agriculture, Nanchang, China, 22–25 October 2010; pp. 630–642.
6. Ji, W.; Zhao, D.; Cheng, F.; Xu, B.; Zhang, Y.; Wang, J. Automatic recognition vision system guided for apple harvesting robot. *Comput. Electr. Eng.* **2012**, *38*, 1186–1195. [CrossRef]
7. Bulanon, D.; Kataoka, T.; Zhang, S.; Ota, Y.; Hiroma, T. Optimal Thresholding for the Automatic Recognition of Apple Fruits. In Proceedings of the 2001 ASAE Annual Meeting, Sacramento, CA, USA, 29 July–1 August 2001. [CrossRef]
8. Yan, B.; Fan, P.; Lei, X.; Liu, Z.; Yang, F. A Real-Time Apple Targets Detection Method for Picking Robot Based on Improved YOLOv5. *Remote Sens.* **2021**, *13*, 1619. [CrossRef]
9. Prasetiyowati, M.I.; Maulidevi, N.U.; Surendro, K. Determining threshold value on information gain feature selection to increase speed and prediction accuracy of random forest. *J. Big Data* **2021**, *8*, 84. [CrossRef]
10. López-Morales, J.A.; Martínez, J.A.; Skarmeta, A.F. Digital transformation of agriculture through the use of an interoperable platform. *Sensors* **2020**, *20*, 1153. [CrossRef]
11. Sun, J.; He, X.; Ge, X.; Wu, X.; Shen, J.; Song, Y. Detection of Key Organs in Tomato Based on Deep Migration Learning in a Complex Background. *Agriculture* **2018**, *8*, 196. [CrossRef]
12. Bulanon, D.; Kataoka, T. Fruit detection system and an end effector for robotic harvesting of Fuji apples. *Agric. Eng. Int. CIGR E-J.* **2010**, *12*, 203–210.
13. Tian, Y.; Duan, H.; Luo, R.; Zhang, Y.; Jia, W.; Lian, J.; Zheng, Y.; Ruan, C.; Li, C. Fast Recognition and Location of Target Fruit Based on Depth Information. *IEEE Access* **2019**, *7*, 170553–170563. [CrossRef]
14. Hu, L. An Improved YOLOv5 Algorithm of Target Recognition. In Proceedings of the 2023 IEEE 2nd International Conference on Electrical Engineering, Big Data and Algorithms (EEBDA), Changchun, China, 24–26 February 2023. [CrossRef]
15. Wang, J.; Su, Y.; Yao, J.; Liu, M.; Du, Y.; Wu, X.; Huang, L.; Zhao, M. Apple rapid recognition and processing method based on an improved version of YOLOv5. *Ecol. Inform.* **2023**, *77*, 102196. [CrossRef]
16. Shang, Y.; Xu, X.; Jiao, Y.; Wang, Z.; Hua, Z.; Song, H. Using lightweight deep learning algorithm for real-time detection of apple flowers in natural environments. *Comput. Electron. Agric.* **2023**, *207*, 107765. [CrossRef]
17. Mirbod, O.; Choi, D.; Heinemann, P.H.; Marini, R.P.; He, L. On-tree apple fruit size estimation using stereo vision with deep learning-based occlusion handling. *Biosyst. Eng.* **2023**, *226*, 27–42. [CrossRef]
18. Gené-Mola, J.; Sanz-Cortiella, R.; Rosell-Polo, J.R.; Escolà, A.; Gregorio, E. PFuji-Size dataset: A collection of images and photogrammetry-derived 3D point clouds with ground truth annotations for Fuji apple detection and size estimation in field conditions. *Data Brief* **2021**, *39*, 107629. [CrossRef] [PubMed]
19. Biffi, L.J.; Mitishita, E.; Liesenberg, V.; Santos, A.A.; Gonçalves, D.N.; Estrabis, N.V.; Silva, J.D.; Osco, L.P.; Ramos, A.P.; Centeno, J.A.; et al. ATSS Deep Learning-Based Approach to Detect Apple Fruits. *Remote Sens.* **2020**, *13*, 54. [CrossRef]
20. Ma, L.; Zhao, L.; Wang, Z.; Zhang, J.; Chen, G. Detection and Counting of Small Target Apples under Complicated Environments by Using Improved YOLOv7-tiny. *Agronomy* **2023**, *13*, 1419. [CrossRef]
21. Chen, J.; Mai, H.; Luo, L.; Chen, X.; Wu, K. Effective Feature Fusion Network in BIFPN for Small Object Detection. In Proceedings of the 2021 IEEE International Conference on Image Processing (ICIP), Anchorage, AK, USA, 19–22 September 2021; pp. 699–703.
22. Hodson, T.O. Root-Mean-Square Error (RMSE) or Mean Absolute Error (MAE): When to Use Them or Not. *Geosci. Model Dev.* **2022**, *15*, 5481–5487. [CrossRef]
23. Hussain, M.; Al-Aqrabi, H.; Munawar, M.; Hill, R.; Alsboui, T. Domain feature mapping with YOLOv7 for automated edge-based pallet racking inspections. *Sensors* **2022**, *22*, 6927. [CrossRef] [PubMed]
24. Wang, J.L.; Li, A.Y.; Huang, M.; Ibrahim, A.K.; Zhuang, H.; Ali, A.M. Classification of white blood cells with pattern net-fused ensemble of convolutional neural networks (pecnn). In Proceedings of the 2018 IEEE International Symposium on Signal Processing and Information Technology (ISSPIT), Louisville, KY, USA, 6–8 December 2018; pp. 325–330.
25. Brock, H.; Rengot, J.; Nakadai, K. Augmenting sparse corpora for enhanced sign language recognition and generation. In Proceedings of the 11th International Conference on Language Resources and Evaluation (LREC 2018) and the 8th Workshop on the Representation and Processing of Sign Languages: Involving the Language Community, Miyazaki, Japan, 7–12 May 2018; pp. 7–12.
26. Yang, H.; Liu, Y.; Wang, S.; Qu, H.; Li, N.; Wu, J.; Yan, Y.; Zhang, H.; Wang, J.; Qiu, J. Improved Apple Fruit Target Recognition Method Based on YOLOv7 Model. *Agriculture* **2023**, *13*, 1278. [CrossRef]

27. Shindo, T.; Watanabe, T.; Yamada, K.; Watanabe, H. Accuracy improvement of object detection in VVC coded video using YOLO-v7 features. *arXiv* **2023**, arXiv:2304.00689v1.
28. Wang, C.-Y.; Bochkovskiy, A.; Liao, H.-Y.M. YOLOv7: Trainable bag-of-freebies sets new state-of-the-art for real-time object detectors. *arXiv* **2022**, arXiv:2207.02696.
29. Hu, J.; Fan, C.; Wang, Z.; Ruan, J.; Wu, S. Fruit Detection and Counting in Apple Orchards Based on Improved Yolov7 and Multi-Object Tracking Methods. *Sensors* **2023**, *23*, 5903. [CrossRef] [PubMed]
30. Xiao, B.; Nguyen, M.; Yan, W.Q. Apple ripeness identification from digital images using transformers. *Multimedia Tools Appl.* **2023**, *83*, 7811–7825. [CrossRef]
31. Chen, X.; Pu, H.; He, Y.; Lai, M.; Zhang, D.; Chen, J.; Pu, H. An Efficient Method for Monitoring Birds Based on Object Detection and Multi-Object Tracking Networks. *Animals* **2023**, *13*, 1713. [CrossRef] [PubMed]
32. Vaswani, A.; Shazeer, N.; Parmar, N.; Uszkoreit, J.; Jones, L.; Gomez, A.N.; Kaiser, L.; Polosukhin, I. Attention Is All You Need. *arXiv* **2017**, arXiv:1706.03762.
33. Thakuria, A.; Erkinbaev, C. Improving the network architecture of YOLOv7 to achieve real-time grading of canola based on kernel health. *Smart Agric. Technol.* **2023**, *5*, 100300. [CrossRef]
34. Andriyanov, N.; Khasanshin, I.; Utkin, D.; Gataullin, T.; Ignar, S.; Shumaev, V.; Soloviev, V. Intelligent System for Estimation of the Spatial Position of Apples Based on YOLOv3 and Real Sense Depth Camera D415. *Symmetry* **2022**, *14*, 148. [CrossRef]
35. Stereolabs Docs: API Reference, Tutorials, and Integration. Available online: https://docs.stereolabs.com/depth-sensing/depth-settings (accessed on 5 December 2023).
36. Wang, H.; Feng, J.; Yin, H. Improved Method for Apple Fruit Target Detection Based on YOLOv5s. *Agriculture* **2023**, *13*, 2167. [CrossRef]
37. Zhao, Z.; Wang, J.; Zhao, H. Research on Apple Recognition Algorithm in Complex Orchard Environment Based on Deep Learning. *Sensors* **2023**, *23*, 5425. [CrossRef]
38. Kumar, S.P.; Naveen Kumar, K. Drone-based apple detection: Finding the depth of apples using YOLOv7 architecture with multi-head attention mechanism. *Smart Agric. Technol.* **2023**, *5*, 100311. [CrossRef]
39. Liu, J.; Wang, C.; Xing, J. YOLOv5-ACS: Improved Model for Apple Detection and Positioning in Apple Forests in Complex Scenes. *Forests* **2023**, *14*, 2304. [CrossRef]
40. Sekharamantry, P.K.; Melgani, F.; Malacarne, J. Deep Learning-Based Apple Detection with Attention Module and Improved Loss Function in YOLO. *Remote Sens.* **2023**, *15*, 1516. [CrossRef]
41. Kong, T.; Sun, F.; Liu, H.; Jiang, Y.; Li, L.; Shi, J. Foveabox: Beyound anchor-based object detection. *IEEE Trans. Image Process.* **2020**, *29*, 7389–7398. [CrossRef]
42. Ren, S.; He, K.; Girshick, R.; Sun, J. Faster R-CNN: Towards Real-Time Object Detection with Region Proposal Networks. *arXiv* **2016**, arXiv:1506.01497. [CrossRef]
43. Bewley, A.; Ge, Z.; Ott, L.; Ramos, F.; Upcroft, B. Simple online and realtime tracking. In Proceedings of the 2016 IEEE International Conference on Image Processing (ICIP), Phoenix, AZ, USA, 25–28 September 2016; pp. 3464–3468.
44. Zhang, Y.; Sun, P.; Jiang, Y.; Yu, D.; Yuan, Z.; Luo, P.; Liu, W.; Wang, X. Track: Multi-Object Tracking by Associating Every Detection Box. *arXiv* **2021**, arXiv:2110.06864.
45. Yu, C.; Feng, Z.; Wu, Z.; Wei, R.; Song, B.; Cao, C. HB-YOLO: An Improved YOLOv7 Algorithm for Dim-Object Tracking in Satellite Remote Sensing Videos. *Remote Sens.* **2023**, *15*, 3551. [CrossRef]
46. Welch, G.; Bishop, G. *An Introduction to the Kalman Filter*; University of North Carolina at chapel hill: Chapel hill, NC, USA, 1995; p. 2.
47. Kuhn, H.W. The Hungarian method for the assignment problem. *Nav. Res. Logist.* **2005**, *52*, 7–21. [CrossRef]
48. Yang, H.; Chang, F.; Huang, Y.; Xu, M.; Zhao, Y.; Ma, L.; Su, H. Multi-object tracking using deep SORT and modified CenterNet in cotton seedling counting. *Comput. Electron. Agric.* **2022**, *202*, 107339. [CrossRef]
49. Fischer, T.; Huang, T.E.; Pang, J.; Qiu, L.; Chen, H.; Darrell, T.; Yu, F. QDTrack: Quasi-Dense Similarity Learning for Appearance-Only Multiple Object Tracking. *arXiv* **2022**, arXiv:2210.06984. [CrossRef] [PubMed]
50. Zhang, Y.; Sun, P.; Jiang, Y.; Yu, D.; Weng, F.; Yuan, Z.; Luo, P.; Liu, W.; Wang, X. ByteTrack: Multi-object Tracking by Associating Every Detection Box. In *Computer Vision—ECCV 2022*; Avidan, S., Brostow, G., Cissé, M., Farinella, G.M., Hassner, T., Eds.; ECCV 2022. Lecture Notes in Computer Science; Springer: Cham, Switzerland, 2022; Volume 13682. [CrossRef]
51. Zheng, Z.; Li, J.; Qin, L. YOLO-BYTE: An efficient multi-object tracking algorithm for automatic monitoring of dairy cows. *Comput. Electron. Agric.* **2023**, *209*, 107857. [CrossRef]
52. Gennari, M.; Fawcett, R.; Prisacariu, V.A. DSConv: Efficient Convolution Operator. In Proceedings of the IEEE/CVF International Conference on Computer Vision, Seoul, Republic of Korea, 27 October–2 November 2019.
53. van Meekeren, A.; Aghaei, M.; Dijkstra, K. Exploring the Effectiveness of Dataset Synthesis: An application of Apple Detection in Orchards. *arXiv* **2013**, arXiv:2306.11763.
54. Gené-Mola, J.; Ferrer-Ferrer, M.; Gregorio, E.; Blok, P.M.; Hemming, J.; Morros, J.-R.; Rosell-Polo, J.R.; Vilaplana, V.; Ruiz-Hidalgo, J. Looking behind occlusions: A study on amodal segmentation for robust on-tree apple fruit size estimation. *Comput. Electron. Agric.* **2023**, *209*, 107854. [CrossRef]

55. Ferrer-Ferrer, M.; Ruiz-Hidalgo, J.; Gregorio, E.; Vilaplana, V.; Morros, J.-R.; Gené-Mola, J. Simultaneous fruit detection and size estimation using multitask deep neural networks. *Biosyst. Eng.* **2023**, *233*, 63–75. [CrossRef]
56. Abeyrathna, R.M.R.D.; Nakaguchi, V.M.; Minn, A.; Ahamed, T. Recognition and Counting of Apples in a Dynamic State Using a 3D Camera and Deep Learning Algorithms for Robotic Harvesting Systems. *Sensors* **2023**, *23*, 3810. [CrossRef]

computers

MDPI

Article

Optimizing Loss Functions for You Only Look Once Models: Improving Object Detection in Agricultural Datasets

Atsuki Matsui [1], Ryuto Ishibashi [1] and Lin Meng [2,*]

[1] Graduate School of Science and Engineering, Ritsumeikan University, 1-1-1, Nojihigashi, Kusatsu 525-8577, Shiga, Japan; ri0106hi@ed.ritsumei.ac.jp (A.M.); ri0097fx@ed.ritsumei.ac.jp (R.I.)
[2] College of Science and Engineering, Ritsumeikan University, 1-1-1, Nojihigashi, Kusatsu 525-8577, Shiga, Japan
* Correspondence: menglin@fc.ritsumei.ac.jp

Abstract: Japan faces a significant labor shortage due to an aging population, particularly in the agricultural sector. The rising average age of farmers and the declining participation of younger individuals threaten the sustainability of farming practices. These trends reduce the availability of agricultural labor and pose a risk to lowering Japan's food self-sufficiency rate. The reliance on food imports raises concerns regarding price fluctuations and sanitation standards. Moreover, the challenging working conditions in agriculture and a lack of technological innovation have hindered productivity and increased the burden on the existing workforce. To address these challenges, "smart agriculture" presents a promising solution. By leveraging advanced technologies such as sensors, drones, the Internet of Things (IoT), and automation, smart agriculture aims to optimize farm operations. Real-time data collection and AI-driven analysis play a crucial role in monitoring crop growth, assessing soil conditions, and improving overall efficiency. This study proposes enhancements to the YOLO (You Only Look Once) object detection model to develop an automated tomato harvesting system. This system uses a camera to detect tomatoes and assess their ripeness for harvest. Our objective is to streamline the harvesting process through AI technology. Our improved YOLO model integrates two novel loss functions to enhance detection accuracy. The first, "VSR", refines the model's ability to classify tomatoes and determine their harvest readiness. The second, "SBCE", enhances the detection of small tomatoes by training the model to recognize a range of object sizes within the dataset. These improvements have significantly increased the system's detection performance. Our experimental results demonstrate that the mean Average Precision (mAP) of YOLOv7-tiny improved from 61.81% to 70.21%. Additionally, the F1 score increased from 0.61 to 0.71 and the mean Intersection over Union (mIoU) rose from 65.03% to 66.44% on the tomato dataset. These findings underscore the potential of our proposed system to enhance efficiency in agricultural practices.

Keywords: object detection; YOLO; loss

1. Introduction

Recently, the labor shortage caused by Japan's aging population has become a critical issue. This challenge is particularly severe in the agricultural sector, where farmers struggle with a significant workforce decline. The sustainability of farming practices is under threat, primarily due to the aging population. According to data from the Ministry of Agriculture, Forestry and Fisheries [1], the number of farmers has decreased from 1.302 million in 2020 to 1.114 million in 2024. In addition, the average age of farmers has increased from 67.8 to 68.7 over the same period.

Furthermore, slow technological innovation has hindered productivity while increasing workloads, which has exacerbated the labor shortage in agriculture. These factors collectively contribute to the steady decline in the agricultural workforce. To address these challenges, "smart agriculture" presents a promising solution. Smart agriculture leverages advanced information technology and data analysis to optimize farming processes. This includes using sensor technology, drones, the Internet of Things (IoT), and automation. For instance, real-time data collection via sensors and AI-based analysis enables precise crop growth and monitoring of soil conditions. Additionally, using Unmanned Aerial Vehicles (UAVs) and automated tractors enhances workflow efficiency.

To further enhance agricultural productivity, AI is being implemented to automate various tasks, such as visual inspection and condition checking [2–4]. In this study, we aim to apply AI for agricultural products [5]. This paper focuses on developing an AI-based system for detecting tomato leaf diseases. This system enables farmers to automatically monitor crop conditions, reducing their workload and allowing for more efficient resource allocation.

We employ an AI model called "You Only Look Once" (YOLO) to automate the detection of tomato leaf diseases. YOLO is a widely recognized object detection model known for its high detection speed, which makes it well suited for industrial applications. Its speed enables the real-time inspection of large volumes of crops, while its lightweight design reduces initial costs and power consumption compared to other AI models. Specifically, we use YOLOv7, a model in the YOLO series that offers a balance of superior detection performance and compact size. Our proposed improvements enhance YOLOv7's effectiveness for agricultural applications. This paper introduces two key enhancements to YOLOv7. First, we propose an improvement to the object loss function ($Loss_{obj}$) that trains the model to better account for the distribution of object sizes in the dataset, placing more emphasis on each object. Second, we introduce a novel classification loss function to train the model's classification head, thereby increasing the reliability of its predictions. By optimizing the separation between class dimensions, this approach reduces classification errors.

These enhancements are integrated into YOLOv7 to improve the performance in detecting tomato leaf diseases, as shown in Figure 1. We evaluate the effectiveness of our proposed methods using the PASCAL VOC dataset, commonly used for benchmarking object detection models. The results highlight the quantitative benefits of our approach, underscoring its potential for improving agricultural efficiency.

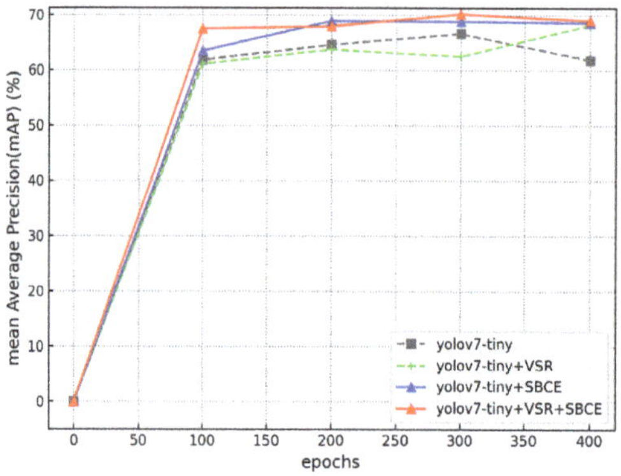

Figure 1. Comparison between our proposal and base model (YOLOv7-tiny).

In summary, the major contributions of this paper are as follows:

- Developing a new loss function to classify the condition of tomatoes more correctly.
- Developing a new loss function to detect small tomato leaf disease efficiently.

The remainder of this paper is structured as follows: Section 2 reviews related work on the current state of tomato leaf disease detection. Section 3 introduces our proposed loss function. Section 4 describes the dataset used in this study. Section 5 presents the results, and Section 6 discusses their implications. Finally, Section 7 concludes this paper and outlines directions for future research.

2. Related Work

This section explains the related works of this study.

2.1. Object Detection

Object detection is a key technology in image processing [6]. It identifies and classifies objects within images, and unlike image recognition, it can detect multiple types of objects in a single image. This versatility enables object detection models to be applied across a wide range of scenarios [7]. For example, automated driving systems rely on onboard cameras to detect pedestrians and vehicles, while manufacturing plants employ object detection to automatically inspect products and parts for external damage.

Object detection models are generally categorized based on their detection workflows. The first category is the two-stage detector, exemplified by models such as R-CNN [8] and Faster R-CNN [9]. These models achieve high detection accuracy but often sacrifice detection speed, making them less suitable for applications that require real-time performance. The second category is the one-stage detector, represented by models like YOLO and SSD [10]. These models prioritize high detection speed but typically offer slightly lower detection accuracy than two-stage detectors. Choosing the appropriate model depends on the specific use case and the dataset's characteristics. Despite its advantages, object detection has a significant drawback: the time-intensive process of creating training data. Each image in the training dataset must be manually annotated with detection targets, which requires substantial effort and time. This challenge makes generating large-scale datasets suitable for training effective object detection models difficult.

2.2. You Only Look Once

YOLO (You Only Look Once) [11] is one of the most popular object detection models, first introduced by Joseph Redmon in 2015. Compared to models such as R-CNN, EfficientDet [12], and DETR [13], YOLO stands out for its lightweight architecture and faster detection speed, making it well suited for real-time applications.

Over the past decade, researchers have continuously enhanced YOLO, resulting in a series of improved versions [14–16]. Various techniques have been employed to refine these models, including advanced feature extraction methods and modifications to training targets. These improvements aim to optimize the training process and further enhance YOLO's detection accuracy, speed, and overall efficiency.

2.2.1. Training

YOLO extracts image features through convolution operations applied to the training dataset. For example, Figure 2 shows the flow of YOLO's object detection on one of the person images of PASCAL VOC dataset. The backbone of YOLO is composed of convolutional blocks that are responsible for extracting these features. These features, known as feature maps, acquire a broader receptive field as the convolutional layers are stacked. However, smaller features may be lost as the receptive field increases.

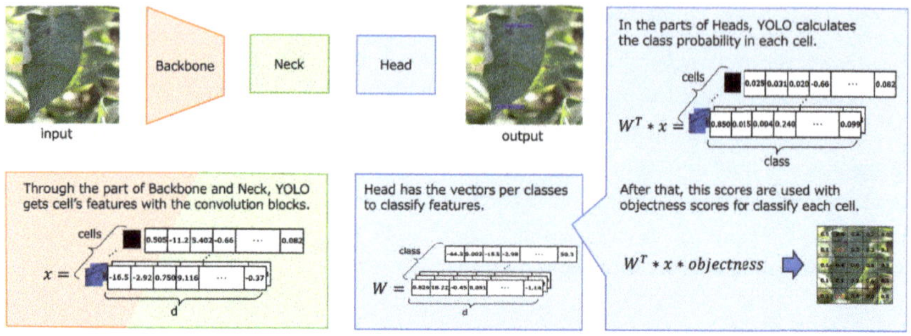

Figure 2. YOLO uses image feature vector (x) and the parameter (W). x is made from the images in the backbone and neck parts. W is the parameter of class representative vectors in the head part. YOLO compares the similarity between these vectors.

To address this issue, the neck component of YOLO is designed to share information among feature maps, combining them to generate feature maps that retain a variety of information. Based on these enriched feature maps, YOLO calculates loss scores and updates the model parameters iteratively. This constitutes the training procedure for YOLO. YOLO employs three key loss functions as the foundation for parameter updates.

L_{IoU} is a score that evaluates the model's ability to predict the object's shape. YOLO predicts the shape of an object for each cell in an image divided into $N \times N$ grids. YOLO assumes that each cell represents the center of an object and predicts the object's height (h) and width (w). To assess the accuracy of the predicted shape, YOLO uses a score called the Intersection over Union (IoU), as shown in Figure 3. IoU is the ratio of the intersection between the Ground Truth (GT) and the Prediction (Pr). IoU can be written as follows:

$$IoU = \sum_{i=1}^{n}\sum_{j=1}^{n} \frac{Intersection_{ij}}{GT + Pr_{ij} - Intersection_{ij}}, \tag{1}$$

L_{IoU} can be written as follows:

$$L_{IoU} = 1 - IoU, \tag{2}$$

Considering various information such as the aspect ratio, many methods are proposed for IoU to predict more correctly [17–19].

L_{obj} is a score that evaluates the model's ability to predict the presence or absence of an object in the image. YOLO predicts the presence or absence of an object for each image cell divided into $N \times N$ grids. YOLO predicts whether an object is present in the image by determining whether a cell contains part of an object. L_{obj} is defined using Binary Cross Entropy (BCE) with the Ground Truth (GT) of each cell and the model's Prediction (Pr). L_{obj} can be written as follows:

$$L_{obj} = \sum_{i=1}^{n}\sum_{j=1}^{n} -(GT_{ij} * \log(Pr_{ij}) + (1 - GT_{ij}) * \log(1 - Pr_{ij})), \tag{3}$$

With various methods such as scaling, BCE is improved as a new $Loss_{obj}$ [20,21].

L_{cls} is a score that evaluates the model's ability to classify objects. YOLO predicts the object class for each image cell divided into $N \times N$ grids. YOLO receives the feature map from the neck, and the head creates a vector x containing d dimensions per cell. The head also has a vector W with d dimensions for each class. By calculating each cell's class information from these two vectors, the head predicts which objects are associated with each cell. L_{cls} is defined using Cross Entropy (CE) with the Ground Truth (GT) of each cell and the model's Prediction (Pr). L_{cls} is written as follows:

$$L_{cls} = \sum_{i=1}^{n}\sum_{j=1}^{n}\sum_{k=1}^{c} -(GT_{ij} * \log(P_{ijk}) + (1 - GT_{ij}) * \log(1 - P_{ijk})), \quad (4)$$

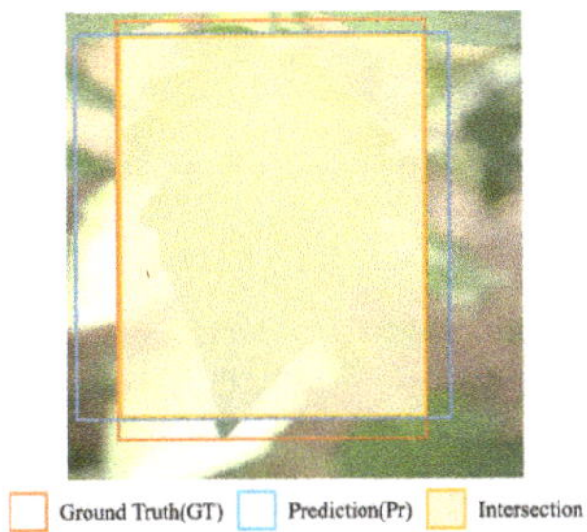

Figure 3. About IoU .

2.2.2. Test

YOLO uses the optimized parameters obtained during training to calculate the final results during testing. For object detection, YOLO combines two outputs, as shown in Figure 4. The first output relates to classification and objectness, which are calculated using the vectors x, the parameter W and the $objectness$ score. YOLO computes this output for each image cell divided into $N \times N$ grids. The second output pertains to the shape of the object. By applying non-maximum suppression to combine the predictions, assuming each cell as the object's center, YOLO accurately predicts the object's shape. By calculating and integrating these outputs simultaneously, YOLO, as a one-stage detector, achieves faster detection speeds.

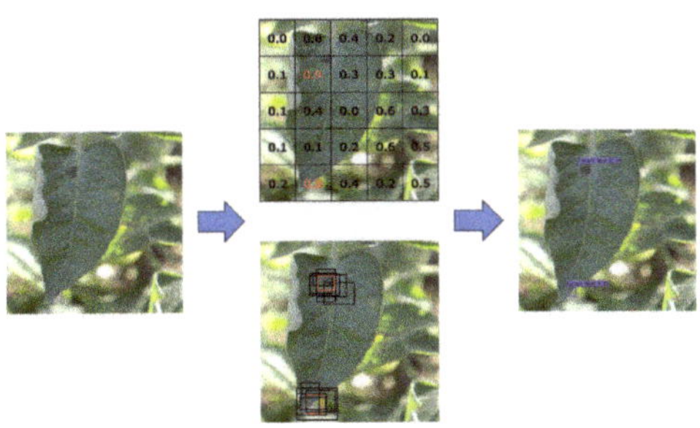

Figure 4. YOLO's output.

3. Method

In this paper, we propose two improvements to the loss function ($Loss$) to train YOLO-based models. By incorporating these new loss components into the training process and optimizing the training targets, our model achieves superior detection performance as an industrial AI compared to baseline models.

In the agricultural sector, where tasks are often large-scale and resource-intensive, smaller model sizes are essential for reducing installation costs and power consumption. However, small AI models face challenges such as limited expressive power and lower detection accuracy due to having fewer parameters. While larger models can enhance expressive power by training on extensive datasets, achieving high accuracy with smaller models requires optimal parameter tuning and advanced loss functions to enhance learning efficiency.

In addition, industrial data sets, particularly in agriculture, are often imbalanced and have limited images due to the challenges associated with data collection and preparation. Training with such datasets presents unique challenges compared to training with large-scale datasets. In this context, each back-propagation step becomes significantly more impactful, highlighting the importance of designing loss functions and training strategies to maximize the effectiveness of small, imbalanced datasets.

3.1. Vector Similarity Regularization

To solve this problem, the first one, referred to as "Vector Similarity Regularization (VSR)", incorporates head parameter into the loss function. As shown in Section 2, the head classifies objects in images using the vectors x and the parameter W. Classification is performed by comparing the similarity between these matrix. Therefore, the parameter W is regarded as the representative class vector. In practice, YOLO compute class probabilities for each $N \times N$ segmented cell of the image. The object's shape and classification are detected simultaneously by predicting which object each cell belongs to. When the values of the parameter W are too similar across classes, the model's classification ability is weakened. Regularization is applied to impose certain constraints and guide the learning process. Such studies have been proposed along with various constraints [22]. Our proposal trains YOLO to improve classification (Precision) by eliminating the similarity of the elements of the parameter W across classes. Cosine similarity, a widely adopted measure for evaluating vector distances, is used to evaluate the similarity between the vector x and the parameter W.

Cosine similarity can be written as follows:

$$\cos(W_i, W_j) = \frac{W_i \cdot W_j}{||W_i||\,||W_j||}, \tag{5}$$

An example of the calculation is shown in Figure 5. When the dataset contains three classes and the head has three dimensions per representative class vector, VSR trains the sum of θ_a, θ_b, and θ_c to increase. The cosine similarity $\cos(W_i, W_j)$ represents the similarity between each pair of dimensions. Since the diagonal elements of a matrix are always 1, the average of the off-diagonal elements is calculated.

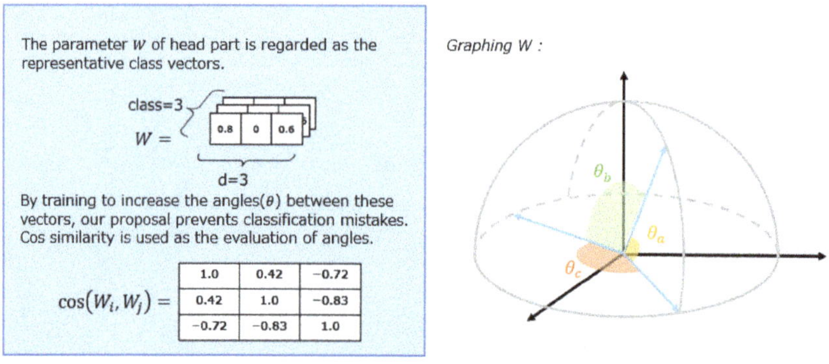

Figure 5. Vector Similarity Regularization (VSR): VSR regards the parameter W as representative class vectors. L_{VSR} trains W to separate representative features between each class.

Algorithm 1 illustrates the flow for calculating L_{VSR}. This proposal uses representative class vectors, with one vector being compared for similarity to the others. The similarity is calculated only for the corresponding dimensions. After computing all similarities, the average of these values is used as the final score.

Algorithm 1 Vector Similarity Regularization

Input: W_{ij}: Head vectors per classes
Output: L_{VSR}

```
l = []
for i in c do
    for j in c do
        if i ≠ j then
            l.append(cos(W_i,W_j))
        end if
    end for
end for
L_VSR = average(l) + 1
```

By training to minimize the cosine similarity between each vector toward -1, our proposal eliminates the similarity of elements between class vectors. Since the loss function requires a non-negative value, we add +1 to ensure that the minimum value is 0 and define L_{VSR} accordingly. L_{VSR} can be written as follows:

$$L_{VSR} = \text{average}(\cos(W_i, W_j)) + 1. \tag{6}$$

This proposal trains YOLO to learn a representative vector for each class, preventing multiple vectors from being similar to vector x. Only one class vector is similar to an object, which can improve classification accuracy. This proposal is classified as "Metric Learning". While various methods have been proposed in the field of "Image Recognition [23–25]", previous YOLO proposals do not adopt it. One reason for this is the training method used in YOLO. YOLO calculates the loss per $N \times N$ cell within the image. Therefore, the entire image feature cannot be treated at one time. This paper incorporates distance learning into YOLO using head vectors instead of image feature vectors. The weights are defined as "$loss_{obj}$:$loss_{cls}$:$loss_{iou}$(:$loss_{aux}$) = 10:1:2(:1)" for the PASCAL VOC dataset. This ratio remains in the open-source code. On the other hand, the $loss_{aux}$ ratio is defined by us. We set the weights such that the auxiliary losses are small compared to the other losses. When this loss is too large, the class information is broken, and detection will be difficult. To achieve this, we carefully choose the weight ratios.

3.2. Scaled Binary Cross Entropy

The second one, referred to as "Scaled Binary Cross Entropy (SBCE)", integrates object size into $Loss_{obj}$. Industrial datasets such as agricultural data often exhibit an imbalanced distribution of object sizes, as shown in Figure 6. This imbalance must be addressed when aiming to train AI models more efficiently. On the other hand, Binary Cross Entropy (BCE) is used to calculate the loss regardless of object size. BCE can be written as follows:

$$BCE = \sum_{i=1}^{n} \sum_{j=1}^{n} -(GT_{ij} * \log(Pr_{ij}) + (1 - GT_{ij}) * \log(1 - Pr_{ij})), \tag{7}$$

BCE is not suitable for training unbalanced and small data because it does not consider an uneven distribution of object sizes. Also, excessive back-propagation with small datasets should be avoided, as it can lead to overfitting. When a user implements AI into industries such as agriculture, users often need to create custom datasets. These original datasets, however, often suffer from imbalances in object size distribution. To address this issue, our proposed Scaled Binary Cross Entropy (SBCE) method incorporates object size into the loss function, emphasizing the importance of each object during training. Adapting the training process to fit the characteristics of the dataset can help to mitigate data imbalance.

As mentioned earlier, these original datasets often contain a large number of small objects. Treating large and small objects equally under these conditions can negatively affect the training process. To remedy this, SBCE scales $Loss_{obj}$ for small objects, prioritizing their detection. Larger loss values lead to greater parameter adjustments, making it easier for the model to detect small objects.

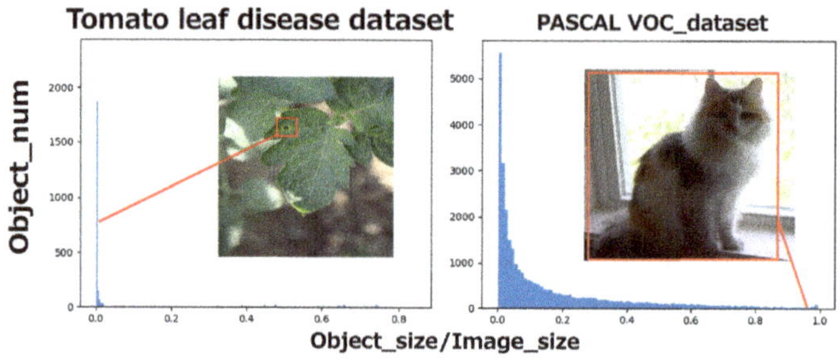

Figure 6. Examples of datasets with poor distributions for training.

SBCE can be written as follows:

$$SBCE = \sum_{i=1}^{n}\sum_{j=1}^{n} -(GT_{ij} * \log(Pr_{ij})^r + (1 - GT_{ij}) * \log(1 - Pr_{ij})^r), \tag{8}$$

To prioritize smaller objects during training, the SBCE scales the BCE using r. It becomes bigger than 1 with sizes below a predefined threshold to scale $Loss_{obj}$. The smaller the object size, the larger the value of r, and the larger the value of $Loss$. Since larger values of $Loss_{obj}$ lead to more significant parameter updates, r indicates the importance of that object in training. To determine this threshold, SBCE needs to define M before training as shown in Algorithm 2. M represents the maximum object size for which the $Loss_{obj}$ is scaled. When YOLO adopts SBCE, the object sizes in the Ground Truth (GT) dataset must be computed. The object size percentage in the images ($w \times h/W \times H$) is pre-calculated and used during training. For GT objects with sizes larger than M, r is set to 1, and the standard BCE is applied. In contrast, for GT objects smaller than M, r is set to a value between 1 and 2, and $Loss_{obj}$ is scaled accordingly.

Algorithm 2 Scaled Binary Cross Entropy

Input: M:max_{size}, GT:Ground Truth, Pr:Prediction
Output: L_{obj}

for image in Dataset **do**
    get image width as W
    get image height as H
    $image_{size} = W * H$
    for object in image **do**
        get object width as w
        get object height as h
        $object_{size} = w * h / image_{size}$
        if $object_{size} < M$ **then**
            $r = 2 - object_{size}/M$
        else if $M \leq object_{size}$ **then**
            $r = 1$
        end if
        $L_{obj} = SBCE(GT, Pr, r)$
    end for
end for

The main advantage of the proposed method is the flexibility to adjust the scaling range according to the characteristics of the dataset. In this paper, we define an appropriate range for datasets that contain many small objects. When the dataset contains many large objects and the user aims to detect larger objects, the suitable range can be specified for the size of the object.

4. Dataset and Hyper-Parameter

In this study, we evaluate our proposed methods using two datasets. First, our model is trained on the PASCAL VOC dataset, which is widely used for quantitative evaluation. Additionally, we train our model on a tomato leaf disease dataset to demonstrate its application in industrial AI.

4.1. PASCAL VOC Dataset

Our proposed methods are evaluated using the PASCAL VOC dataset [26], which enables quantitative evaluation. The dataset contains 8069 training images and 997 test images, providing a reliable basis for assessing the proposed methods. Additionally, the dataset includes 20 object classes (e.g., airplane, person, dog, etc.) , as shown in Figure 7, further supporting the quantitative evaluation of the proposed approaches.

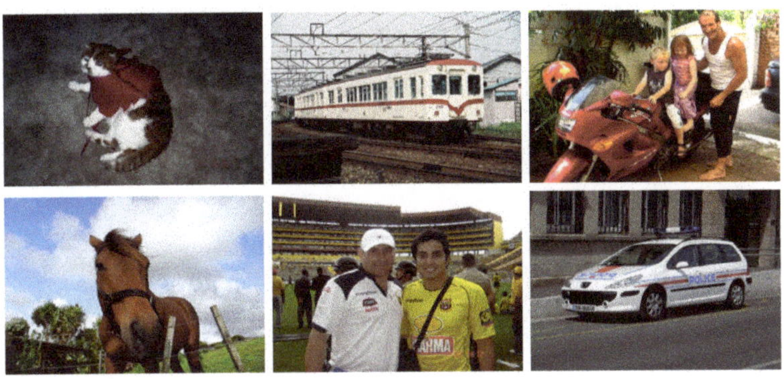

Figure 7. PASCAL VOC dataset.

4.2. Tomato Leaf Disease Dataset

This dataset consists of images of diseased tomato leaves [27]. These diseases are classified into six types (bacterial spot, black spot, early blight, late blight, leaf mold, and target spot). Leaves without disease symptoms are labeled as healthy , as shown in Figure 8. The model is trained using 645 images, with the results evaluated on 61 inference images and 31 test images. All image sizes are 640 × 640 pixels.

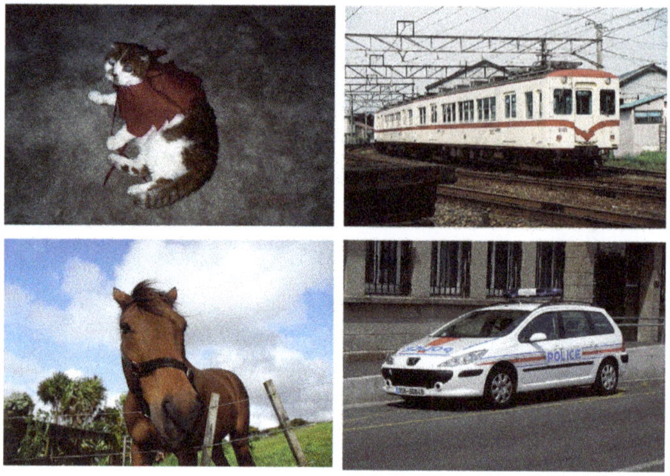

Figure 8. Tomato leaf disease dataset.

4.3. Hyper-Parameter

YOLO has various hyper-parameters for training, which are determined based on the size of the training data and the model. For the tomato leaf disease dataset, we set the batch size to 8, the number of epochs to 400, and the input shape to 640 × 640 pixels. For the PASCAL VOC dataset, the batch size is set to 64, the number of epochs to 500, and the input shape to 640 × 640 pixels. The optimizer used is Adam, and weight decay is adjusted from 1×10^{-3} to 1×10^{-5} using a cosine annealing function.

5. Results

In this paper, YOLOv7 is used as the baseline model due to its optimal dimensionality for representing vectors. When the dimensionality is too large, the VSR may easily produce a cosine similarity of −1. Conversely, when the dimensionality is too small, the VSR cannot achieve a cosine similarity of −1 without distorting the vector. To achieve these conditions, we balance YOLOv7.

As mentioned earlier, this paper trains and evaluates the proposed method on two datasets: the PASCAL VOC dataset and the tomato leaf dataset. Table 1 presents the evaluation results of the proposed method using the PASCAL VOC dataset.

Table 1. Results of PASCAL VOC dataset.

Model	mAP50 (%)	F1	mIoU (%)
YOLOv7-tiny	81.51	0.766	52.91
+VSR	**83.53**	0.802	**54.32**
+SBCE$_{maxobj}$	81.96	0.787	53.47
+VSR+SBCE$_{maxobj}$	83.53	0.806	54.24
YOLOv7	97.68	0.966	64.87
+VSR	97.71	0.967	64.77
+SBCE$_{maxobj}$	97.56	0.966	64.62
+VSR+SBCE$_{maxobj}$	97.57	0.965	64.83

Additionally, Tables 2 and 3 present the evaluation results of the proposed method using the tomato leaf disease dataset. Table 2 defines the size of the largest object in the dataset as M for SBCE. Table 3 also defines the largest object size as M for SBCE, focusing on the detection of smaller disease symptoms that are more critical to identify, as shown in Figure 9. Tables 4 and 5 present the evaluation results between proposed method and existing method on the tomato leaf disease dataset. Finaly, Table 6 present the ablation study about w_{VSR}, and Table 7 compares between our model and existing models on tomato leaf disease dataset.

Table 1 shows that the loss improvement of our proposed methods is effective for the PASCAL VOC dataset. Compared to the base model (YOLOv7-tiny and YOLOv7), VSR improved the mAP of YOLOv7-tiny from 81.51% to 83.53% and the mAP of YOLOv7 from 97.68% to 97.71%. Additionally, SBCE improved the map of YOLOv7-tiny from 81.51% to 81.96%. When both proposed methods are applied together, the mAP of YOLOv7-tiny improved from 81.51% to 83.53%.

Table 2 demonstrates that the loss improvement achieved by the proposed method is effective for the tomato leaf disease dataset. Compared to the base models (YOLOv7-tiny and YOLOv7), VSR improved the mAP of YOLOv7-tiny from 61.81% to 68.16%. Additionally, SBCE improved the mAP of YOLOv7-tiny from 61.81% to 68.55% and the mAP of YOLOv7 from 70.60% to 74.27%. When both proposed methods are applied together, the mAP of YOLOv7-tiny improved from 61.81% to 68.95%, and the mAP of YOLOv7 improved from 70.60% to 73.24%.

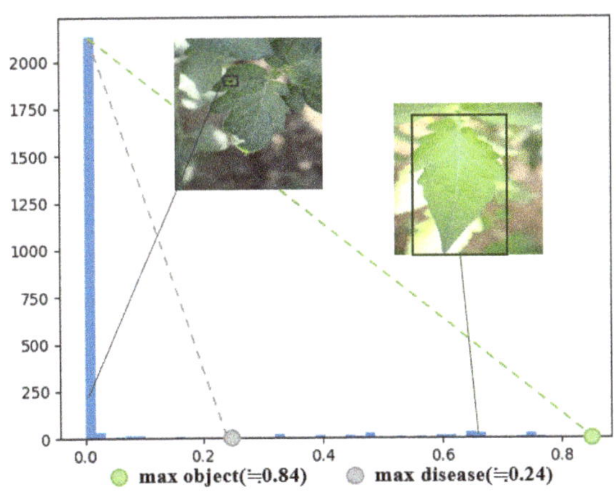

Figure 9. The distribution of tomato leaf disease dataset.

Table 2. Results of tomato leaf disease dataset, which defines max object size as M.

Model	mAP50 (%)	F1	mIoU (%)
YOLOv7-tiny	61.81	0.61	65.03
+VSR	68.16	0.71	63.83
+SBCE$_{maxobj}$	68.55	0.64	65.80
+VSR+SBCE$_{maxobj}$	68.95	0.70	65.30
YOLOv7	70.60	0.66	65.98
+VSR	69.35	0.70	48.83
+SBCE$_{maxobj}$	74.27	0.75	64.58
+VSR+SBCE$_{maxobj}$	73.24	0.73	65.69

Table 3 demonstrates that the loss improvement achieved by the proposed method is effective for the tomato leaf disease dataset. Compared to the base models (YOLOv7-tiny and YOLOv7), VSR improved the mAP of YOLOv7-tiny from 68.16% to 61.81%. Additionally, SBCE improved the mAP of YOLOv7-tiny from 63.16% to 61.81% and the mAP of YOLOv7 from 70.60% to 71.95%. When both proposed methods are applied together, the mAP of YOLOv7-tiny improved from 61.81% to 70.21%, and the mAP of YOLOv7 improved from 70.60% to 73.09%.

Table 3. Results of tomato leaf disease dataset, which defines max disease size as M.

Model	mAP50 (%)	F1	mIoU (%)
YOLOv7-tiny	61.81	0.61	65.03
+VSR	68.16	0.71	63.83
+SBCE$_{maxdis}$	63.16	0.58	65.67
+VSR+SBCE$_{maxdis}$	70.21	0.71	66.44
YOLOv7	70.60	0.66	65.98
+VSR	69.35	0.70	64.20
+SBCE$_{maxdis}$	71.95	0.74	65.47
+VSR+SBCE$_{maxdis}$	73.09	0.75	64.00

Figures 10 and 11 show the results of disease detection in the image. Our proposed methods enable the detection of diseases on leaves in the background of the images, which YOLOv7-tiny fails to detect.

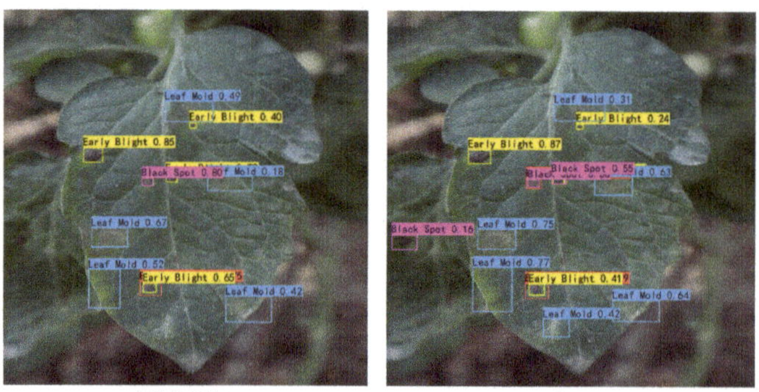

YOLOv7-tiny Ours

Figure 10. Comparison of image results on YOLOv7-tiny.

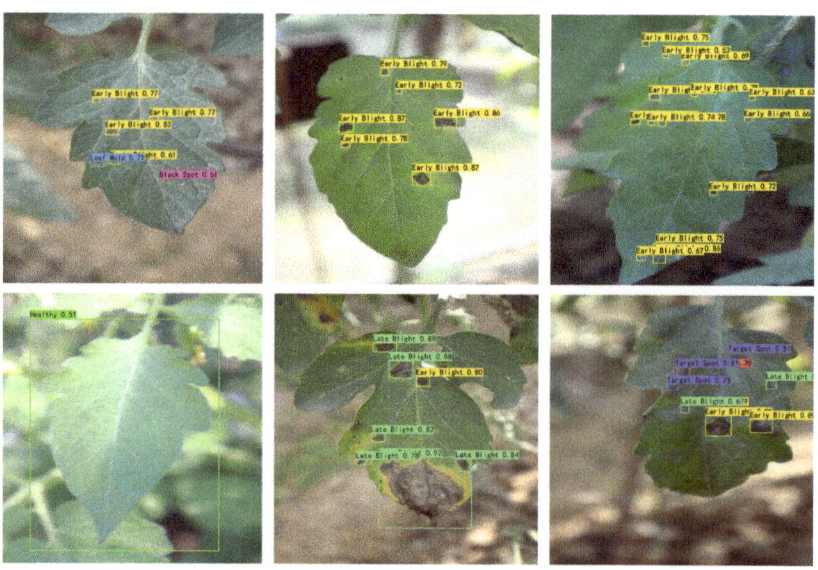

Figure 11. Detection results on YOLOv7 with our proposal.

As shown in Table 4, our proposed method achieves higher detection performance compared to existing methods. While focal loss reduces the mAP from 61.81% to 49.42%, our proposed method improves the mAP from 61.81% to 68.55%. Additionally, as shown in Table 5, the detection accuracy for leaf mold is particularly improved with both SBCE_{maxdis} and SBCE_{maxobj} on YOLOv7.

Table 4. Comparison results of tomato Leaf disease dataset with existing loss functions.

Model	mAP50 (%)	F1	mIoU (%)
YOLOv7-tiny	61.81	0.610	65.03
+Focal Loss	49.42	0.376	64.81
+SBCE_{maxdis}	63.16	0.580	65.67
+SBCE_{maxobj}	68.55	0.640	65.80

Table 5. Evaluation results of SBCE_{maxobj} and SBCE_{maxdis} on tomato leaf disease dataset.

Model	Class	AP50 (%)	F1	Recall (%)	Precision (%)
YOLOv7	Bacterial Spot	50.00	0.67	50.00	100.00
	Black Spot	59.68	0.50	35.71	83.33
	Early Blight	84.33	0.86	84.85	87.50
	Healthy	100.00	1.00	100.00	100.00
	Late Bright	80.21	0.73	60.00	92.31
	Leaf Mold	30.00	0.40	33.33	50.00
	Target Spot	90.00	0.89	100.00	80.00
+SBCE_{maxobj}	Bacterial Spot	50.00 (±0)	0.67 (±0)	50.00 (±0)	100.00 (±0)
	Black Spot	52.67 (−7.01)	0.55 (+0.05)	42.86 (+7.15)	75.00 (−8.33)
	Early Blight	79.36 (−4.97)	0.79 (−0.07)	81.82 (−3.03)	77.14 (−10.36)
	Healthy	100.00 (±0)	1.00 (± 0)	100.00 (±0)	100.00 (±0)
	Late Bright	77.89 (−2.32)	0.78 (+0.05)	70.00 (+10.00)	87.50 (−4.81)
	Leaf Mold	60.00 (+30.00)	0.73 (+0.33)	66.67 (+33.34)	80.00 (+30.00)
	Target Spot	100.00 (+10.00)	0.73 (−0.16)	100.00 (±0)	57.14 (−22.86)
+SBCE_{maxdis}	Bacterial Spot	50.00 (±0)	0.50 (−0.17)	50.00 (±0)	50.00 (−50.00)
	Black Spot	52.77 (−6.91)	0.57 (+0.07)	42.86 (+7.15)	85.71 (+2.38)
	Early Blight	82.99 (−1.34)	0.86 (±0)	81.82 (−3.03)	90.00 (+2.50)
	Healthy	100.00 (±0)	0.92 (−0.08)	85.71 (−14.29)	100.00 (±0)
	Late Bright	77.86 (−2.35)	0.78 (+0.05)	70.00 (+10.00)	87.50 (−4.81)
	Leaf Mold	56.67 (+26.67)	0.73 (+0.33)	66.67 (+33.34)	80.00 (+30.00)
	Target Spot	83.33 (−6.67)	0.80 (−0.09)	100.00 (±0)	66.67 (−13.33)

Table 6 presents the ablation results for the L_{aux} weight. With a weight of 0.2, our VSR achieves an mAP from 81.51% to 83.53% on the PASCAL VOC dataset. Other weight values also achieve higher mAP, such as 82.42% and 82.20%. In addition, all weights show a better mAP with SBCE on yolov7-tiny.

Table 7 presents the results of our proposed methods and existing YOLO series models. When compared to other YOLO models with similar architectures, our proposed methods achieve higher mAP and $F1$ scores.

Table 6. Ablation study of L_{aux} weight on PASCAL VOC dataset.

Model	mAP50 (%)	F1	mIoU (%)
YOLOv7-tiny	81.51	0.766	52.91
+VSR(w = 0.1)	82.42	0.786	54.29
+VSR(w = 0.1)+SBCE	82.71	0.804	54.05
+VSR(w = 0.2)	83.53	0.802	54.32
+VSR(w = 0.2)+SBCE	83.53	0.806	54.24
+VSR(w = 0.3)	82.20	0.770	52.78
+VSR(w = 0.3)+SBCE	82.60	0.794	53.47

Table 7. Comparison results of our proposed methods with existing models on PASCAL VOC dataset.

Model	mAP50 (%)	F1
YOLOX-tiny	64.57	0.548
YOLOX-nano	79.47	0.747
YOLOv7-tiny	81.51	0.766
YOLOv8-nano	79.73	0.768
YOLOv8-s	82.70	0.813
Ours (VSR+SBCE)	83.53	0.802

6. Discussion

Our proposed methods demonstrate improved performance on the PASCAL VOC and tomato leaf disease datasets. As shown in Table 1, YOLOv7-tiny shows better performance on the PASCAL VOC dataset with our proposed enhancements. However, applying SBCE slightly reduces the performance of YOLOv7. This result suggests that, with sufficiently large datasets and model sizes, YOLOv7 can achieve satisfactory performance without additional training adjustments, such as head vector optimization using VSR. Furthermore, the 20-class configuration of the PASCAL VOC dataset increases the complexity of VSR training. For SBCE, the wide variation in object sizes within a single class, combined with a large number of training samples, makes weighted back-propagation less effective. These factors explain the limited improvements observed with our methods on the PASCAL VOC dataset.

Conversely, as shown in Table 2, our proposed methods are highly effective when applied to smaller datasets and models. Smaller models, such as YOLOv7-tiny, naturally struggle with expressive power due to their limited number of parameters. However, VSR facilitates the creation of more optimal parameters, compensating for this limitation. Additionally, SBCE effectively weights back-propagation, which is especially beneficial for datasets with limited training samples, where each back-propagation step carries greater significance.

For these reasons, YOLOv7-tiny, with its smaller model size, achieved a significant improvement in mean Average Precision (mAP) of 7.14%. Similarly, YOLOv7 also showed an improvement in mAP of 2.64%. These results emphasize the efficacy of our proposed methods, especially in scenarios involving small models and limited datasets.

Table 3 presents the results of adjusting the scaling range of SBCE from the maximum object size in the dataset to the maximum disease size. Reducing the scaling range makes the weighted values relatively more significant, which helps to clarify the training target and leads to more efficient training. Compared to the results in Table 2, this adjustment improved the mean Average Precision (mAP) for YOLOv7 from 68.95% to 70.21%.

This improvement is likely influenced by inadequate annotations, as illustrated in Figure 12. For example, detecting multiple diseases in a single annotated image, as shown in the "Train Image" example, can lead to false positives, which negatively impact the training process.

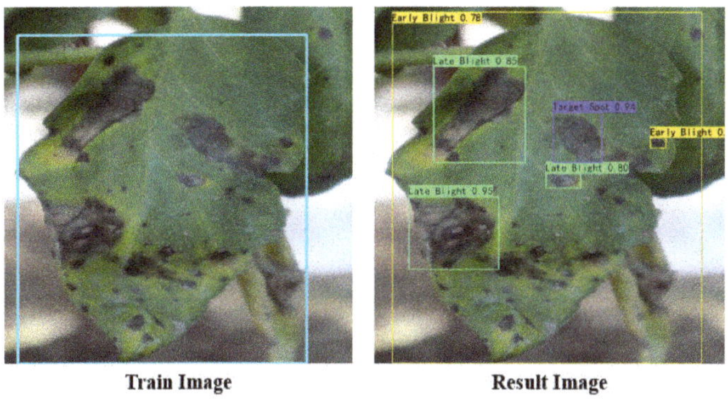

Figure 12. An example of poor annotation in tomato leaf disease dataset.

As shown in Table 4, our proposed methods achieve higher detection results compared to existing methods. Focal loss is a method that considers confidence for training. However, focal loss may not be suitable for training datasets that contain multiple similar classes, such as different disease types.

Additionally, Table 5 compares the results across different classes. SBCE enhances L_{obj}, allowing the model to detect more objects. However, the smaller scaling range and the lack of scaling for the healthy (leaf) loss contribute to inadequate training and lower accuracy in some cases. These challenges highlight the challenges of improving detection performance with limited and unbalanced datasets.

Table 6 presents the ablation results of L_{aux} weight. The results highlight the importance of selecting an appropriate value. Values that are too small reduce the effectiveness of VSR, while values that are too high increase the difficulty of training VSR. Therefore, it is crucial to define an optimal value for the L_{aux} weight. To prevent parameter breakdowns as shown in Figure 13 during YOLO training, this weight should be set to its optimal value.

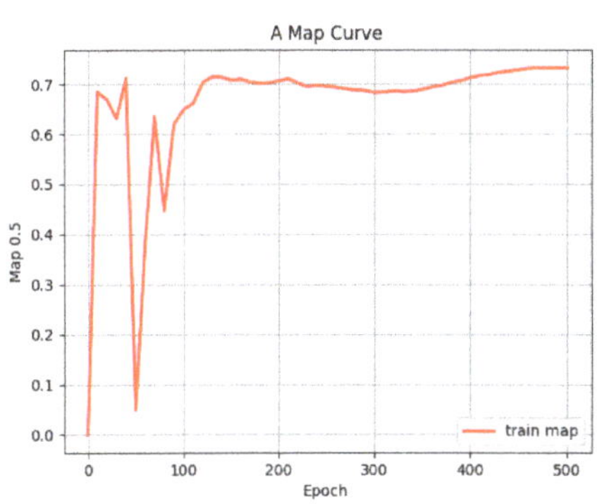

Figure 13. When YOLO trains with high L_{aux} weight like 0.50, head parameter become unstable.

Based on these findings, we conclude that our proposed method is most effective when applied to YOLOv7-tiny, as shown in Table 7. This model benefits the most from the optimized training process, leading to significant improvements in both detection efficiency and accuracy.

7. Conclusions

This paper proposes two loss improvement methods to enhance detection performance on industrial datasets. Industrial datasets are often imbalanced and contain a limited number of images due to challenges in data preparation. Training on such datasets requires careful optimization, as each back-propagation step is more significant than training on large-scale datasets. Additionally, small AI models, favored for agricultural applications due to their lower cost and energy requirements, have fewer parameters compared to large-scale AI models. This limitation requires more precise parameter tuning to achieve satisfactory performance. To address these challenges, we propose the following improvements: "VSR" optimizes class classification by separating the head vector values for each class, thereby reducing false positives and improving prediction accuracy; "SBCE" incorporates object size into the training process, ensuring that the training is appropriately tailored to the specific characteristics of the dataset. This approach enhances the model's ability to detect objects of varying sizes in imbalanced datasets.

By integrating these improvements, our proposed method enhances the detection accuracy of compact models on imbalanced industrial datasets, making it particularly suitable for applications in agriculture and other industries where data constraints are common. In future work, we plan to further validate the effectiveness of our methods through quantitative comparisons across various model architectures and datasets. This will provide deeper insights into the broader applicability of our approach.

Author Contributions: Conceptualization, L.M. and A.M.; methodology, A.M.; software, A.M.; validation, A.M. and R.I.; formal analysis, A.M. and R.I.; investigation, A.M.; resources, A.M.; data curation, A.M.; writing—original draft preparation, A.M.; writing—review and editing, R.I. and L.M.; visualization, A.M.; supervision, L.M.; project administration, L.M.; funding acquisition, L.M. All authors have read and agreed to the published version of the manuscript.

Funding: This research received no external funding.

Data Availability Statement: The PASCAL VOC dataset is widely used for object detection tasks, which is created by Visual Object Classes Challenge (VOC Challenge) concludes Everingham, L. et al. The dataset contains 8069 training images and 997 test images. It is available at [26]. The Tomato Leaf Disease dataset is created by Sylhet Agricultural University. The dataset contains 645 training images, 61 inference images and 31 test images. It is available at [27].

Conflicts of Interest: The authors declare no conflict of interest.

References

1. Research of the Ministry of Agriculture, Forestry, and Fisheries. Statistics on Agricultural Labor Force. Available online: https://www.maff.go.jp/j/tokei/sihyo/data/08.html (accessed on 20 January 2025).
2. Li, Q.; Wang, M.; Gu, W. Computer vision based system for apple surface defect detection. *Comput. Electron. Agric.* **2002**, *36*, 215–223. [CrossRef]
3. Wang, Q.; Qi, F.; Sun, M.; Qu, J.; Xue, J. Identification of tomato disease types and detection of infected areas based on deep convolutional neural networks and object detection techniques. *Comput. Intell. Neurosci.* **2019**, *2019*, 9142753. [CrossRef] [PubMed]
4. Tian, Y.; Yang, G.; Wang, Z.; Li, E.; Liang, Z. Detection of apple lesions in orchards based on deep learning methods of cyclegan and YOLOv3-dense. *J. Sens.* **2019**, *2019*, 7630926. [CrossRef]
5. Matsui, A.; Meng, L.; Hattori, K. Enhanced YOLO using Attention for Apple grading. In Proceedings of the 2023 International Conference on Advanced Mechatronic Systems (ICAMechS), Melbourne, Australia, 4–7 September 2023; pp. 1–5.
6. Wu, X.; Sahoo, D. Recent advances in deep learning for object detection. *Neurocomputing* **2020** , *396*, 39–64. [CrossRef]
7. Ishibashi, R.; Kaneko, H.; Meng, L. Enhancing DETR with Attention-Based Thresholding for Efficient Early Japanese Book Reorganization. In Proceedings of the 2023 International Conference on Advanced Mechatronic Systems (ICAMechS), Melbourne, Australia, 4–7 September 2023; pp. 1–7.

8. Girshick, R.; Donahue, J.; Darrell, T.; Malik, J. Rich feature hierarchies for accurate object detection and semantic segmentation. In Proceedings of the IEEE Conference on Computer Vision and Pattern Recognition, Columbus, OH, USA, 23–28 June 2014; pp. 580–587.
9. Ren, S.; He, K.; Girshick, R.; Sun, J. Faster R-CNN: Towards real-time object detection with region proposal networks. *IEEE Trans. Pattern Anal. Mach. Intell.* **2016**, *39*, 1137–1149. [CrossRef] [PubMed]
10. Liu, W.; Anguelov, D.; Erhan, D.; Szegedy, C.; Reed, S.; Fu, C.Y.; Berg, A.C. Ssd: Single shot multibox detector. In Proceedings of the Computer Vision–ECCV 2016: 14th European Conference, Amsterdam, The Netherlands, 11–14 October 2016; Proceedings, Part I 14; Springer: Berlin/Heidelberg, Germany, 2016; pp. 21–37.
11. Redmon, J. You only look once: Unified, real-time object detection. In Proceedings of the IEEE Conference on Computer Vision and Pattern Recognition, Las Vegas, NV, USA, 27–30 June 2016.
12. Tan, M.; Pang, R.; Le, Q.V. Efficientdet: Scalable and efficient object detection. In Proceedings of the IEEE/CVF Conference on Computer Vision and Pattern Recognition, Seattle, WA, USA, 13–19 June 2020; pp. 10781–10790.
13. Carion, N.; Massa, F.; Synnaeve, G.; Usunier, N.; Kirillov, A.; Zagoruyko, S. End-to-end object detection with transformers. In Proceedings of the European Conference on Computer Vision, Glasgow, UK, 23–28 August 2020; pp. 213–229.
14. Redmon, J.; Farhadi, A. YOLO9000: Better, faster, stronger. In Proceedings of the IEEE Conference on Computer Vision and Pattern Recognition, Honolulu, HI, USA, 21–26 July 2017; pp. 7263–7271.
15. Wang, C.Y.; Bochkovskiy, A.; Liao, H.Y.M. YOLOv7: Trainable bag-of-freebies sets new state-of-the-art for real-time object detectors. In Proceedings of the IEEE/CVF Conference on Computer Vision and Pattern Recognition, Vancouver, BC, Canada, 17–24 June 2023; pp. 7464–7475.
16. Wen, H.; Dai, F.; Yuan, Y. A Study of YOLO Algorithm for Target Detection. In Proceedings of the 2021 International Conference on Artificial Life and Robotics (ICAROB2021), Online, 21–24 January 2021; pp. 287–290.
17. Rezatofighi, H.; Tsoi, N.; Gwak, J.; Sadeghian, A.; Reid, I.; Savarese, S. Generalized intersection over union: A metric and a loss for bounding box regression. In Proceedings of the IEEE/CVF Conference on Computer Vision and Pattern Recognition, Long Beach, CA, USA, 15–20 June 2019; pp. 658–666.
18. Zheng, Z.; Wang, P.; Liu, W.; Li, J.; Ye, R.; Ren, D. Distance-IoU loss: Faster and better learning for bounding box regression. In Proceedings of the AAAI Conference on Artificial Intelligence, New York, NY, USA, 7–12 February 2020; Volume 34, pp. 12993–13000.
19. Zheng, Z.; Wang, P.; Ren, D.; Liu, W.; Ye, R.; Hu, Q.; Zuo, W. Enhancing geometric factors in model learning and inference for object detection and instance segmentation. *IEEE Trans. Cybern.* **2021**, *52*, 8574–8586. [CrossRef] [PubMed]
20. Lin, T. Focal Loss for Dense Object Detection. *arXiv* **2017**, arXiv:1708.02002.
21. Zhang, H.; Wang, Y.; Dayoub, F.; Sunderhauf, N. Varifocalnet: An iou-aware dense object detector. In Proceedings of the IEEE/CVF Conference on Computer Vision and Pattern Recognition, Nashville, TN, USA, 20–25 June 2021; pp. 8514–8523.
22. Kaneko, H.; Ishibashi, R.; Meng, L. Deteriorated characters restoration for early Japanese books using enhanced cyclegan. *Heritage* **2023**, *6*, 4345–4361. [CrossRef]
23. Hoffer, E.; Ailon, N. Deep metric learning using triplet network. In Proceedings of the Similarity-Based Pattern Recognition: Third International Workshop, SIMBAD 2015, Copenhagen, Denmark, 12–14 October 2015; Proceedings 3; Springer: Berlin/Heidelberg, Germany, 2015; pp. 84–92.
24. Qi, C.; Su, F. Contrastive-center loss for deep neural networks. In Proceedings of the 2017 IEEE International Conference on Image Processing (ICIP), Beijing, China, 17–20 September 2017; pp. 2851–2855.
25. Deng, J.; Guo, J.; Xue, N.; Zafeiriou, S. Arcface: Additive angular margin loss for deep face recognition. In Proceedings of the IEEE/CVF Conference on Computer Vision and Pattern Recognition, Long Beach, CA, USA, 15–20 June 2019; pp. 4690–4699.
26. Everingham, M.; Van Gool, L.; Williams, C.K.; Winn, J.; Zisserman, A. The pascal visual object classes (voc) challenge. *Int. J. Comput. Vis.* **2010**, *88*, 303–338. [CrossRef]
27. Sylhet Agricultural University Tomato Leaf Diseases Detect Dataset. 2024. Sylhet Agricultural University, Tomato Leaf DIseases Detect Computer Vision Project. Available online: https://universe.roboflow.com/sylhet-agricultural-university/tomato-leaf-diseases-detect (accessed on 20 January 2025).

computers

Article

Commutative Quaternion Algebra with Quaternion Fourier Transform-Based Alpha-Rooting Color Image Enhancement †

Artyom M. Grigoryan * and Alexis A. Gomez

Electrical and Computer Engineering, The University of Texas at San Antonio, San Antonio, TX 78249, USA; alexis.gomez@utsa.edu

* Correspondence: artyom.grigoryan@utsa.edu

† This article is a revised and expanded version of authors' conference paper which was presented at *SPIE 13033 Conference, Defense + Commercial Sensing 2024*, National Harbor, MD 20745, USA, 22 April 2024.

Abstract: In this paper, we describe the associative and commutative algebra or the (2,2)-model of quaternions with application in color image enhancement. The method of alpha-rooting, which is based on the 2D quaternion discrete Fourier transform (QDFT) is considered. In the (2,2)-model, the aperiodic convolution of quaternion signals can be calculated by the product of their QDFTs. The concept of linear convolution is simple, that is, it is unique, and the reduction of this operation to the multiplication in the frequency domain makes this model very attractive for processing color images. Note that in the traditional quaternion algebra, which is not commutative, the convolution can be chosen in many different ways, and the number of possible QDFTs is infinite. And most importantly, the main property of the traditional Fourier transform that states that the aperiodic convolution is the product of the transform in the frequency domain is not valid. We describe the main property of the (2,2)-model of quaternions, the quaternion exponential functions and convolution. Three methods of alpha-rooting based on the 2D QDFT are presented, and illustrative examples on color image enhancement are given. The image enhancement measures to estimate the quality of the color images are described. Examples of the alpha-rooting enhancement on different color images are given and analyzed with the known histogram equalization and Retinex algorithms. Our experimental results show that the alpha-rooting method in the quaternion space is one of the most effective methods of color image enhancement. Quaternions allow all colors in each pixel to be processed as a whole, rather than individually as is done in traditional processing methods.

Keywords: color image enhancement; quaternion convolution; quaternion Fourier transform; alpha-rooting; quaternion pyramids

1. Introduction

In recent years, many articles have been published on color image processing, wherein image enhancement plays an important role. Many color images are low quality and require enhancement as the first stage of processing. [1–5]. Examples of such images can be found among underwater images, thermal images, and medical images. Decades ago, we divided methods of image enhancement into two classes, namely spatial and traditional, or complex, frequency domains; now, a new class has been added to them. Here, we mention methods of image enhancement in the quaternion algebras. Color and grayscale images can be processed in the quaternion space with good results not only in image enhancement but in filtration, face recognition, neural networks, and other applications. The first class of methods includes contrast stretching techniques and logarithmic models [4] and the very effective and simple histogram equalization with its different modifications [6–10]. The Retinex algorithm can also be classified into this class [11,12]. In the second class, we should note the Fourier transform-based alpha-rooting [13], which is the most effective method for enhancing grayscale and color images. The advantage of enhancing color images in the quaternion space is in the fact that the primary colors plus the gray are processed as one unit, not separately. Therefore, quaternion image processing does not introduce false color artifacts [14].

In this paper, we focus on the commutative quaternion algebra, or the (2,2)-model. In this model, the concepts of the 1D and 2D QDFT are considered, and their properties are described. This model of quaternion uses the color image enhancement alpha-rooting by the 2D QDFT. A comparison with the traditional quaternion algebra is also given.

The main contributions of this work are the following:

- The separable alpha-rooting method of color image enhancement;
- New two-parameter alpha-rooting methods of color image enhancement;
- The effectiveness of using the 2D QDFT-based alpha-rooting in the (2,2)-model;
- Illustrative examples showing the effectiveness of using the (2,2)-model in color image enhancement.

The rest of the paper is organized in the following way. Section 2 describes two models of quaternions, namely the (2,2)- and (1,3)-models. The first model is commutative, and the second one is not. Section 3 describes the exponential functions of the (2,2)-model. The concepts of the QDFTs are considered in Section 4 for both models. The methods of alpha-rooting in these models are described in Section 5. The comparison of the 2D QDFT-based alpha-rooting methods in the (2,2)- and (1,3)-models are given. Results and illustrative examples of color images are presented in Section 6.

2. Quaternion Numbers: Two Arithmetics

In this section, we describe quaternion numbers in two algebras, non-commutative and commutative. The concept of the quaternion, or quadruple of numbers (a, b, c, d), as a vector in the 4-dimensional (4D) space was introduced by Gauss in 1819 [15]. As complex numbers, quaternions have one real part and one imaginary part. Only the imaginary part presents a triplet of numbers or a 3D vector. Therefore, quaternions can be considered as an extension of complex numbers [16–18]. It is not possible for us to draw quaternions in 4D space, but we will show how such numbers can be embedded in geometric figures in 3D space. There are different types of arithmetic of quadruples of numbers, or quaternions, because they define the main operation—multiplication—differently. We consider two arithmetics, or models, in which the operation of multiplication is commutative and non-commutative. The second arithmetic attracted much attention from researchers in the field of signal and image processing. However, the fact that the multiplication of quaternions is a non-commutative operation leads to large uncertainties in such important operations as the convolution, correlation, and Fourier transform, especially in processing color images. Therefore, we think it is necessary to pay more attention to the commutative operation of the multiplication of quaternions and the corresponding arithmetic, or the commutative algebra of quaternions.

2.1. The (1,3)-Model of Quaternions

Consider three units i, j, and k with the following multiplication laws:

$$ij = -ji = k,\ jk = -kj = i,\ ki = -ik = j,\ i^2 = j^2 = k^2 = ijk = -1. \tag{1}$$

A quaternion is defined as the number $q = a + bi + cj + dk$ with real numbers a, b, c, and d. The number $q' = bi + cj + dk$ is the imaginary part q' of the quaternion and can be considered as the vector (a, b, c) in the 3D space. Therefore, we can write $q = a + q' = a + (bi + cj + dk)$. This model of representation of quaternions as $q = (a, q')$ is called the (1,3)-model [14]. A quaternion has one real part, a, and the three-component imaginary part, q'. If the imaginary part $a = 0$, then the quaternion is called a pure quaternion number. If $c = d = 0$, the quaternion $q = a + bi$ is a complex number. Similar to the complex numbers, the conjugate of the quaternion q is defined as $\bar{q} = (a, -q')$, or $\bar{q} = a - q' = a - bi - cj - dk$.

The multiplication of two quaternions $q_1 = a_1 + q_1' = a_1 + (ib_1 + jc_1 + kd_1)$ and $q_2 = a_2 + q_2' = a_2 + (ib_2 + jc_2 + kd_2)$ is defined according to the laws in Equation (1). Thus, the quaternion $q = q_1q_2 = (a + q')$ is calculated by

$$a = a_1a_2 - [b_1b_2 + c_1c_2 + d_1d_2], \text{ and } q' = [a_1q_2' + a_2q_1'] + \begin{vmatrix} i & j & k \\ b_1 & c_1 & d_1 \\ b_2 & c_2 & d_2 \end{vmatrix} \tag{2}$$

It is important to note, that the number $q\bar{q}$ is real and non-negative, $q\bar{q} = a^2 + (b^2 + c^2 + d^2)$; it is denoted by $|q_1|^2$. The number $|q_1|$ is called the length of the quaternion.

The sum of quaternions is calculated component-wise, $q_1 + q_2 = (a_1 + a_2) + (q_1' + q_2')$. In the multiplication of imaginary units, $ij \neq ji$, $jk \neq kj$, and $ik \neq ki$. The multiplication in the (1,3)-model is not commutative. That is, for different q_1 and q_2, the product $q_1q_2 \neq q_2q_1$ or $q_1q_2 = q_2q_1$.

Considering the quaternions q_1 and q_2 as the 4D vectors, $\mathbf{q}_1 = (a_1, b_1, c_1, d_1)'$ and $\mathbf{q}_2 = (a_2, b_2, c_2, d_2)'$, the above operation of multiplication can be written in the matrix form as follows:

$$\mathbf{q} = \mathbf{A}_1 \begin{bmatrix} a_2 \\ b_2 \\ c_2 \\ d_2 \end{bmatrix} = \begin{bmatrix} a_1 & -b_1 & -c_1 & -d_1 \\ b_1 & a_1 & -d_1 & c_1 \\ c_1 & d_1 & a_1 & -b_1 \\ d_1 & -c_1 & b_1 & a_1 \end{bmatrix} \begin{bmatrix} a_2 \\ b_2 \\ c_2 \\ d_2 \end{bmatrix} \tag{3}$$

The determinant of the matrix equals $|q_1|^4 = \left(a_1^2 + b_1^2 + c_1^2 + d_1^2\right)^2$. For the case when $|q_1| = 1$, the matrix $\mathbf{A}_1$ is unitary and its determinant $\det\mathbf{A}_1 = 1$. The coefficients of this matrix are components of the quaternion q_1. The first column of the matrix is the quaternion q_1. A similar matrix of multiplication can be defined by the components of the quaternion q_2 (for details, see [14]).

Unlike traditional arithmetic, where the exponential function is defined uniquely, in the (1,3)-model, the number of such functions is infinite. Given a pure unit quaternion $\mu = im_1 + jm_2 + km_3$, $|\mu| = 1$, $\mu^2 = -1$, the quaternion exponential function at the angle x is defined as $e^{\mu x} = \cos x + \mu \sin x$. In the next sections, we will discuss the concept of the quaternion discrete Fourier transforms, which are different analogues of the traditional DFT. This transform is defined by the system of basis functions, which are calculated by the single complex exponential function e^{ix}. In the (1,3)-model, we are faced with the problem of which exponential function to use as the base function for the QDFT. In other words, if in the traditional representation each signal or image has the unique representation in the frequency domain, in the (1,3)-model, there are an infinite number of such representations. How to choose, namely which quaternion number μ is best for the QDFT, is unknown today. And it is this model that has been widely used in the last two decades in many applications in signal and image processing [14,19–21].

2.2. The (2,2)-Model of Quaternions

In this section, we consider the arithmetic of quaternions with the associative and commutative operation of multiplication introduced by Grigoryan in 2022 [22]. This is the so-called (2,2)-model of representation of quaternions.

In the (2,2)-model, the complex arithmetic is used in the following way. Given two complex numbers a_1 and a_2, the quaternion q is considered to be a pair of them and is written as

$$q = [a_1, a_2],\ a_1 = (a_{1,1}, a_{1,2}),\ a_2 = (a_{2,1}, a_{2,2}). \tag{4}$$

Here, the numbers $a_{1,1}$, $a_{1,2}$, $a_{2,1}$, and $a_{2,2}$ are real. We use the round brackets for 2D vectors a_1 and a_2, which represent the complex numbers $(a_{1,1} + ia_{1,2})$ and $(a_{2,1} + ia_{2,2})$, respectively. In this model, the quaternion is a pair of two complex numbers, or the pair of two 2-D vectors.

The quaternions include the complex and real numbers. Indeed, a quaternion $q = [a_1, 0]$ is a complex number. If a complex number $a_1 = (a_{1,1}, 0)$, that is, a_1 is real, then $q = [a_1, 0] = [(a_{1,1}, 0), (0, 0)]$ is a real number. We call the quaternion numbers $q = [0, a_2]$ the second complex numbers. Only complex numbers are used with the traditional unit i. The conjugate of the quaternion q is the quaternion $\overline{q} = [\overline{a}_1, \overline{a}_2] = [(a_{1,1}, -a_{1,2}), (a_{2,1}, -a_{2,2})]$. One can see that the conjugates of the unit quaternions are $\overline{e}_2 = -e_2$, $\overline{e}_3 = e_3$, and $\overline{e}_4 = -e_4$. The second conjugate $\overline{\overline{q}} = q$.

The operation of sum of two quaternions $q_1 = [a_1, a_2]$ and $q_2 = [b_1, b_2]$ is defined component-wise. That is, the sum $q = q_1 + q_2 = [a_1 + b_1, a_2 + b_2]$. The multiplication of quaternions q_1 and q_2 is defined by

$$q = q_1q_2 = [a_1, a_2]\,[b_1, b_2] \triangleq [a_1b_1 - a_2b_2, a_1b_2 + a_2b_1]. \tag{5}$$

Here, the complex numbers are written as $a_1 = (a_{1,1}, a_{1,2})$, $a_2 = (a_{2,1}, a_{2,2})$, $b_1 = (b_{1,1}, b_{1,2})$, and $b_2 = (b_{2,1}, b_{2,2})$. It should be noted that the similar operation over 4D elements was described by Clyde Davenport [23]; the multiplication was defined by using the complex conjugates as

$$q = q_1q_2 \triangleq \left[a_1b_1 - a_2\overline{b}_2, a_1b_2 + a_2\overline{b}_1\right].$$

It directly follows from Equation (5) that if the quaternions are complex numbers, $q_1 = [a_1, 0] = a_1$ and $q_2 = [b_1, 0] = b_1$, then the multiplication $q = q_1q_2$ is the multiplication of complex numbers, that is,

$$q = q_1q_2 = [a_1, 0]\,[b_1, 0] = [a_1b_1, 0] = a_1b_1.$$

The operation of multiplication in Equation (5) can also be written in the matrix form. For this, we consider the quaternions as 4D vectors $\boldsymbol{q}_1 = (a_{1,1}, a_{1,2}, a_{2,1}, a_{2,2})'$ and $\boldsymbol{q}_2 = (b_{1,1}, b_{1,2}, b_{2,1}, b_{2,2})'$. In the matrix form, the product $q = q_1q_2$ can be written as

$$q = \begin{bmatrix} q_{1,1} \\ q_{1,2} \\ q_{2,1} \\ q_{2,2} \end{bmatrix} = \boldsymbol{M}_1 \begin{bmatrix} b_{1,1} \\ b_{1,2} \\ b_{2,1} \\ b_{2,2} \end{bmatrix} = \begin{bmatrix} a_{1,1} & -a_{1,2} & -a_{2,1} & a_{2,2} \\ a_{1,2} & a_{1,1} & -a_{2,2} & -a_{2,1} \\ a_{2,1} & -a_{2,2} & a_{1,1} & -a_{1,2} \\ a_{2,2} & a_{2,1} & a_{1,2} & a_{1,1} \end{bmatrix} \begin{bmatrix} b_{1,1} \\ b_{1,2} \\ b_{2,1} \\ b_{2,2} \end{bmatrix}. \tag{6}$$

As in the matrix $\boldsymbol{A}_1$ in the (1,3)-model, the first column of the matrix $\boldsymbol{M}_1$ is the quaternion q_1. This matrix has a block structure, that is,

$$\boldsymbol{M}_1 = \begin{bmatrix} A & -B \\ B & A \end{bmatrix}, \; A = \begin{bmatrix} a_{1,1} & -a_{1,2} \\ a_{1,2} & a_{1,1} \end{bmatrix}, \; B = \begin{bmatrix} a_{2,1} & -a_{2,2} \\ a_{2,2} & a_{2,1} \end{bmatrix}. \tag{7}$$

Here, the matrices A and B are matrices of multiplication of complex numbers a_1 and a_2, respectively. The matrix $\boldsymbol{A}_1$ also has the same block structure, but it is orthogonal, and the matrix $\boldsymbol{M}_1$ is not orthogonal.

To compare these two algebras visually, namely the operations of multiplication, we consider the following representation of quadruples of numbers in the 3D space. We call this representation the 4-in-3 representation. Any 4D vector can be represented in the form of four triplets, as follows:

$$q = (a, b, c, d) \to (a, b, c),\ (b, c, d),\ (c, d, a),\ (d, a, b).$$

The geometry of these four coordinates can be described by the quadrangular pyramid. It is clear that not every pyramid can have such a quaternion representation. Therefore, we will call such pyramids the quaternion pyramids (*QP*). As example, Figure 1 shows the quaternion pyramid, $QP(q)$, for the quaternion $q = (1, -2, 8, 5)$ in part (a) and the pyramid $QP(\bar{q})$, for the conjugate quaternion $\bar{q} = (1, 2, -8, -5)$, in part (b), and the conjugate quaternion $\bar{q} = (1, 2, 8, -5)$ in the (2,2)-model in part (c). The first point (the vertex) of each pyramid is marked as an asterisk, '*'. The vertex of the pyramid should be considered, that is, the $QP(q)$ is the pyramid with the top point $v = (a, b, c)$. Therefore, we consider that $QP(q) = QP(q; v)$. Otherwise, we need to introduce concepts of equivalent pyramids. For instance, the figures of pyramids for four quaternion units, $1 = (1, 0, 0, 0)$, $i = (0, 1, 0, 0)$, $j = (0, 0, 1, 0)$, and $k = (0, 0, 0, 1)$, are the same. Such a vertex can also be considered the point (b, c, d), which corresponds to the imaginary part of the quaternion, $q' = (bi + cj + dk)$. Quaternion pyramids can be added, subtracted, multiplied, and divided, and the inverse pyramids exist. In other words, the set of all quaternion-pyramids is the space with the complete arithmetic as the quaternions.

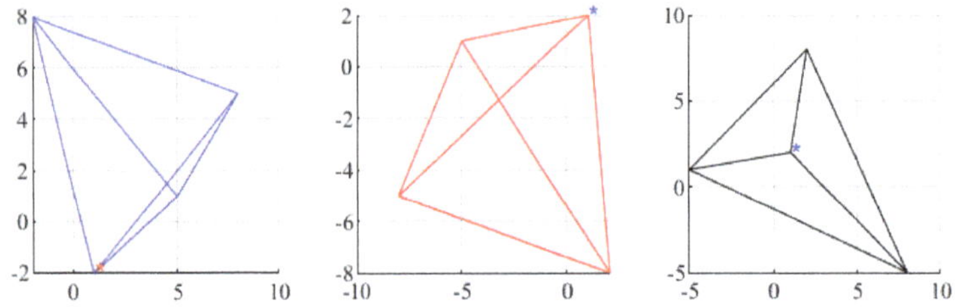

Figure 1. Quaternion-pyramids for (**a**) the quaternion q and its conjugates $\bar{q}$ in (**b**) the (1,3)-model and (**c**) the (2,2)-model.

Figure 2 shows the following four pyramids. Two quaternions are considered, $q_1 = (1, 2, 8, 4)/\sqrt{85}$ and $q_2 = (-2, 1, 1, 2)/\sqrt{10}$. The figure shows two pyramids $QP(q_1)$ and $QP(q_2)$ together with two pyramids for the quaternion multiplications $q = q_1 q_2$. The first pyramid $QP(q)$ is calculated in the non-commutative (1,3)-model, $g = q_2(A_{q_1})' = (4, -23, -23, 4)/\sqrt{850}$, and another $QP(p)$ in the commutative (2,2)-model, $p = q_2(M_{q_1})' = (-20, 9, -15, -12)/\sqrt{850}$.

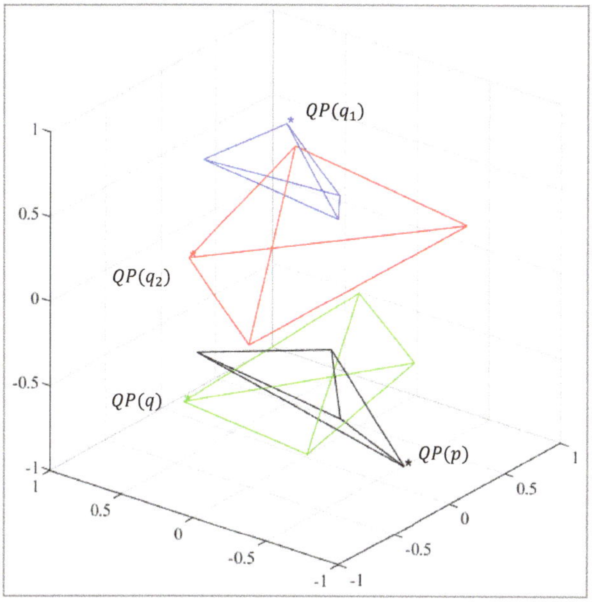

Figure 2. Four quaternion-pyramids.

The following properties hold for the multiplication.

1. The multiplication is commutative, $q_1q_2 = q_2q_1$.
2. The multiplication unit is the quaternion $e_1 = [(1,0),(0,0)] = (1,0) = 1$. For this real unit $e_1q = qe_1 = q$ for any quaternion q.
3. The multiplication rules of four quaternion units e_1, $e_2 = [(0,1),(0,0)]$, $e_3 = [(0,0),(1,0)]$, and $e_4 = [(0,0),(0,1)]$ are given in Table 1. It should be noted that for two quaternion units e_2 and e_3, the square is $-e_1 = -1$. For the other two units e_1 and e_4, the square is $e_1 = 1$.

Table 1. Multiplication table, $T(e_1, e_2, e_3, e_4)$.

	e_1	e_2	e_3	e_4
e_1	e_1	e_2	e_3	e_4
e_2	e_2	$-e_1$	e_4	$-e_3$
e_3	e_3	e_4	$-e_1$	$-e_2$
e_4	e_4	$-e_3$	$-e_2$	e_1

4. The multiplication is associative, that is, $(q_1q_2)q_3 = q_1(q_2q_3)$, for any quaternions q_1, q_2, and q_3.
5. The multiplication is distributive, that is, $q_1(q_2 + q_3) = q_1q_2 + q_1q_3$.
6. The zero quaternion $q = 0$ has "divisors." For instance, the multiplication of two quaternions $q_1 = (1 + e_4)$ and $q_2 = (1 - e_4)$ is equal to $q_1q_2 = 1 - e_4^2 = 0$.
7. The inverse to the non-zero quaternion $q_1 = [a_1, a_2]$ is calculated by

$$q_1^{-1} = \left[\frac{a_1}{a_1^2 + a_2^2}, \frac{-a_2}{a_1^2 + a_2^2}\right] = \frac{1}{a_1^2 + a_2^2}[a_1, -a_2], \text{ if } a_1^2 + a_2^2 \neq 0. \tag{8}$$

8. The inverse operation exists for all q, except the quaternions of the form $q = a_1(1 \pm e_4)$. For quaternion exponential numbers, the inverse exists. As mentioned in [24], the absence of some inverse numbers is not an obstacle when using quaternions to process signals and color images.
9. The division $q = q_2/q_1$ of quaternions $q_2 = [b_1, b_2]$ and $q_1 = [a_1, a_2]$ is calculated by $q \triangleq q_2 q_1^{-1}$.
10. The multiplication of a quaternion q on its conjugate $\bar{q}$ is equal to the following quaternion:

$$q\bar{q} = [a_1, a_2][\bar{a}_1, \bar{a}_2] = \left[|a_1|^2 - |a_2|^2, 2a_1 \cdot a_2\right] \tag{9}$$

11. In the general case, $q\bar{q}$ is not a real number and cannot be used to define the modulus of the quaternion in the traditional sense. For example, $e_4\overline{e_4} = e_4(-e_4) = -e_4e_4 = -1$.
12. The length, or modulus, of the quaternion is defined as $|q| = \sqrt{E[q]}$, where the energy of the quaternion number q is calculated by

$$E[q] = E[a_1] + E[a_2] = |a_1|^2 + |a_2|^2 = \left(\left|a_{1,1}\right|^2 + \left|a_{1,2}\right|^2\right) + \left(\left|a_{2,1}\right|^2 + \left|a_{2,1}\right|^2\right). \tag{10}$$

Table 2 shows the main properties of quaternion numbers in the (1,3)- and (2,2)-models.

Table 2. Main operations and properties of quaternions in two quaternion models.

	The (2,2)-Model				The Traditional (1,3)-Model			
Representation	$q_1 = [a_1, a_2] = [(a_{1,1}, a_{1,2}), (a_{2,1}, a_{2,2})]$				$q_1 = a_1 + q_1' = a_1 + (b_1 i + c_1 j + d_1 k)$			
Multiplication q_1q_2	$q_1q_2 = [a_1b_1 - a_2b_2, a_1b_2 + a_2b_1]$				$[a_1 q_2' + a_2 q_1'] + a_1a_2 - q_1' \cdot q_2' + q_1' \times q_2'$			
Multiplication rules	$e_1 = 1$	e_2	e_3	e_4	1	i	j	k
	e_2	-1	e_4	$-e_3$	i	-1	k	$-j$
	e_3	e_4	-1	$-e_2$	j	$-k$	-1	i
	e_4	$-e_3$	$-e_2$	1	k	j	$-i$	-1
Multiplication matrix	$(a_1 = a_{11}, b_1 = a_{12}, c_1 = a_{21}, d_1 = a_{22})$ $M_1 = \begin{bmatrix} a_1 & -b_1 & -c_1 & d_1 \\ b_1 & a_1 & -d_1 & -c_1 \\ c_1 & -d_1 & a_1 & -b_1 \\ d_1 & c_1 & b_1 & a_1 \end{bmatrix}$				$A_1 = \begin{bmatrix} a_1 & -b_1 & -c_1 & -d_1 \\ b_1 & a_1 & -d_1 & c_1 \\ c_1 & d_1 & a_1 & -b_1 \\ d_1 & -c_1 & b_1 & a_1 \end{bmatrix}$			
Orthogonality	Not				Yes			
Commutativity	Yes : $q_1q_2 = q_2q_1$				Not : $q_1q_2 \neq q_2q_1$ or $q_1q_2 = q_2q_1$			
Zero "divisors"	Yes : $(1 + e_4)(1 - e_4) = 0$				None : $q_1q_2 = 0 \rightarrow q_1 = 0$, or q_2=0.			
Conjugate	$\bar{q}_1 = [(a_{1,1}, -a_{1,2}), (a_{2,1}, -a_{2,2})]$				$\bar{q}_1 = a_1 - b_1 i - c_1 j - d_1 k,$			
Quaternion inverse	$q_1^{-1} = \frac{1}{a_1^2 + a_2^2}[a_1, -a_2],\ a_1^2 + a_2^2 \neq 0$				$q_1^{-1} = \frac{a_1 - b_1 i + c_1 j - d_1 k}{\lvert q_1 \rvert^2},\ q_1 \neq 0$			
Division $q = \frac{q_1}{q_2}$	$q = q_2[a_1, -a_2]\frac{1}{a_1^2 + a_2^2},\ a_1^2 + a_2^2 \neq 0.$				$q = \frac{\bar{q}_2 q_1}{\lvert q_2 \rvert^2}$ (from left) $q = \frac{q_1 \bar{q}_2}{\lvert q_2 \rvert^2}$ (from right)			

3. The Quaternion Exponents in the (2,2)-Model

In this section, we describe the exponential functions in the (2,2)-model. For two pairs of quaternions $\mu = \pm e_3$ and $\pm e_2$, the square $\mu^2 = -1$. There are only two pairs of quaternions with the square equal to -1. For each of these quaternions, the exponential function is defined by the following series [22]:

$$\begin{aligned} e^{\mu\varphi} &= 1 + \mu\varphi + \frac{(\mu\varphi)^2}{2!} + \frac{(\mu\varphi)^3}{3!} + \frac{(\mu\varphi)^4}{4!} + \frac{(\mu\varphi)^5}{5!} + \ldots + \frac{(\mu\varphi)^n}{n!} + \ldots \\ &= \left[1 - \frac{\varphi^2}{2!} + \frac{\varphi^4}{4!} - \frac{\varphi^6}{6!} + \ldots\right] + \mu\left[\varphi - \frac{\varphi^3}{3!} + \frac{\varphi^5}{5!} - \frac{\varphi^7}{7!} + \ldots\right] = \cos\varphi + \mu\sin\varphi. \end{aligned} \tag{11}$$

Thus, there are four different exponential functions, or we can say two pair of quaternion exponential functions. The fundamental multiplicative property holds for these exponents, that is,

$$\exp(\mu[\varphi+\vartheta]) = \exp(\mu\varphi)\exp(\mu\vartheta) \tag{12}$$

Now, we consider these two pairs of quaternion exponents.

1. The first pair of exponents is defined for the conjugate quaternions $\mu = \pm e_2 = [(0,\pm 1),(0,0)]$. The quaternion exponents are the following conjugate functions:

$$e^{\mu\varphi} = \cos\varphi \pm e_2 \sin\varphi = [(\cos\varphi, \pm\sin\varphi), 0] = (\cos\varphi, \pm\sin\varphi). \tag{13}$$

In the matrix form, the multiplication of a quaternion $q = [a_1, a_2]$ by the exponent $q_1 = e^{\mu\varphi}$ is described as follows:

$$qq_1 = qe^{\mu\varphi} = (\cos\varphi, \pm\sin\varphi)q = \begin{bmatrix} c & -s & 0 & 0 \\ s & c & 0 & 0 \\ 0 & 0 & c & -s \\ 0 & 0 & s & c \end{bmatrix} q = \begin{bmatrix} R_\varphi & \mathbf{0} \\ \mathbf{0} & R_\varphi \end{bmatrix} q. \tag{14}$$

Here, we denote $c = \cos\varphi$ and $s = \pm\sin\varphi$. With the operation of the Kronecker product of matrices, the above matrix of multiplication can be written as $A_{q_1} = I_2 \otimes R_\varphi$. The matrix R_φ is the matrix of elementary rotation by the angle $\pm\varphi$. Thus, the operation $qe^{\mu\varphi}$ is reduced to separate rotations of two components of the quaternion, a_1 and a_2, by the same angle.

2. The second pair of exponents is defined by the quaternion $\mu = \pm e_3 = [(0,0),(\pm 1,0)]$. The corresponding pair of quaternion exponential functions is

$$e^{\mu\varphi} = \exp(\mu\varphi) = \cos\varphi \pm e_3 \sin\varphi = [(\cos\varphi, 0), (\pm\sin\varphi, 0)]. \tag{15}$$

These two exponential functions are not conjugate but inverse to each other. The inverse of the exponent is $(e^{\mu\varphi})^{-1} = [(\cos\varphi, 0), (-\sin\varphi, 0)] = e^{-\mu\varphi}$. In the matrix form, the multiplication of the exponent $q_1 = e^{\mu\varphi}$ by a quaternion q can be written as follows:

$$qq_1 = q_1 q = e^{\mu\varphi} q = \begin{bmatrix} c & 0 & -s & 0 \\ 0 & c & 0 & s \\ s & 0 & c & 0 \\ 0 & -s & 0 & c \end{bmatrix} q. \tag{16}$$

The matrix of the multiplication is the tensor product of the rotation matrix and the identity matrix, $A_{q_1} = R_\varphi \otimes I_2$.

It should be noted that if we consider the symmetric matrix $P_{(1,2)}$ of the permutation (1,2), then the above two pairs of quaternion exponents can be derived from each as

$$[(\cos\varphi, 0), (\pm\sin\varphi, 0)] = [(\cos\varphi, \pm\sin\varphi), (0,0)] \begin{bmatrix} 1 & 0 & 0 & 0 \\ 0 & 0 & 1 & 0 \\ 0 & 1 & 0 & 0 \\ 0 & 0 & 0 & 1 \end{bmatrix}. \tag{17}$$

4. Quaternion Discrete Fourier Transforms

In this section, we consider the concept of the quaternion discrete Fourier transform (QDFT) in the (1,3)- and (2,2)-models. In the first model, the N-point QDFT of the quaternion signal $q = \{q_n; n = 0 : (N-1)\}$ is defined by

$$Q_p = \sum_{n=0}^{N-1} q_n W_\mu^{np} = \sum_{n=0}^{N-1} q_n \left[\cos\left(\frac{2\pi}{N}np\right) - \mu\sin\left(\frac{2\pi}{N}np\right)\right],\ p = 0 : (N-1). \tag{18}$$

Here, μ is a pure quaternion unit number, such that $\mu^2 = -1$, $|\mu| = 1$. As mentioned above, the number of such quaternions is infinite. For instance, this number can be taken as $\mu = i, j, k$, and $(i \pm j \pm k)/3$. The multiplication is not commutative; therefore, this QDFT is the left-sided transform. The right-sided QDFT is defined as the sum of $W_\mu^{np} q_n$. The inverse N-point QDFT is calculated by

$$q_n = \frac{1}{N}\sum_{p=0}^{N-1} Q_p W_\mu^{-np} = \frac{1}{N}\sum_{p=0}^{N-1} Q_p \left[\cos\left(\frac{2\pi}{N}np\right) + \mu\sin\left(\frac{2\pi}{N}np\right)\right],\ n = 0 : (N-1). \tag{19}$$

The fast algorithms to calculate the QDFT exist for both types of transform in the 1D and 2D cases. For 2D signals, the QDFT can be defined as the right-, left-, or both-sided transform [14,24]. These transforms do not have one of the basic properties of the traditional Fourier transform, namely, the cyclic convolution of signals is not reduced to the operation of multiplication in the frequency domain. In the 1D case, the cyclic convolution of two periodic quaternion signals $q_n = [f_n, g_n]$ and $h_n = [h_{1,n}, h_{2,n}]$ is defined as

$$y_n = q_n \circledast h_n = \sum_{k=0}^{N-1} q_{n-k} h_k,\ n = 0 : (N-1). \tag{20}$$

Here, we need to consider that $q_n \circledast h_n \neq h_n \circledast q_n$, because the products $q_{n-k}h_k \neq h_k q_{n-k}$. Thus, in the (1,3)-model, two different linear convolutions can be used.

Now, we consider these concepts in the (2,2)-model with two pairs of quaternion exponential functions, namely $e^{\mu\varphi}$, when $\mu = \pm e_2$ and $\pm\, e_3$. Each pair of these functions is used for the direct and inverse QDFTs. Thus, in the (2,2)-model there are only two pairs of the direct and inverse QDFTs. The (2,2)-model is commutative; therefore, the transform of the N-point quaternion signal $[f_n, g_n]$ is defined as

$$Q_p = \sum_{n=0}^{N-1} q_n W_\mu^{np} = \sum_{n=0}^{N-1} W_\mu^{np} q_n,\ W_\mu = \exp\left(-\frac{\mu 2\pi}{N}\right) e^{-\mu\frac{2\pi}{N}}. \tag{21}$$

Two different N-point QDFTs are described in the following way.

1. When the quaternion μ is $e_2 = [(0,1),(0,0)]$ and the angle is $\varphi = 2\pi/N$, the basis exponential functions are

$$\psi_p(n) = W_{e_2}^{np} = \exp(-e_2\varphi np)[(\cos np\varphi, -\sin np\varphi),(0,0)]\ \left[e^{-inp\varphi}, 0\right], \tag{22}$$

$p, n = o = 0 : (N-1)$. The N-point direct QDFT is defined as

$$Q_p = \sum_{n=0}^{N-1} q_n \psi_p(n) = \sum_{n=0}^{N-1} [f_n, g_n][e^{-i\varphi np}, 0] = \sum_{n=0}^{N-1} \left[f_n e^{-i\varphi np}, g_n e^{-i\varphi np}\right].$$

or

$$Q_p = \left[\sum_{n=0}^{N-1} f_n e^{-i\varphi np}, \sum_{n=0}^{N-1} g_n e^{-i\varphi np}\right] = [F_p, G_p]. \tag{23}$$

Here, F_p and G_p are the traditional N-point DFTs of the complex signal f_n and g_n, respectively,

$$F_p = \sum_{n=0}^{N-1} f_n e^{-i\varphi np},\ G_p = \sum_{n=0}^{N-1} g_n e^{-i\varphi np},\ p = 0 : (N-1).$$

This N-point QDFT is called the N-point e_2-QDFT and it requires two N-point DFTs [22]. The inverse N-point e_2-QDFT is calculated by

$$q_n = [f_n, g_n] = \frac{1}{N}\sum_{p=0}^{N-1} Q_p W_\mu^{-np} = \frac{1}{N}\sum_{p=0}^{N-1} [F_p, G_p]\left[e^{inp\varphi}, 0\right],\ n = 0 : (N-1). \quad (24)$$

2. In the $\mu = e_3$ case, the basis exponential functions for the QDFT are

$$\psi_p(n) = W_{e_3}^{np} = \exp(-e_3\varphi np) = [(\cos(np\varphi), 0),\ (-\sin(np\varphi), 0)],\ p, n = 0 : (N-1). \quad (25)$$

The N-point QDFT which is called the *N-point e_3-QDFT* is defined as [22]

$$Q_p = \sum_{n=0}^{N-1} [f_n, g_n] W_{e_3}^{np} = \sum_{n=0}^{N-1} [f_n \cos(\varphi np) + g_n \sin(\varphi np), -f_n \sin(\varphi np) + g_n \cos(\varphi np)].$$

In the matrix form, this transform can be written with the rotation matrices as

$$Q_p = \sum_{n=0}^{N-1} [f_n, g_n] R_{\varphi np} = \sum_{n=0}^{N-1} [f_n, g_n] \begin{bmatrix} \cos(\varphi np) & -\sin(\varphi np) \\ \sin(\varphi np) & \cos(\varphi np) \end{bmatrix},\ p = 0 : (N-1). \quad (26)$$

The inverse N-point e_3-QDFT $Q_p = [A_p, B_p]$ is calculated by

$$q_n = [f_n, g_n] = \frac{1}{N}\sum_{p=0}^{N-1} Q_p W_\mu^{-np} = \frac{1}{N}\sum_{p=0}^{N-1} [A_p, B_p] R_{-\varphi np},\ n = 0 : (N-1). \quad (27)$$

Thus, in the (2,2)-model, we can work with only two N-point QDFT, namely, e_2-QDFT and e_3-QDFT.

As an example, Figure 3 shows the color image 'leonardo9.jpg' of 744 × 526 pixels in part (a) and the quaternion signal composed from column number 101 in part (b). The signals b_n, c_n, and d_n are the red, green, and blue channels of the image column, respectively. The signal a_n is the average of these signals.

The e_2-QDFT and e_3-QDFT of this quaternion signal are plotted in absolute scale, $|Q_p|$, $p = 0 : 733$, in Figure 4 in parts (a) and (b), respectively. The difference between these two plots is shown in part (c).

As shown in [22], in the (2,2)-model, the aperiodic convolution of quaternion signals can be calculated by multiplying the QDFTs. This statement is valid for both types of QDFT. The convolution of a periodic quaternion signal $q_n = [f_n, g_n]$ with another one $h_n = [h_{1,n}, h_{2,n}]$ is unique,

$$y_n = q_n \circledast h_n = \sum_{k=0}^{N-1} q_{n-k} h_k = \sum_{k=0}^{N-1} q_k h_{n-k},\ n = 0 : (N-1). \quad (28)$$

Here, the subscripts $n - k$ are considered by modulo N. This convolution is calculated by four complex convolutions as follows:

$$y_n = \left[y_{1,n}, y_{2,n}\right],\ y_{1,n} = f_n \circledast h_{1,n} - g_n \circledast h_{2,n}\ y_{2,n} = f_n \circledast h_{2,n} + g_n \circledast h_{1,n}. \quad (29)$$

For $k = 2$ and 3, the N-point e_k-QDFT of the convolution y_n is calculated by $Y_p = Q_p H_p$, $p = 0 : (N-1)$. Here, Q_p and H_p are components of the corresponding N-point e_k-QDFT of signals q_n and h_n, respectively. What type of QDFT is used for computing the aperiodic convolution is irrelevant. We think that the calculation of the quaternion convolution by the e_2-QDFT is simple. According to the multiplication, the e_2-QDFT of the aperiodic convolution is calculated by

$$Y_p = Q_p H_p = [F_p, G_p][H_{1,p}, H_{2,p}] = [F_p H_{1,p} - G_p H_{2,p}, F_p H_{2,p} + G_p H_{1,p}]. \quad (30)$$

Therefore, the task of calculating the quaternion aperiodic convolution in the frequency domain is solved in the (2,2)-model. In the traditional (1,3)-model of quaternions, this problem does not have such a simple solution—it is unsolvable. Table 3 summarizes the above considerations.

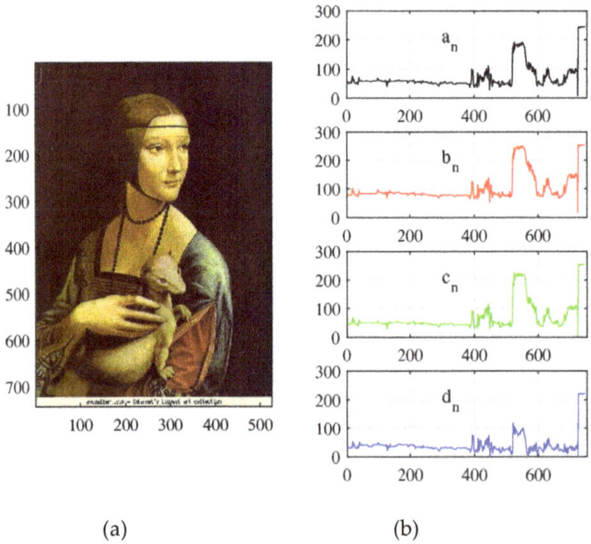

Figure 3. (**a**) The color image and (**b**) the quaternion signal of length 744 composed from one image column.

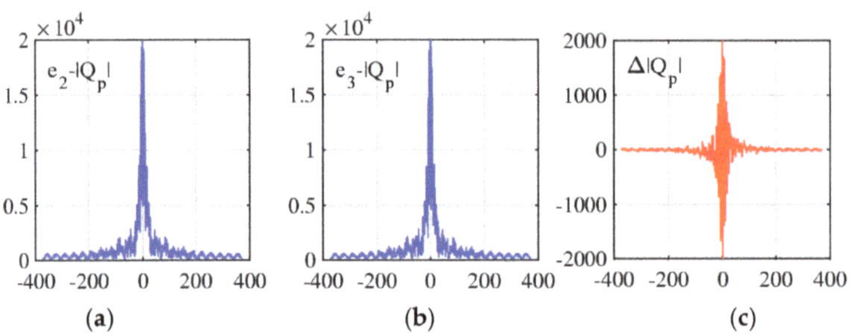

Figure 4. The magnitude of (**a**) the e_2-QDFT, (**b**) the e_3-QDFT, and (**c**) the difference of these transforms.

Table 3. Properties of aperiodic convolution and QDFT.

	The (2,2)-Model	The (1,3)-Model
Aperiodic convolution	$q = q_1 \circledast q_2 = q_2 \circledast q_1$	$q = q_1 \circledast q_2 \neq q_2 \circledast q_1$
Exponential functions	Only two pairs	Infinite number
The pair of the QDFT	Only two	Infinite number
Convolution property	$Q_p(q_1 \circledast q_2) = Q_p(q_1) \cdot Q_p(q_1)$	$Q_p(q_1 \circledast q_2) \neq Q_p(q_1) \cdot Q_p(q_1)$

5. Processing Images in the (2,2)-Model

In this section, we describe the concept of the 2D QDFT of images, which will be used in color image enhancement, namely, in the method which is called alpha-rooting. A color image in the RGB model will be presented by the quaternion image $q_{n,m} = [f_{n,m}, g_{n,m}]$ and then transformed to the frequency domain. Let $(r_{n,m}, g_{n,m}, b_{n,m})$ be components of the primary colors, red (R), green (G), and blue (B), in the image of $N \times M$ pixels. To compose the quaternion image $q_{n,m}$, we add the real component $a_{n,m}$. Thus, $q_{n,m} = (a_{n,m}, r_{n,m}, g_{n,m}, b_{n,m})$. The real part of this image is usually considered zero, $a_{n,m} = 0$, or the gray-scale component $a_{n,m} = (r_{n,m} + g_{n,m} + b_{n,m})/3$ at each pixel (n, m). The brightness of the image can also be considered, $a_{n,m} = 0.3r_{n,m} + 0.59g r_{n,m} + 0.11b_{n,m}$. In the (2,2)-model, the quaternion image $q_{n,m} = [f_{n,m}, g_{n,m}]$ is the pair of 2D data $f_{n,m} = (a_{n,m}, r_{n,m})$ and $g_{n,m} = (g_{n,m}, b_{n,m})$. In many applications, processing color images in quaternion space is efficient, since at each pixel the color triplet (plus the gray) is treated as one number, quaternion. Note that in the traditional approach, each color component of the image is processed separately. And this causes many unwanted effects on colors in the processed images [5,14].

The two-dimension $N \times M$-point QDFT in the frequency-point (p, s) is calculated by

$$Q_{p,s} = \sum_{n=0}^{N-1} \sum_{m=0}^{M-1} q_{n,m} W_{\mu}^{np} W_{\mu}^{ms} = \sum_{n=0}^{N-1} \sum_{m=0}^{M-1} q_{n,m} W_{\mu}^{np+ms}, \tag{31}$$

where $p,\ s = 0, 1, \ldots,\ (N-1), (M-1)$. In the (1,3)-model, two sums in this equation are different transforms; the first one is called the separable right-sided 2D QDFT [21,24].

We consider the 2D QDFT, which is calculated by the 1D e_2-QDFTs. This 2D transform is called the 2D $N \times M$-point e_2-QDFT—the case when $\mu = e_2$ [22,25]. As in the 1D case, the 2D e_2-QDFT has a simple form, when compared with the 2D e_3-QDFT. The 2D e_2-QDFT of the quaternion image $q_{n,m} = [f_{n,m}, g_{n,m}]$ is calculated by

$$Q_{p,s} = \sum_{n=0}^{N-1} \sum_{m=0}^{M-1} [f_{n,m}, g_{n,m}] W_N^{np} W_M^{ms} = [F_{p,s}, G_{p,s}]. \tag{32}$$

Here, $F_{p,s}$ and $G_{p,s}$ are the $N \times M$-point 2-D DFTs of the complex components $f_{n,m}$ and $g_{n,m}$, respectively,

$$F_{p,s} = \sum_{n=0}^{N-1} \sum_{m=0}^{M-1} f_{n,m} e^{-i\frac{2\pi}{N}np} e^{-i\frac{2\pi}{M}ms},\ G_{p,s} = \sum_{n=0}^{N-1} \sum_{m=0}^{M-1} g_{n,m} e^{-i\frac{2\pi}{N}np} e^{-i\frac{2\pi}{M}ms}.$$

Thus, the calculation of the $N \times M$-point e_2-QDFT is reduced to two 2D DFTs. The inverse $N \times M$-point e_2-QDFT is calculated by

$$q_{n,m} = \mathcal{F}^{-1}[Q]_{n,m} = \frac{1}{NM} \sum_{p=0}^{N-1} \sum_{s=0}^{M-1} [F_{p,s}, G_{p,s}] W_N^{-np} W_M^{-ms},\ n, m = 0 : (N-1), (M-1).$$

5.1. Method of Alpha-Rooting by the 2D QDFT

The absolute value, or the module, of the quaternion $Q_{p,s} = [F_{p,s}, G_{p,s}]$ is defined as $|Q_{p,s}| = \sqrt{|F_{p,s}|^2 + |G_{p,s}|^2}$. In the alpha-rooting [26,27], the image is enhanced by changing its absolute value at each frequency point to $|Q_{p,s}| \to |Q_{p,s}|^\alpha$, where the parameter α is from the interval (0,1). Given value α, the 2D e_2-QDFT of the quaternion image $q_{n,m}$ is processed as follows:

$$q_{n,m} \to Q_{p,s} \to \underbrace{V_{p,s} = Q_{p,s}|Q_{p,s}|^{\alpha-1}} \to \underbrace{(q_\alpha)_{n,m} = \mathcal{F}^{-1}[V_{p,s}]_{n,m}} \to A[q_\alpha]_{n,m}. \quad (33)$$

Here, $A > 1$ is a necessary constant, since the alpha-rooting method reduces the transforms in absolute scale.

The main steps of the algorithm:

1. Compose the quaternion image $q_{n,m}$ from the given RGB color image, $q_{n,m} = (a_{n,m}, r_{n,m}, g_{n,m}, b_{n,m})$.
2. Calculate the 2D e_2-QDFT of the quaternion image, $Q_{p,s} = \mathcal{F}[q]_{p,s} = [F_{p,s}, G_{p,s}]$.
3. Calculate the module of the transform, $|Q_{p,s}|$.
4. Process the transform modules by the alpha-rooting, $V_{p,s} = Q_{p,s}|Q_{p,s}|^{\alpha-1}$.

Thus, the 2D e_2-QDFT of the quaternion image changes by the non-negative coefficients $c(p,s) = |Q_{p,s}|^{\alpha-1}$,

$$Q_{p,s} = [F_{p,s}, G_{p,s}] \to V_{p,s} = c(p,s)[F_{p,s}, G_{p,s}] = [c(p,s)F_{p,s}, c(p,s)G_{p,s}]. \quad (34)$$

5. Calculate the inverse 2D e_2-QDFT, $(q_\alpha)_{n,m} = \mathcal{F}^{-1}[V]_{n,m}$.
6. Multiply the image by the constant $A > 1$ to raise the range of the image.
   The output of the alpha-rooting is the quaternion image $(v_\alpha)_{n,m} = A(q_\alpha)_{n,m}$. Rounding to integers is required.
7. Compose the new color image, $(v_c)_{n,m}$, as the three-component imaginary part of the quaternion image $(v_\alpha)_{n,m}$.
8. Extract the new grayscale image from the quaternion image $(v_\alpha)_{n,m}$, as its real part. Note that this grayscale image is not the gray or brightness of the new color image $(v_c)_{n,m}$.

The new image $v_{n,m}$ is parameterized by α. Therefore, the question arises as to how to choose the value of this parameter to better enhance the color image. As our preliminary examples have shown, the choice of the best values of α for enhancing color and quaternion images can be based on the known measure of color image enhancement (EMEC) [5,13]. This measure is used before and after image processing. The EMEC is the generalization of the enhancement measure that was used for grayscale images.

A. ***Enhancement measures for grayscale images***

To estimate the quality of grayscale images, we effectively developed and used the concept of the quantitative estimated measure of enhancement (EME). This measure was selected after analyzing the Weber and Fechner laws of the human visual system [28,29]. The measure is defined as the average of the range of image intensity in the logarithm scale when it is divided by blocks of the same size $L_1 \times L_2$, for example, 7×7. Only the full blocks are considered. Therefore, the number of blocks inside a discrete image $f = \{f_{n,m}\}$

of $N \times M$ pixels is calculated as k_1k_2, where $k_1 = \lfloor N/L_1 \rfloor$, $k_2 = \lfloor M/L_2 \rfloor$, and $\lfloor . \rfloor$ denotes the rounding floor function. The EME of the image is

$$EME(f) = \frac{1}{k_1k_2}\sum_{k=1}^{k_1}\sum_{l=1}^{k_2} 20\ln\left[\frac{\max\limits_{k,l}(f)}{\min\limits_{k,l}(f)}\right] = \frac{1}{k_1k_2}\sum_{k=1}^{k_1}\sum_{l=1}^{k_2} 20\left[\ln\max_{k,l}(f) - \ln\min_{k,l}(f)\right]. \quad (35)$$

Here, inside the (k,l)th block, the maximum, $\max_{k,l}(f)$, and minimum, $\min_{k,l}(f)$, of the image $f_{n,m}$ are calculated. Thus, the EME of the image is estimated block-wise by using the logarithm range of the image. If all values of the image in a block are 0, this block can be removed from the measure calculation. To avoid such cases, $EME(f+1)$ can be calculated instead. The change $f \to (f+1)$ does not change the quality of the image unless it is binary.

Together with EME, other contrast measures also can be used, including [14]:

1. The estimated measure of enhancement entropy measure (EMEE)

$$EMEE(f) = \frac{1}{k_1k_2}\sum_{k=1}^{k_1}\sum_{l=1}^{k_2} \frac{\max\limits_{k,l}(f)}{\min\limits_{k,l}(f)}\ln\left[\frac{\max\limits_{k,l}(f)}{\min\limits_{k,l}(f)}\right]. \quad (36)$$

2. The Michelson enhancement measure (MEM)

$$MEM(f) = -\frac{1}{k_1k_2}\sum_{k=1}^{k_1}\sum_{l=1}^{k_2} [MVR_{k,l}(f)]\ln[MVR_{k,l}(f)], \quad (37)$$

where the Michelson visibility ratio is calculated by

$$MVR_{k,l}(f) = \frac{\left|\max\limits_{k,l}(f) - \min\limits_{k,l}(f)\right|}{\min\limits_{k,l}(f) + \min\limits_{k,l}(f)}.$$

3. The signal-noise ratio (or the ratio of the mean of the image and standard deviation)

$$SNR(f) = \frac{E[f]}{\sqrt{E[f^2] - E^2[f]}} = \frac{1}{\sqrt{E[f^2]/E^2[f] - 1}}, \quad (38)$$

where

$$E[f] = \frac{1}{NM}\sum_{n=0}^{N-1}\sum_{m=0}^{M-1} f_{n,m} \text{ and } E\left[f^2\right] = \frac{1}{NM}\sum_{n=0}^{N-1}\sum_{m=0}^{M-1} f_{n,m}^2.$$

Our experimental results show that the EME and EMEE measures can be effectively used in enhancing images. After processing the image, $f_{n,m} \to g_{n,m}$, the EME of the enhanced image is calculated and compared with the EME of the original image. The range of the alpha-rooting image is usually smaller than [0,255]. Therefore, the obtained image should be multiplied by a coefficient. The new image and its quality depend on the value of parameter α, i.e., $g = g_\alpha$ and the measure is a function of a, that is, $EME(g_a) = EME(\alpha)$. The parameters of interest for alpha-rooting are in the range $R\{\alpha \in (0,1);\ EME(\alpha) > EME(g_\alpha) > EME(f)\}$. The degree of enhancement is determined by the EME measure. The best or optimal values of the enhancement are considered to be the values α_0, for which $EME(g_{\alpha_0}) = \max\limits_{a\in R} EME(g_\alpha)$ or $\min\limits_{a\in R} EME(g_\alpha)$.

To illustrate the introduced above measures of image enhancement, we consider the image of 512×512 pixels shown in Figure 5 in part (a). The histogram of the image is given in part (b). The enhancement by the Fourier transform-based alpha-rooting was used when changing the parameter α in the interval [0,1] with a step of 0.01. The graph of the measure of this image, $EME = EME(\alpha)$, as the function of α is shown in part (c). Blocks of size 7×7 were used to calculate the EME. For the original image, the measure of enhancement equals 7.63. The maximum of the function $EME(\alpha)$ is at point $\alpha = 0.83$ and equals $EME(0.83) = 20.69$. The image enhanced by the 0.83-rooting is shown in part (d). It was multiplied by the coefficient 19 to scale the image. In parts (e) and (f), the graph of the measure $EMEE(\alpha)$ and the enhanced image by the 0.83-rooting (and multiplied by 17) are shown, respectively. This measure has the maximum 1071.26 at point $\alpha = 0.84$. The measure of the original image equals $EMEE(1) = 0.68$. The best parameters $\alpha = 0.83$ and 0.84 for these two measures are very close to each other, as well as the results of the enhancement, which are shown in parts (d) and (f). The $EME(\alpha)$ function is much smoother than the $EMEE(\alpha)$ measure, and its graph has a distinct peak. For other images, the optimal values of the parameter α may be very different, but the smoothness of the function $EME(\alpha)$ is preserved and easier to work with.

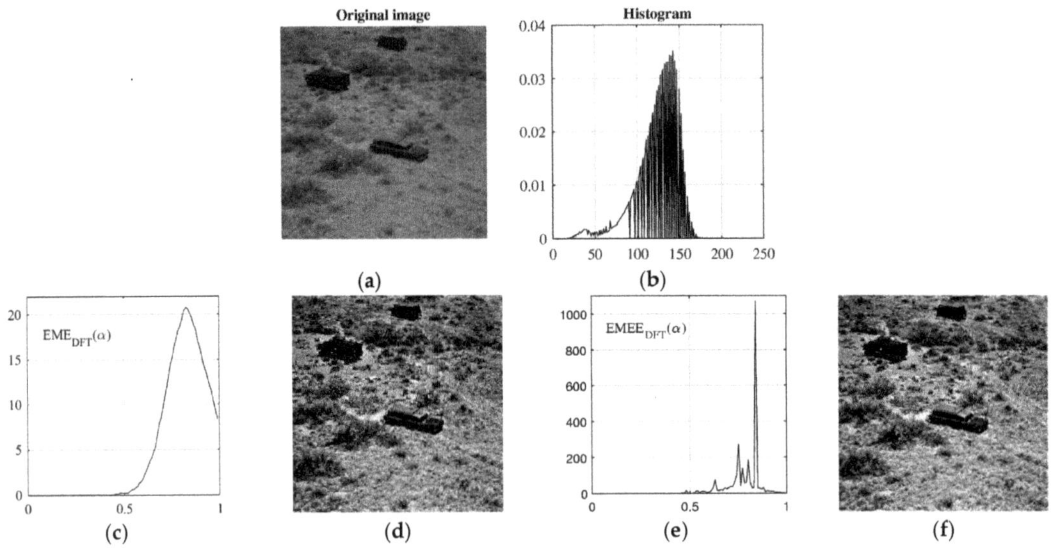

Figure 5. (**a**) The image '7.1.10.tiff' (from http://sipi.usc.edu/database, accessed on 22 January 2025), (**b**) the histogram of the image, (**c**) the EME function, (**d**) the enhanced image by the 0.83-rooting. (**e**) The graph of the EMEE function and (**f**) the image enhanced by the 0.84-rooting method.

In Figure 6a, the image of 440×750 pixels is shown, as well as the result of the histogram equalization (HE) of the image in part (b). The graph of the enhancement measure $EME(\alpha)$, when processing by the alpha-rooting, is given in part (c). The measure function $EME(\alpha)$ was calculated by dividing the image by blocks of sizes 5×5 and 7×7. The parameter α for the α-rooting method of enhancement varies in the interval [0.4,1] with a step of 0.005. Two graphs of the enhancement measure EME have pikes at the point 0.84 and 0.855, for the 5×5 and 7×7 block sizes, respectively. These values are almost the same, and we consider $\alpha_0 = 0.855$ for the best visual estimation of the enhancement. The EME of the original image equals 8.30 and 25.76 for the 0.855-rooting enhancement, which is shown in part (d). There, the enhancement can be estimated as $EME(g_{0.855}) - EME(f) = 25.76 - 8.30 = 17.46$. One can note the high quality of the 0.855-rooting image in comparison with the HE image in part (b).

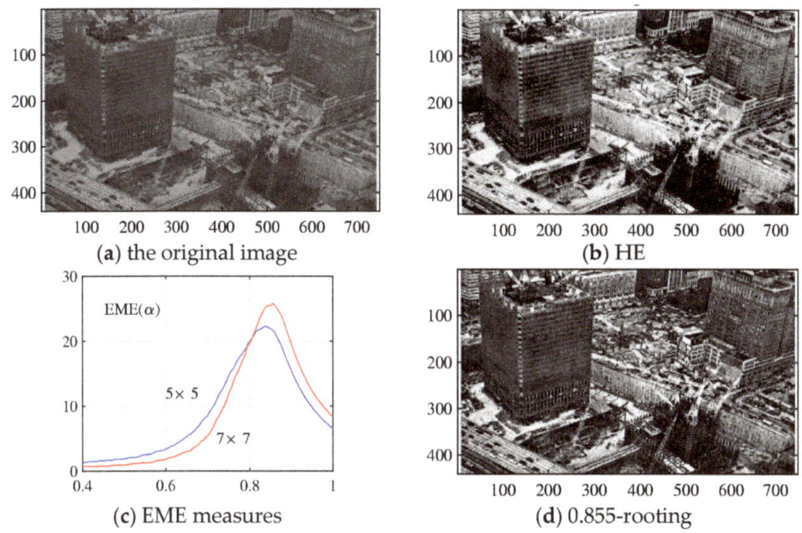

Figure 6. (**a**) The original grayscale image and (**b**) enhanced image by (**b**) histogram equalization. (**c**) Two EME measures of alpha-rooting method, and (**d**) the 0.855-rooting of the image.

To estimate the quality of color images, we consider the color image enhancement measure (EMEC). For a color image $f_{n,m} = (r_{n,m}, g_{n,m}, b_{n,m})$ after division by blocks of size $L_1 \times L_2$ each, for instance 7×7, the measure is calculated by

$$EMEC(f) = \frac{1}{k_1 k_2} \sum_{k=1}^{k_1} \sum_{l=1}^{k_2} 20\log_{10} \left[\frac{\max_{k,l}(r_{n,m}, g_{n,m}, b_{n,m})}{\min_{k,l}(r_{n,m}, g_{n,m}, b_{n,m})} \right]. \tag{39}$$

Here, $k_1 k_2$ is the number of blocks, and $\max_{k,l}(\ldots)$ and $\min_{k,l}(\ldots)$ are the maximum and minimum values in the (k,l)-th image block, respectively.

B. *Alpha-rooting components-wise*

Color images in the RGB color model can be separately processed by red, green, and blue colors. This is the traditional method of processing color images. In the alpha-rooting enhancement, each color component can be processed by alpha-rooting with different or the same values of parameters α_1, α_2, and α_3. We call this method $(\alpha_1, \alpha_2, \alpha_3)$-rooting of the color image For images in the HSI color model, with hue (H), saturation (S), and intensity (I) components, only the last component, intensity, will be only processed by alpha-rooting. The first two components, hue and saturation will stay the same.

To choose values of these parameters, we can use, for instance, the EME measure. As an example, Figure 7 shows the 1516×2012-pixel underwater RGB image in part (a) with EMEC of 38.77, which was calculated by blocks of size 5×7. In part (b), the graphs of functions $EME(\alpha)$ of the red, green, and blue channels are shown. The parameter of α runs the interval [0.2,1]. The maximum values of these functions are at points $\alpha = 0.94$, 0.83, and 0.84. The color image composed of 0.94-rooting of red, 0.83-rooting of green, and 0.84-rooting of blue components is shown in part (c). The enhancement measure of this image equals EMEC = 44.08.

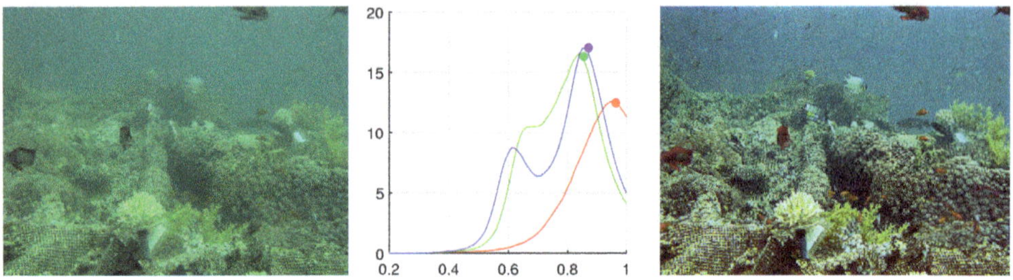

(**a**) EMEC 38.77 (**b**) (**c**) EMEC 44.08

Figure 7. (**a**) The original image, (**b**) EMEs of red, green, and blue components, and (**c**) enhanced image.

Since the color components are processed separately, it is not possible to state that the above (094,0.84,0.83)-rooting results in the highest enhanced image. It is possible to select other triplets of the vector parameter $\boldsymbol{\alpha} = (\alpha_1, \alpha_2, \alpha_3)$ and obtain images that we can consider the best. As examples, Figure 8 shows two enhanced images together with the graphs of the EMEs of three color channels, R, B, and B. The values of alpha parameters for these channels are marked on the graphs. The case with equal EME for all color channels is shown in part (a). The EMEC of the color image is of 59.62, which is the highest number for all considered cases. Also, a good, enhanced color image is shown in part (b) for the vector parameter (0.9,0.8,0.7).

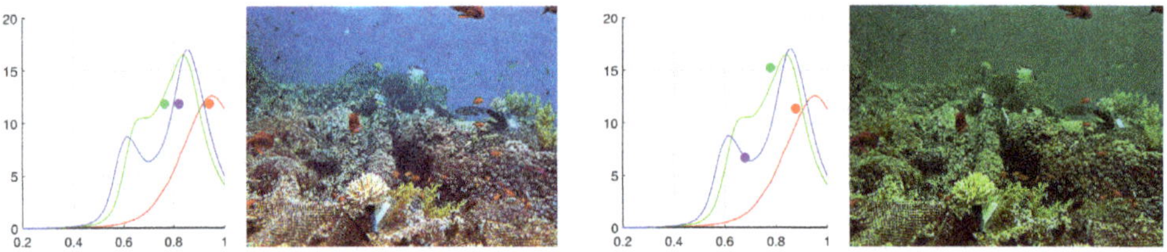

(**a**) (0.92,0.75,0.80)-rooting (EMEC = 59.62) (**b**) (0.9,0.8,0.7)-rooting (EMEC = 55.71)

Figure 8. (**a**) and (**b**) Two enhanced images.

C. *Comparison with HE and Retinex*

The methods of histogram equalization (HE) [30–32] and Retinex [33–37] are widely used in color image enhancement. We consider these methods together with the method of alpha-rooting. The underwater RGB color image of 192 × 262 pixels is shown in Figure 9 in part (a). This image has a measured EMEC of 11.26, which was calculated by blocks 5 × 5. The graphs of EME of three colors are given in part (b), with maximum values at points 0.85, 0.82, and 0.82, for the red, green, and blue channels, respectively. The corresponding (0.85,0.82,0.82)-rooting of this image with an EMEC of 35.46 is shown in part (c). In part (d), the (0.82,0.82,0.82)-rooting is shown with an EMEC of 36.37.

Figure 10 shows the result of the histogram equalization with a measured EMEC of 44.29 in part (a). The result of image enhancement by the multi-retinex is shown in part (b). The image was normalized, and sizes of the Gaussian filters were taken 7, 15, and 21 as suggested [33]. The retinex enhancement has an EMEC of 16.96. One can see that the enhancement of the color image was not achieved in these two methods. For comparison, we also add the result of the color image enhancement by the 0.82-rooting. The result is shown in part (c). One can see good enhancement of the image; the color measure of enhancement equals 33.50. Measures of EMEC and EME were calculated by blocks of 5 × 5 pixels.

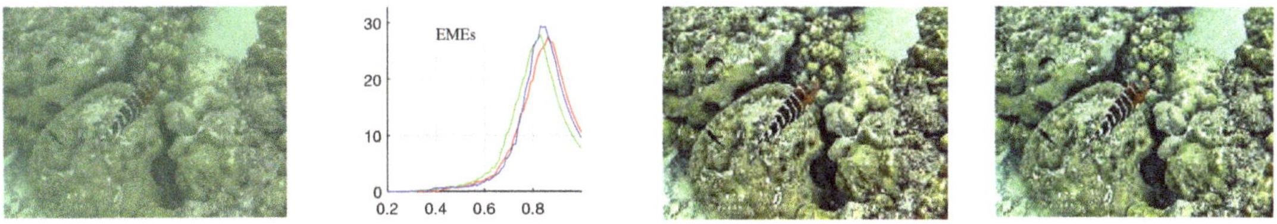

(**a**) EMEC 14.28 (**b**) (**c**) EMEC 35.46 (**d**) EMEC 36.37

Figure 9. (**a**) The original image, (**b**) EMEs of red, green, and blue components, and enhanced images by (**c**) (0.85,0.82,0.82)-rooting and (**d**) (0.82,0.82,0.82)-rooting.

histogram equalization multiscale retinex 0.82-rooting

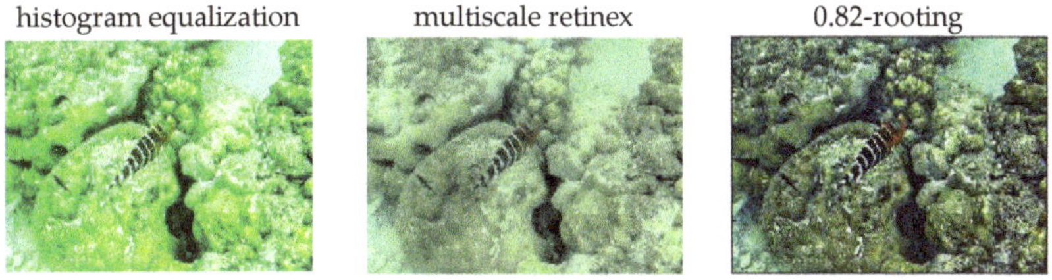

(**a**) EMEC 44.29 (**b**) EMEC 16.96 (**c**) EMEC 33.50

Figure 10. Color image enhancement by (**a**) histogram equalization (MATLAB's version), (**b**) multi-retinex algorithm (the original version [33]), and (**c**) method of 0.82-rooting.

The quaternion image enhancement (EMEQ) measure for a quaternion image $q_{n,m} = (a_{n,m}, r_{n,m}, g_{n,m}, b_{n,m})$ is calculated similarly [27],

$$EMEQ(q) = \frac{1}{k_1 k_2}\sum_{k=1}^{k_1}\sum_{l=1}^{k_2} 20\log_{10}\left[\frac{\max_{k,l}(a_{n,m}, r_{n,m}, g_{n,m}, b_{n,m})}{\min_{k,l}(a_{n,m}, r_{n,m}, g_{n,m}, b_{n,m})}\right]. \tag{40}$$

This measure includes the real part of the quaternion image. The measure EMEQ is calculated for the input quaternion image $q_{n,m}$ and the processed image $v_{n,m}$. In most cases, the best parameter for color enhancement is considered the value of α with a maximum of $EMEC(q)$ and $EMEQ(v)$ (or minimum). Our experimental results show that the measures EMEC and EMEQ are effective in selecting the best parameters to receive color images with high quality [27]. Other measures for selecting the best values of α and estimating color image quality after image processing can also be used. We mention the color image contrast and quality measures [14].

As an example, Figure 11 shows the quaternion image of 877 $\times$ 1024 pixels in part (a). The grayscale image is the real part, and the color image is the imaginary part of the quaternion image. The graph of the EMEC measure as the function of α is shown in part (b). The maximum of this function is at point 0.879. In part (c), the graphs of the measured EME of the color channels are given. The point $\alpha = 0.82$ was selected, at which these graphs roughly intersect. The quaternion images after 0.879 and 0.82-rooting enhancements are shown in parts (d) and (e), respectively.

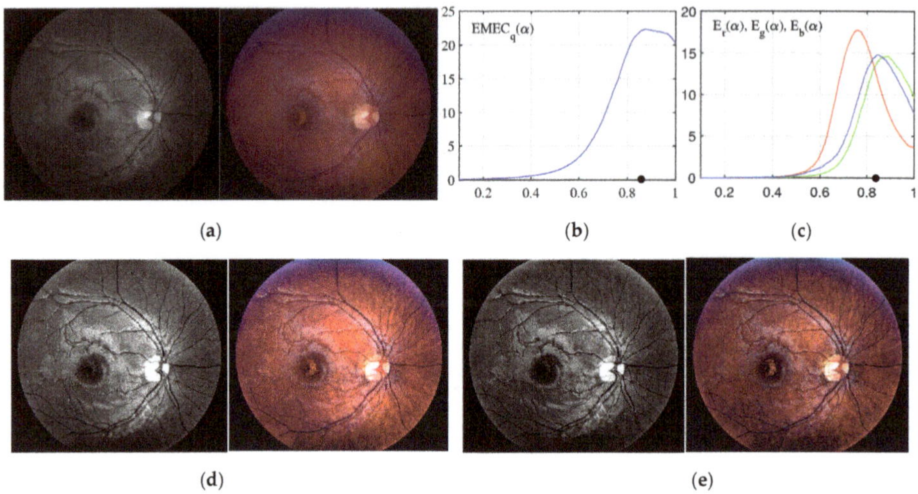

Figure 11. (**a**) The quaternion fundus image, (**b**) the graph of the EMEC function calculated for α-rooting by the 2-D QDFT, (**c**) the graphs of EME functions calculated for red, green, and blue channels of the α-rooting. The enhanced quaternion after (**d**) 0.879-rooting and (**e**) 0.82-rooting.

5.2. The Separable Alpha-Rooting

The alpha-rooting method by the QDFT can be modified in the following two ways.

1. The separable 1-parameter alpha-rooting of the quaternion image $q_{n,m} = [f_{n,m}, g_{n,m}]$ is the method of processing the 2D e_2-QDFT of the image as

$$Q_{p,s} = [F_{p,s}, G_{p,s}] \to \left[F_{p,s}\Big|F_{p,s}|^{\alpha-1}, G_{p,s}\Big|G_{p,s}|^{\alpha-1}\right],\ \alpha \in (0,1). \tag{41}$$

2. The 2-parameter alpha-rooting of the quaternion image uses two parameters α_1 and α_2 from the interval $[0,1]$ to process the 2D e_2-QDFT of the quaternion image as follows:

$$Q_{p,s} = [F_{p,s}, G_{p,s}] \to \left[F_{p,s}\Big|F_{p,s}|^{\alpha_1-1}, G_{p,s}\Big|G_{p,s}|^{\alpha_2-1}\right]. \tag{42}$$

In the $\alpha_1 = \alpha_2 = \alpha$ case, the 2-parameter alpha-rooting coincides with the 1-parameter alpha-rooting.

5.3. Alpha-Rooting of Color Images and the (1,3)-Model

In the (1,3)-model, we consider one of the 2D QDFTs, namely, the separable right-sided 2D QDFT [27]. This transform of the quaternion image $q_{n,m} = (a_{n,m}, r_{n,m}, g_{n,m}, b_{n,m})$ is calculated by

$$Q_{p,s} = \sum_{n=0}^{N-1}\left(\sum_{m=0}^{M-1} q_{n,m} W_{\mu_1}^{ms}\right) W_{\mu_2}^{np},\ p,s = 0:(N-1),(M-1). \tag{43}$$

Here, μ_1 and μ_2 are pure quaternion units. The transform uses N 1D QDFTs by rows and then M 1D QDFT by columns. Given quaternion signal $q_n = (a_n, r_n, g_n, b_n)$ and a pure quaternion $\mu = (0, m_1, m_2, m_3)$, the 1D QDFT, Q_p, with the basis exponential functions

$W_\mu^{np} = \cos(2\pi np/N) - \mu\sin(2\pi np/N)$ requires four traditional DFTs since it is calculated by [14]

$$Q_p = \text{Re}\begin{bmatrix} A_p \\ R_p \\ G_p \\ B_p \end{bmatrix} + M_\mu \times \text{Im}\begin{bmatrix} A_p \\ R_p \\ G_p \\ B_p \end{bmatrix} = \text{Re}\begin{bmatrix} A_p \\ R_p \\ G_p \\ B_p \end{bmatrix} + \begin{bmatrix} 0 & m_1 & m_2 & m_3 \\ -m_1 & 0 & -m_3 & m_2 \\ -m_2 & m_3 & 0 & -m_1 \\ -m_3 & -m_2 & m_1 & 0 \end{bmatrix} \text{Im}\begin{bmatrix} A_p \\ R_p \\ G_p \\ B_p \end{bmatrix}. \quad (44)$$

A_p, R_p, G_p, and B_p are the DFTs of the components a_n, r_n, g_n, and b_n, respectively. $\text{Re}(z)$ and $\text{Im}(z)$ denote the operations of real and imaginary parts of the complex number z, respectively. The multiplication of the 4D vector by the matrix M_μ requires a maximum of 12 real multiplications. In the case, when $\mu_1 = (0,0,1,0) = j$ and $\mu_2 = (0,0,0,1) = k$, the exponential basis functions are $W_k^{ms} = \cos(2\pi ms/M) - k\sin(2\pi ms/M)$ and $W_j^{np} = \cos(2\pi np/N) - j\sin(2\pi np/N)$. The matrices of multiplication have simple forms,

$$M_j = \begin{bmatrix} 0 & 0 & 1 & 0 \\ 0 & 0 & 0 & 1 \\ -1 & 0 & 0 & 0 \\ 0 & -1 & 0 & 0 \end{bmatrix} \text{ and } M_k = \begin{bmatrix} 0 & 0 & 0 & 1 \\ 0 & 0 & -1 & 0 \\ 0 & 1 & 0 & 0 \\ -1 & 0 & 0 & 0 \end{bmatrix}.$$

and the corresponding 1D QDFTs are calculated by

$$Q_p = \begin{bmatrix} Re(A_p) + Im(G_p) \\ Re(R_p) + Im(B_p) \\ Re(G_p) - Im(A_p) \\ Re(B_p) - Im(R_p) \end{bmatrix} \text{ and } Q_p = \begin{bmatrix} Re(A_p) + Im(B_p) \\ Re(R_p) - Im(G_p) \\ Re(G_p) + Im(R_p) \\ Re(B_p) - Im(A_p) \end{bmatrix}.$$

These N-point QDFTs require four 1D DFTs plus $4N$ additions. In this case, the right-sided 2D QDFT of the quaternion image $q_{n,m}$ is calculated by

$$Q_{p,s} = \sum_{n=0}^{N-1}\left(\sum_{m=0}^{M-1} q_{n,m}W_k^{ms}\right)W_j^{np}, \; p = 0:(N-1), \; s = 0:(M-1). \quad (45)$$

A total of $4(N+M)$ 1D QDFTs plus $4(NM) + (4M)N = 8NM$ additions are used to calculate the 2D QDFT. The inverse 2D right-sided QDFT is calculated by

$$q_{n,m} = \frac{1}{NM}\sum_{p=0}^{N-1}\left(\sum_{s=0}^{M-1} Q_{p,s}W_k^{-ms}\right)W_j^{-np}, \quad (46)$$

The complexity of the QDFTs in the (1,3) and (2,2)-models for images of $N \times N$ pixels is described in Table 4.

Table 4. Complexity of the calculations for the two algebras.

Model	Transforms	Number of 1D DFTs	Number of Additional Multiplications	Number of Additional Additions
The (1,3)-model:				
General case of μ	1D QDFT	4 (real)	$12N$	$12N$
	2D QDFT	$4(2N) = 8N$	$12N(2N) = 24N^2$	$12N(2N) = 24N^2$
Case $\mu = j, k$	1D QDFT	4 (real)	-	$4N$
	2D QDFT	$4(2N) = 8N$	-	$4N(2N) = 8N^2$
The (2,2)-model:				
1D e_2-QDFT	1D QDFT	2 (complex)	-	-
2D e_2-QDFT	2D QDFT	$2(2N) = 4N$	-	-

The main steps of the algorithm for α-rooting in the (1,3)-model:

1. Compose the quaternion image $q_{n,m} = (a_{n,m}, r_{n,m}, g_{n,m}, b_{n,m})$ from the color RGB image $(r_{n,m}, g_{n,m}, b_{n,m})$.
2. Calculate the right-sided 2D QDFT, $Q_{p,s}$, of the quaternion image.
3. Given $\alpha \in (0,1)$, calculate the coefficients $c(p,s) = |Q_{p,s}|^{\alpha-1}$.
4. Modify the 2D QDFT as $Q_{p,s} \to V_{p,s} = c(p,s)Q_{p,s}$.
5. Calculate the inverse 2D QDFT $v_{n,m} = v_{n,m}(\alpha)$.
6. Select the best value α for color image enhancement by using the measures EMEQ or EMEC.

6. Experimental Results with Color Images

In this section, a few illustrative examples of the 2D QDFT-based alpha-rooting are presented. Many color images of art in this paper are from Olga's Gallery—Free Art Print Museum by address https://www.freeart.com/gallery/ (accessed on 22 January 2025) with permission to use them in our research. Figure 12 shows the RGB color image 'rembrandt195.jpg' in part (a) and the enhanced image in part (b). The enhanced image was calculated by the alpha-rooting with e_2-QDFT, when the parameter $\alpha = 0.9143$. This value of the parameter is considered optimal, or best, according to the EMEC measure calculated by Equation (39) with block size 7×7. This measure as the function EMEC(α) has a maximum of 36.54 at this point. The measure of the original image is EMEC(1) = 34.74.

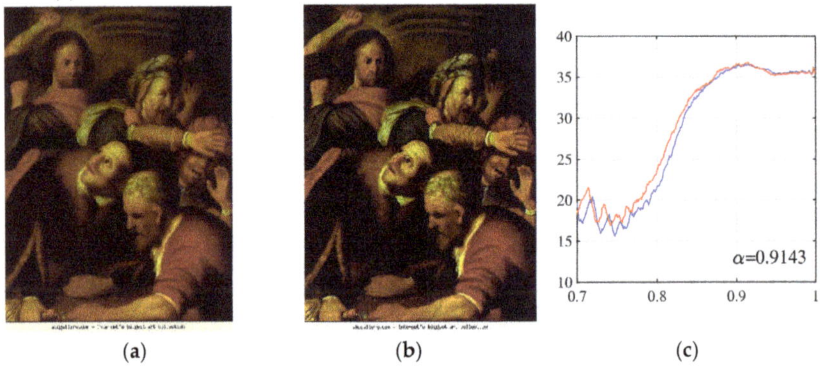

Figure 12. (**a**) The original image, (**b**) 2D e2-QDFT based 0.9143-rooting (with the scaling factor of $A = 4$), and (**c**) the two curves of the EMEC.

Two EMEC functions are shown in Figure 12 in part (c); they are close to each other, and both achieve the maximum at the same point. The first graph (which is a little higher than the other one) was calculated by the 2D e_2-QDFT-based alpha-rooting described in Section 5.1, when the transform is modified as $Q_{p,s} = [F_{p,s}, G_{p,s}] \to |Q_{p,s}|^{\alpha-1}[F_{p,s}, G_{p,s}]$, $\alpha \in [0.7, 1]$. The second graph is for the EMEC measure calculated from the 1-parameter alpha-rooting described in Section 5.2, when the e_2-QDFT of the images is processed as follows: $Q_{p,s} = [F_{p,s}, G_{p,s}] \to [F_{p,s}|F_{p,s}|^{\alpha-1}, G_{p,s}|G_{p,s}|^{\alpha-1}]$, $\alpha \in [0.7, 1]$. Figure 13 shows the enhanced image by 1-parameter 0.9143-rooting in part (a). For comparison, the 0.9143-rooting of the image by the 2D QDFT in the (1,3)-model is shown in part (b).

Below are a few results of processing other color images by the alpha-rooting and separate algorithms of the alpha-rooting in the commutative (2,2)-model. The results of image enhancement by the alpha-rooting in the non-commutative (1,3)-model are also shown. Figure 14 shows the results of the 0.92-rootings, when processing the image of San Antonio. The values of the color image enhancement EMEC are shown.

Figure 15 shows the results of the same methods of the 0.92-rootings, when processing another image of San Antonio. One can note that the images processed in the (2,2)-model have higher values of EMEC.

Figure 16 shows the results of processing image 'image13-2.jpg.' The method of alpha-rooting works well in both models for many images. It means that the (2,2)-model does not perform any worse but in fact better than another model, that is, the (1,3)-model.

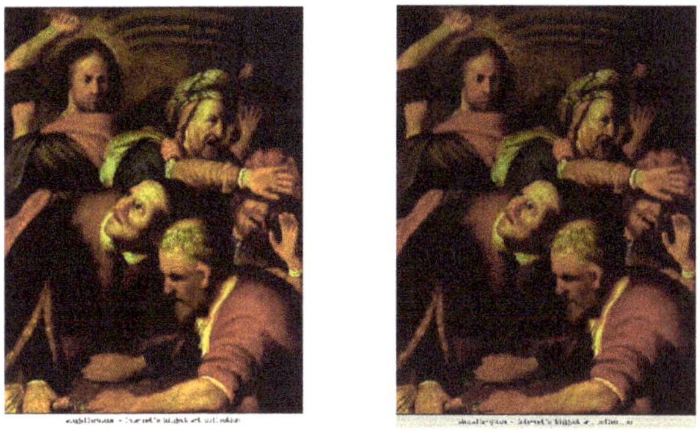

(a) (b)

Figure 13. The enhanced images of the 0.9143-rooting: (**a**) in the (2,2)-model and (**b**) in the (1,3)-model.

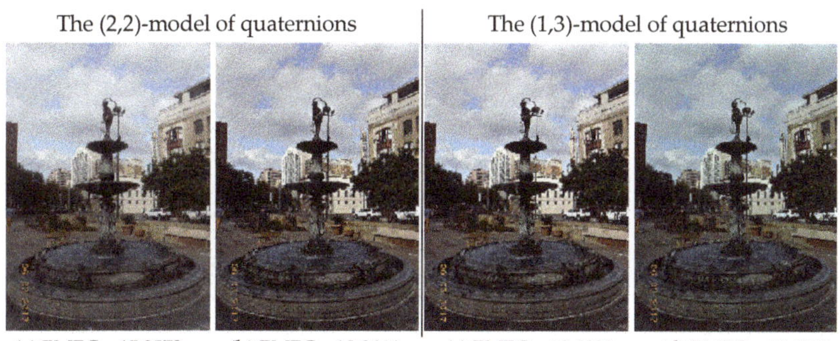

(**a**) EMEC = 15.2572 (**b**) EMEC = 18.9644 (**c**) EMEC = 18.6932 (**d**) EMEC = 18.6892

Figure 14. (**a**) The original color image. The enhanced images in the (2,2)-model by (**b**) the main 0.92-rooting and (**c**) separable 1-parameter 0.92-rooting. (**d**) The 0.92-rooting in the (1,3)-model.

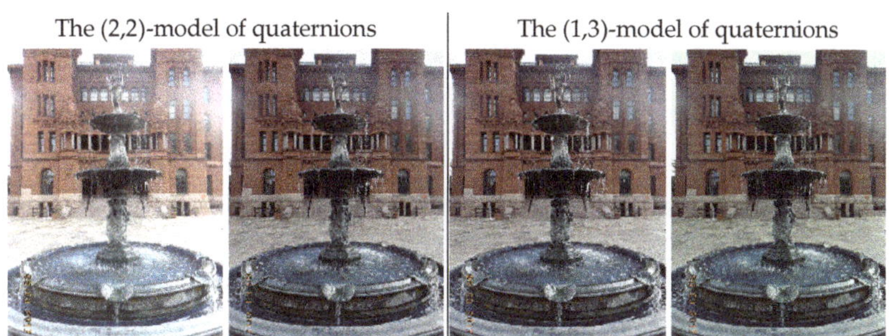

(**a**) EMEC = 8.4645 (**b**) EMEC = 16.5311 (**c**) EMEC = 16.5174 (**d**) EMEC = 16.5005

Figure 15. (**a**) The original color image. The enhanced images in the (2,2)-model by (**b**) the main 0.92-rooting and (**c**) separable 1-parameter 0.92-rooting. (**d**) The 0.92-rooting in the (1,3)-model.

The results of processing the well-known "flowers" image are shown in Figure 17 in parts (a)–(d).

Now we apply the method of alpha-rooting in the (2,2)-model, when two parameters α_1 and α_2 are used and the 2D QDFT of the color image is processed as

$$Q_{p,s} = \left[F_{p,s}, G_{p,s}\right] \to \left[F_{p,s}\Big|F_{p,s}\Big|^{\alpha_1 - 1}, G_{p,s}\Big|G_{p,s}\Big|^{\alpha_2 - 1}\right],\ \alpha_1, \alpha_2 \in (0,1]. \tag{47}$$

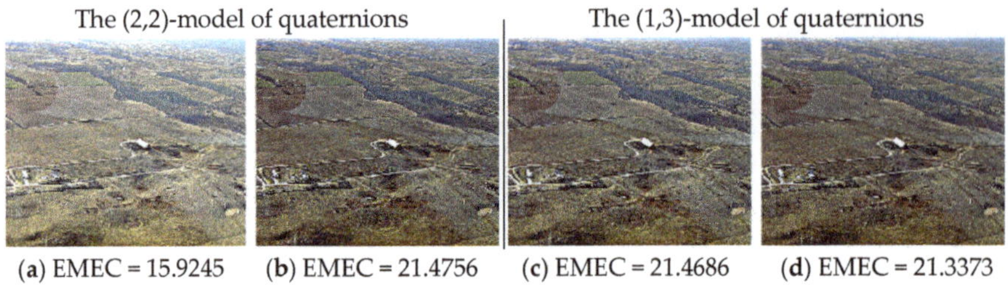

Figure 16. (**a**) The original color image. The enhanced images in the (2,2)-model by (**b**) the main 0.92-rooting and (**c**) separable 1-parameter 0.92-rooting. (**d**) The 0.92-rooting in the (1,3)-model.

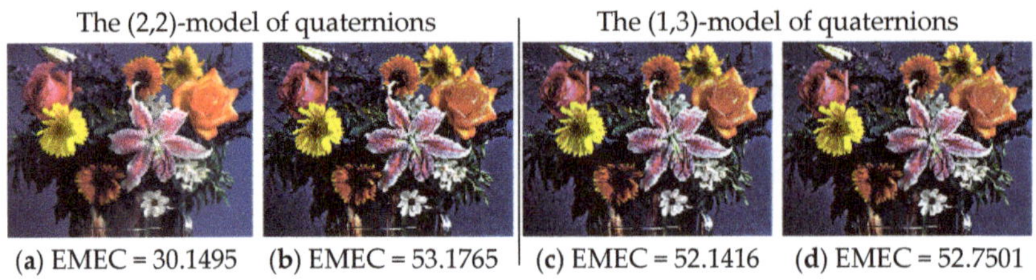

Figure 17. (**a**) The original color image. The enhanced images in the (2,2)-model by (**b**) the main 0.92-rooting and (**c**) separable 1-parameter 0.92-rooting. (**d**) The 0.92-rooting in the (1,3)-model.

Figure 18 shows results of the color image enhancement processing by the 2-parameter alpha-rooting with different sets of parameters α_1 and α_2. In part (b), the image of San Antonio was processed by the parameters $\alpha_1 = \alpha_2 = 0.92$. The enhancement by parameters $\alpha_1 = 0.92$ and $\alpha_2 = 0.93$ is shown in part (c).

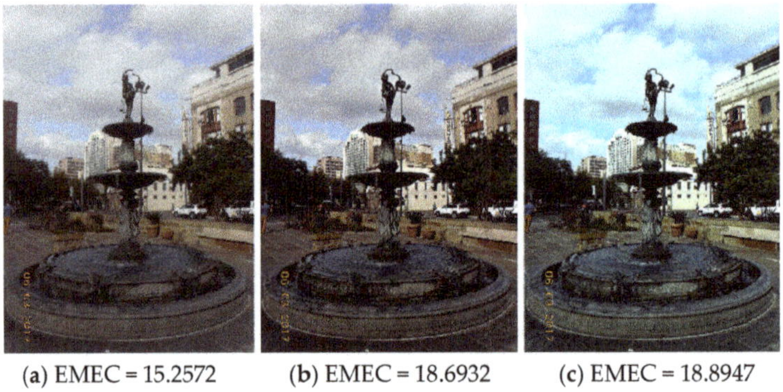

Figure 18. (**a**) The original color image, and (**b**) the [0.92,0.92]-rooting, and (**c**) the [0.92,0.93]-rooting in the (2,2)-model.

It should be noted that when processing color images in the quaternion models, the color image is only the imaginary part of the quaternion image. The enhancement of quaternion image includes two images, the color one and the gray one. They are processed together. The first component of the quaternion image, which is referred to as the grayscale image is not the grayscale image of the processed color image. The enhancement of quaternion image results in the enhancement of both images. As examples, we consider a few color images processed in the (2,2)-model by the 2-D e_2-QDFT-based alpha-rooting.

Figure 19 shows the color image 'raphael155.jpg' in part (a), which was embedded in the quaternion image as its imaginary part. The imaginary component (the new color image) of the enhanced quaternion image by the 0.92-rooting is shown in part (b). The grayscale image of the original color image is shown in part (c). The real part of the processed quaternion image is shown in part (d). This image is not the average of colors in the image in part (b). Thus, both grayscale and color images were enhanced when processing the quaternion image.

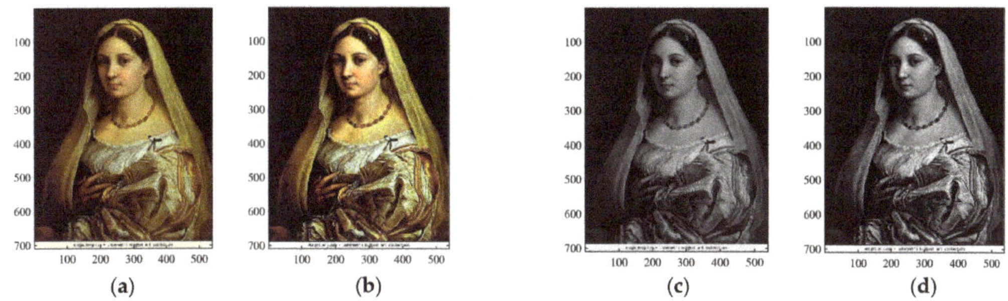

Figure 19. (**a**) The original color image and (**c**) its grayscale image. The processed (**b**) imaginary and (**d**) real components of the enhanced quaternion image by the e_2-QDFT 0.92-rooting.

Figures 20 and 21 show the results of enhancement of the quaternion images when the color images 'leonardo9.jpg' and 'flowers' were used, respectively.

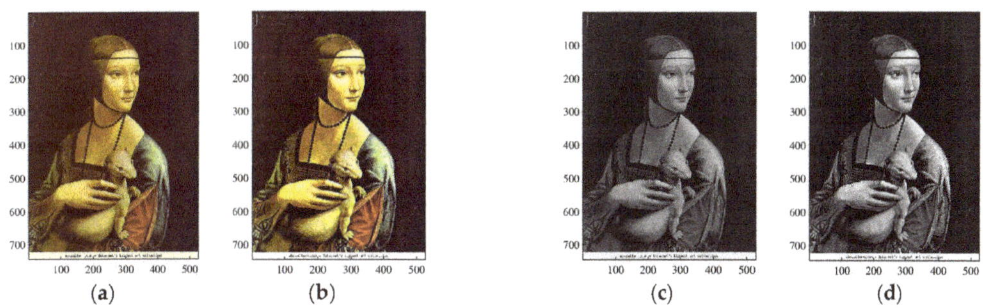

Figure 20. (**a**) The original color image 'leonardo9.jpg' and (**c**) its grayscale image. The processed (**b**) imaginary and (**d**) real components of the enhanced quaternion image by the e_2-QDFT 0.92-rooting ($\times 4$).

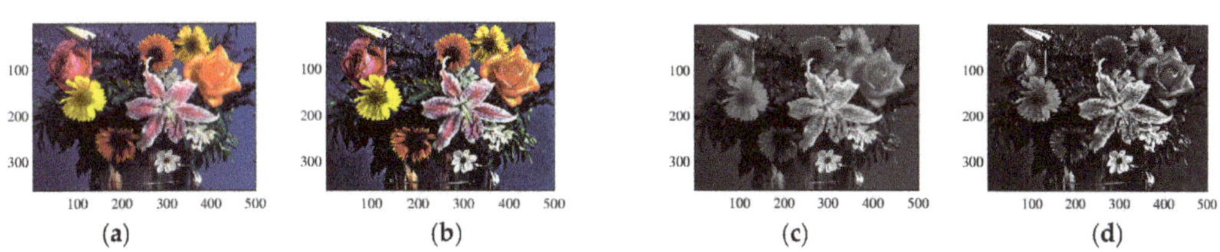

Figure 21. (**a**) The original color flowers image and (**c**) its grayscale image. The processed (**b**) imaginary and (**d**) real components of the enhanced quaternion image by the e_2-QDFT 0.80-rooting ($\times 20$).

7. Conclusions

New quaternion algebra, the (2,2)-model, was presented, and new methods of alpha-rooting by the quaternion discrete Fourier transform (QDFT) were described and analyzed in this model. The main properties of this model were considered. This model of quaternions is commutative and associative and allows to calculate the aperiodic convolution of quaternion images in the frequency domain. The results of the image enhancement of color images in this model were compared with the alpha-rooting in the traditional (1,3)-model. The comparison with the known methods of histogram equalization and Retinex is also provided with examples. The preliminary experimental examples show the effectiveness of the proposed methods for color image enhancement by the 2D QDFT. We believe that the commutative (2,2)-model together with the non-commutative (1,3)-model can be effectively used in color image enhancement, as well as other areas of color imaging. The proposed methods of alpha-rooting are fast, because of fast 1D and 2D QDFTs, and do not require much memory, as well as machine learning algorithms, which require much time and memory and do not work well on many images presented in this work.

Author Contributions: Conceptualization, A.M.G.; methodology, A.M.G.; software, A.M.G. and A.A.G.; validation, A.M.G.; formal analysis, A.M.G. and A.A.G.; investigation, A.M.G.; resources, A.M.G.; data curation, A.M.G.; writing—original draft preparation, A.M.G.; writing—review and editing, A.M.G. and A.A.G.; visualization, A.M.G. and A.A.G.; supervision, A.M.G.; project administration, A.M.G. All authors have read and agreed to the published version of the manuscript.

Funding: This research received no external funding.

Data Availability Statement: The original contributions presented in this study are included in the article. Further inquiries can be directed to the corresponding author(s).

Acknowledgments: This article is a revised and expanded version of Ref. [25], which was presented at *SPIE 13033 Conference, Defense + Commercial Sensing 2024*, National Harbor, MD 20745, USA, 22 April 2024.

Conflicts of Interest: The authors declare no conflicts of interest.

References

1. Harris, J.L. Constant variance enhancement: A digital processing technique. *Appl. Opt.* **1977**, *16*, 1268. [CrossRef] [PubMed]
2. Wang, D.C.; Vagnucci, A.H.; Li, C.C. Digital image enhancement: A survey. *Comput. Vis. Graph. Image Process.* **1983**, *24*, 363–381. [CrossRef]
3. Trussell, H.J.; Saber, E.; Vrhel, M. Color image processing [basics and special issue overview]. *IEEE Signal Process. Mag.* **2005**, *22*, 14–22. [CrossRef]
4. Gonzalez, R.C.; Woods, R.E. *Digital Image Processing*, 4th ed.; Pearson: New York, NY, USA, 2018.
5. Grigoryan, A.M.; Agaian, S.S. Image processing contrast enhancement. In *Wiley Encyclopedia of Electrical and Electronics Engineering*; Webster, J.G., Ed.; Wiley: Hoboken, NJ, USA, 2017; pp. 1–22.
6. Nithyananda, C.R.; Ramachandra, A.C.; Preethi. Survey on histogram equalization method-based image enhancement techniques. In Proceedings of the 2016 International Conference on Data Mining and Advanced Computing (SAPIENCE), Ernakulam, India, 16–18 March 2016; IEEE: New York, NY, USA, 2016; pp. 150–158.
7. Han, J.-H.; Yang, S.; Lee, B.-U. A novel 3-D color histogram equalization method with uniform 1-D gray scale histogram. *IEEE Trans. Image Process.* **2011**, *20*, 506–512. [CrossRef] [PubMed]
8. Trahanias, P.E.; Venetsanopoulos, A.N. Color image enhancement through 3-D histogram equalization. In Proceedings of the 11th IAPR International Conference on Pattern Recognition, The Hague, The Netherlands, 30 August–3 September 1992; IEEE Comput. Soc. Press: Washington, DC, USA, 1992; Volume IV, pp. 545–548.
9. Pitas, I.; Kiniklis, P. Multichannel techniques in color image enhancement and modeling. *IEEE Trans. Image Process.* **1996**, *5*, 168–171. [CrossRef] [PubMed]
10. Mlsna, P.A.; Zhang, Q.; Rodriguez, J.J. 3-D histogram modification of color images. In Proceedings of the 3rd IEEE International Conference on Image Processing, Lausanne, Switzerland, 16–19 September 1996; IEEE: New York, NY, USA, 1996; Volume 3, pp. 1015–1018.
11. Land, E.H.; McCann, J.J. Lightness and retinex theory. *J. Opt. Soc. Am.* **1971**, *61*, 1–11. [CrossRef]
12. Land, E. An alternative technique for the computation of the designator in the retinex theory of color vision. *Proc. Natl. Acad. Sci. USA* **1986**, *83*, 3078–3080. [CrossRef] [PubMed]
13. Agaian, S.S.; Panetta, K.; Grigoryan, A.M. Transform-based image enhancement algorithms with performance measure. *IEEE Trans. Image Process.* **2001**, *10*, 367–382. [CrossRef] [PubMed]
14. Grigoryan, A.M.; Agaian, S.S. *Quaternion and Octonion Color Image Processing with MATLAB*; SPIE Press: Bellingham, WA, USA, 2018.
15. Gauss, C.F. Mutationen des raumes [transformations of space] (c. 1819). In *Carl Friedrich Gauss Werke*, 8th ed.; Brendel, M., Ed.; Teubner: Stuttgart, Germany, 1900; pp. 357–361.
16. Hamilton, W.R. On a new species of imaginary quantities connected with a theory of quaternions. *Proc. R. Ir. Acad.* **1844**, *2*, 424–434. Available online: https://www.emis.de/classics/Hamilton/Quatern1.pdf (accessed on 27 December 2024).

17. Hamilton, W.R. *Elements of Quaternions*; Longmans, Green & Co.: London, UK, 1866.
18. Kantor, I.L.; Solodovnikov, A.S. *Hypercomplex Numbers*; Nauka: Moscow, Russia, 1973.
19. Bülow, T. *Hypercomplex Spectral Signal Representations for the Processing and Analysis of Images*; Christian-Albrechts-Univ.: Kiel, Germany, 1999; Volume 9903, p. 171.
20. Yin, Q.; Wang, J.; Luo, X.; Zhai, J.; Jha, S.K.; Shi, Y.-Q. Quaternion convolutional neural network for color image classification and forensics. *IEEE Access* **2019**, *7*, 20293–20301. [CrossRef]
21. Sangwine, S.J. Fourier transforms of colour images using quaternion, or hypercomplex, numbers. *Electron. Lett.* **1996**, *32*, 1979–1980. [CrossRef]
22. Grigoryan, A.M.; Agaian, S.S. Commutative quaternion algebra and DSP fundamental properties: Quaternion convolution and Fourier transform. *Signal Process.* **2022**, *196*, 108533. [CrossRef]
23. Davenport, C. Commutative Hypercomplex Mathematics. Unpublished Work, 2008. Available online: https://swissenschaft.ch/tesla/content/T_Library/L_Theory/EM%20Field%20Research/Hypercomplex%20Commutative%20Mathematics.pdf (accessed on 22 January 2025).
24. Ell, T.A.; Sangwine, S.J. Hypercomplex Fourier transforms of color images. *IEEE Trans. Image Process.* **2007**, *16*, 22–35. [CrossRef]
25. Grigoryan, A.M.; Gomez, A.A. Quaternion Fourier transform-based alpha-rooting color image enhancement in 2 algebras: Commutative and non-commutative. In Proceedings of the SPIE 13033 Conference, Defense + Commercial Sensing 2024, National Harbor, MD, USA, 21–25 April 2024; SPIE: Bellingham, WA, USA, 2024; p. 12. [CrossRef]
26. McClellan, J.H. Artifacts in alpha-rooting of images. In Proceedings of the IEEE International Conference on Acoustics, Speech, and Signal Processing, Denver, CO, USA, 9–11 April 1980; pp. 449–452.
27. Grigoryan, A.M.; Jenkinson, J.; Agaian, S.S. Quaternion Fourier transform-based alpha-rooting method for color image measurement and enhancement. *Signal Process.* **2015**, *109*, 269–289. [CrossRef]
28. Fechner, G.T. *Elements of Psychophysics*; Rinehart & Winston: New York, NY, USA, 1960; Volume 1.
29. Gordon, I.E. *Theory of Visual Perception*; John Wiley & Sons: New York, NY, USA, 1989.
30. Zuiderveld, K. Contrast limited adaptive histogram equalization. In *Graphics Gems IV*; Academic Press: San Diego, CA, USA, 1994; pp. 474–485.
31. Kim, Y.T. Contrast enhancement using brightness preserving bi-histogram equalization. *IEEE Trans. Consum. Electron.* **1997**, *43*, 1–8.
32. Zhu, H.; Chan, F.H.; Lam, F.K. Image contrast enhancement by constrained local histogram equalization. *Comput. Vis. Image Underst.* **1999**, *73*, 281–290. [CrossRef]
33. Jabson, D.J.; Rahmann, Z.; Woodell, G.A. A multiscale retinex for bridging the gap between color images and the human observations of scenes. *IEEE Trans. Image Process.* **1997**, *6*, 897–1056. [CrossRef] [PubMed]
34. Chen, S.; Beghdadi, A. Nature rendering of color image based on Retinex. In Proceedings of the IEEE International Conference on Image Processing, Cairo, Egypt, 7–10 November 2009; pp. 1813–1816.
35. Huang, K.-Q.; Wang, Q.; Wu, Z.-Y. Natural color image enhancement and evaluation algorithm based on human visual system. *Comput. Vis. Image Underst.* **2006**, *103*, 52–63. [CrossRef]
36. Struc, V.; Pavei, N. Photometric normalization techniques for illumination invariance. In *Advances in Face Image Analysis: Techniques and Technologies*; Zhang, Y.J., Ed.; IGI Global: Hershey, PA, USA, 2011; pp. 279–300.
37. Struc, V.; Pavei, N. Gabor-based kernel-partial-least-squares discrimination features for face recognition. *Informatica* **2009**, *20*, 115–138. [CrossRef]

computers

Article

Number Recognition Through Color Distortion Using Convolutional Neural Networks

Christopher Henshaw [1,2,*], Jacob Dennis [1], Jonathan Nadzam [2] and Alan J. Michaels [1,2,*]

1 Virginia Tech National Security Institute, Blacksburg, VA 24060, USA; heeroyuy@vt.edu
2 Bradley Department of Electrical and Computer Engineering, Virginia Tech, Blacksburg, VA 24061, USA
* Correspondence: chenshaw@vt.edu (C.H.); ajm@vt.edu (A.J.M.)

Abstract: Machine learning applied to image-based number recognition has made significant strides in recent years. Recent use of Large Language Models (LLMs) in natural language search and generation of text have improved performance for general images, yet performance limitations still exist for data subsets related to color blindness. In this paper, we replicated the training of six distinct neural networks (MNIST, LeNet5, VGG16, AlexNet, and two AlexNet modifications) using deep learning techniques with the MNIST dataset and the Ishihara-Like MNIST dataset. While many prior works have dealt with MNIST, the Ishihara adaption addresses red-green combinations of color blindness, allowing for further research in color distortion. Through this research, we applied pre-processing to accentuate the effects of red-green and monochrome colorblindness and hyper-parameterized the existing architectures, ultimately achieving better overall performance than currently published in known works.

Keywords: machine learning; optical character recognition (OCR); color blindness; Ishihara

1. Introduction

While there has been extensive research of character recognition in the field of Machine Learning (ML) in the past 30 years, most of the research has been centered around creating and analyzing less than ideal datasets representing handwritten numbers and letters [1]. This application has many uses, such as increasing performance with vision-based systems, transcribing and understanding old texts, and using the combination of steganography and cryptography to hide information within images [2]. A decent portion of early optical character recognition (OCR) research was centered around using the Modified National Institute of Standards and Technology (MNIST) dataset in conjunction with convolutional neural networks (CNNs) [3,4]. Examples of this work include expanding the MNIST dataset in 2017 to letters [5] and creating a dataset around standard clothing items (Fashion MNIST) [6].

In this paper, we present the idea, procedure, and results of ML-based evaluation of red-green color blindness distortions similar to [7] that is intended to create and train a neural network model that can succeed through the variations in human writing to detect the visual character in a nonideal color distorted environment. Essentially, instead of simply trying to detect characters with heavy distortion due to their writing style, this research seeks to augment prior research by evaluating a distorted letter in an environment that would cause the information to become more diluted. To do this, the Ishihara-Like MNIST [8] dataset was used. This dataset comprises the characters from the MNIST dataset, but they are placed inside an Ishihara circle. Ishihara circles [9], more commonly known as color blindness circles, are used to detect which category of color deficiency a person may possess. In this dataset, as opposed to MNIST, the characters are no longer cohesive in nature as the entire circle is comprised of varying sized circles in different colors. In comparison, a standard Ishihara circle has a near perfect character in the center. Examples of a standard Ishihara circle and a MNIST Ishihara circle for the numbers 6 and 8 are shown in Figures 1 and 2.

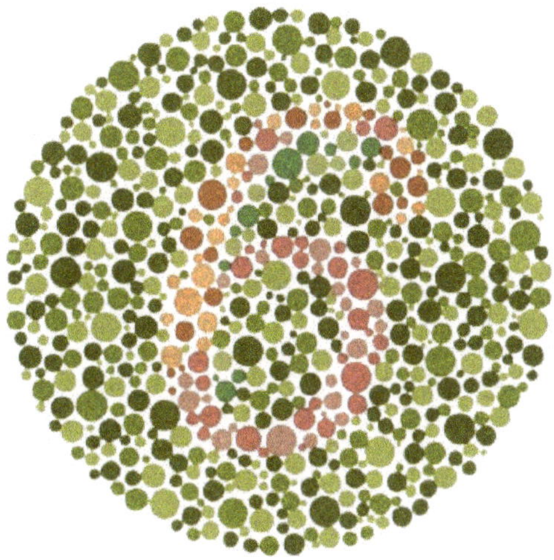

Figure 1. Standard Ishihara Circle [10].

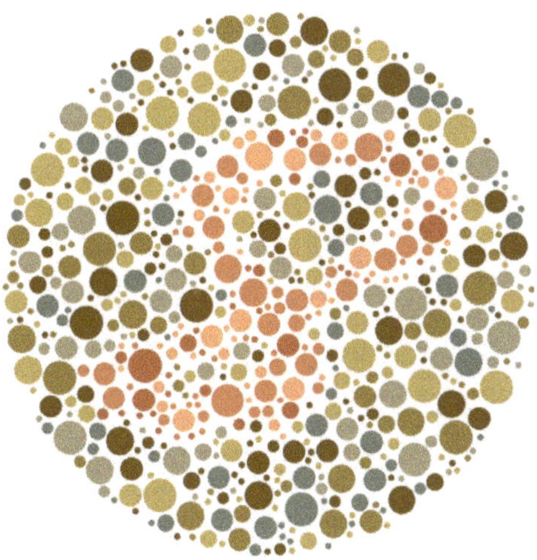

Figure 2. MNIST Ishihara Circle [8].

1.1. Prevalence

Color blindness, or rather *color vision deficiency*, affects nearly 8% of men and 0.5% of women, for a total of roughly 4% of the population [11]. This deficiency is caused by the absence of one or more of the three types of cone cells (a type of photoreceptor cell) in the retina of the eyes. These cells are responsible for our color vision as well as our color sensitivity. Human eyes are comprised of approximately 6 million cones, wherein 60% are red sensing, 30% are green sensing, and 10% are blue sensing [12]. This deficiency can be caused due to genetic disorders (most common), injury to the eyes, or cancer and tumors that affect the optical nerve [13]. Additionally, color blindness can be caused by medications, the deterioration of the eyes from aging, and diseases such as Alzheimer's or Parkinson's [14]. There is no known cure for color blindness, but mitigation techniques exist in the form of special glasses and contact lenses or visual aids [13].

While there are seven official diagnoses of color deficiency, the most common is red-green [11]. Red-green color deficiency encapsulates four of the seven diagnoses: deuteranomaly, protanomaly, protanopia, and deuteranopia. Deuteranomaly is the most common and causes shades of green to appear more red, while protanomaly causes shades of red to appear more green. Protanopia is the absence of red cones, while deuteranopia is the absence of green cones. The next two deficiencies are blue-yellow: tritanomaly and tritanopia. Tritanomaly makes it difficult to distinguish between blue and green and also between yellow and red. This is due to malfunctioning blue cones. Tritanopia, on the other hand, makes the patient unable to distinguish between blue and green, purple and red, and yellow and pink. Due to this, all colors appear less bright. This deficiency is caused by the lack of blue cones. The last type of color deficiency is known as monochromacy, monocromacia, or Aachromatopsia. This is the lack of color cones entirely and causes all color to appear in grayscale [15]. Figure 3 attempts to highlight the distinction between the various types of color deficiency. While this image shows the comparison of the scale of colors, it fails to show exactly how the world appears for those with a given deficiency. Figure 4 shows the seven different deficiencies when considering a colorful image of fruit.

Name	Color Scale	Description of effect	Percentage of population
Normal	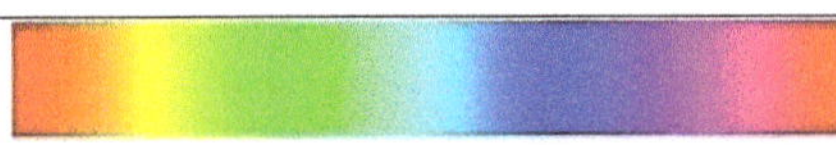	Normal vision	92%
Deuteranomaly	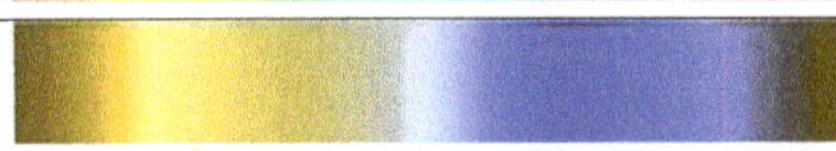	Dull Green	4.6%
Deuteranopia		No Green	1.27%
Protanomaly		Dull Red	1.08%
Protanopia		No Red	1.01%
Tritanomaly	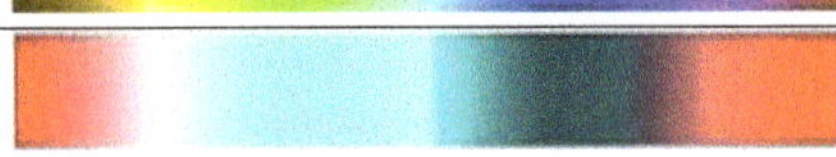	Blue = Green, Yellow = Red	0.02%
Tritanopia	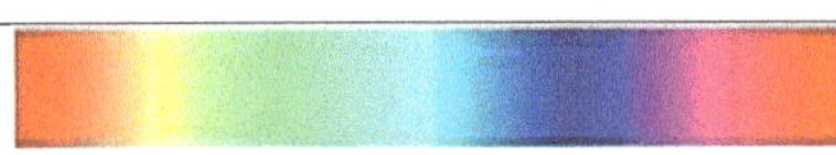	Blue = Green, Yellow = Pink, Red = Purple	0.03%
Achromatopsia	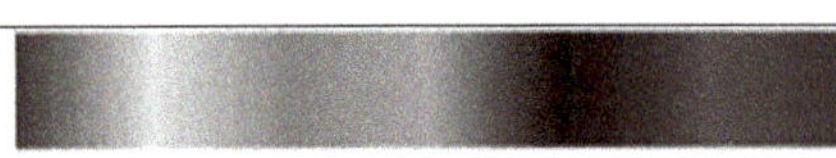	All Gray	0.0033%

Figure 3. Color Blindness Spectrum [11,15–17].

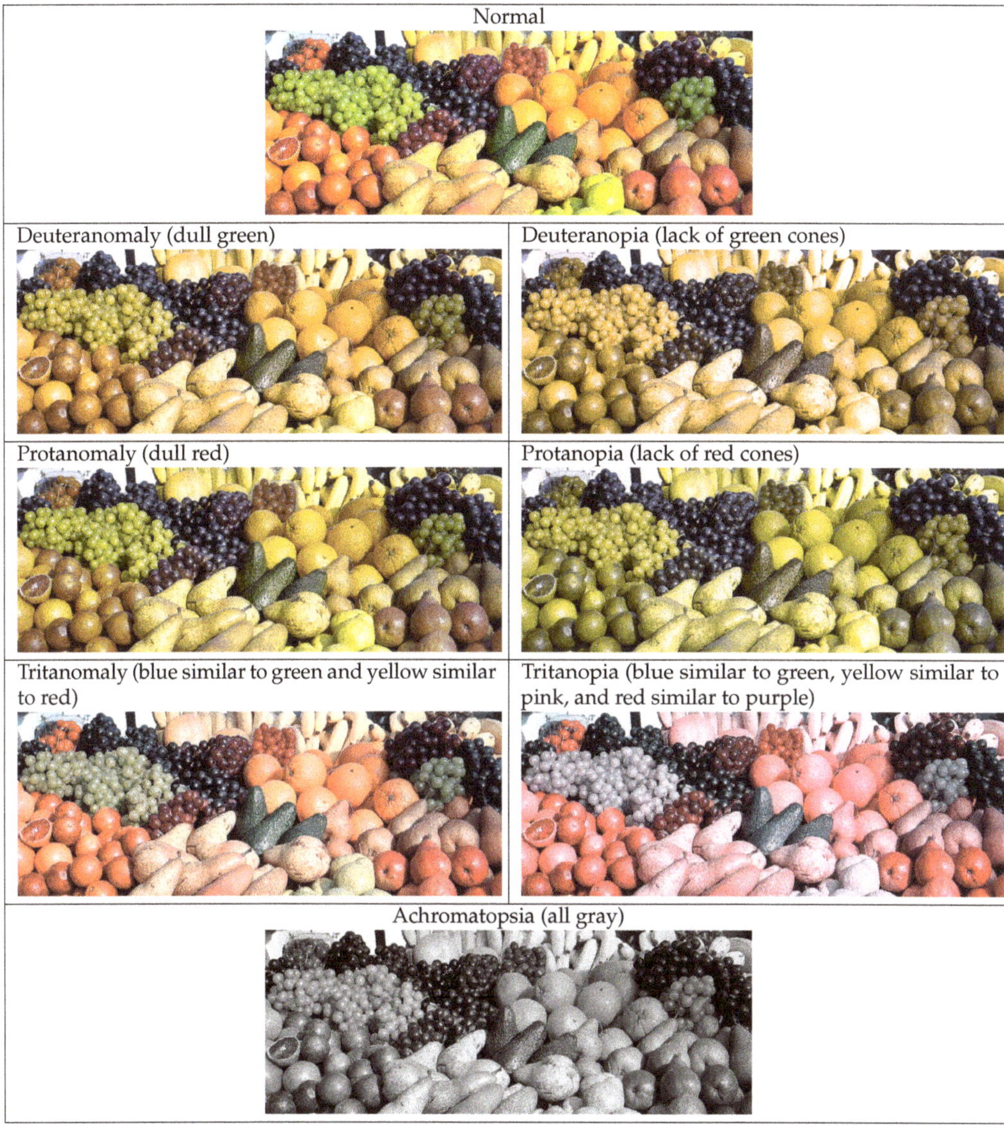

Figure 4. A normal color image followed by the image modified as to emulate the seven different types of color blindness [18,19].

1.2. Motivation

This may seem like an arbitrary topic to model research after, but most models in ML for color correction are based on the physiological models on how people with color blindness perceive the world [20]. Most research in this field tends to focus on correcting the images for those with the deficiency [21–24]. Therefore, we think it is important to explore training a neural network model with images that have color distortion with the intent not of modifying the image, but instead modifying the architecture of the model to bypass or see through the distortion. In doing so, we may work towards a better understanding of how the brain (or CNN) learns when presented with distorted data inputs.

The real world application of this research is to create a model that processes an image with heavy distortion in near real time such that the machine can read the image but a human cannot. This is achieved by training on data that has heavy artificial color distortion in the particular targeted color scheme. A significant amount of research has been conducted to use color theory and color segmentation to help CV algorithms in detection of characters. In [25,26], this research was used to correct the distortion that dirt and fading has on traffic signs. Additionally, more research has been performed with color transformation to increase the detection of the traffic sign as seen in [27]. The goal of this paper is to use the theory behind research to use the color gradients in these images such that they become indistinguishable to humans but clear to a machine. Additional work could also be done in the realm of ML if models understand the information presented as proposed in [28] because fragmented color filters could be used to hide more information.

1.3. Background

The basis for this research started with replicating [29], in which Solonko attempted to modify traditional Ishihara circles to make them look more like MNIST. The goal was to train a model on MNIST and then test it with his custom Ishihara circles, evaluating the character in the center of the circle. However, to achieve high validation results, the images underwent heavy image modification. This included median blurring, k-means clustering, erosion, thresholding, and morphology [29]. All of these pre-processing techniques were used to isolate the character inside the circle, essentially eliminating the distortion from the background. By the end, only a white skeletonized version of the image on a black background was left. An example of his process on the images can be shown in Figure 5. It should be noted that before feeding the image into pre-processing, some processing had already been performed, as the character in the foreground was separated from its background in terms of color. To increase the reach in this research, we sought to limit the modifications to the image.

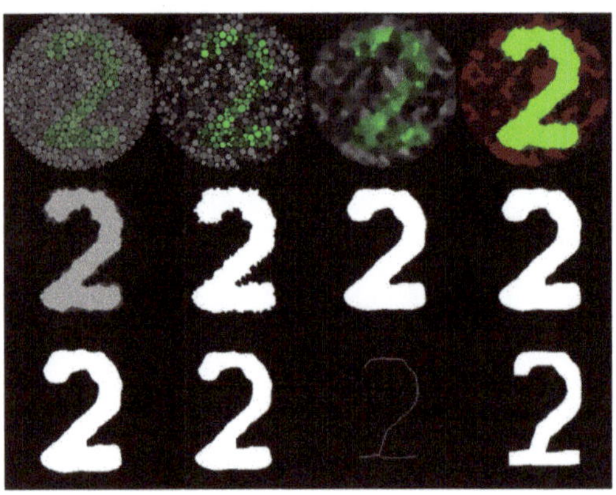

Figure 5. The modifications the image undertook when pre-processing with Solonko's work [29].

In 1998, the MNIST dataset was presented by LeCun et al. [3]. It comprised 60,000 training images and 10,000 testing images of handwritten digits from 0 to 9. These digits were handwritten from 500 different writers (divided into two sets) and then shuffled together. The first set was from high school students and the second set was from Census Bureau employees. These handwritten digits were scanned into digital form, normalized to 20×20 pixels, converted to grayscale, and then padded to increase their size to 28×28 [3,4,30]. Today, the original dataset is used mainly as a baseline for training OCR models and CV models, similar to an ML-based "hello world" program [4]. Outside of research and construction of ML models, the original MNIST dataset is used in various business sectors such as banks for reading checks, postal services when reading addresses and zip codes, and documentation management for sorting hand written documents [31]. As previously stated, the MNIST dataset has since been expanded to many other areas. The focus here is to encapsulate more domains into an MNIST-like form so that research can be performed on those areas as well. Expansions within the realm of language include making datasets similar to the original comprised of English letters instead of digits (EMIST) [5], Kuzushiji (cursive Japanese) [32], and even ancient Sumerian characters [33]. Outside of language, the Fashion-MNIST, for example, seeks to help train neural networks in recognizing various clothing pieces such as shirts, blouses, dresses, and shoes. This dataset is intended to be the modern replacement for MNIST [34]. Using these more detailed datasets could help with the problem of overfitting in Deep Neural Networks (DNNs) as shown in [35] and help with recognition of everyday objects as seen in [6]. Figures 6–8, show the original MNIST with the indicated expansions. The images were created using the datasets from Keras.

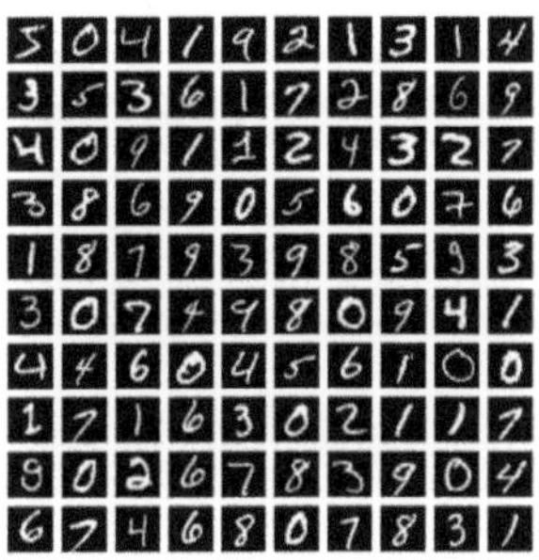

Figure 6. Original MNIST.

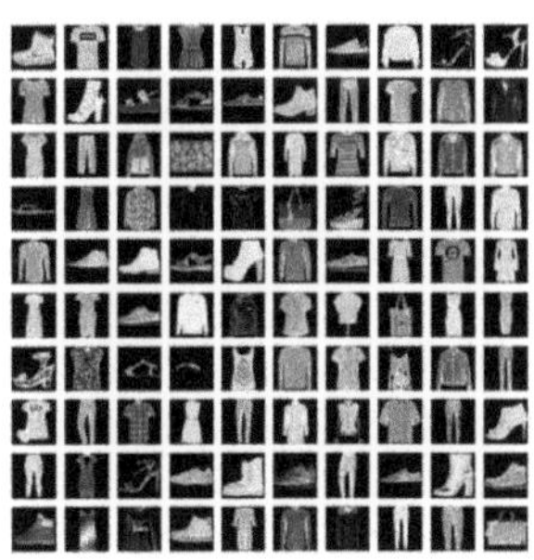

Figure 7. Fashion MNIST.

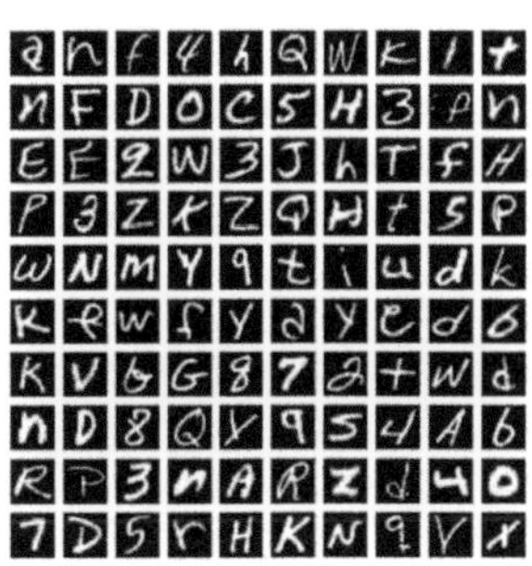

Figure 8. EMNIST.

However, as pertaining to this research, the Ishihara-Like MNIST dataset was not created for the purposes of character recognition. It was created and used for the exploration of explainable AI, the notion that humans should be able to trust the evaluation of a computer-based system for its validity. For this, an assessment framework was made for a human-centric evaluation. To do this, Ishihara-Like MNIST circles were created and tested on color blind individuals, wherein they would need an explanation to determine if their interpretation of the images were correct. Therefore, they would have to rely on the validity of a machine in that assessment [36]. With the current limitations of ML, this was a perfect use for MNIST, where a non-biased question could be asked that most individuals could not answer correctly. This provided for a uniform distribution of samples and would allow for a control by using those that were not color blind.

To create these Ishihara circles, the following process was used. First, the original MNIST images were loaded and the character was separated from its background. To do this, the image was binarized and a monochrome reduction was applied. Once the digit was extracted, the inner and outer outlines of the character were placed on a blank background. While not explicitly stated in the documentation, the images were resized at some point as the end result was a 128 × 128 image. Using a Monte Carlo simulation, a circle was then generated with varying circles inside it, and the extracted MNIST frame was placed in the circle. Edge detection was used to correct the circles inside the digit and the background to ensure all circles were fully formed. Then, coloring was applied to the background and character according to the plate [36]. Figure 9 depicts this process.

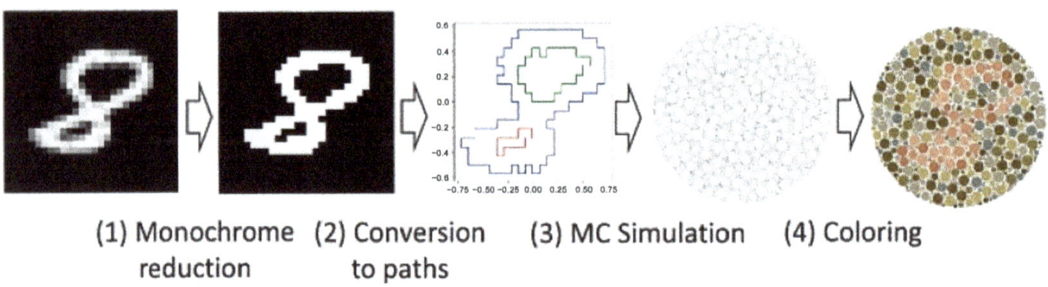

Figure 9. The process to convert an MNIST character to an Ishihara-Like MNIST circle [36].

In 1917, Dr Shinobu Ishihara from the University of Tokyo created and introduced the color blindness test [9]. This test consisted of a series of "plates" or images, usually 14, 24, or 38 at a time. The plates contained closely packed circles that varied in size and color to hide a number. The patient who was being tested for color deficiency was given these plates and asked to identify them correctly. The score of correct plates out of the total number identified the severity of the deficiency. To distinguish the different types of color blindness, the numerated plates held different meanings [37]. The Ishihara-Like MNIST dataset comprises 8 of those plates (numerical 2–9) and one additional plate containing random colors. Each folder of this dataset contains 10,000 training images and 2000 testing images. While it is not explicitly shared what the breakdown of each plate contains, it is stated that the generation of these plates "reasonable [sic] reproduces the themes of the original Ishihara plates" [36]. By this statement, it is assumed the same nomenclature and color scheming was followed. The only discrepancy stated is that plate 2 was the normal plate instead of plate 1. In Figure 10, each image shows what the image should depict and what red-green individuals see in the form of (actual answer, color deficient answer). It should be noted that only red-green color blindness is covered in these images as the other deficiencies are represented in plates greater than 9. Additionally, when researching this topic, there are some deviations in the listing of plates, wherein plates are out of order or changed. Therefore, not every test had the images in the exact same order. Finally, plates were created that only color blind individuals could see. Figure 11 shows an example of one of these plates.

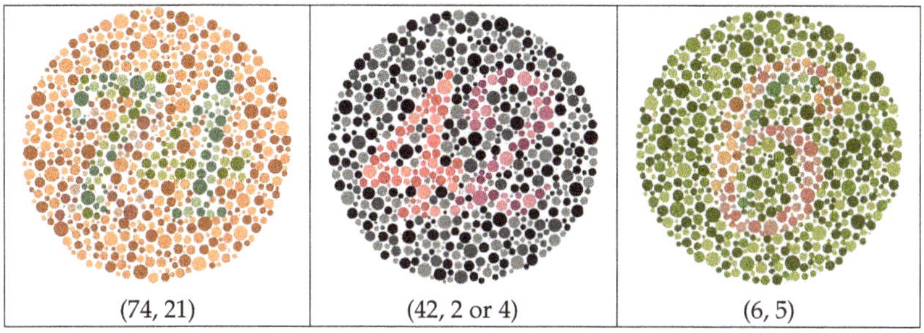

Figure 10. Sample Ishihara plates from the Ishihara test. The first number inside the parenthesizes is the correct number, followed by what an individual with red-green color blindness would see [38,39].

While many other fields have used the Ishihara circles in their research, no other research or articles are known using this particular dataset without expert modification. Other published work as seen in [40] use the standard Ishihara circles in the training and evaluation of models. However, it should be noted that the images used in [40] were also heavily modified to achieve a high validation accuracy and the characters inside the circle were not handwritten variations. Similar types of research are also seen in [41], where a model is trained on character images that were taken at obscure angles or with difficult font styles, or in [42], where a model is trained on images taken of old documents or texts where time has degraded the images. The goal of these two articles is to extrapolate the character from the image despite the color distortion.

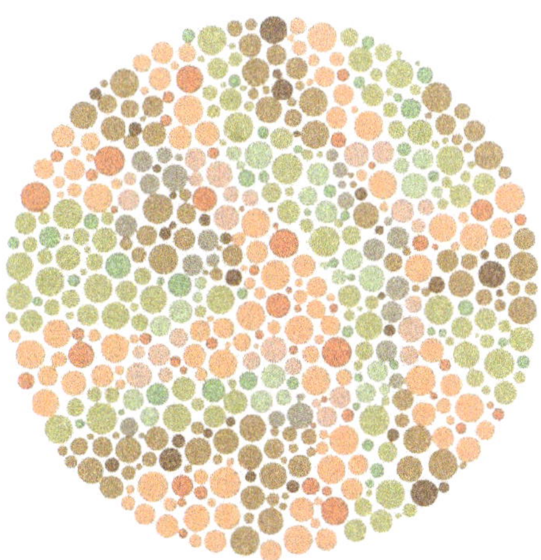

Figure 11. A plate that only red-green color-blind individuals can decipher. The value inside the circle is 73 [38].

For this research, we used LeNet [43], VGG16 [44], Alexnet [45], and two modification of the AlexNet architecture in evaluating the Ishihara circles. Since the Ishihara-Like MNIST dataset was created using the original MNIST dataset, the standard model used to train MNIST was also used. This sets a baseline to see if the original model used to train the MNIST characters could be used to evaluate the circles. The reasoning behind the other previously mentioned models is because they were all significant improvements of the original MNIST model and showed greater accuracy with OCR training [46,47]. While more advanced models such as YOLO [48] could have been used, the goal was to optimize a small architecture that would improve the amount of time required to train the model. In testing, various permutations of the data were used. This included training and testing the models on the color Ishihara-Like MNIST circles, training and testing on the Grayscale Ishihara-Like MNIST circles, and cross-testing the two sets.

An example of a grayscale Ishihara-Like MNIST circle and its color counterpart is shown in Figure 12. The color image in this figure was generated using matplotlib, wherein the colors are not exactly as they should appear due to color mapping. The character inside the circle is a "2".

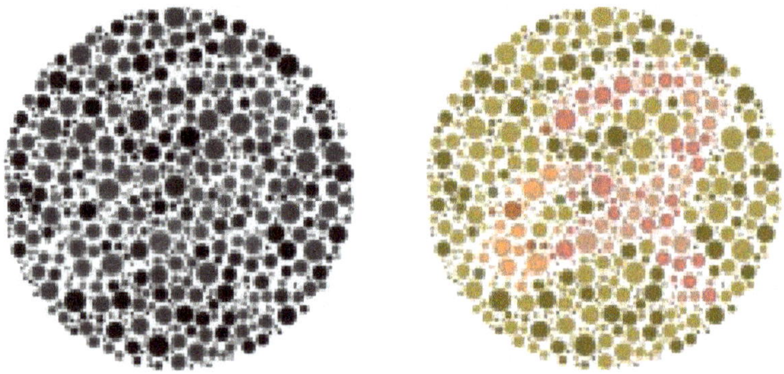

Figure 12. Grayscale (**left**) and Color MNIST Ishihara Circle (**right**).

1.4. Outline

Section 2 lays out the experimental design for this research. It begins in Section 2.1 by stating the tools that were used to perform this research. Then in Section 2.2, the process of how each of the datasets are loaded, processed, and ingested into the neural network models is provided. In Section 2.3, the models used to evaluate the datasets, why they were selected, and the modifications made are shown. In Section 2.4, the metrics by which these models were judged for their effectiveness with the datasets are given. Then in Section 2.5, the complete list of test cases performed are described. Finally, Section 2.5 ends with our initial assumptions on how each test case would perform. Section 3 quantifies the results of our research. This includes comprehensive tables showing the output of each test with each tested metric. Included with these results is our analysis on how each test performed. Additionally, confusion matrices are shown for the models that were trained and tested with the entire MNIST-Like Ishihara dataset. Section 4 summarizes the results of our entire research and concludes with our findings.

2. Experimental Design

In the following section, the methodology used for testing this research is described. This includes the tools that were used for the creation of the Python script, the process by which it was tested, the model selection, and how the evaluation was performed. Furthermore, the section lists the hardware that was used to perform the aforementioned tests.

2.1. Tools Used

This research used Python as the programming language, Keras and Tensorflow for the ML aspects, and OpenCV for the image processing. These selections were mainly due to the compatibility with Solonko's prior work. By using common tools, this allowed for easy modification to the architecture for further testing.

2.2. Testing Process

To perform adequate testing, a program was constructed in Python with two parent classes: the Data Loader and the Model Wrapper. These two wrappers served as the starting point for selecting between the two different datasets and the four distinct models. The Data Loader was broken into two pieces. One piece dealt with loading and processing the Ishihara-Like MNIST set, and the other loaded and processed the MNIST dataset. While the two parts operated in the same manner, they were separated due to the differences in form between the two datasets. The Model Wrapper then uses the specified images and labels and perform the training, testing, and evaluation.

MNIST was pulled directly from Keras through an API call in the form of an array. While not necessary in testing, the ability to resize the MNIST dataset so that it matched the size of the Ishihara set was implemented. Additionally, a function was implemented using OpenCV to apply a color filter to the MNIST dataset to determine if adding color had any effect on the training of the model. The possible color masks applied to the MNIST dataset were as follows: viridis, magma, plasma, inferno, cividis, mako, rocket, and turbo. An example of a modified MNIST image along with its original is displayed in Figure 13.

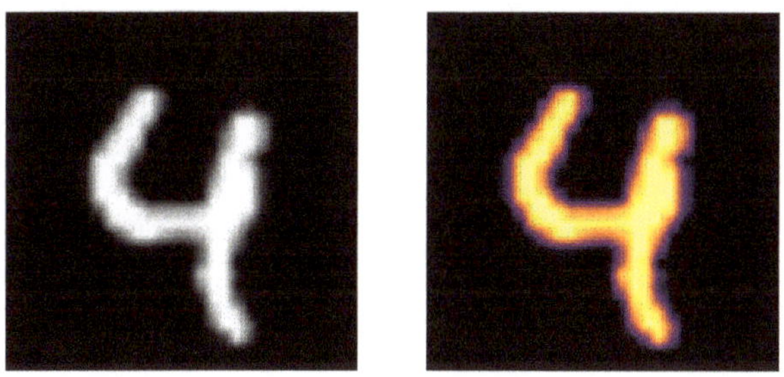

Figure 13. Original (**left**) and Colorized (**right**) version of an MNIST digit using the "inferno" color mask.

The Ishihara-Like MNIST set was downloaded from Kaggle [49] and was provided as a folder containing 9 sub-folders (or plates), each containing a Training and Testing set in the form of Printer Command Language (.pcl) files. Each of these sub-folders contained 10 k training images and 2 k testing images. Due to the Ishihara set being stored in files, these files had to be loaded, processed to tensors, and added to an array. To contain the amount of memory required to run the program, the option to load a specific amount of images or plates was implemented. Additionally, to test the images in grayscale, a color modification was performed using OpenCV. It should be noted that the original color scheme of these images was BGR, and not the standard RGB. Other than the conversion of the images from color to grayscale, no other preprocessing techniques were applied.

Once the images were loaded and processed, the model was then built and training began. Using a parent structure for model selection allowed each of the separate models to share in using the built-in functions from Keras without the re-implementation of code. When training the model, the amount of epochs to train on, the training accuracy threshold, validation accuracy threshold, and the validation split could be set. By default, for each of the datasets, a standard 80%/20% split was used for the separation of the training and validation sets.

For each of the runs, the amount of epochs was defaulted to 50; however, the training could stop if the training and validation accuracies were met. As a general notion, anywhere between 50 and 200 epochs are used for medium sized datasets, wherein medium is defined as any set between 10 GB and 1 TB [50]. For our research purposes, this value was based on the amount of epochs needed to stabilize training grayscale Ishihara in preliminary training. For training/testing of MNIST, 99% was used for both training and validation accuracy. Likewise, for color Ishihara and grayscale Ishihara, 99% was used for training and testing. Figure 14 shows the dataflow and program operation.

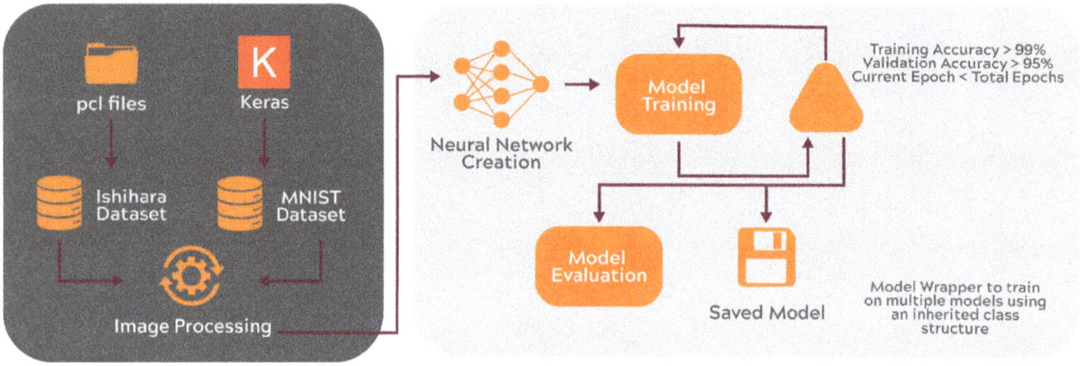

Figure 14. Program Description.

2.3. Model Training and Selection

As previously stated, each of the following models were used due to their significance in OCR. Specifically, each model was picked due to its significance in training on the MNIST dataset. Given that the Ishihara-Like MNIST dataset was created from the original MNIST dataset, a standard model architecture to train MNIST was used as the baseline for this research. This model, as shown in [51], is a simple architecture that comprises of two Conv2d layers and two Dense layers. In particular, the "ReLu" activation function was used for its ability to speed up gradient computation and its ability to introduce non-linearity to the dataset [52]. While this model does not have a formal name, we will refer to it as the MNIST model for the remainder of this paper. For this model and the sequential models listed, the "Adam" optimizer was used due to it being a leading adaptive stochastic gradient descent optimizer. For loss, the "Sparse Categorical Cross Entropy" was used due to how well it works for predicting models with multiple classes.

For the second model, LeNet5 was used. LeNet is a convolutional neural network that was introduced by Yann LeCun and his colleagues at Bell Labs in 1998. It "is considered the classic model that laid the foundation for deep learning" [43,53]. It was proposed to be used for hand written images. Since the architecture is small, it is also easy and fast to run. Given that this research runs the MNIST dataset and a derivative of MNIST, this model was consistent with showing progress with a more efficient architecture. The difference in this model and models used prior to its creation, outside of the number of parameters, was the change from the "Sigmoid" to the "TanH" activation function. This change allowed for higher gradient values when training neural networks [54].

While the first two models are relatively small in size, the third model dwarfs them both and is much more heavily involved. VGG16 is a CNN that was introduced and developed by K. Simonyan and A. Zisserman from the University of Oxford in 2014. It gained notoriety because it achieved an accuracy of 92.7% on ImageNet, which was not matched at the time. Additionally, this model started a change in newer architectures by showing that a model could learn with a reduced size of the convolutional kernels to (3, 3) as opposed to the (11, 11) used at the time [44,55]. Like the previous models, VGG16 is used in image classification, image recognition, and object detection tasks. The potential downside to using this model is its size. VGG16 is composed of 13 convolutional layers, 5 max-pooling layers, and 3 fully connected layers. It should be noted that this is the model that was used to train the Ishihara-Like MNIST. From their documentation, it appears that [36] used the standard model without any modifications except for the addition of a Batch Normalization after each Conv2d layer [36].

AlexNet was the fourth choice for a standard OCR model. AlexNet was introduced by Alex Krizhevsky, Ilya Sutskever, and Geoffrey E. Hinton at the university of Toronto in 2012. It was developed as a faster method for image recognition and classification tasks than previous models. The purpose of this model was to rectify the previous issues of Deep Learning by solving the gradient descent issue with Dropout, setting the activation function from Tanh to ReLu, and allowing overlapping pooling of the layers [45,56].

On top of the four distinct models, we decided to branch off and modify the architecture of AlexNet to be more efficient in terms of its size. In initial research and training, we found that AlexNet seemed to perform the best with the fewest amount of epochs and time required to run on the Ishihara dataset. This allowed us to leverage the use of a much smaller model than VGG16. In the fifth model, we reduced the size of AlexNet's filters by 4, reduced the kernel size from (11, 11) to (5, 5), and reduced the dropout from 0.5 to 0.1. By reducing the number of filters, the model size also decreases by this factor. With a smaller kernel size, the model would hopefully be able to generalize features better. Finally, by decreasing the dropout, less neurons are dropped out during training. In the remainder of this paper, this model will be known as Custom 1. In the sixth model, we reduced the filters by 8, but kept all of the other parameters the same. This model will be referred to as Custom 2. The goal of these two models was to run faster than either VGG16 or the original AlexNet, while minimizing the performance loss of using a smaller model. Table 1 shows a summary of each of the models chosen for this research. To allow for replication of our process, the compiler and architectures of the two custom models in Python are shown in Figures 15 and 16. For the other models (MNIST, LeNet5, and VGG16), the standard architectures with the addition of a Batch Normalization layer after each Conv2D layer were used.

```
self.model = Sequential([
    Input(shape = self.input_shape),

    Conv2D(24, (5, 5), strides = (4, 4), activation = 'relu', padding = 'same'),
    BatchNormalization(),
    MaxPooling2D((3, 3), strides = (2, 2)),

    Conv2D(64, (5, 5), activation = 'relu', padding = 'same', groups = 2),
    BatchNormalization(),
    MaxPooling2D((3, 3), strides = (2, 2)),

    Conv2D(96, (3, 3), activation = 'relu', padding = 'same'),
    BatchNormalization(),

    Conv2D(96, (3, 3), activation = 'relu', padding = 'same', groups = 2),
    BatchNormalization(),

    Conv2D(64, (3, 3), activation = 'relu', padding = 'same', groups = 2),
    BatchNormalization(),
    MaxPooling2D((3, 3), strides = (2, 2)),

    Flatten(),

    Dense(1024, activation = 'relu'),
    Dropout(rate = 0.1),

    Dense(1024, activation = 'relu'),
    Dropout(rate = 0.1),

    Dense(self.num_classes, activation = 'softmax')
])
```

Figure 15. Custom 1 model in Python.

```
self.model = Sequential([
    Input(shape = self.input_shape),

    Conv2D(12, (5, 5), strides = (4, 4), activation = 'relu', padding = 'same'),
    BatchNormalization(),
    MaxPooling2D((3, 3), strides = (2, 2)),

    Conv2D(32, (5, 5), activation = 'relu', padding = 'same', groups = 2),
    BatchNormalization(),
    MaxPooling2D((3, 3), strides = (2, 2)),

    Conv2D(48, (3, 3), activation = 'relu', padding = 'same'),
    BatchNormalization(),

    Conv2D(48, (3, 3), activation = 'relu', padding = 'same', groups = 2),
    BatchNormalization(),

    Conv2D(32, (3, 3), activation = 'relu', padding = 'same', groups = 2),
    BatchNormalization(),
    MaxPooling2D((3, 3), strides = (2, 2)),

    Flatten(),

    Dense(512, activation = 'relu'),
    Dropout(rate = 0.1),

    Dense(512, activation = 'relu'),
    Dropout(rate = 0.1),

    Dense(self.num_classes, activation = 'softmax')
])
```

Figure 16. Custom 2 model in Python.

Table 1. A comparison of each of the models by number of parameters and model size.

Model Name	Number of Trainable Parameters	Number of Layers	Conv2d Layers	Dense Layers
MNIST	2,416,330	8	3	2
Lenet	1,214,006	8	2	3
VGG16	50,415,434	22	13	3
AlexNet	23,357,514	19	5	3
Custom 1	1,469,466	19	5	3
Custom 2	371,154	19	5	3

2.4. Metrics of Success

To compare each of the models in their evaluation of the datasets, a quantitative basis was made. For this basis, we used multiple metrics to determine which models performed the best in each test case. For each of the models and test cases ran, the following metrics were recorded for evaluation:

- Performance: the overall accuracy percentage the model achieved when predicting new images. This is the value that matters the most. The goal is to have the model evaluate with a high accuracy on images it has never seen before. This will be the metric we compare to previous research.
- Precision: the percentage of correctly predicted positives out of all instances by the models.
- Recall (TPR): the percentage of actual positives that are correctly identified by the models.
- Training Time (in seconds): The amount of time it took for the model to train. Likewise with the number of epochs, the goal is to run the model as quickly as possible.
- Evaluation Time (in seconds): the amount of time it took for the model to evaluate on a new image or batch of images. In the real world, this is the value that matters the most when incorporating the model in a OCR sensor.

It should be noted that [36] achieved a 99% performance accuracy using VGG16 on the color Ishihara-Like MNIST. It was not stated what percentage of the dataset was used to train this model or how long it took to train. However, in our research, we will be training with the color and grayscale versions of the dataset. When training and testing these models, an NVIDIA A100 80GB PCIe GPU was used.

Before testing, our assumptions were that the MNIST dataset would perform well on all of the models. Given that each of these models were trained on MNIST previously, we would expect nothing less than 99% or 98% evaluation accuracy. With the Ishihara-Like MNIST dataset, we expect that the accuracy could be significantly lower with the smaller models (MNIST and LeNet) due to the complexity of the dataset but on par with MNIST with the larger models (VGG16 and AlexNet). However, the grayscale version of the Ishihara is expected to perform significantly worse than the colored version due to the reduction of training information. For the cross testing of the datasets, it is presumed that the models will perform on par with random guessing as the models are trained and tested with two different datasets. However, our hope is that it will be slightly better than chance due to the incorporation of MNIST in the Ishihara-Like MNIST dataset.

2.5. Test Cases

With each of the models above, we sought to try a few variations with testing. While the end goal of this research was to find and perform better with the Ishihara-Like MNIST dataset than previous research, we thought it would be enlightening to compare the variations and analyze the output. By expanding the testing into two categories (color and grayscale), and by cross-testing the two datasets, we hoped to understand what features were being learned with these datasets. Additionally, if the datasets performed the same with grayscale as they did with color, this would show that the expansion of information from one channel to three had little or no effect on the ability of the neural networks to learn and extract features from these datasets. The test cases performed on each of the above models is shown in Figure 17.

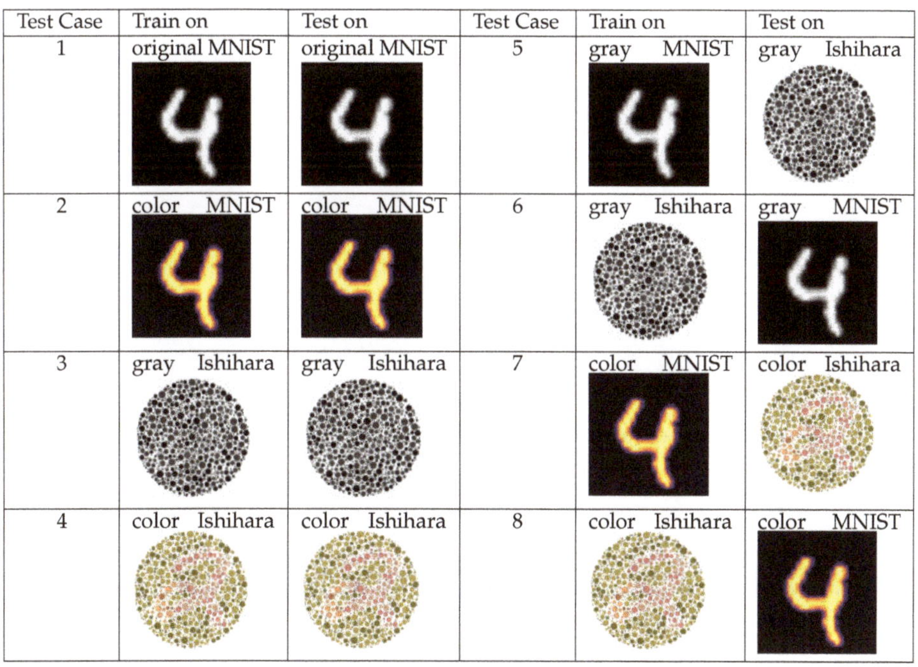

Figure 17. Test cases performed on the datasets.

In the first two test cases, the goal is to see how MNIST trains on the architecture which will provide initial assumptions on how well the Ishihara-Like MNIST will perform. However, MNIST is a much simpler dataset to work with and has cohesive characters. While the colored version of MNIST is not needed, we want to observe if there are any changes in the training output of MNIST when expanded from one channel to three. The next two test cases (Ishihara) are the crux of this research, wherein we will try to exceed performance values of previous research. For test cases 5–8, we seek to determine if the model has learned any feature extractions or feature spaces that will allow it to cross-test on a completely different dataset. Even though the Ishihara-Like MNIST dataset was created using the MNIST, the dataset is different enough that it is unlikely for the models to perform extremely well.

3. Results

In the following section, the results from each of the tests are listed. In each table, the performance accuracy, the precision of the model, the recall of the model, the time it took for the model to train (in seconds), and the time it took for evaluation (in seconds) are listed as (accuracy, epochs, training time, evaluation time). To note, the training time is the total amount of time it took to train the model and the evaluation time is the amount of time it took to correctly predict the amount of testing images. Therefore, to calculate the time required to determine one image, divide the listed evaluation time by the total number of testing images. Additionally, only the Ishihara tests have associated confusion matrices since they are most pertinent to this research.

To set a baseline for the entire evaluation, the original MNIST dataset was trained and tested against each of the models. As shown in Table 2, it performed reasonably well as expected. We expected higher performance on the first two models (MNIST and LeNet5), but this decline could have been due to the resizing of the original dataset from (28, 28, 1) to (112, 112, 1). The image resizing was performed so that the MNIST dataset was the same size as the Ishihara-Like MNIST dataset. As shown in Table 3, injecting color in the MNIST images seemed to have little effect on the performance of the models. To reiterate, the performance was as expected, but slightly under the target value of 99% in half of the models.

Table 2. For the above test, the original MNIST dataset was used to train and evaluate each model.

Test 1—Original MNIST (Accuracy, Precision, Recall Training Time, Evaluation Time)—60 k Training Images, 10 k Testing Images	
Model	**Results**
MNIST	(98.37%, 98.38%, 98.36%, 835 s, 6.33 s)
LeNet5	(98.21%, 98.21%, 98.20%, 820 s, 7.45 s)
VGG16	(99.14%, 99.13%, 99.15%, 493 s, 8.28 s)
AlexNet	(99.22%, 99.23%, 99.22%, 221 s, 6.39 s)
Custom 1	(99.12%, 99.11%, 99.12%, 199 s, 6.69 s)
Custom 2	(99.21%, 99.21%, 99.20%, 333 s, 6.12 s)

In each of the models, the performance accuracy was within 1% or 2% of the others. While these results are what was expected, the LeNet5 model performed the worst on both versions of the dataset. We believe this is due to the "TanH" activation function being used instead of the modern "Relu" function. The anomaly from these two tests is the performance of Custom 1 and Custom 2 as compared to the MNIST and LeNet5 models. Custom 1 and 2 were able to perform better than either of the other two models with less parameters. In the case of Custom 2, the architecture is roughly eight times smaller than MNIST but was able to outperform it. We believe this is due to the addition of more convolutional layers in conjunction with a larger kernel size.

Table 3. In this test, the colored version of the MNIST dataset was used to train and evaluate each model.

Test 2—Color MNIST (Accuracy, Precision, Recall, Training Time, Evaluation Time)—60 k Training Images, 10 k Testing Images	
Model	**Results**
MNIST	(98.68%, 98.68%, 98.66%, 957 s, 6.12 s)
LeNet5	(97.90%, 97.91%, 97.87%, 938 s, 8.23 s)
VGG16	(99.10%, 99.10%, 99.09%, 566 s, 8.30 s)
AlexNet	(99.24%, 99.26%, 99.23%, 276 s, 7.51 s)
Custom 1	(98.98%, 98.99%, 98.96%, 189 s, 10.00 s)
Custom 2	(99.16%, 99.17%, 99.16%, 247 s, 8.66 s)

Tables 4 and 5 show the results for training and evaluating on the Ishihara-Like MNIST dataset with each of the models. Table 4 uses the grayscale version of the images and Table 5 uses the color version of the images. These tests were broken into several parts. First, each plate was tested individually on each of the models wherein each plate contained 10 k training images and 2 k testing images. It should be noted that we believe this is not an adequate amount of images to use for the training phase of a model, however this was the maximum amount of images per plate from [8]. For the last test, all of the plates were combined into one array such that the array contained 90 k training images and 18 k testing images. In the case where the models resulted in a 10% performance accuracy, this means that the model performed on par with chance as there were ten classes in this dataset.

In the early phases of testing with this dataset, the first three models (MNIST, LeNet5, and VGG16) performed very poorly with this dataset in both grayscale and in color. It was only when testing with all 90k images together that better results were obtained. This prompted further investigation given that VGG16 was used in the original training of this dataset. After analyzing the difference between these three models and AlexNet, we concluded that this was due to a lack of data normalization. Therefore, this was the reason a Batch Normalization layer was inserted after each Con2d layer in each model. This theory was further confirmed after reviewing [36], finding that they inserted this layer in their training with VGG16. After the insertion of the layer, performance drastically increased.

As shown in Table 4, there is quite a variation in results between all of the models with the grayscale version of the images. We believe the decrease in performance is due to the small amount of training images and the reduction of information with one channel, as opposed to three channels with color images. While VGG16 was the largest model with the most parameters, it was not able to consistently perform better than the rest of the models with the individual plates. AlexNet was able to consistently perform on average around 70–80% whereas VGG16's performance dips quite heavily on plates four through eight. When examining the reduction of size to AlexNet, it appears that this had a sizable effect on the evaluation of the grayscale images as the performance accuracy was consistently lower on average with Custom 1 and Custom 2. Even with this reduction in performance, the results were still consistent and stable across all of the tests as was the case with the original AlexNet model.

When all of the plates were combined, all of the models were able to perform significantly better. In the case of VGG16, this resulted in a substantially higher performance than every other model. We presume this is due to the increased size of the model that allowed for the extraction of features that would not be picked up in the smaller models. While we argue that a larger model is not the best pick for every dataset, it did perform quite well with the lack of information in these images. Even with a reduced architecture, AlexNet and the two custom architectures were able to achieve roughly 90% accuracy when using all of the grayscale images. On the other end of the scale of performance, LeNet5 performed very poorly in almost every test in comparison to the other models, similarly as it did with Tests 1 and 2. Given that the LeNet model is very similar to the MNIST model, we attribute this failure to the "TanH" activation function. The results from the MNIST model were in between that of LeNet5 and AlexNet, therefore resulting in no meaningful conclusions. The one anomaly to this test was the results from VGG16 on the rand plate. While the other models were able to adequately train on this plate on par with the other plates, VGG16 was not able to be trained. It is unclear why this occurred. For this test, it should be noted that these images are very hard for a human to read. Therefore, it is promising that a ML model is able to correctly evaluate these images. Figure 18 shows the performance accuracy for each plate for each of the models with the grayscale images. As shown in this image, AlexNet has an overall higher evaluation than the other models while also maintaining a relatively straight line resulting in more stable training. The "rand" or random plate was removed from this graphic due to its low results.

Table 4. Training/Testing results of the grayscale Ishihara-Like MNIST images on each of the models with each of the plates followed by a run with all of the plates combined.

Test 3: Grayscale Ishihara (Accuracy, Precision, Recall, Training Time, Evaluation Time)—10 k Training Images, 2 k Testing Images Per Plate			
Plate	**MNIST**	**LeNet5**	**VGG16**
2	(43.00%, 78.18%, 43.00%, 113 s, 0.74 s)	(33.85%, 53.03%, 33.85%, 152 s, 0.84 s)	(84.85%, 88.25%, 84.85%, 391 s, 1.44 s)
3	(65.35%, 78.47%, 65.35%, 149 s, 0.77 s)	(42.00%, 64.12%, 42.00%, 153 s, 1.07 s)	(93.65%, 94.15%, 93.65%, 388 s, 1.07 s)
4	(50.90%, 72.67%, 50.90%, 152 s, 0.92 s)	(40.75%, 49.52%, 40.75%, 147 s, 0.90 s)	(75.90%, 83.55%, 75.90%, 383 s, 0.85 s)
5	(41.50%, 73.07%, 41.50%, 148 s, 0.88 s)	(25.95%, 57.72%, 25.95%, 151 s, 0.91 s)	(78.35%, 85.23%, 78.35%, 383 s, 1.03 s)
6	(45.20%, 73.90%, 45.20%, 152 s, 0.90 s)	(31.40%, 61.03%, 31.40%, 129 s, 0.87 s)	(43.95%, 66.19%, 43.95%, 383 s, 1.11 s)
7	(42.50%, 62.24%, 42.50%, 151 s, 0.72 s)	(32.45%, 61.74%, 32.45%, 151 s, 0.76 s)	(75.50%, 82.82%, 75.50%, 362 s, 0.95 s)
8	(82.65%, 82.88%, 82.65%, 152 s, 0.80 s)	(50.55%, 64.38%, 50.55%, 151 s, 0.59 s)	(68.30%, 81.07%, 68.30%, 359 s, 0.90 s)
9	(82.40%, 82.92%, 82.40%, 151 s, 0.79 s)	(41.20%, 62.24%, 41.20%, 149 s, 0.73 s)	(91.60%, 91.93%, 91.60%, 384 s, 0.89 s)
rand	(80.30%, 80.54%, 80.30%, 152 s, 0.72 s)	(60.45%, 60.83%, 60.45%, 150 s, 0.71 s)	(10.00%, 1.00%, 10.00%, 382 s, 0.95 s)
all	91.16%, 91.35%, 91.16%, 1238 s, 6.08 s)	(78.43%, 78.55%, 78.43%, 1214 s, 5.84 s)	(98.53%, 98.53%, 98.53%, 732 s, 7.49 s)
Plate	**AlexNet**	**Custom 1**	**Custom 2**
2	(57.70%, 77.69%, 57.70%, 177 s, 0.91 s)	(81.00%, 85.56%, 81.00%, 166 s, 0.87 s)	(55.35%, 76.27%, 55.35%, 173 s, 0.91 s)
3	(85.75%, 87.47%, 85.75%, 177 s, 0.80 s)	(76.85%, 81.76%, 76.85%, 167 s, 0.93 s)	(69.60%, 75.39%, 69.60%, 165 s, 0.82 s)
4	(87.05%, 89.04%, 87.05%, 174 s, 0.94 s)	(69.70%, 80.16%, 69.70%, 172 s, 0.85 s)	(61.10%, 76.24%, 61.10%, 167 s, 0.91 s)
5	(82.45%, 88.81%, 82.45%, 179 s, 0.89 s)	(72.50%, 81.78%, 72.50%, 172 s, 0.89 s)	(69.20%, 76.53%, 69.20%, 170 s, 0.88 s)
6	(83.55%, 87.31%, 83.55%, 177 s, 0.86 s)	(67.10%, 79.72%, 67.10%, 175 s, 0.90 s)	(74.60%, 77.64%, 74.60%, 172 s, 0.95 s)
7	(78.75%, 83.65%, 78.75%, 175 s, 0.70 s)	(68.50%, 81.56%, 68.50%, 173 s, 0.74 s)	(67.80%, 74.95%, 67.80%, 172 s, 0.75 s)
8	(85.00%, 86.97%, 85.00%, 174 s, 0.75 s)	(68.85%, 77.39%, 68.85%, 172 s, 0.77 s)	(66.65%, 74.87%, 66.65%, 170 s, 0.75 s)
9	(67.85%, 81.03%, 67.85%, 177 s, 0.70 s)	(76.65%, 81.07%, 76.65%, 173 s, 0.69 s)	(75.35%, 76.99%, 75.35%, 169 s, 0.68 s)
rand	(78.25%, 81.50%, 78.25%, 175 s, 0.73 s)	(72.50%, 75.84%, 72.50%, 169 s, 0.73 s)	(68.30%, 74.57%, 68.30%, 169 s, 0.79 s)
all	(89.84%, 90.9%, 89.84%, 1413 s, 5.81 s)	(90.29%, 90.83%, 90.29%, 1391 s, 6.10 s)	(88.06%, 88.67%, 88.06%, 1395 s, 5.94 s)

Table 5. Training/Testing results of the color Ishihara-Like MNIST images on each of the models with each of the plates followed by a run with all of the plates combined.

Test 4: Color Ishihara (Accuracy, Precision, Recall, Training Time, Evaluation Time)—10 k Training Images, 2 k Testing Images Per Plate			
Plate	**MNIST**	**LeNet5**	**VGG16**
2	(94.25%, 94.28%, 94.25%, 162 s, 1.44 s)	(92.45%, 92.44%, 92.45%, 172 s, 1.42 s)	(98.25%, 98.27%, 98.25%, 413 s, 1.60 s)
3	(94.30%, 94.31%, 94.30%, 172 s, 1.45 s)	(93.35%, 93.38%, 93.35%, 166 s, 1.44 s)	(97.75%, 97.83%, 97.75%, 406 s, 1.35 s)
4	(95.90%, 95.91%, 95.90%, 171 s, 1.42 s)	(93.45%, 93.44%, 93.45%, 166 s, 1.38 s)	(97.50%, 97.58%, 97.50%, 401 s, 1.60 s)
5	(94.60%, 94.63%, 94.60%, 174 s, 1.43 s)	(92.25%, 92.32%, 92.25%, 171 s, 1.44 s)	(97.95%, 97.99%, 97.95%, 403 s, 1.77 s)
6	(95.40%, 95.42%, 95.40%, 171 s, 1.41 s)	(92.80%, 92.86%, 92.80%, 171 s, 1.47 s)	(97.45%, 97.50%, 97.45%, 392 s, 2.79 s)
7	(96.45%, 96.45%, 96.45%, 171 s, 1.55 s)	(93.00%, 93.01%, 93.00%, 169 s, 0.98 s)	(99.00%, 99.00%, 99.00%, 402 s, 0.92 s)
8	(94.75%, 94.76%, 94.75%, 171 s, 1.00 s)	(92.15%, 92.19%, 92.15%, 171 s, 1.03 s)	(99.10%, 99.11%, 99.10%, 398 s, 1.17 s)
9	(95.15%, 95.16%, 95.15%, 170 s, 0.94 s)	(92.80%, 92.83%, 92.80%, 168 s, 0.89 s)	(98.55%, 98.56%, 98.55%, 401 s, 1.06 s)
rand	(78.95%, 79.08%, 78.95%, 171 s, 1.19 s)	(44.20%, 43.83%, 44.20%, 168 s, 1.21 s)	(10.00%, 1.00%, 10.00%, 404 s, 0.92 s)
all	(92.30%, 92.40%, 92.30%, 1328 s, 10.74 s)	(82.26%, 83.68%, 82.26%, 1319 s, 8.85 s)	(98.31%, 98.32%, 98.31%, 572 s, 11.73 s)
Plate	**AlexNet**	**Custom 1**	**Custom 2**
2	(94.10%, 95.10%, 94.10%, 194 s, 1.41 s)	(95.75%, 95.95%, 95.75%, 191 s, 1.44 s)	(95.95%, 96.01%, 95.95%, 190 s, 1.36 s)
3	(96.30%, 96.43%, 96.30%, 196 s, 1.50 s)	(96.55%, 96.62%, 96.55%, 182 s, 1.51 s)	(94.55%, 94.84%, 94.55%, 190 s, 1.43 s)
4	(89.95%, 91.19%, 89.95%, 190 s, 1.42 s)	(96.85%, 96.92%, 96.85%, 190 s, 1.46 s)	(96.40%, 96.45%, 96.40%, 188 s, 1.41 s)
5	(95.25%, 95.43%, 95.25%, 195 s, 1.44 s)	(97.25%, 97.27%, 97.25%, 186 s, 1.46 s)	(96.20%, 96.26%, 96.20%, 190 s, 1.45 s)
6	(96.85%, 96.89%, 96.85%, 196 s, 1.45 s)	(96.65%, 96.84%, 96.65%, 190 s, 1.48 s)	(97.10%, 97.13%, 97.10%, 182 s, 1.47 s)
7	(94.40%, 95.04%, 94.40%, 193 s, 0.86 s)	(97.40%, 97.43%, 97.40%, 191 s, 0.94 s)	(96.55%, 96.69%, 96.55%, 188 s, 0.89 s)
8	(93.70%, 94.49%, 93.70%, 195 s, 0.97 s)	(95.75%, 96.05%, 95.75%, 192 s, 1.07 s)	(96.20%, 96.33%, 96.20%, 192 s, 0.91 s)
9	(95.70%, 95.92%, 95.70%, 199 s, 0.85 s)	(92.50%, 93.81%, 92.50%, 191 s, 0.94 s)	(96.95%, 97.00%, 96.95%, 192 s, 1.46 s)
rand	(83.70%, 85.24%, 83.70%, 196 s, 1.02 s)	(76.50%, 78.74%, 76.50%, 194 s, 0.91 s)	(76.20%, 77.45%, 76.20%, 194 s, 0.94 s)
all	(96.77%, 96.78%, 96.77%, 1512 s, 9.07 s)	(94.38%, 94.54%, 94.38%, 1484 s, 10.36 s)	(90.81%, 90.92%, 90.81%, 1472 s, 9.48 s)

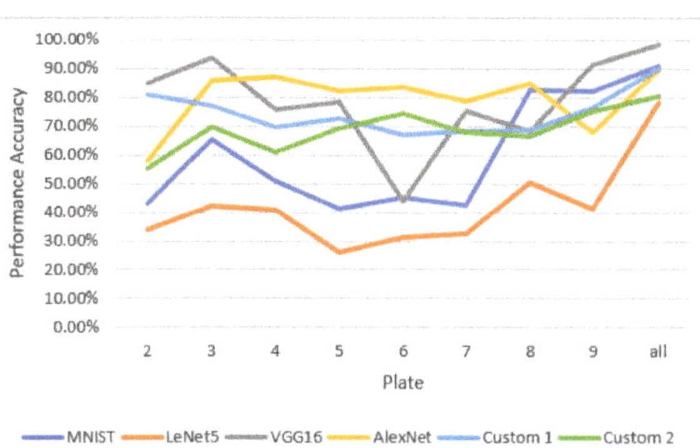

Figure 18. The performance accuracy for each of the models with the grayscale Ishihara plates. The rand plate was not used in this graphic.

The confusion matrices from the training of the grayscale images are shown in Figure 19. In each picture, the classes are listed from left to right and top to bottom. When reading these pictures, the rows represent the ground truth labels while the column represent the predicted labels. For example, in the first confusion matrix with the MNIST model, the model predicted the image as the value "0" incorrectly four times when the correct label was actually "9" (this value is in the lower left-hand corner of the plot). In an ideal case, the matrices would show a solid diagonal line (representing 100% performance accuracy).

Confusion Matrices for training/testing Grayscale Ishihara

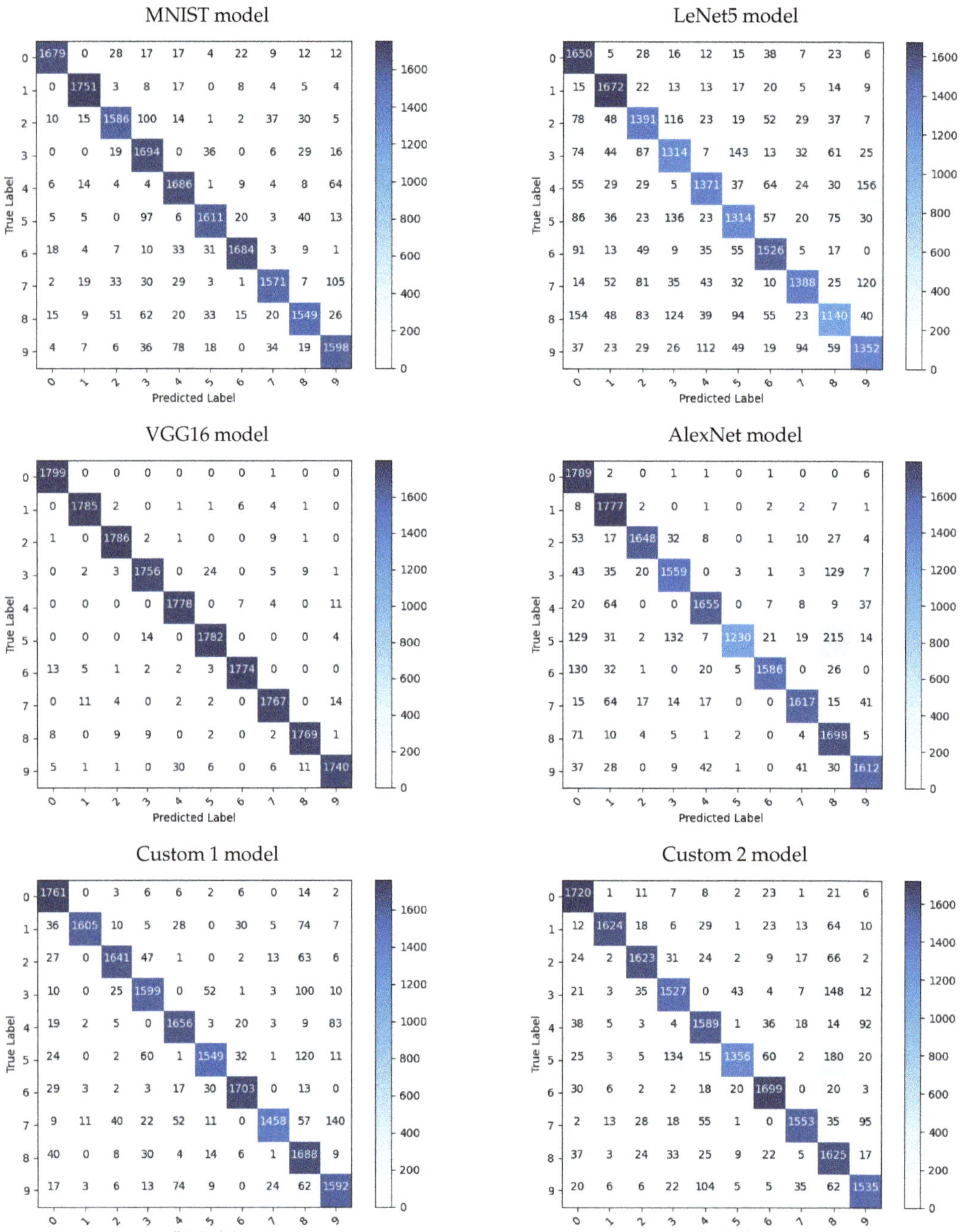

Figure 19. Confusion matrices for the Grayscale Ishihara-Like MNIST dataset showing the correct evaluation of the 10 distinct classes. Each class contained 1800 testing images in these matrices.

Examining the matrices from the grayscale testing shows results that are consistent with errors in the evaluation of MNIST or standard OCR characters when the model's performance is sub-par. As shown, a few of the classes were misidentified as another class due to their similarity. LeNet5 is able to show the results the most. In this case, it incorrectly predicted a "9" as a "4" 5.61% , a "5" as an "8" 6.11%, and a "7" as a "9" 9.94% of the time. Also it should be noted that it predicted the value "1" as an "8" 13.39% of the time. This is an abnormal mis-classification.The next highest incorrect value is a "3" being predicted an an "8" which is consistent with incorrect predictions in the numerical system with handwritten numbers. Given that the Ishihara-Like MNIST dataset was created using the original MNIST and MNIST was created using handwriting from many different people, it is not uncommon for there to be many variations of each class potentially causing errors in training.

As shown in Table 5, the models performed significantly better on the color versions of the dataset. Given the expansion of data from one channel into three channels with color, we anticipated that the training would fare significantly better. Even with the individual plates, the models were able to extract enough features to distinguish the ten distinct classes with only 10 k training images. In the case of using all of the images together, each of the models performed in the upper decile except for LeNet5. Again, we attribute the poor performance of LeNet5 to its activation function. When analyzing the training and evaluation times, AlexNet was able to perform within 5% of VGG16 in almost all cases but was able to train in half the required time and evaluate slightly faster. A significant difference in this test is the combination of all of the plates into one set only performed slightly better the the plates individually. Figure 20 shows the performance accuracy for each plate on each of the models and Figure 21 shows the confusion matrices for this test. When examining the matrices of the color version of the Ishihara images, the results were on par with what was shown in the table above. In each model except for LeNet5, the matrices resulted in at least a 93% accuracy for each of the ten classes as expected.

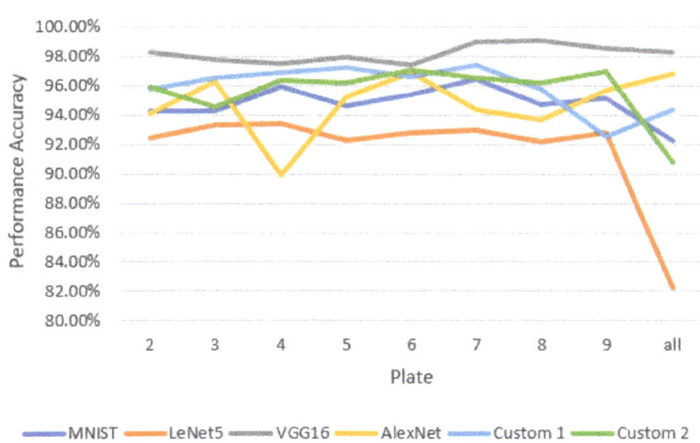

Figure 20. The performance accuracy for each of the models with each of the colored Ishihara plates. The rand plate was not used in this graphic.

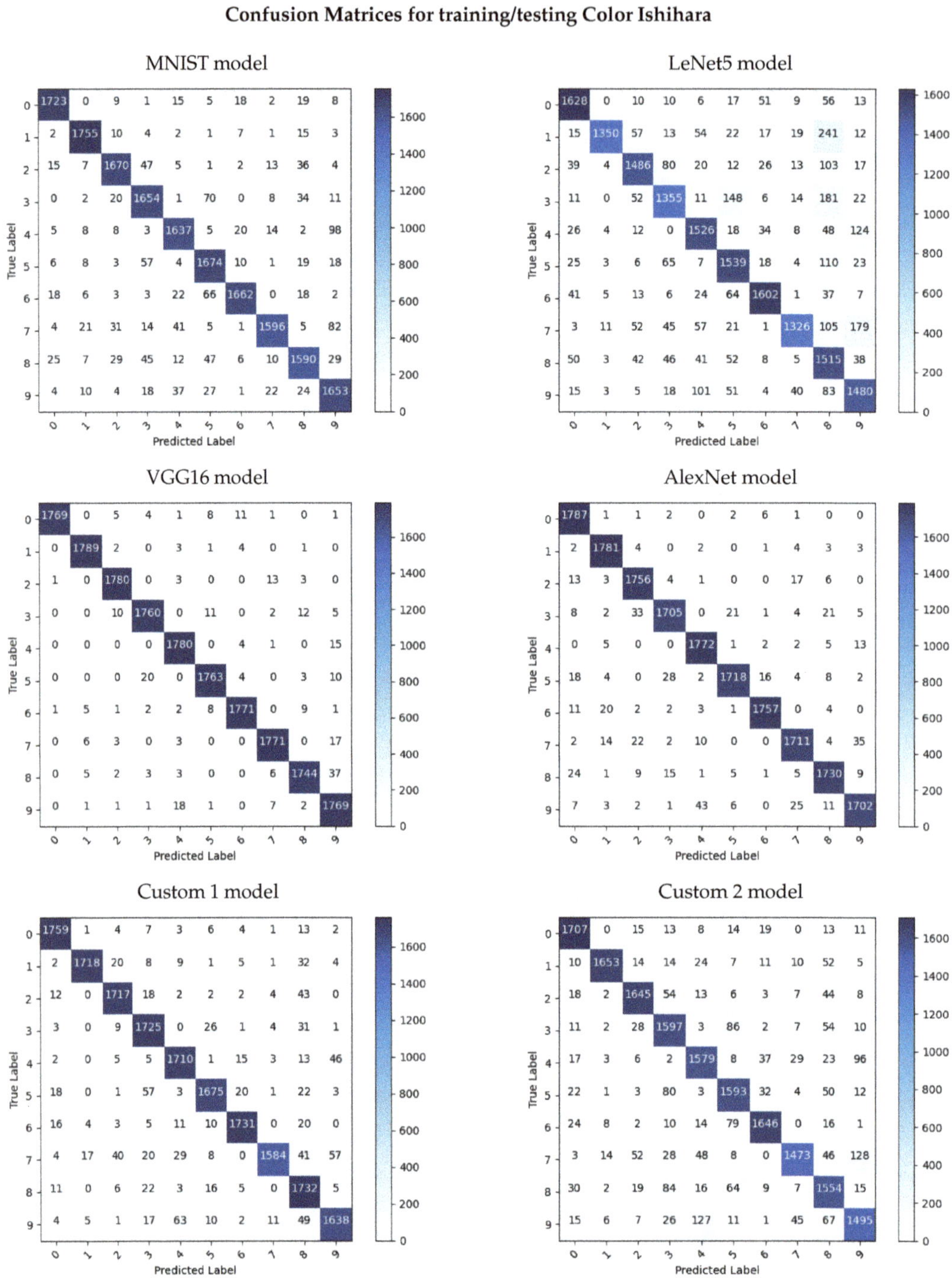

Figure 21. Confusion matrices for the Color Ishihara-Like MNIST dataset showing the correct evaluation of the 10 distinct classes. Each class contained 1800 testing images in these matrices.

In both grayscale and in color, the "rand" or random plate had an abnormal effect on the ability of the models to train. This plate had a drastically lower performance on each of the models than the rest of the plates. On each of the other plates with all of the models, the results were in the upper decile with color but this plate caused as low as 10% evaluation in the case of VGG16. While the difference in evaluation with the grayscale images is not noticeable outside of VGG16, it becomes quite noticeable with the color images. To deduce the reasoning behind this, we took a close look at the images. Figure 22 shows two examples of images from this plate. After reviewing the images, it became abundantly clear why the models had poor performance. The image on the left is a 7 and the image on the right is an 8. However, without the labels, we would not have been able to decipher the contents of these two circles. Realizing this, it warranted a test case wherein each of the models are trained on all of the color plates except the Random plate. Table 6 shows the results of this training. As shown, without the inclusion of the Random colors plate in the combination of all the other plates, the models were able to produce higher performance accuracy. In this run, we were able to match the results with VGG16 with prior research. Therefore, we conclude that the inclusion of this plate had a overall negative effect on the training of these models. The confusion matrices for this test have been provided in Figure 23.

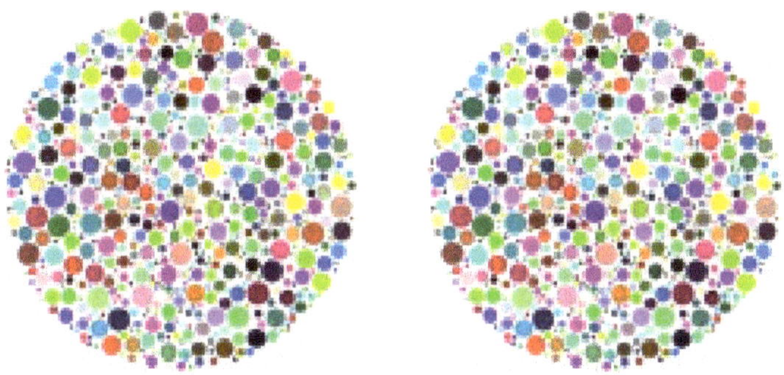

Figure 22. Sample images from the "random" Ishihara plate. The image on the left is 7 and the image on the right is 8.

Table 6. This test trained each of the models with all of the plates combined except for the Random plate.

Ishihara Color—Test Case Without the Random Plate (Accuracy, Precision, Recall, Training Time, Evaluation Time)	
Model	**Results**
MNIST	(97.19%, 97.20%, 97.19%, 1395 s, 9.87 s)
LeNet5	(96.11%, 96.11%, 96.11%, 1382 s, 10.48 s)
VGG16	(98.88%, 98.89%, 98.88%, 640 s, 11.54 s)
AlexNet	(98.55%, 98.56%, 98.55%, 493 s, 10.00 s)
Custom 1	(98.45%, 98.46%, 98.45%, 852 s, 11.49 s)
Custom 2	(98.09%, 98.11%, 98.09%, 1537 s, 9.28 s)

To further examine the reasoning behind decline in performance evaluation with this plate, the confusion matrices from both the grayscale and color trainings of this plate have been provided in Figures 24 and 25. In these matrices, only 200 images from each of the 10 distinct classes were evaluated upon. This was due to the limited number of images in the rand plate. As shown with the Random plate, each of the models struggled to identify the correct class for each of the ten classes in all of the matrices. This was likely the cause of the low performance in the test with all plates combined for both grayscale and color. It should be noted that it is unclear why VGG16 was unable to train at all on this plate. When looking at the training process, the training accuracy and validation accuracy did not rise above 10%.

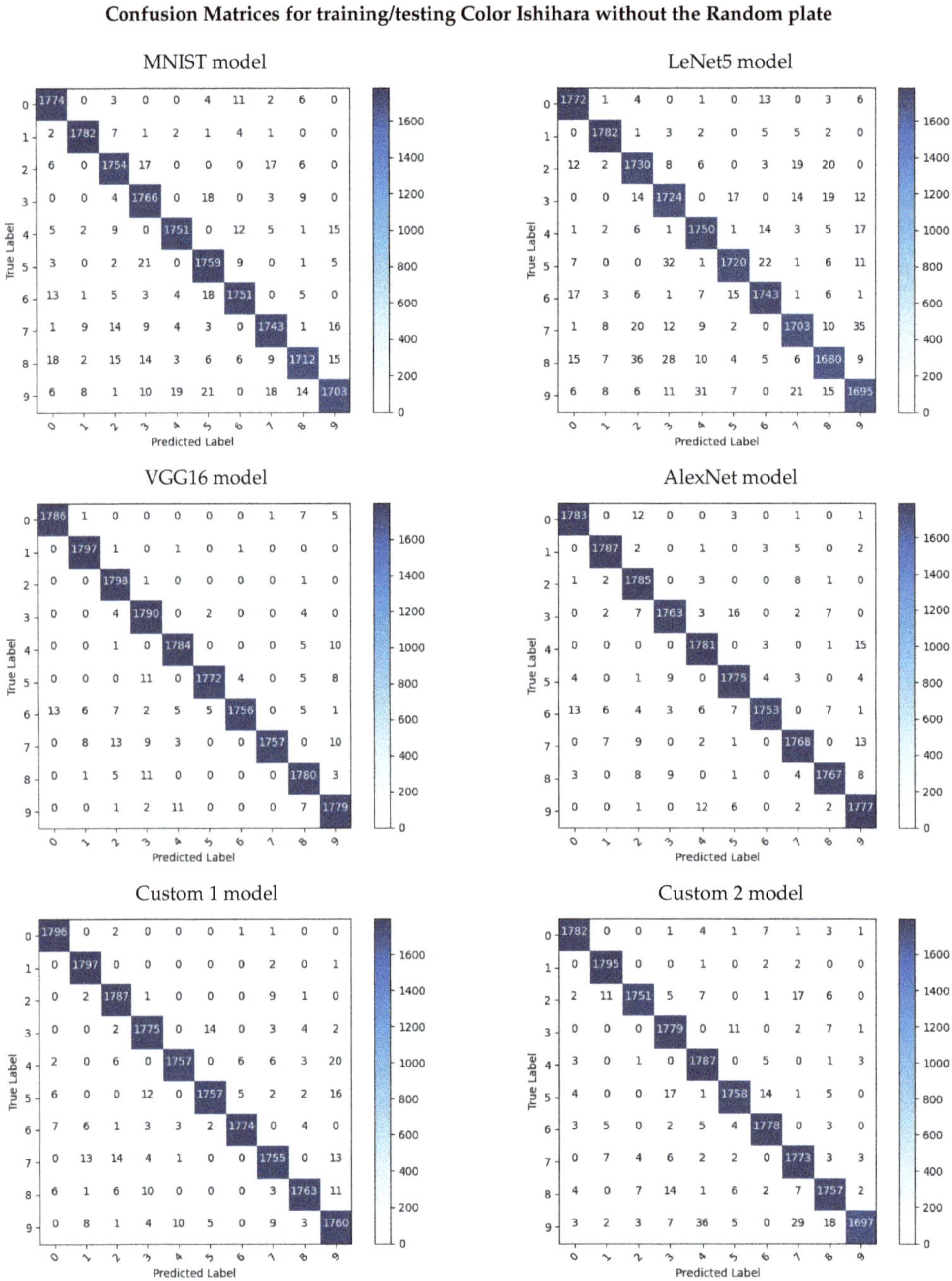

Figure 23. Confusion matrices for the Color Ishihara-Like MNIST dataset without the Random plate showing the correct evaluation of the 10 distinct classes. Each class contained 1800 testing images in these matrices.

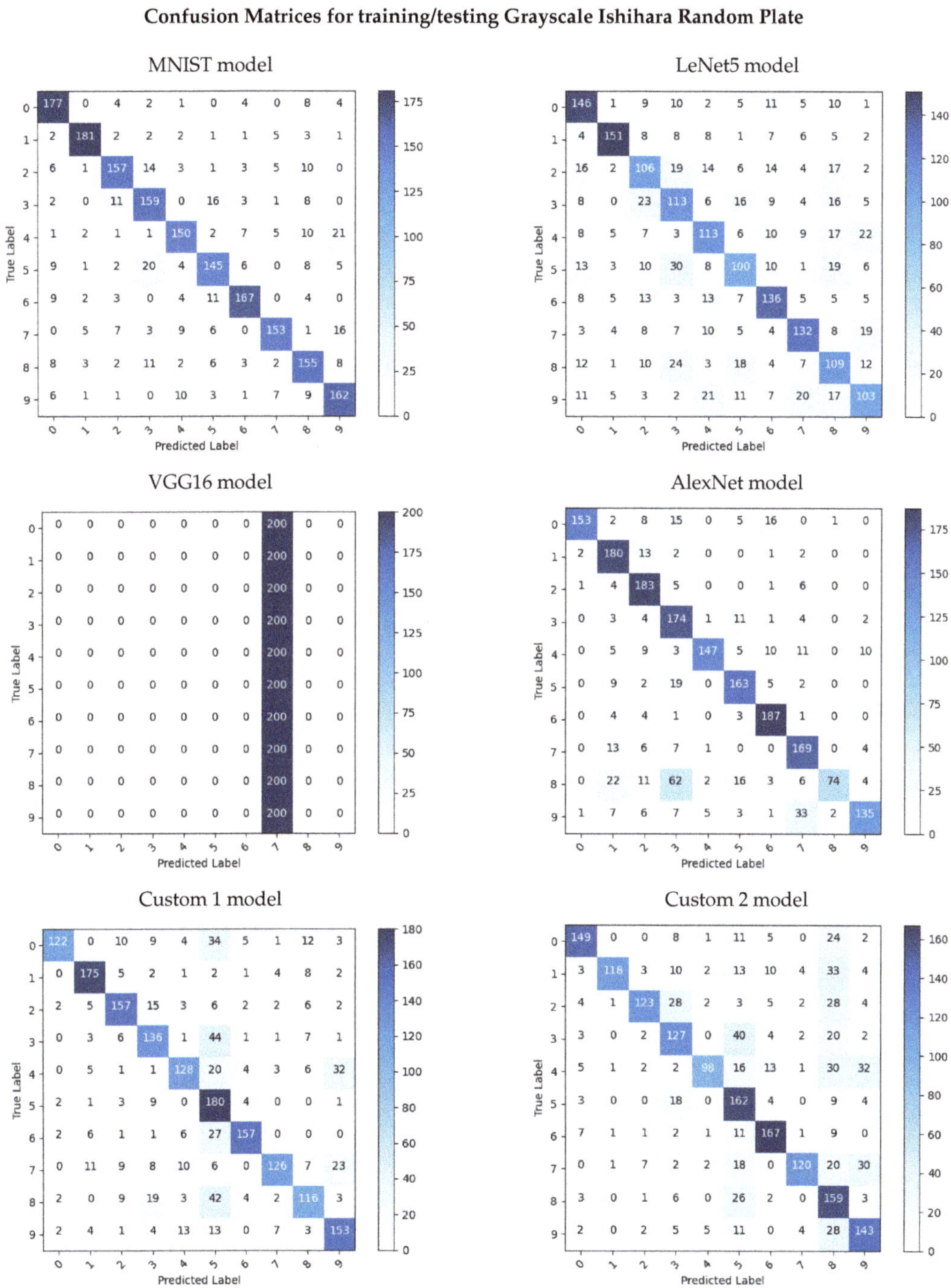

Figure 24. Confusion matrices for the Grayscale Ishihara-Like MNIST Random plate showing the correct evaluation of the 10 distinct classes. Each class contained 200 testing images in these matrices.

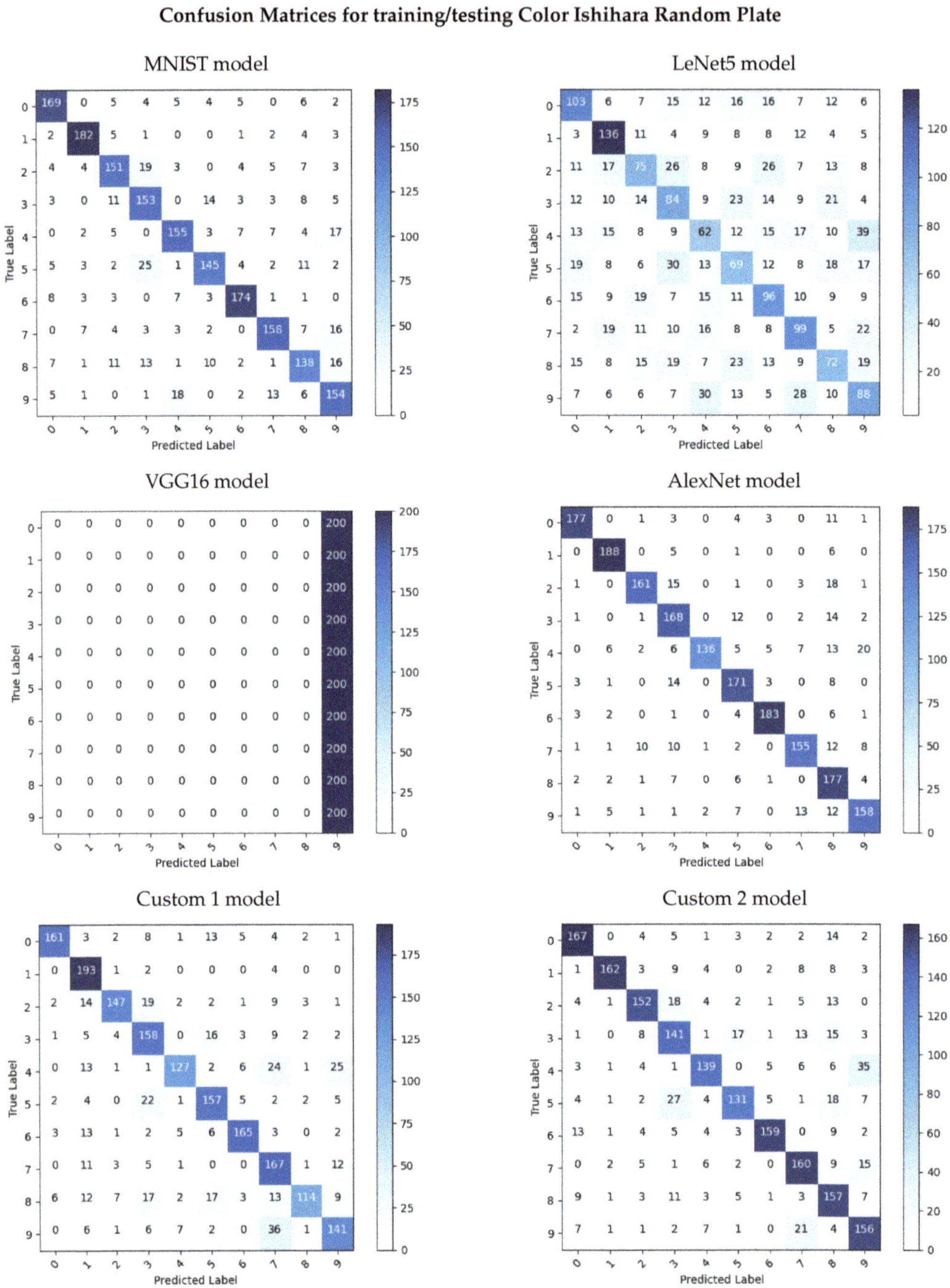

Figure 25. Confusion matrices for the Color Ishihara-Like MNIST Random plate showing the correct evaluation of the 10 distinct classes. Each class contained 200 testing images in these matrices.

In Tables 7–10, the results from cross training the two sets is shown. In these test cases, each of the models are trained on the first dataset and then evaluated on the second dataset.

Our initial hopes were that the training of MNIST and evaluation on Ishihara-Like MNIST would have performed slightly better but the results are not surprising given the difference in the datasets. As shown, all of the models performed within the realm of chance for their output. In some cases, the models performed worse than chance. To note, the MNIST and LeNet5 models were able to perform better than chance when trained on the grayscale version of the Ishihara dataset and evaluated with MNIST. It is unclear why these models were able to perform 20–25% better than their counterparts. However with only a 20% increase in a set of ten classes, we believe this does not warrant further research. In the case where the models were trained on MNIST and evaluated on the Ishihara-Like MNIST, we believe the performance would have been significantly better if the images underwent some form of preprocessing. Such is the case with Solonko's work wherein the images underwent heavy modifications before they were evaluated by the neural network resulting in high performance. However, there seems to be no correlation between these two models when training with a neural network even though the latter was created using the first.

Table 7. Training each of the models with the original version of the MNIST dataset and then testing on the grayscale version of the Ishihara-Like MNIST dataset.

Test 5—Original MNIST with Gray Ishihara (Accuracy, Precision, Recall, Training Time, Evaluation Time)–60 k Training Images, 10 k Testing Images	
Model	**Results**
MNIST	(10.00%, 1.00%, 10.00%, 805 s, 4.77 s)
LeNet	(10.01%, 2.67%, 10.01%, 821 s, 5.55 s)
VGG16	(12.48%, 12.51%, 12.48%, 536 s, 7.83 s)
AlexNet	(10.02%, 4.06%, 10.02%, 182 s, 5.35 s)
Custom 1	(9.95%, 4.56%, 9.95%, 158 s, 5.95 s)
Custom 2	(10.23%, 4.13%, 10.23%, 267 s, 6.26 s)

Table 8. Training each of the models with a colored version of the MNIST dataset and then testing on the original version of the Ishihara-Like MNIST dataset.

Test 7—Color MNIST with Color Ishihara (Accuracy, Precision, Recall, Training Time, Evaluation Time)–60 k Training Images, 10 k Testing Images	
Model	**Results**
MNIST	(9.93%, 5.64%, 9.93%, 950 s, 8.65 s)
LeNet	(10.49%, 2.22%, 10.49%, 934 s, 9.62 s)
VGG16	(10.00%, 19.12%, 10.00%, 523 s, 9.49 s)
AlexNet	(10.06%, 5.05%, 10.06%, 209 s, 8.27 s)
Custom 1	(10.02%, 2.62%, 10.02%, 249 s, 10.36 s)
Custom 2	(10.06%, 7.17%, 10.06%, 246 s, 10.57 s)

Table 9. Training each of the models with the grayscale version of the Ishihara-Like MNIST dataset and then testing on the original version of the MNIST dataset.

Test 6—Grayscale Ishihara with Original MNIST (Accuracy, Precision, Recall, Training Time, Evaluation Time)–60 k Training Images, 10 k Testing Images	
Model	**Results**
MNIST	(32.13%, 31.14%, 32.94%, 785 s, 5.84 s)
LeNet	(35.81%, 51.21%, 35.46%, 819 s, 5.70 s)
VGG16	(9.84%, 11.98%, 10.02%, 1104 s, 6.56 s)
AlexNet	(10.28%, 1.03%, 10.00%, 944 s, 5.34 s)
Custom 1	(9.68%, 1.59%, 9.94%, 959 s, 6.08 s)
Custom 2	(10.32%, 1.03%, 10.00%, 912 s, 6.63 s)

Table 10. Training each of the models with the original version of the Ishihara-Like MNIST dataset and then testing on the colored version of the MNIST dataset.

Test 8—Color Ishihara with Color MNIST (Accuracy, Precision, Recall, Training Time, Evaluation Time)—60 k Training Images, 10 k Testing Images	
Model	**Results**
MNI sT	(11.20%, 7.21%, 10.95%, 938 s, 7.04 s)
LeNet	(25.55%, 55.60%, 24.57%, 901 s, 7.15 s)
VGG16	(11.48%, 13.30%, 10.13%, 1126 s, 7.80 s)
AlexNet	(9.74%, 0.97%, 10.00%, 1058 s, 8.19 s)
Custom 1	(9.05%, 1.48%, 9.22%, 1029 s, 7.77 s)
Custom 2	(12.29%, 6.49%, 12.05%, 1026 s, 8.60 s)

4. Future Works

While only a small portion of the population are affected by color blindness, this research could be used to understand how ML models interpret images with color distortion. Additionally, the random plate and grayscale version of these images show that a ML model can learn to extract features from images that are not human readable. We believe there is still much work that could be completed with this dataset.

4.1. Improvements

Keras and Tensorflow are very good tools for ML, however if this project were to be expanded, PyTorch would be used. This is due to its ability to create more complex models. This would allow for a more systematic approach for adding more models to test on. Additionally, in terms of performance and stability, using Pytorch would allow more diagnostic tools to be implemented into the program to help determine why a particular model was suffering in terms of accuracy and what improvements could be made. Following this idea, more models like ResNet and Inception could be added to the list of models above to analyze their performance in association with the other models.

As stated earlier, the Ishihara-Like MNIST dataset only reasonably recreated the red-green plates from the color blindness test. This only included using 8 of the 39 plates available. In future applications, we would like to follow the process of creating these circles for the other forms of red-green color blindness and create plates for blue-yellow color blindness. Given that each folder of this dataset only contained 10 k training images and 2 k testing images, more images would allow for an easier training process. Additionally, this generation of new images would include plates that are only able to be seen by individuals with these deficiencies. Finally, this type of research could be used to determine how easily readable a picture is for someone who is color blind or used to build a program that could create an Ishihara circle from any image (not just MNIST).

4.2. Extensions

While our paper focused on the training of models with color distortion, future applications of this research could use federated and split learning based-methods as seen in [57]. This would allow for the analysis of images that have possible corruption wherein the privacy or security of the dataset is a concern.

5. Conclusions

In this paper, we presented our research and findings with correctly identifying numerical characters in images with color distortion. While much work has been performed on this topic previously, we sought to use, expand, and improve upon the overall performance of correctly identifying the Ishihara-Like MNIST dataset. While prior work has only analyzed performance on the color (original) versions of the images, we sought to train models on the grayscale version as well. In our research, we did not perform any preprocessing to the images other than conversion of color to grayscale. To do this analysis, we performed our tests with a standard model architecture used to train MNIST, LeNet5, VGG16, AlexNet, and two small custom modifications of AlexNet. In each model, we trained the neural network models with each plate of images individually followed by a combination of all of the images in one set.

In our findings, we concluded that all of the aforementioned models had lower than expected performance accuracy when trained on the grayscale version of the Ishihara-Like MNIST images (averaging around 60%). However, VGG16 was still able to perform the overall better overall than the rest of the presented models. We believe this low performance with the grayscale images is due to the lack of information found in a monotone image as compared to the 3 channels in a color image. Therefore, a larger model is able to extract more features from the images. Even though VGG16's performance was good overall, the results were not consistent with every plate whereas AlexNet provided stable results. To examine this in the future, multiple runs of each model on each of the individual grayscale plates would be required.

With the color version of the images, each of the models except LeNet5 performed very well, achieving results on average above 90%. This occurred with the individual plates and the test case where all of the plates were combined. During the evaluation of the colored Ishihara images, we discovered that the rand plate (which is a randomly colored Ishihara circle) had significantly lower performance than the other colored plates. After analyzing the images, it was found that these images are very similar in their appearance to the grayscale versions, thus resulting in a lower performance. In the case of the grayscale images, the images are hard for humans to distinguish. With the rand plate, we found them to be illegible.

We concluded that this dataset could be trained faster and perform nearly as well using an architecture that is at least 100 times smaller than previously researched. While not explicitly stated how VGG16 was trained, what percentage of the dataset was used, and what steps were taken to pre-process the data in former research, we believe that our results conclude with an overall increase in performance due to the reduction in size of the model and an increase in evaluation time. Using a smaller model on a dataset of this size may result in a small performance loss, but would allow the user to run the model significantly faster. As shown in the performance graphs above, the reduction of size in AlexNet caused a slight drop in performance in each test case but caused the models to become more stable with their results. The curve of performance accuracy was more smooth with Custom 1 and Custom 2 than with the original AlexNet. With more hyper-tuning of the parameters of the model, we believe that the performance of models like AlexNet and smaller could be increased to match that of VGG16 while also maintaining the benefits of using a smaller model. Additionally, we believe that by understanding how the distortion of color affects images such as these, ML models could be improved to extract features more easily from everyday images.

Author Contributions: Conceptualization, C.H. and J.N.; methodology, C.H. and J.N.; software, C.H., J.N. and J.D.; validation, J.D. and A.J.M.; investigation, C.H.; writing—original draft preparation, C.H.; writing—review and editing, A.J.M.; supervision, A.J.M. All authors have read and agreed to the published version of the manuscript.

Funding: This research received no external funding.

Data Availability Statement: The code repository for this research is available at: https://github.com/vtnsi/ishihara-mnist.git, accessed on 12 December 2024).

Acknowledgments: Thank you to Lisha Henshaw for her support in proofreading the draft manuscript. Thank you to Chelsy Ables for creating Figure 14 and the cover figure to this paper.

Conflicts of Interest: The authors declare no conflicts of interest.

References

1. Memon, J.; Sami, M.; Khan, R.A.; Uddin, M. Handwritten Optical Character Recognition (OCR): A Comprehensive Systematic Literature Review (SLR). *IEEE Access* **2020**, *8*, 142642–142668. [CrossRef]
2. Tseng, Y.C.; Pan, H.K. Secure and invisible data hiding in 2-color images. In Proceedings of the Proceedings IEEE INFOCOM 2001. Conference on Computer Communications. Twentieth Annual Joint Conference of the IEEE Computer and Communications Society (Cat. No.01CH37213), Anchorage, AK, USA, 22–26 April 2001; Volume 2, pp. 887–896. [CrossRef]
3. LeCun, Y.; Cortes, C.; Burges, C. MNIST Handwritten Digit Database. ATT Labs [Online]. Available online: http://yann.lecun.com/exdb/mnist (accessed on 12 December 2024).
4. Baldominos, A.; Saez, Y.; Isasi, P. A Survey of Handwritten Character Recognition with MNIST and EMNIST. *Appl. Sci.* **2019**, *9*, 3169. [CrossRef]
5. Cohen, G.; Afshar, S.; Tapson, J.; van Schaik, A. EMNIST: Extending MNIST to handwritten letters. In Proceedings of the 2017 International Joint Conference on Neural Networks (IJCNN), Anchorage, AK, USA, 14–19 May 2017; pp. 2921–2926. [CrossRef]
6. Nocentini, O.; Kim, J.; Bashir, M.Z.; Cavallo, F. Image Classification Using Multiple Convolutional Neural Networks on the Fashion-MNIST Dataset. *Sensors* **2022**, *22*, 9544. [CrossRef] [PubMed]
7. Gerónimo, D.; Serrat, J.; López, A.M.; Baldrich, R. Traffic Sign Recognition for Computer Vision Project-Based Learning. *IEEE Trans. Educ.* **2013**, *56*, 364–371. [CrossRef]
8. Shaker, A.; Saralajew, S.; Gashteovski, K.; Faust, I.; Xu, Z.; Kotnis, B.; Ben-Rim, W.; Lawrence, C. Ishihara Like MNIST. 2022. Available online: https://www.kaggle.com/datasets/ammarshaker/ishihara-mnist (accessed on 12 December 2024).
9. Ishihara, S. Tests for colour-blindness, 1951.
10. Picryl. Available online: https://picryl.com/media/eight-ishihara-charts-for-testing-colour-blindness-europe-wellcome-l00591 55-cf3385 (accessed on 12 December 2024).
11. We Are Colorblind. 2019. Available online: https://wearecolorblind.com/articles/a-quick-introduction-to-color-blindness/ (accessed on 12 December 2024).
12. American Academy of Ophthalmology. 2018. Available online: https://www.aao.org/eye-health/anatomy/cones#:~:text=There%20are%20three%20types%20of,%2Dsensing%20cones%20(10%20percent) (accessed on 12 December 2024).
13. National Eye Institute. Color Blindness. Available online: https://www.nei.nih.gov/learn-about-eye-health/eye-conditions-and-diseases/color-blindness (accessed on 12 December 2024).
14. Mayo Clinic. Color Blindness. Available online: https://www.mayoclinic.org/diseases-conditions/poor-color-vision/symptoms-causes/syc-20354988 (accessed on 12 December 2024).
15. National Eye Institute. Types of Color Vision Deficiency. Available online: https://www.nei.nih.gov/learn-about-eye-health/eye-conditions-and-diseases/color-blindness/types-color-vision-deficiency (accessed on 12 December 2024).
16. GavinAdmin. Available online: https://doctorofeye.com/colour-blindness/ (accessed on 12 December 2024).
17. MedlinePlus. Available online: https://medlineplus.gov/genetics/condition/achromatopsia/#frequency (accessed on 12 December 2024).
18. PickPik. Available online: https://www.pickpik.com/fruit-mixed-color-food-assorted-variety-62464 (accessed on 12 December 2024).
19. Pilestone Inc. Color Blind Vision Simulator. Available online: https://pilestone.com/pages/color-blindness-simulator-1 (accessed on 12 December 2024).
20. Petrovic, G.; Fujita, H. *Deep Correct: Deep Learning Color Correction for Color Blindness*; IOS Press: Amsterdam, The Netherlands, 2017. [CrossRef]
21. Lin, H.Y.; Chen, L.Q.; Wang, M.L. Improving Discrimination in Color Vision Deficiency by Image Re-Coloring. *Sensors* **2019**, *19*, 2250. [CrossRef] [PubMed]
22. Jefferson, L.; Harvey, R. Accommodating color blind computer users. In Proceedings of the 8th International ACM SIGACCESS Conference on Computers and Accessibility, Portland, OR, USA, 23–25 October 2006; pp. 40–47. [CrossRef]
23. Jefferson, L.; Harvey, R. An interface to support color blind computer users. In Proceedings of the SIGCHI Conference on Human Factors in Computing Systems, San Jose, CA, USA, 28 April–3 May 2007; pp. 1535–1538. [CrossRef]
24. Tsekouras, G.E.; Rigos, A.; Chatzistamatis, S.; Tsimikas, J.; Kotis, K.; Caridakis, G.; Anagnostopoulos, C.N. A Novel Approach to Image Recoloring for Color Vision Deficiency. *Sensors* **2021**, *21*, 2740. [CrossRef] [PubMed]
25. de la Escalera, A.; Moreno, L.; Salichs, M.; Armingol, J. Road traffic sign detection and classification. *IEEE Trans. Ind. Electron.* **1997**, *44*, 848–859. [CrossRef]

26. Bahlmann, C.; Zhu, Y.; Ramesh, V.; Pellkofer, M.; Koehler, T. A system for traffic sign detection, tracking, and recognition using color, shape, and motion information. In Proceedings of the IEEE Proceedings. Intelligent Vehicles Symposium, Las Vegas, NV, USA, 6–8 June 2005; pp. 255–260. [CrossRef]
27. Creusen, I.; Hazelhoff, L.; de With, P. Color transformation for improved traffic sign detection. In Proceedings of the 2012 19th IEEE International Conference on Image Processing, Orlando, FL, USA, 30 September–3 October 2012; pp. 461–464. [CrossRef]
28. Xie, Z.; Lyu, R. Whether pattern memory can be truly realized in deep neural network? *Research Square* **2024**. [CrossRef]
29. Solonko, M. Reading Color Blindness Charts: Deep Learning and Computer Vision. Available online: https://towardsdatascience.com/reading-color-blindness-charts-deep-learning-and-computer-vision-a8c824dd71cd (accessed on 12 December 2024).
30. Bottou, L.; Cortes, C.; Denker, J.; Drucker, H.; Guyon, I.; Jackel, L.; LeCun, Y.; Muller, U.; Sackinger, E.; Simard, P.; et al. Comparison of classifier methods: A case study in handwritten digit recognition. In Proceedings of the 12th IAPR International Conference on Pattern Recognition, Vol. 3—Conference C: Signal Processing (Cat. No.94CH3440-5), Jerusalem, Israel, 9–13 October 1994; Volume 2, pp. 77–82. [CrossRef]
31. GeeksforGeeks. MNIST Dataset: Practical Applications Using Keras and PyTorch. 2024. Available online: https://www.geeksforgeeks.org/mnist-dataset/ (accessed on 12 December 2024).
32. Clanuwat, T.; Bober-Irizar, M.; Kitamoto, A.; Lamb, A.; Yamamoto, K.; Ha, D. Deep Learning for Classical Japanese Literature. *arXiv* **2018**, arXiv:1812.01718. [CrossRef]
33. Al-Noori, A.H.; Talib, M.; Harbi S., J. The Classification of Ancient Sumerian Characters using Convolutional Neural Network. In Proceedings of the 1st International Conference on Computing and Emerging Sciences, Lahore, Pakistan, 26–27 May 2023; SciTePress: Setúbal, Portugal, 2020. [CrossRef]
34. Zalando Research; Crawford Company. Fashion Mnist. 2017. Available online: https://www.kaggle.com/datasets/zalando-research/fashionmnist (accessed on 12 December 2024).
35. Xhaferra, E.; Cina, E.; Toti, L. Classification of Standard FASHION MNIST Dataset Using Deep Learning Based CNN Algorithms. In Proceedings of the 2022 International Symposium on Multidisciplinary Studies and Innovative Technologies (ISMSIT), Ankara, Turkey, 20–22 October 2022; pp. 494–498. [CrossRef]
36. Rim, W.B.; Shaker, A.; Xu, Z.; Gashteovski, K.; Kotnis, B.; Lawrence, C.; Quittek, J.; Saralajew, S. A Human-Centric Assessment of the Usefulness of Attribution Methods in Computer Vision. In Proceedings of the Joint European Conference on Machine Learning and Knowledge Discovery in Databases, Vilnius, Lithuania, 9–13 September 2024. [CrossRef]
37. Potjewyd, G. The Color Code. 2022. Available online: https://theophthalmologist.com/business-profession/the-color-code (accessed on 12 December 2024).
38. Welcome Collection. Available online: https://wellcomecollection.org/search/works (accessed on 12 December 2024).
39. Ishihara, S. Ishihara Instructions. Available online: https://web.stanford.edu/group/vista/wikiupload/0/0a/Ishihara.14.Plate.Instructions.pdf (accessed on 12 December 2024).
40. Dhawale, K.; Vohra, A.S.; Jain, P.; Kumar, T. A Framework to Identify Color Blindness Charts Using Image Processing and CNN. In *Communication, Networks and Computing: Second International Conference (CNC 2020), Gwalior, India, 29–31 December 2020*; Revised Selected Papers 2; Springer: Singapore, 2021; pp. 100–109. [CrossRef]
41. Ye, Q.; Doermann, D. Text Detection and Recognition in Imagery: A Survey. *IEEE Trans. Pattern Anal. Mach. Intell.* **2015**, *37*, 1480–1500. [CrossRef]
42. Imran, F.; Hossain, D.M.A.; Mamun, M.A. Identification and Recognition of Printed Distorted Characters Using Proposed DCR Method. In Proceedings of the 2020 IEEE Region 10 Symposium (TENSYMP), Dhaka, Bangladesh, 5–7 June 2020; pp. 1478–1481. [CrossRef]
43. paravisionlab.co.in. LeNet-5: A Simple Yet Powerful CNN for Image Classification. Available online: https://paravisionlab.co.in/lenet-5-architecture/ (accessed on 12 December 2024).
44. Boesch, G. Very Deep Convolutional Networks (VGG) Essential Guide. Available online: https://viso.ai/deep-learning/vgg-very-deep-convolutional-networks/ (accessed on 12 December 2024).
45. Krizhevsky, A.; Sutskever, I.; Hinton, G.E. ImageNet Classification with Deep Convolutional Neural Networks. *Commun. ACM* **2017**, *60*, 84–90. [CrossRef]
46. Wang, Y.; Li, F.; Sun, H.; Li, W.; Zhong, C.; Wu, X.; Wang, H.; Wang, P. Improvement of MNIST Image Recognition Based on CNN. *IOP Conf. Ser. Earth Environ. Sci.* **2020**, *428*, 012097. [CrossRef]
47. Cheng, S.; Shang, G.; Zhang, L. Handwritten digit recognition based on improved VGG16 network. In Proceedings of the Tenth International Conference on Graphics and Image Processing (ICGIP 2018), Chengdu, China, 12–14 December 2018; Volume 11069, pp. 954–962. [CrossRef]
48. Redmon, J.; Divvala, S.; Girshick, R.; Farhadi, A. You Only Look Once: Unified, Real-Time Object Detection. In Proceedings of the 2016 IEEE Conference on Computer Vision and Pattern Recognition (CVPR), Las Vegas, NV, USA, 27–30 June 2016; pp. 779–788. [CrossRef]
49. Kaggle. Available online: https://www.kaggle.com/ (accessed on 12 December 2024).

50. GeeksforGeeks. How to Choose Batch Size and Number of Epochs When Fitting a Model? 2024. Available online: https://www.geeksforgeeks.org/how-to-choose-batch-size-and-number-of-epochs-when-fitting-a-model/ (accessed on 12 December 2024).
51. Kaggle, A.J. Available online: https://www.kaggle.com/code/amyjang/tensorflow-mnist-cnn-tutorial/ (accessed on 12 December 2024).
52. Thakur, A. ReLU vs. Sigmoid Function in Deep Neural Networks. 2020. Available online: https://wandb.ai/ayush-thakur/dl-question-bank/reports/ReLU-vs-Sigmoid-Function-in-Deep-Neural-Networks--VmlldzoyMDk0MzI#:~:text=The%20model%20trained%20with%20ReLU,better%20when%20trained%20with%20ReLU (accessed on 12 December 2024).
53. Lecun, Y.; Bottou, L.; Bengio, Y.; Haffner, P. Gradient-based learning applied to document recognition. *Proc. IEEE* **1998**, *86*, 2278–2324. [CrossRef]
54. Kumar, S. Comparison of Sigmoid, Tanh and Relu Activation Functions. 2023. Available online: https://www.aitude.com/comparison-of-sigmoid-tanh-and-relu-activation-functions/ (accessed on 12 December 2024).
55. Melanie. Unveiling the Secrets of the VGG Model: A Deep Dive with Daniel. Available online: https://datascientest.com/en/unveiling-the-secrets-of-the-vgg-model-a-deep-dive-with-daniel#:~:text=A%20little%20history,Recognition%20Challenge)%20competition%20in%202014 (accessed on 12 December 2024).
56. Wei, J. AlexNet: The Architecture That Challenged CNNs. Available online: https://towardsdatascience.com/alexnet-the-architecture-that-challenged-cnns-e406d5297951 (accessed on 12 December 2024).
57. Taheri, R.; Arabikhan, F.; Gegov, A.; Akbari, N. Robust Aggregation Function in Federated Learning. In *International Conference on Information and Knowledge Systems*; Springer: Cham, Switzerland, 2023; pp. 168–175.

computers

Article

Leveraging Scene Geometry and Depth Information for Robust Image Deraining

Ningning Xu and Jidong J. Yang *

Smart Mobility and Infrastructure Lab, College of Engineering, University of Georgia, Athens, GA 30602, USA; ningning.xu@uga.edu
* Correspondence: jidong.yang@uga.edu

Abstract: Image deraining holds great potential for enhancing the vision of autonomous vehicles in rainy conditions, contributing to safer driving. Previous works have primarily focused on employing a single network architecture to generate derained images. However, they often fail to fully exploit the rich prior knowledge embedded in the scenes. Particularly, most methods overlook the depth information that can provide valuable context about scene geometry and guide more robust deraining. In this work, we introduce a novel learning framework that integrates multiple networks: an AutoEncoder for deraining, an auxiliary network to incorporate depth information, and two supervision networks to enforce feature consistency between rainy and clear scenes. This multi-network design enables our model to effectively capture the underlying scene structure, producing clearer and more accurately derained images, leading to improved object detection for autonomous vehicles. Extensive experiments on three widely used datasets demonstrated the effectiveness of our proposed method.

Keywords: image deraining; AutoEncoder; prior knowledge; supervision networks; feature consistency; depth information; autonomous driving

1. Introduction

Image deraining is a critical preprocessing step in computer vision applications due to its significant impact on visual clarity and accuracy. Rain on images can obscure the visibility of objects, leading to substantial degradation in image quality. This can adversely affect the performance of object detection [1], recognition [2], and tracking algorithms [3], which are essential in various domains such as surveillance and navigation. In autonomous driving [4], clear vision is paramount for safety and robust decision making; rain-induced artifacts can compromise the accuracy of perception systems, potentially leading to hazardous situations. Therefore, effective image deraining techniques are vital to enhance the reliability and functionality of vision-based systems.

In general, a rainy image can be represented as a superimposition of two layers: a clean image layer and a rain layer. The rain layer encompasses various artifacts such as rain streaks, raindrops, and fog, which make rain removal a challenging task. These rain-induced artifacts obscure objects and scenes, not only blurring visual data but also partially concealing critical features necessary for accurate image interpretation. Moreover, spatial factors further complicate the process. For objects are closer to the camera, rain is the primary occluding element, making its removal relatively easier. In contrast, distant objects are more challenging to recover due to additional occlusions from fog and other atmospheric conditions. This intricacy underscores the challenges of deraining in computer

 https://doi.org/10.3390/computers14010011

vision. Garg and Nayar [5] illustrated this phenomenon by demonstrating how the intensity of rain effects transitions into fog as the distance to the scene increases. Recent deep learning approaches for single-image rain removal have predominantly concentrated on the removal of rain streaks, often neglecting the broader physical characteristics of rain itself. The existing training datasets for rain removal typically include images featuring artificial rain streaks, raindrops, or a combination of both, with some datasets even containing indoor scenes. This limitation significantly hampers the effectiveness of these methods when applied to real-world outdoor scenarios, where the intricate interplay between rain patterns and environmental factors differs substantially from the synthetic conditions represented in these datasets.

In this study, we proposes a novel method for the automatic removal of rain streaks, raindrops, and fog in real-world photographs, with an emphasis on achieving real-time performance. The primary objective is to improve image quality for environmental monitoring and vision-based autonomous driving, thereby enhancing the accuracy and reliability of these applications under challenging weather conditions. To achieve this, we introduce an AutoEncoder model equipped with a consistent feature extraction module that processes both rainy and clear images while incorporating depth information. This approach allows the model to capture the underlying shared features between rain and clear images, thereby preserving the essential scene information obscured by rain and fog. Furthermore, the integration of depth information enables the extraction of global image features, ensuring the retention of key structural details across entire images.

In summary, this work provides the following contributions:

- Firstly, we constructed a Derain AutoEncoder (DerainAE) model to effectively handle various rain-related artifacts and atmospheric disturbances.
- Secondly, we designed a consistent feature extraction module with a supervision network during training to effectively capture shared features between rain and clear images.
- Thirdly, we developed a depth network (DepthNet) to extract depth information, which aids in capturing global structure of scenes. By leveraging these shared and global features, our deraining model is capable of generating more accurate and visually coherent results.
- Lastly, we conducted extensive experiments to evaluate our approach on various outdoor datasets. The results showed that our method effectively removes rain artifacts while preserving critical image details. The efficacy of our model was further validated through its performance on an object detection task.

2. Related Work

Image deraining methods can be broadly categorized into model-based methods [6–8] and deep learning methods [9–12]. Model-based methods often approach deraining as a filtering problem, using various filters to restore a rain-free image. While this can effectively remove rain effects, it also tends to eliminate important structures within the image. Many model-based approaches develop various image priors based on the statistical properties of rain and clear images. These methods include image decomposition [3], low-rank representation [6,13], discriminative sparse coding [14], and Gaussian mixture models [15]. Although these techniques have achieved improved results, they still struggle to effectively handle complex and varying rainy conditions.

In contrast, deep learning-based methods have significantly advanced image deraining by learning data-driven representations of rain and clear images. These approaches utilize powerful architectures and novel mechanisms to achieve superior performance. Early works such as [16] demonstrated substantial improvements in rain removal across benchmark datasets using convolutional neural networks (CNNs). Generative adversarial networks (GANs) [17] have also been employed to restore perceptually superior rain-free images, as demonstrated by [18]. The introduction of transformers, such as [19], enabled effective modeling of non-local dependencies, further enhancing image reconstruction quality. Inspired by the success of recent diffusion models [20] in generating high-quality images, diffusion-based approaches [21] have shown great potential in improving image deraining performance across complex scenarios. Recent advancements include the integration of additional data modalities and novel priors into the learning process. For instance, Hu et al. [22] introduced depth information via an attention mechanism, achieving promising results on synthetic rainy datasets. Zhang et al. [9] exploited both stereo images and semantic information for improved image deraining performance. Guo et al. [23] proposed the use of Fourier priors to improve model generalization in rain removal tasks.

In summary, model-based methods have historically provided a solid foundation for image deraining, emphasizing handcrafted priors and optimization frameworks. However, their limitations in handling complex rainy conditions and preserving image details have led to a growing focus on deep learning approaches. Deep learning methods, driven by CNNs, GANs, transformers, and diffusion models, continue to achieve state-of-the-art results by leveraging large datasets, powerful architectures, and innovative priors. With the rapid evolution of data-driven techniques, deep learning is poised to dominate future advancements in image deraining, offering scalable solutions for complex and diverse real-world scenarios.

3. Methods

In this section, we introduce our multi-network approach for effective image deraining, as depicted in Figure 1. The core of this framework is the Deraining AutoEncoder (DerainAE), which serves as the primary network for the deraining task. To enhance its performance, we introduce a supplementary Depth Network (DepthNet) that integrates depth information to assist in rain removal. Additionally, we utilize pretrained networks to provide supervisory signals, ensuring multiscale feature consistencies between clear and rainy images. The detailed architecture and loss functions are discussed subsequently.

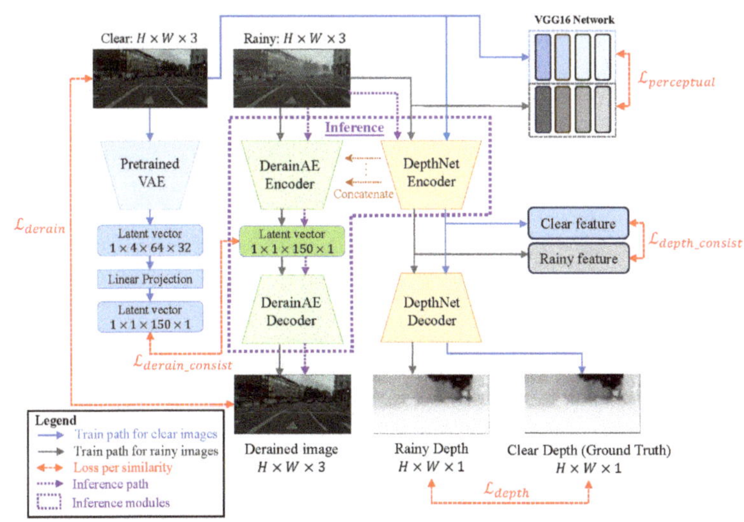

Figure 1. The overall architecture of our model. A pretrained VAE extracts clear features, while the DerainAE and DepthNet modules handle rainy images. Latent space comparison between clear and rainy features improves depth estimation and deraining images prediction.

3.1. Network Architecture

For image deraining, the commonality between clear and rainy images lies in their depiction of the same scene, meaning the depth map should remain consistent between them. Apart from the rain artifacts, the feature map of the clear and rainy images should also be identical. Therefore, our approach employs two forms of supervision: one from the depth map and one from the feature map. This dual supervision ensures that the model not only learns to remove the rain but also retains the intrinsic features of the scene, leveraging the consistency between the depth and feature information to enhance the deraining process.

Our DerainAE model (see Figure 2, left) adopts an AutoEncoder architecture to tackle the image deraining task by learning both the latent representation and the restored derained image. The AutoEncoder is designed to effectively capture the underlying structure and intrinsic features of rain-affected images through an encoding–decoding process. The encoder compresses the input image into a lower-dimensional latent space, extracting critical high-level information necessary for rain removal while filtering out irrelevant noise. The decoder then reconstructs the derained image from this latent representation, ensuring the preservation of essential details and textures. This dual functionality enables the model to efficiently map rain-degraded images to their rain-free counterparts.

To enhance the learning capacity of the DerainAE model and enable it to capture more comprehensive scene information, we integrate a DepthNet (see Figure 2, right) that also adopts an encoder–decoder architecture. Features from the DepthNet encoder are concatenated with the corresponding feature levels of the DerainAE encoder, establishing a shared learning mechanism that effectively leverages depth information for improved deraining performance. In our implementation, the DepthNet encoder employs the VGG16 architecture, allowing the model to leverage depth information to better understand the spatial structure and geometry of the scene, which is crucial for accurate rain removal. The decoder employs transposed convolutions to progressively upsample the feature maps, restoring them to the original input resolution. To preserve high-resolution details, skip connections are implemented between the encoder's convolutional blocks and their corresponding layers in the decoder, following the design principles of the U-Net architecture. Additionally, the decoder incorporates multiple convolutional layers to effectively fuse information across different spatial resolutions. The network predicts disparity maps at multiple scales and resolutions using convolutional layers with sigmoid activation functions.

During training, we use the DerainAE for image deraining while simultaneously leveraging the DepthNet to predict the depth maps of both clear and rainy images. The feature maps from the DepthNet encoder are concatenated with the corresponding feature maps in the DerainAE encoder, enabling depth-aware deraining. Additionally, a pretrained Variational AutoEncoder (VAE) is used to obtain a latent vector of the clear image, which serves as a supervisory signal during during training to ensure high-level feature consistency. Feature consistency is further enforced at multiple levels via a pretrained VGG16. Depth consistency is also maintained in the latent space of the DepthNet. During inference, our method requires only the rainy image as input, which is processed by DerainAE and the DepthNet encoder to produce the derained output, where the DepthNet encoder extracts depth information, which is then passed to the DrainAE encoder to aid in the deraining process.

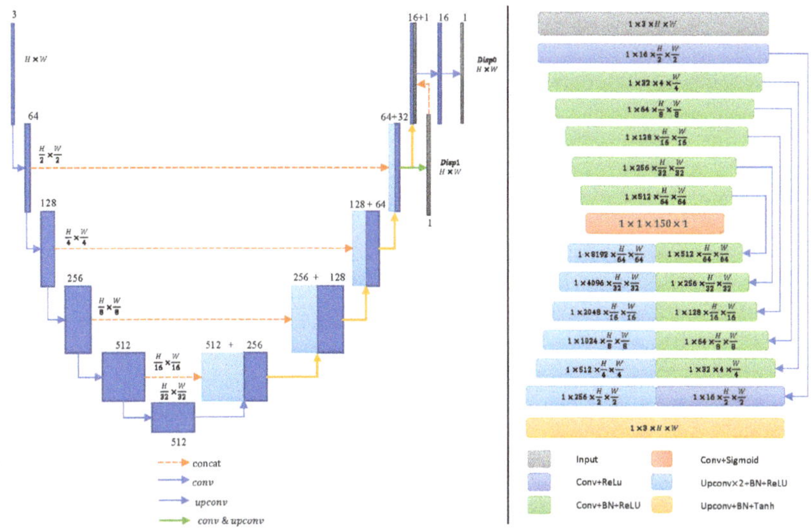

Figure 2. An overview of our DepthNet and DerainAE architecture. **Left**: DepthNet, this model employs a U-Net structure, with skip connections from each encoder layer to the corresponding decoder layers. The network outputs two disparity maps with Disp0 used as the final predicted depth map. **Right**: DerainAE; this model is a simple convolutional network with skip connections at corresponding feature levels between the encoder and decoder.

3.2. Loss Function

To jointly train DerainAE and DepthNet, we introduce a composite loss function that considers multiple complementary loss components. Building on the perceptual loss $\mathcal{L}_{\text{perceptual}}$ proposed by Johnson et al. [24], we measure the discrepancy between clear images and corresponding rain images in a manner more consistent with human visual perception. Specifically, we utilize a pretrained VGG16 network to capture discrepancies at various feature levels, which is computed by Equation (1).

$$\mathcal{L}_{perceptual} = \sum_{l} \lambda_l \cdot |\phi_l(y) - \phi_l(\hat{y})|_2^2 \tag{1}$$

where ϕ_l denotes the activation map of the l-th layer in VGG16.

We employ cosine similarity losses (Equations (2) and (3)) to measure the consistency of latent representations of clear images and corresponding rain images for both DerainAE and DepthNet.

$$\mathcal{L}_{depth\_consist} = \cos(D_R, D_C) \tag{2}$$

$$\mathcal{L}_{derain\_consist} = \cos(R_L, C_L) \tag{3}$$

where $\cos(\cdot,\cdot)$ denotes the cosine similarity function.

Additionally, we use mean squared error (MSE) losses for reconstruction of the depth map $\hat{D}$ and the derained image $\hat{C}$:

$$\mathcal{L}_{derain} = MSE(\hat{C}, C) \tag{4}$$

$$\mathcal{L}_{depth} = MSE(\hat{D}, D) \tag{5}$$

The loss function used to train our model is a weighted sum of these individual loss terms by Equation (6):

$$\mathcal{L} = \lambda_1 \mathcal{L}_{perceptual} + \lambda_2 \mathcal{L}_{depth\_consist} + \lambda_3 \mathcal{L}_{derain\_consist} + \lambda_4 \mathcal{L}_{derain} + \lambda_5 \mathcal{L}_{depth} \quad (6)$$

where $\lambda_1, \ldots, \lambda_5$ are hyperparameters that control the relative importance of each loss component during training. This hybrid loss function enables the joint optimization of DerainAE and DepthNet, ensuring robust performance across both deraining and depth estimation tasks.

4. Experimental Results

In this section, we begin by introducing the datasets and evaluation metrics, which is followed by a discussion of the implementation details and results. Ablation studies are conducted to evaluate the contributions of key components. Additionally, the effectiveness of our model is validated through an object detection task, highlighting the benefits of deraining for enhanced vision.

4.1. Datasets and Evaluation Metrics

Due to the challenge of obtaining paired rain and clear images, various rain models have been developed to synthetically generate rain streaks from clear images. In the linear model proposed by [15], the observed rain image $\mathbf{O} \in \mathbb{R}^{M\times N}$ is represented as a combination of a desired background layer $\mathbf{B} \in \mathbb{R}^{M\times N}$ and a rain streak layer $\mathbf{R} \in \mathbb{R}^{M\times N}$, such that $\mathbf{O} = \mathbf{B} + \mathbf{R}$. Building upon this model, ref. [25] proposed a more generalized formulation: $\mathbf{O} = \mathbf{B} + \mathbf{R}\tilde{\mathbf{R}}$, where $\tilde{\mathbf{R}}$ is a new region-dependent variable that indicates the locations of individually visible rain streaks. The elements of $\tilde{\mathbf{R}}$ take binary values, with 1 indicating rain regions and 0 indicating non-rain regions. Further, refs. [22,26] modeled a rain image as a composite of a rain-free image, a rain layer, and a fog layer, formulating the observed rain image as below,

$$\mathbf{O} = \mathbf{B}(1 - \mathbf{R} - \mathbf{F}) + \mathbf{R} + f_0\mathbf{F}$$

where $\mathbf{F}$ is a fog layer, and f_0 is the atmospheric light, which is assumed to be a global constant following [27].

RainKITTI2012 and RainKITTI2015 Datasets: These two synthetic datasets were created by Zhang et al. [9] using Photoshop to introduce synthetic rain effects on the publicly available KITTI stereo datasets 2012 and 2015 [28]. The RainKITTI2012 dataset consists of a training set with 4062 image pairs and a testing set with 4085 image pairs, each having a resolution of 1242 × 375 pixels. Similarly, the RainKITTI2015 dataset contains 4200 pairs of training images and 4189 pairs of testing images, all maintaining the same resolution.

RainCityScapes Dataset: This synthetic dataset, developed by Hu et al. [22], is based on the Cityscapes dataset [29]. It is generated by the aforementioned rain models and consists of a rain layer, a fog layer, and a rain-free image. It includes a training set of 9432 paired rainy and clear images, which is accompanied by ground truth depth information. The testing set consists of 1188 images.

Evaluation Metrics: We use PSNR [30] and SSIM [31] as the evaluation metrics.

4.2. Implementation Details

In model training, we set the hyperparameters $\lambda_1, \lambda_2, \lambda_3, \lambda_4, \lambda_5$ to [1, 0.5, 0.5, 10, 2], respectively. For the pretrained Variational AutoEncoder (VAE) model, we adopt the VAE component from the Stable Diffusion framework [20], employing Mean Squared Error (MSE) as the loss function. The latent space of the VAE is sampled to produce a latent vector of the same size (length 150) as that used in our DerainAE model. During training, we keep the VAE model weights frozen and only fine-tune the final output layer. For depth reconstruction, we use the pretrained VGG16 model as the encoder, which is frozen during training, and train the decoder from scratch. Our entire model is implemented in PyTorch [32] and is trained on a workstation with an NVIDIA RTX A6000 GPU. All datasets in our experiments share the same training configuration: a batch size of 4, and the ADAM optimizer [33] with an initial learning rate of 5×10^{-3} and a weight decay of 0.9.

4.3. Evaluation on Different Datasets

Table 1 presents the evaluation metrics for the three datasets. The SSIM demonstrates that our model can restore most of the clear image's information, while the PSNR indicates better overall clarity in the predictions. Figure 3 shows results of exemplar images from the RainCityScapes and RainKITTI2012 datasets. It is clear that besides rain streaks, the foggy effect has been removed as well.

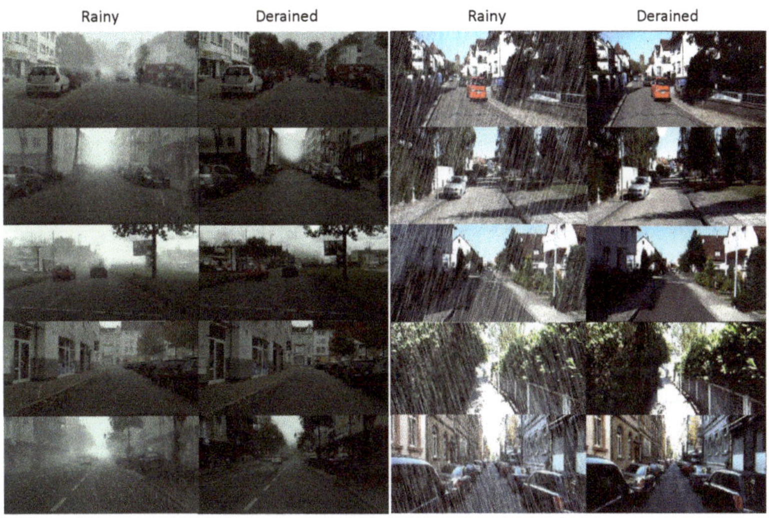

Figure 3. Visualization results of RainCityScapes and RainKITTI2012 dataset. The first two columns are exemplar images from the RainCityScapes dataset and corresponding derained outputs; the last two columns are exemplar images from the RainKITTI2012 dataset and corresponding derained outputs.

Table 1. Model evaluation on three outdoor datasets—RainCityScapes, RainKITTI2012 and RainKITTI2015—Average (Ave), Maximum (Max), and Minimum (Min) values of PSNR and SSIM.

Datasets	PSNR			SSIM		
	Ave	Max	Min	Ave	Max	Min
RainCityScapes	28.45243	33.58215	19.07696	0.93726	0.97048	0.85108
RainKITTI2012	25.73460	29.70556	22.32341	0.87256	0.92983	0.80549
RainKITTI2015	26.33563	29.74982	22.95045	0.87402	0.91881	0.79097

4.4. Comparsion with Other Methods

We evaluate two additional deraining models, DID-MDN [34] and PReNet [10], on the RainCityscapes testing dataset. For the DID-MDN model, we utilize the pretrained weights provided by the authors on GitHub. Since the DID-MDN model accepts an input size of 512×512, while RainCityscapes images are sized at 2028×1024, we resize the RainCityscapes images to 512×512 for processing and then resize the derained outputs back to the original resolution for evaluation. For PReNet, we leverage all the pretrained models available for the Rain100H, Rain100L, and Rain1400 datasets, selecting the best-performing results on the RainCityscapes testing dataset as the final outputs. As we can see in Table 2, our model can perform better that other methods. Table 3 presents the running times of DID-MDN, PReNet, and our method on an NVIDIA RTX A6000 GPU. As shown, our method achieves greater efficiency compared to the other approaches, which is attributed to its simpler backbone architecture.

Table 2. Comparsion results on the RainCityscapes testing dataset. We report the average, minimum and maximum of PSNR and SSIM mertrics on PReNet, DID-MDN and our model.

Methods	PSNR			SSIM		
	Ave	**Max**	**Min**	**Ave**	**Max**	**Min**
DID-MDN	16.82741	24.30264	11.12157	0.77786	0.86142	0.65167
PRENET	15.75766	23.40013	10.55631	0.80006	0.94088	0.61976
OURS	28.45243	33.58215	19.07696	0.93726	0.97048	0.85108

Table 3. Comparison of inference times on RainCityscapes dataset (image size: 512 × 512).

Method	Inference Time
DID-MDN	0.0322
PReNet	0.0899
Ours	0.0044

4.5. Ablation Studies

All ablation studies are performed on the RainCityscapes, RainKITTI2012, and RainKITTI2015 datasets. To evaluate the effectiveness of our model architecture, we calculate PSNR and SSIM on the respective testing sets. These metrics provide a quantitative assessment of the quality of the generated images with higher PSNR and SSIM values indicating better image restoration and alignment with ground truth. By comparing different configurations of our model, referred to as Settings A, B, C, D, E, and Full in Table 4, we demonstrate the contributions of each component to the overall performance.

Table 4. Ablation settings (A–E). Compared to our full model, we conduct an ablation study by removing component(s) to evaluate their respective contributions.

Component	A	B	C	D	E	Full
Depth Latent		✓	✓	✓	✓	✓
Derain Latent	✓		✓	✓	✓	✓
Ground Truth Depth	✓	✓	✓			✓
Concatenation of Depth Features	✓	✓		✓		✓

Loss Functions: To evaluate the impact of the depth latent and derain latent constraints on our model's performance, we conducted ablation studies on loss components. Table 1 presents the results of the full model, while Tables 5 and 6 show that where the depth latent constraint and derain latent constraint are excluded, we observe a noticeable drop in both PSNR and SSIM across all datasets.

Table 5. PSNR and SSIM results of the model trained without depth latent constraint (WO depth latent) on three outdoor datasets: RainCityScapes, RainKITTI2012, and RainKITTI2015.

Setting A		PSNR			SSIM	
Datasets	**Ave**	**Max**	**Min**	**Ave**	**Max**	**Min**
RainCityScapes	25.17939	32.74820	12.38616	0.89550	0.95628	0.75533
RainKITTI2012	25.16171	28.75597	21.98756	0.87104	0.92994	0.80130
RainKITTI2015	25.62023	29.53999	22.13033	0.86560	0.91456	0.78444

Table 6. PSNR and SSIM results of the model trained without derain latent constraint (WO derain latent) on three outdoor datasets: RainCityScapes, RainKITTI2012, and RainKITTI2015.

Setting B		PSNR			SSIM	
Datasets	**Ave**	**Max**	**Min**	**Ave**	**Max**	**Min**
RainCityScapes	26.49246	30.54199	21.31583	0.92993	0.96342	0.80553
RainKITTI2012	24.80499	28.64988	21.50745	0.86331	0.92666	0.78119
RainKITTI2015	25.56248	29.41232	22.47581	0.87237	0.91106	0.80080

Ground Truth Depth: Table 7 shows the performance of the model when trained without using the ground truth depth map (WO GT depth). The results reveal a moderate drop in both PSNR and SSIM across all datasets when the ground truth depth information is removed.

Table 7. PSNR and SSIM results of the model trained without the ground truth depth map (WO GT depth) on three outdoor datasets: RainCityScapes, RainKITTI2012, and RainKITTI2015.

Setting C		PSNR			SSIM	
Datasets	**Ave**	**Max**	**Min**	**Ave**	**Max**	**Min**
RainCityScapes	27.25449	32.11505	19.81718	0.93005	0.96428	0.84685
RainKITTI2012	24.04377	27.61285	21.22836	0.84602	0.91315	0.76548
RainKITTI2015	25.04490	28.21179	22.28209	0.85778	0.90852	0.77175

Depth Feature Concatenation: Table 8 shows the results of removing depth feature connection between the DerainAE encoder and DepthNet encoder. We found that the concatenation of depth features improves the performance.

Table 8. PSNR and SSIM results of the model trained without depth feature concatenation (WO concatenation) on three outdoor datasets: RainCityScapes, RainKITTI2012, and RainKITTI2015.

Setting D		PSNR			SSIM	
Datasets	**Ave**	**Max**	**Min**	**Ave**	**Max**	**Min**
RainCityScapes	21.09265	27.61965	15.57796	0.84027	0.93656	0.69801
RainKITTI2012	22.04879	25.26042	19.11878	0.79373	0.88923	0.68814
RainKITTI2015	21.74929	24.87100	19.52019	0.81088	0.86397	0.71841

GT Depth and Depth Feature Concatenation Table 9 presents the results when both the ground truth depth map and depth feature concatenation are removed from the model during training. The performance is notably impacted across all datasets, as reflected by the lower PSNR and SSIM values compared to the full model.

Table 9. PSNR and SSIM results of the model trained without both ground truth depth map and depth feature concatenation (WO gt depth and concatenation) on three outdoor datasets: RainCityScapes, RainKITTI2012, and RainKITTI2015.

Setting E	PSNR			SSIM		
Datasets	Ave	Max	Min	Ave	Max	Min
RainCityScapes	24.52006	32.31414	14.92033	0.89442	0.95443	0.74023
RainKITTI2012	22.11384	25.00253	19.25391	0.78867	0.88489	0.68008
RainKITTI2015	23.69155	26.68006	21.29122	0.82113	0.87281	0.74432

4.6. Vehicle Detection

Image deraining can be integrated into outdoor vision systems to enhance object visibility during complex weather conditions, which is particularly beneficial for autonomous driving. By improving visibility, it can aid in critical tasks like vehicle detection and navigation, making autonomous vehicles safer and more reliable, especially in regions prone to heavy rainfall. For this evaluation, the focus is on detecting other vehicles in the scene. We implemented YOLOv11 [35] on both rainy and derained images. Figure 4 shows that derained images significantly improve vehicle detection accuracy on the RainKITTI2015 dataset. Similarly, Figure 5 demonstrates the ability of our model in enhancing vehicle detection performance under more challenging rainy scenarios in the RainCityscapes dataset, which closely approximate real-world rainy and foggy conditions. The vehicle detection performance metrics, summarized in Table 10, show that our deraining model significantly improves vehicle detection recall. It achieved a 67% improvement on recall (from 0.5415 to 0.9036) for the RainKITTI2015 dataset and a 19% improvement on recall (from 0.628 to 0.747) for the RainCityscapes dataset. This demonstrates enhanced visibility with significantly reduced false negative (missed) detections, which is critical for the safe driving of autonomous vehicles, particularly in low-visibility environments.

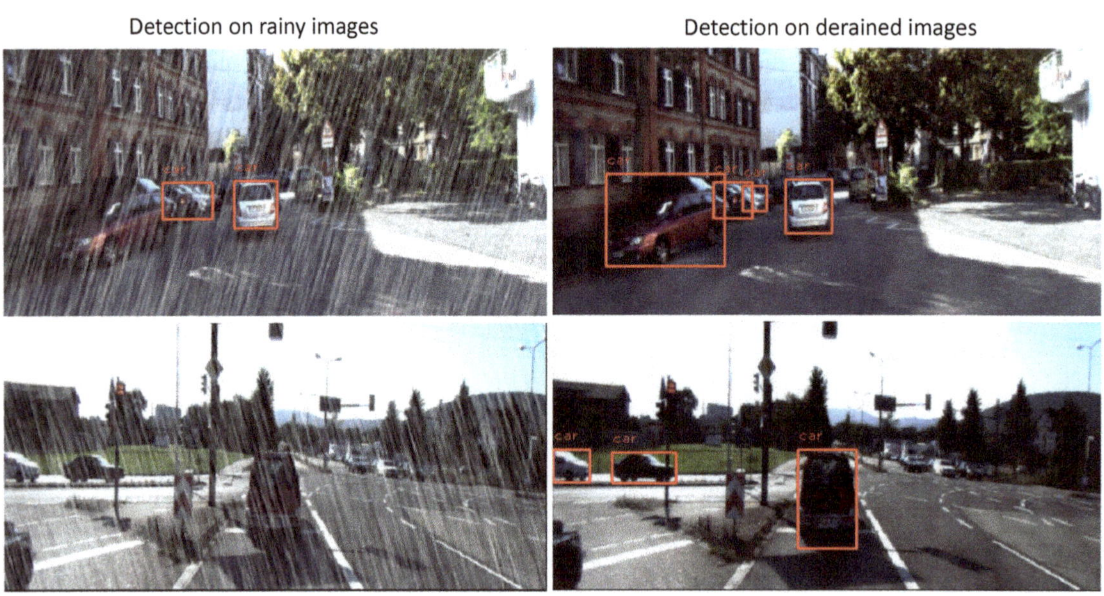

Figure 4. Vehicle detection results using YOLOv11 on the RainKITTI2015 dataset. Red bounding boxes denote the detected vehicles.

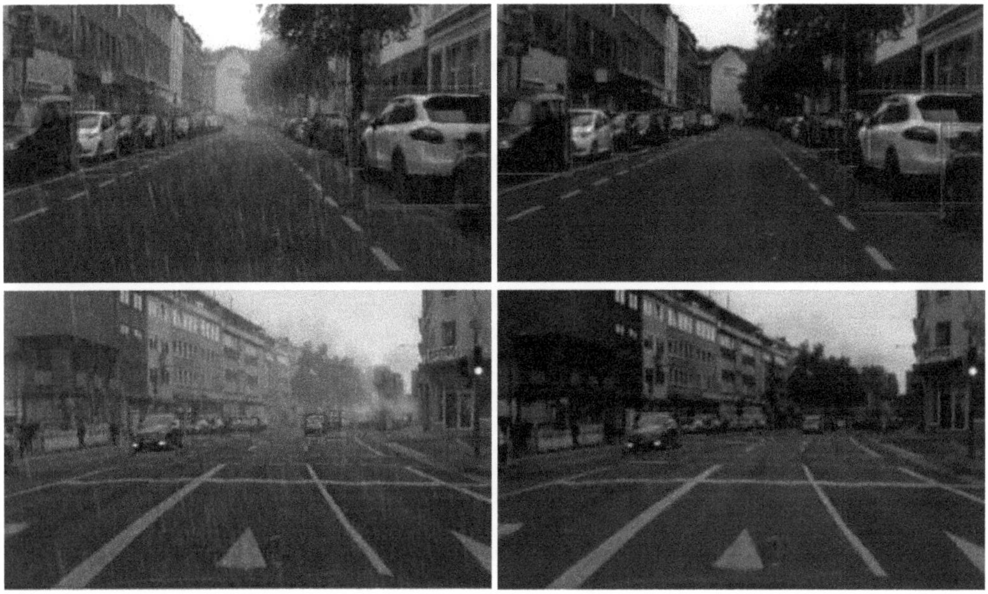

Figure 5. Vehicle detection results using YOLOv11 on the RainCityScapes dataset. Red bounding boxes denote the detected vehicles.

Table 10. Vehicle detection results of RainKITTI2015 test dataset. We calculate mean precision and mean recall on 4189 images. The results shows that our deraining model significantly improves object detection recall.

RainKITTI2015	Mean Precision	Mean Recall
Rainy Image	0.9685	0.5415
Derain Image	0.9533	0.9036
RainCityscapes	Mean precision	Mean recall
Rainy	0.823	0.628
Derain	0.840	0.747

5. Conclusions

In this study, we introduced a novel learning framework that integrates multiple networks, including an AutoEncoder for deraining, an auxiliary network to incorporate depth information, and two supervision networks to enforce feature consistency between rainy and clear scenes. Our approach demonstrates that even with a design based solely on simple convolutional layers, the integration of depth information and feature consistency constraints enables the network to produce high-quality derained images. Our method was evaluated on three public datasets with results demonstrating its efficacy and robustness under diverse rainy conditions. Furthermore, applying our model to an object detection task revealed significant improvement on recall when using derained images.

Despite the efficacy of our approach, we acknowledge several limitations that present opportunities for future research. It is important to note that the primary focus of this study was not on identifying the optimal model architecture but rather on examining the impact of different supervisory signals and training strategies. Future efforts could explore more advanced network architectures to further enhance the deraining performance. While our approach effectively removes rain steaks, it does not directly address other weather-related challenges, such as raindrops on windshields or splashes from preceding vehicles, which can also impair visibility. Expanding the scope to tackle these challenges would be another valuable direction for future investigation.

Additionally, like most existing studies, this work focuses on single-image deraining. Accounting for temporal dynamics across consecutive image frames, such as through direct sequential frame modeling, holds great potential to further improve performance. Finally, leveraging real-world driving datasets that capture a wide range of weather scenarios is expected to enhance the robustness and adaptability of deraining models in practical applications.

Author Contributions: Conceptualization, J.J.Y. and N.X.; methodology, J.J.Y. and N.X.; software, N.X.; validation, N.X. and J.J.Y.; formal analysis, N.X.; investigation, N.X. and J.J.Y.; resources, J.J.Y.; data curation, N.X.; writing—original draft preparation, N.X.; writing—review and editing, J.J.Y.; visualization, N.X. and J.J.Y.; supervision, J.J.Y.; project administration, J.J.Y. All authors have read and agreed to the published version of the manuscript.

Funding: This research received no external funding.

Institutional Review Board Statement: Not applicable.

Informed Consent Statement: Not applicable.

Data Availability Statement: Three publicly accessible datasets were used, including RainKITTI2012, RainKITTI2015 Datasets, and RainCityScapes.

Conflicts of Interest: The authors declare no conflicts of interest.

References

1. Zhao, Z.Q.; Zheng, P.; Xu, S.t.; Wu, X. Object detection with deep learning: A review. *IEEE Trans. Neural Netw. Learn. Syst.* **2019**, *30*, 3212–3232. [CrossRef] [PubMed]
2. Logothetis, N.K.; Sheinberg, D.L. Visual object recognition. *Annu. Rev. Neurosci.* **1996**, *19*, 577–621. [CrossRef] [PubMed]
3. Kang, L.W.; Lin, C.W.; Fu, Y.H. Automatic single-image-based rain streaks removal via image decomposition. *IEEE Trans. Image Process.* **2011**, *21*, 1742–1755. [CrossRef] [PubMed]
4. Yurtsever, E.; Lambert, J.; Carballo, A.; Takeda, K. A survey of autonomous driving: Common practices and emerging technologies. *IEEE Access* **2020**, *8*, 58443–58469. [CrossRef]
5. Garg, K.; Nayar, S.K. Vision and rain. *Int. J. Comput. Vis.* **2007**, *75*, 3–27. [CrossRef]
6. Chen, Y.L.; Hsu, C.T. A generalized low-rank appearance model for spatio-temporally correlated rain streaks. In Proceedings of the IEEE International Conference on Computer Vision, Sydney, Australia, 1–8 December 2013; pp. 1968–1975.
7. Gu, S.; Meng, D.; Zuo, W.; Zhang, L. Joint convolutional analysis and synthesis sparse representation for single image layer separation. In Proceedings of the IEEE International Conference on Computer Vision, Venice, Italy, 22–29 October 2017; pp. 1708–1716.
8. Luo, Y.; Xu, Y.; Ji, H. Removing rain from a single image via discriminative sparse coding. In Proceedings of the IEEE International Conference on Computer Vision, Santiago, Chile, 7–13 December 2015; pp. 3397–3405.
9. Zhang, K.; Luo, W.; Yu, Y.; Ren, W.; Zhao, F.; Li, C.; Ma, L.; Liu, W.; Li, H. Beyond monocular deraining: Parallel stereo deraining network via semantic prior. *Int. J. Comput. Vis.* **2022**, *130*, 1754–1769. [CrossRef]
10. Ren, D.; Zuo, W.; Hu, Q.; Zhu, P.; Meng, D. Progressive image deraining networks: A better and simpler baseline. In Proceedings of the IEEE/CVF Conference on Computer Vision and Pattern Recognition, Long Beach, CA, USA, 15–20 June 2019; pp. 3937–3946.
11. Chen, X.; Pan, J.; Dong, J. Bidirectional multi-scale implicit neural representations for image deraining. In Proceedings of the IEEE/CVF Conference on Computer Vision and Pattern Recognition, Seattle, WA, USA, 16–22 June 2024; pp. 25627–25636.
12. Hou, Z.; Torkamani, M.; Krim, H.; Liu, X. Robustness Reprogramming for Representation Learning. *arXiv* **2024**, arXiv:2410.04577.
13. Zhang, H.; Patel, V.M. Convolutional sparse and low-rank coding-based rain streak removal. In Proceedings of the 2017 IEEE Winter conference on applications of computer vision (WACV), Santa Rosa, CA, USA, 24–31 March 2017; IEEE: Piscataway, NJ, USA, 2017; pp. 1259–1267.
14. Zhu, L.; Fu, C.W.; Lischinski, D.; Heng, P.A. Joint bi-layer optimization for single-image rain streak removal. In Proceedings of the IEEE International Conference on Computer Vision, Venice, Italy, 22–29 October 2017; pp. 2526–2534.

15. Li, Y.; Tan, R.T.; Guo, X.; Lu, J.; Brown, M.S. Rain streak removal using layer priors. In Proceedings of the IEEE Conference on Computer Vision and Pattern Recognition, Las Vegas, NV, USA, 27–30 June 2016; pp. 2736–2744.
16. Fu, X.; Huang, J.; Ding, X.; Liao, Y.; Paisley, J. Clearing the skies: A deep network architecture for single-image rain removal. *IEEE Trans. Image Process.* **2017**, *26*, 2944–2956. [CrossRef] [PubMed]
17. Goodfellow, I.; Pouget-Abadie, J.; Mirza, M.; Xu, B.; Warde-Farley, D.; Ozair, S.; Courville, A.; Bengio, Y. Generative adversarial networks. *Commun. ACM* **2020**, *63*, 139–144. [CrossRef]
18. Yadav, S.; Mehra, A.; Rohmetra, H.; Ratnakumar, R.; Narang, P. DerainGAN: Single image deraining using wasserstein GAN. *Multimed. Tools Appl.* **2021**, *80*, 36491–36507. [CrossRef]
19. Zamir, S.W.; Arora, A.; Khan, S.; Hayat, M.; Khan, F.S.; Yang, M.H. Restormer: Efficient transformer for high-resolution image restoration. In Proceedings of the IEEE/CVF Conference on Computer Vision and Pattern Recognition, New Orleans, LA, USA, 18–24 June 2022; pp. 5728–5739.
20. Rombach, R.; Blattmann, A.; Lorenz, D.; Esser, P.; Ommer, B. High-resolution image synthesis with latent diffusion models. In Proceedings of the IEEE/CVF Conference on Computer Vision and Pattern Recognition, New Orleans, LA, USA, 18–24 June 2022; pp. 10684–10695.
21. Liu, J.; Wang, Q.; Fan, H.; Wang, Y.; Tang, Y.; Qu, L. Residual denoising diffusion models. In Proceedings of the IEEE/CVF Conference on Computer Vision and Pattern Recognition, Seattle, WA, USA, 16–22 June 2024; pp. 2773–2783.
22. Hu, X.; Fu, C.W.; Zhu, L.; Heng, P.A. Depth-attentional features for single-image rain removal. In Proceedings of the IEEE/CVF Conference on Computer Vision and Pattern Recognition, Long Beach, CA, USA, 15–20 June 2019; pp. 8022–8031.
23. Guo, X.; Fu, X.; Zhou, M.; Huang, Z.; Peng, J.; Zha, Z.J. Exploring Fourier Prior for Single Image Rain Removal. *IJCAI* **2022**, 935–941.
24. Johnson, J.; Alahi, A.; Fei-Fei, L. Perceptual losses for real-time style transfer and super-resolution. In Proceedings of the Computer Vision–ECCV 2016: 14th European Conference, Amsterdam, The Netherlands, 11–14 October 2016; Proceedings, Part II 14; Springer: Berlin/Heidelberg, Germany, 2016; pp. 694–711.
25. Yang, W.; Tan, R.T.; Feng, J.; Liu, J.; Guo, Z.; Yan, S. Deep joint rain detection and removal from a single image. In Proceedings of the IEEE Conference on Computer Vision and Pattern Recognition, Honolulu, HI, USA, 21–26 July 2017; pp. 1357–1366.
26. Hu, X.; Zhu, L.; Wang, T.; Fu, C.W.; Heng, P.A. Single-image real-time rain removal based on depth-guided non-local features. *IEEE Trans. Image Process.* **2021**, *30*, 1759–1770. [CrossRef]
27. Sakaridis, C.; Dai, D.; Van Gool, L. Semantic foggy scene understanding with synthetic data. *Int. J. Comput. Vis.* **2018**, *126*, 973–992. [CrossRef]
28. Geiger, A.; Lenz, P.; Urtasun, R. Are we ready for Autonomous Driving? The KITTI Vision Benchmark Suite. In Proceedings of the Conference on Computer Vision and Pattern Recognition (CVPR), Providence, RI, USA, 16–21 June 2012.
29. Cordts, M.; Omran, M.; Ramos, S.; Rehfeld, T.; Enzweiler, M.; Benenson, R.; Franke, U.; Roth, S.; Schiele, B. The cityscapes dataset for semantic urban scene understanding. In Proceedings of the IEEE Conference on Computer Vision and Pattern Recognition, Las Vegas, NV, USA, 27–30 June 2016; pp. 3213–3223.
30. Huynh-Thu, Q.; Ghanbari, M. Scope of validity of PSNR in image/video quality assessment. *Electron. Lett.* **2008**, *44*, 800–801. [CrossRef]
31. Wang, Z.; Bovik, A.C.; Sheikh, H.R.; Simoncelli, E.P. Image quality assessment: From error visibility to structural similarity. *IEEE Trans. Image Process.* **2004**, *13*, 600–612. [CrossRef] [PubMed]
32. Paszke, A.; Gross, S.; Chintala, S.; Chanan, G.; Yang, E.; DeVito, Z.; Lin, Z.; Desmaison, A.; Antiga, L.; Lerer, A. Automatic Differentiation in Pytorch. 2017. Available online: https://openreview.net/forum?id=BJJsrmfCZ (accessed on 29 November 2024).
33. Kingma, D.P. Adam: A method for stochastic optimization. *arXiv* **2014**, arXiv:1412.6980.
34. Zhang, H.; Patel, V.M. Density-aware single image de-raining using a multi-stream dense network. In Proceedings of the IEEE Conference on Computer Vision and Pattern Recognition, Salt Lake City, UT, USA, 18–23 June 2018; pp. 695–704.
35. Khanam, R.; Hussain, M. YOLOv11: An Overview of the Key Architectural Enhancements. *arXiv* **2024**, arXiv:2410.17725.

computers

MDPI

Article

Atrial Fibrillation Type Classification by a Convolutional Neural Network Using Contrast-Enhanced Computed Tomography Images

Hina Kotani [1], Atsushi Teramoto [2,*], Tomoyuki Ohno [3], Yoshihiro Sobue [4], Eiichi Watanabe [4] and Hiroshi Fujita [5]

[1] Graduate School of Health Sciences, Fujita Health University, Toyoake 470-1192, Japan; hina.0306rv@gmail.com
[2] Faculty of Information Engineering, Meijo University, Nagoya 468-8502, Japan
[3] Department of Radiation, Fujita Health University Bantane Hospital, Nagoya 454-8509, Japan
[4] Department of Internal Medicine, Fujita Health University Bantane Hospital, Nagoya 454-8509, Japan
[5] Faculty of Engineering, Gifu University, Gifu 501-1193, Japan
* Correspondence: teramoto@meijo-u.ac.jp

Abstract: Catheter ablation therapy, which is a treatment for atrial fibrillation (AF), has a higher recurrence rate as AF duration increases. Compared to paroxysmal AF (PAF), sustained AF is known to cause progressive anatomic remodeling of the left atrium, resulting in enlargement and shape changes. In this study, we used contrast-enhanced computed tomography (CT) to classify atrial fibrillation (AF) into paroxysmal atrial fibrillation (PAF) and long-term persistent atrial fibrillation (LSAF), which have particularly different recurrence rates after catheter ablation. Contrast-enhanced CT images of 30 patients with PAF and 30 patients with LSAF were input into six pretrained convolutional neural networks (CNNs) for the binary classification of PAF and LSAF. In this study, we propose a method that can recognize information regarding the body axis direction of the left atrium by inputting five slices near the left atrium. The classification was visualized by obtaining a saliency map based on score-class activation mapping (CAM). Furthermore, we surveyed cardiologists regarding the classification of AF types, and the results of the CNN classification were compared with the results of physicians' clinical judgment. The proposed method achieved the highest correct classification rate (81.7%). In particular, models with shallow layers, such as VGGNet and ResNet, are able to capture the overall characteristics of the image and therefore are likely to be suitable for focusing on the left atrium. In many cases, patients with an enlarged left atrium tended to have long-lasting AF, confirming the validity of the proposed method. The results of the saliency map and survey of physicians' basis for judgment showed that many patients tended to focus on the shape of the left atrium in both classifications, suggesting that this method can classify atrial fibrillation more accurately than physicians, similar to the judgment criteria of physicians.

Keywords: atrial fibrillation; catheter ablation; classification; convolutional neural network; contrast-enhanced computed tomography; deep learning

1. Introduction

The number of patients with atrial fibrillation (AF) is increasing annually, and this trend is naturally related to the aging of the population [1]. In recent years, the aging of patients with AF has brought to light clinical problems that were previously invisible. The European Society of Cardiology (ESC) notes that six main problems are closely associated with AF: mortality, stroke, hospitalization, reduced quality of life, left ventricular dysfunction/heart failure, and cognitive decline/vascular dementia [2]. Therefore, the early detection and treatment of AF are important to prevent complications. AF is a disease that gradually shortens the interval between attacks over time, eventually becoming persistent, long-lasting, and permanent. Thus, atrial fibrillation can be viewed as a disease that progresses through various stages [3]. Catheter ablation therapy, which is a treatment for AF, has been shown to be effective for paroxysmal atrial fibrillation (PAF). However, its efficacy is not well established in non-pharmacological guidelines for persistent atrial fibrillation and long-standing persistent atrial fibrillation (LSAF), for which the recommended level is Class IIa or Class IIb [4]. In other words, it is very important to determine which patients with persistent atrial fibrillation will benefit from catheter ablation therapy based on the results and possible complications of catheter ablation therapy for persistent AF, as described above [5]. However, it is difficult to predict postoperative recurrence, and the indications for catheter ablation therapy are currently determined based on the surgeon's empirical judgment and the patient's self-reported AF duration.

AF recurrence after catheter ablation therapy and its predictors have been the subject of many studies [6–9]. Njoku et al. showed that left atrial diameter predicts AF recurrence after radiofrequency catheter ablation treatment in a meta-analysis of the difference in left atrial volume between patients with and without recurrent AF after radiofrequency catheter ablation [6]. Other factors, such as the duration of AF, structural changes in the left atrium and pulmonary veins, and age, may also affect the outcome of catheter ablation therapy.

In recent years, many methods have been reported to classify AF types [10,11], and Nuria Ortigosa et al. proposed a method to classify AF subtypes with feature extraction from a general Fourier time-frequency transform using ECG waveforms and classification using a support vector machine [8]. The classification accuracy of the test data was approximately 77%. However, classification using ECG waveforms is often limited by the possibility of significant changes in the waveform characteristics when other diseases coexist.

Therefore, we attempted to classify AF types by extracting image features, such as left atrial diameter and structural changes in pulmonary veins due to persistent AF, from contrast-enhanced computed tomography (CT) images using convolutional neural networks (CNNs), which have been applied in medical practice in recent years [12–18]. Although previous studies using electrocardiogram waveforms have been reported in the classification of AF type, no method using contrast-enhanced CT images has been proposed. Furthermore, although there are research papers on the relationship between left atrial volume and AF type, there are no reported cases of applying that method to the classification of the type of disease. In this study, we propose a clinically novel method of classifying paroxysmal AF and long-term persistent AF on contrast-enhanced CT images using conventional CNN models, focusing on structural remodeling changes in the left atrium. The purpose of this study is to enable a standardized assessment using a deep learning approach that considers the information physicians need to evaluate the structural remodeling of the left atrium, including left atrial enlargement, poor contrast, structural changes in the pulmonary veins, the presence of thrombi in the left atrium, and coronary artery calcification. Based on this objective, contrast-enhanced CT imaging has an advantage over other dynamic modalities in that it can accurately capture the shape and focus on the structures around the left atrium. Furthermore, we hypothesize that the method using contrast-enhanced CT images will enable standardized evaluation with reduced subjective bias, even in cases in which the ECG waveform cannot detect sudden attacks, such as paroxysmal AF, or when there are concomitant diseases that may affect the ECG waveform. With the application of these systems to clinical workflows, it will be possible to evaluate the load on the atrial muscle when AF is first detected and, if signs of long-term persistence are confirmed, to begin treatment early.

In this study, we also compared the results of the CNN classification with those of physicians' clinical judgment by surveying cardiologists regarding AF type classification. Physicians estimate the type of atrial fibrillation based on factors such as the size of the left atrium, enlargement of the pulmonary veins, thrombus formation in the left atrial appendage, and fibrosis of the atrial septum. Focusing on these features, we looked at images similar to those entered into the CNN to predict the corresponding disease type.

2. Materials and Methods

2.1. Outline

In this study, target slices were selected from contrast-enhanced CT images. The number of images was increased using data augmentation and then input into a CNN model. The output images were classified into two classes, PAF and LSAF, and the saliency map, which emphasized the pixels that contributed to the classification result using score-CAM according to their importance, was used to compare what each model focused on in the image to make its judgment. Persistent atrial fibrillation was excluded because its duration varies widely from 7 days to less than 1 year, making it difficult to accurately identify through the evaluation of the left atrial shape. This study was conducted with the approval of the ethics committee of the first author's institution (approval number HM22-095).

2.2. Image Dataset

This study included 60 patients with AF who underwent CE-CT at Fujita Health University Bantane Hospital between May 2021 and July 2022. A total of 162 contrast-enhanced CT scans were performed during the period, including 116 patients with paroxysmal atrial fibrillation and 46 patients with long-standing persistent atrial fibrillation. From these, 30 patients of each disease type were randomly selected, and only those patients who did not undergo CT examinations due to contrast medium allergy or impaired renal function were excluded. The patients' disease types were diagnosed as defined in the guidelines [4]. Specifically, PAF was defined as AF that returns to sinus rhythm within 7 days of onset, and LSAF was defined as AF that persists beyond 1 year. The percentages of PAF and LSAF were each half of all patients. Basic patient information is shown in Table 1. An Aquilion ONE CT system (Canon Medical Systems, Inc., Tochigi, Japan) was used to obtain the images. The details of the imaging protocol are shown in Table 2. We used transaxial images with a matrix size of 512 × 512 pixels and a pixel size of 0.625 mm. The images were stored in DICOM format, and all images were converted to 8-bit PNG images with a window level of 30HU and a window width of 1000 HU.

Table 1. Basic patient information.

Variables	PAF(N = 30)	LSAF(N = 30)	*p*-Value
Age (years) (mean ± SD)	65.3 ± 12.4	69.5 ± 8.6	0.093
Gender (male, %)	19(63.3%)	25(83.3%)	0.082
Height (cm) (mean ± SD)	164.23 ± 10.2	168.2 ± 8.75	0.131
Body weight (kg) (mean ± SD)	63.7 ± 12.4	68.7 ± 11.1	0.104
BMI (mean ± SD)	23.5 ± 3.35	24.3 ± 3.42	0.309
Hypertension (cases, %)	13(43.3%)	14(46.7%)	0.799
Diabetes mellitus (cases, %)	5(16.7%)	5(16.7%)	1.000
Heart failure (cases, %)	3(10.0%)	12(40.0%)	0.007
Cerebral infarction (cases, %)	4(13.3%)	5(16.7%)	0.723

Table 2. Imaging protocols.

Parameter		Value
Imaging protocols	kV	120 kV
	mAs	CT-AEC
	Slice thickness	0.5 mm
	Scan time	0.35 s
	Scan method	ECG gated volume scan

Table 2. *Cont.*

Parameter		Value
Reconstruction condition	Reconstruction method	AIDR-3D
	FOV	200 mm
	Slice thickness	0.5 mm
	Slice spacing	0.25 mm
	Reconstruction function	FC14
	Reconstruction cardiac phase	Systolic
Angiographic method	Iodine concentration	375 mgI/kg
	Injection time	15 s
	Imaging timing	Bolus tracking

2.3. *Atrial Fibrillation Type Classification Using Contrast-Enhanced CT Images*

The flow of this study is shown in Figure 1, and the details of each process are described below.

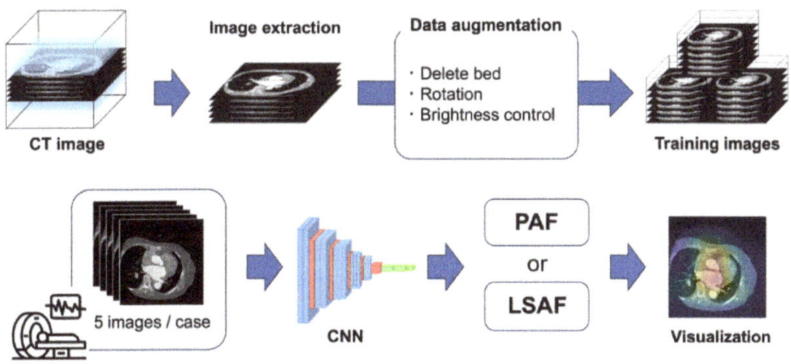

Figure 1. Process of this study.

2.3.1. Image Pre-Processing

Images centered on the slice, with the largest left atrium in the contrast-enhanced CT image and located 5 and 10 mm above and below, were selected, and five images per patient were used for analysis. If a bed was depicted in the image, it was removed by manually setting the CT value of the bed area to −1000 HU.

2.3.2. Data Augmentation

Data augmentation is a method of increasing data by "transforming" image data for training. For example, by rotating, flipping, shifting horizontally, scaling, distorting, adjusting brightness and contrast, and adding noise to an image, various variations can be created. In this study, the number of images increased nine times through data augmentation [19]. CT examinations are usually performed in the supine position; however, in some facilities, the patient is positioned so that the heart, which is located on the left side of the body, is centered in the FOV. In such cases, the curvature of the bed may cause the body to rotate about 10°. To simulate this, the heart was rotated by −10° and +10° for each image, aligning the heart's tilt to match that observed in the actual CT image. In contrast-enhanced CT examinations, since the density of the contrast agent varies depending on the case, we augmented the pixel values to be robust to changes in pixel values. The CT values of the left atrium were observed across the entire dataset, and the window level (WL) and window width (WW) were adjusted so that the CT values after augmentation fell within the range of real CT images. As a result, in addition to the initial condition of WL = 30, WW = 1000, two variations, including WL = −50, WW = 950 and WL = 160, WW = 1500, were added to increase the number of images threefold. An example of the created image is shown in Figure 2.

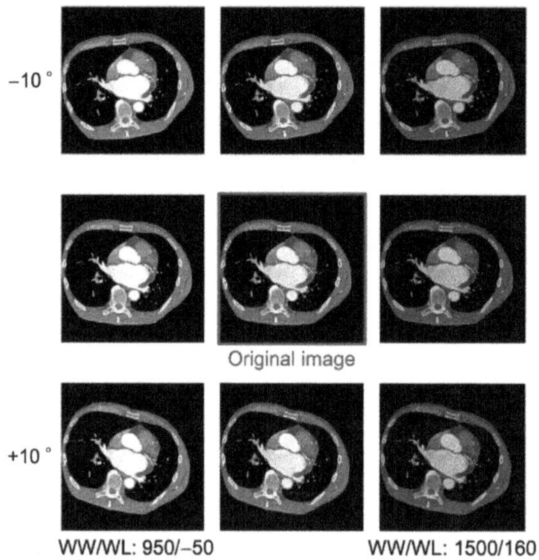

Figure 2. Examples of an original image and images created using data augmentation.

2.3.3. Classification by CNN

In this study, we used six network models (VGG16, VGG19, Resnet50, DenseNet121, DenseNet169, and DenseNet201). These networks were trained on 1.2 million images across 1000 categories in the ImageNet database [20–22]. To adapt these networks to PAF and LSAF classification, we removed the fully connected layers in each of the pretrained network models and replaced them with three new fully connected layers (the final layer being the output layer). The number of units in each layer was set to 1024, 256, and 2. In this study, finetuning was employed. Finetuning is a method to perform transfer learning using a different dataset for a different target task than the one used during pre-training that involves using a network model that has been pretrained from a large dataset as the initial parameters. Finetuning facilitates the learning of highly accurate models for each task from small datasets by simply recalibrating pretrained CNNs. In this case, the weights of the convolutional layer were initialized with the pretrained weights, and both the convolutional and fully connected layers were retrained (finetuning) using real images. The average of five continuous values obtained from the outputs of five slices output from the CNN was used as the patient's evaluation. In this evaluation, the cutoff value was fixed at 0.5.

For the CNN training conditions, we used a learning coefficient of 0.000001, early stopping (maximum number of epochs: 100) as the training frequency, a batch size of eight, and Adam as the optimization algorithm. The categorical cross entropy was employed for the loss function in the training of CNN. The training environment used was Windows 10 Pro OS, an AMD Ryzen 7 2700X CPU, and an NVIDIA TITAN RTX GPU.

2.4. *Saliency Map*

In this study, we used score-class activation mapping (CAM) to visualize the points of interest by highlighting the pixels that contributed to the classification results according to their importance. Score-CAM eliminates the dependence on gradients by obtaining the weight of each activation map through its forward passing score on the target class; the final result is obtained using a linear combination of weights and activation maps [23]. It visualizes the importance based on the results obtained by providing the generated images to the CNN using the feature map obtained when the trained CNN infers a specific image. The resulting feature map was enlarged to the size of the input, normalized to a value between 0 and 1, and multiplied by the input image to generate a heatmap. The output of CAM is shown as a heatmap overlaid on the image. This heatmap is called a saliency map in CAM. The input and saliency map images are shown in Figure 3.

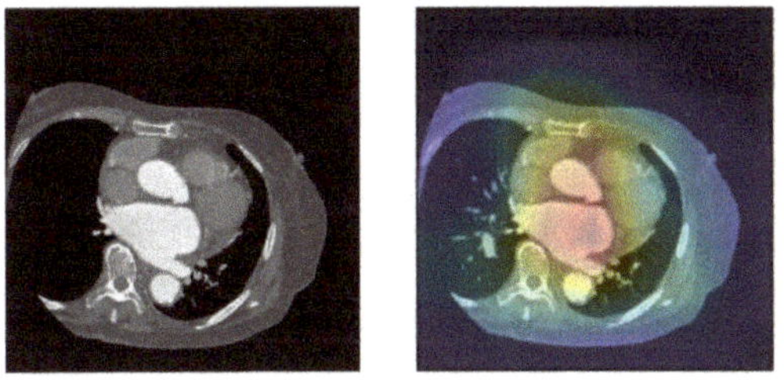

(a) (b)

Figure 3. An example of visualization of decision basis in CNN (score-CAM). (**a**) Input image; (**b**) saliency map image.

2.5. Validation and Evaluation Metrics

In this study, cross-validation was used to assess the generalizability of the model. We also increased the number of folds and chose 10-fold cross-validation to improve generalization performance and reduce bias. The 10-fold cross-validation method divides the dataset into 10 subsets, 70% of which are training data and 20% of which are validation data, 10% of which are test data. Figure 4 shows a schematic of the 10-part cross-validation method.

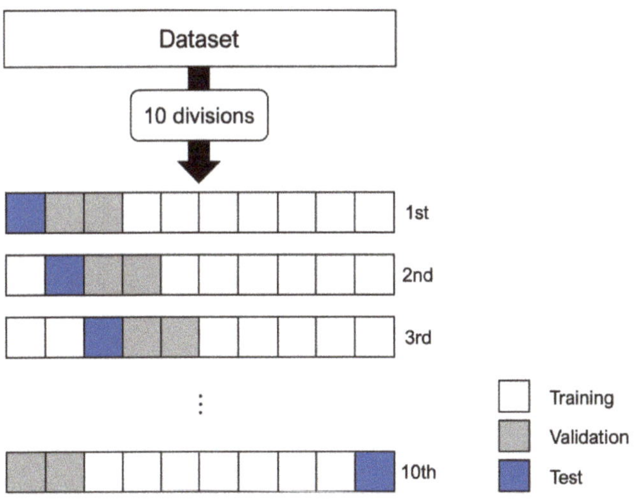

Figure 4. Data assignment in the 10-part cross-validation method.

Using this method, the prediction results were compared based on patient-specific accuracy, sensitivity, specificity, and precision. The final classification performance evaluation was performed by determining the overall accuracy rate using the CNN classification results. The overall accuracy rate was calculated using the following Equation (1). TP,

TN, FP, and FN are the numbers of true positives, true negatives, false positives, and false negatives, respectively.

$$\text{accuracy} = \frac{\text{TP} + \text{TN}}{\text{TP} + \text{TN} + \text{FP} + \text{FN}} \times 100[\%] \tag{1}$$

The ROC curve represents the relationship between the true positive fraction (TP/TP + FN) and the false positive fraction (FP/FP + TN). It was created by plotting the false positive rate on the horizontal axis and the true positive rate on the vertical axis and continuously varying the cutoff value to separate positive and negative results. To smooth the ROC curve, the false positive fraction (FPF) and true positive fraction (TPF) were plotted on both normal probability papers to obtain an approximately straight line, and the curve depicted the relationship between the two.

The CNN was trained and evaluated thrice for each model, with the median value and standard deviation used as the final classification result. In this study, the slice with the largest left atrium and the two slices above and below it were used for training and evaluation to enable continuous evaluation of the left atrium in the direction of the body axis. In addition, the number of images used for training increased with data augmentation. To demonstrate the effectiveness of these methods, we performed an additional validation using only one central slice for training and evaluation (Additional Study 1) and a validation using an evaluation without data augmentation (Additional Study 2).

2.6. *Classification by Physicians*

In this study, we administered the same questionnaire to physicians regarding the classification of atrial fibrillation types based on only five images entered into the CNN classification, and the results were compared with the correct response rate and focus of the CNN classification.

2.6.1. Participants

A questionnaire survey was conducted among physicians in the Department of Cardiovascular Medicine at Fujita Health University Bantane Hospital, and responses were obtained from 18 physicians. In this survey, we asked patients to evaluate the type of AF in terms of structural changes around the left atrium. The purpose of this questionnaire was to compare the results of this study's classification with those of the physicians' clinical judgments.

2.6.2. Questionnaire Items

Questions included: (1) years of experience as a physician, (2) specialty, (3) number of catheter ablation procedures performed per year, (4) whether preoperative CT imaging could predict the efficacy of catheter ablation, and (5) type classification of atrial fibrillation (20 cases) and the basis for decision.

(3) The number of catheter ablation procedures performed in a year and (4) whether preoperative CT images could predict the efficacy of catheter ablation procedures were optional answers for physicians performing catheter ablation procedures. For AF classification (5), 10 cases of paroxysmal PAF and 10 cases of LSAF were randomly selected from the cases used in the CNN classification, and the results were tabulated on a 6-point scale. In addition, the basis for judgment was asked, e.g., "Please tell us the reason why you answered that way", for the answer of the disease type classification, and the answer was left open-ended. This question aimed to compare the points of interest of the CNN with those of physicians.

3. Results

3.1. Classification Results by CNN

First, we describe the results of the AF type classification using a CNN. The classification results and AUC for the six CNN models are listed in Table 3, and the ROC curves are shown in Figure 5. ResNet50 exhibited the highest accuracy for all classification results.

Table 3. Classification results for each CNN model (proposed method).

Model	Sensitivity	Specificity	Precision	Accuracy	AUC
VGG16	80.0 ± 1.56	63.3 ± 4.71	68.6 ± 3.28	71.7 ± 2.84	0.80 ± 0.03
VGG19	80.0 ± 1.56	76.7 ± 4.15	77.4 ± 2.54	78.3 ± 1.56	0.79 ± 0.00
ResNet50	83.3 ± 5.65	80.0 ± 4.15	80.6 ± 3.27	81.7 ± 3.60	0.88 ± 0.07
DenseNet121	76.7 ± 4.71	66.7 ± 3.16	69.7 ± 2.68	71.7 ± 3.45	0.80 ± 0.02
DenseNet169	80.0 ± 2.74	63.3 ± 4.15	68.6 ± 2.59	71.7 ± 2.08	0.76 ± 0.03
DenseNet201	83.3 ± 3.11	63.3 ± 4.16	69.4 ± 2.63	73.3 ± 2.36	0.82 ± 0.01

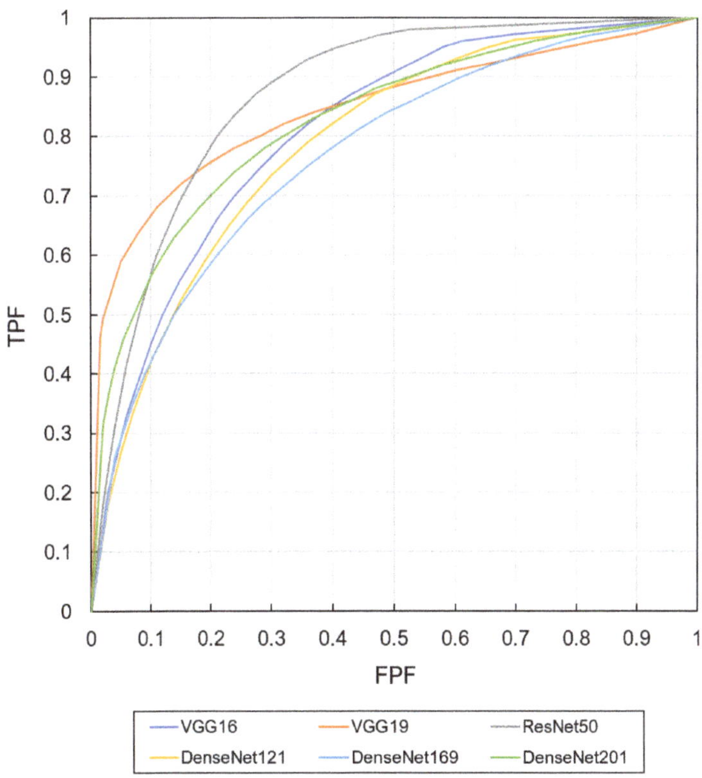

Figure 5. ROC curves of CNN models.

The results of the additional validation are presented in Tables 4 and 5. In addition, Figure 6 shows a comparison of the classification correctness rate between the proposed method and Additional Studies 1 and 2. When learning and evaluation were performed on the central slice only (Additional Study 1), the classification correctness increased for VGG16, VGG19, and ResNet50 but decreased for the other three DenseNet models. Without augmentation of the training data (Additional Study 2), the accuracy remained the same or decreased for models other than DenseNet169.

Table 4. Classification results for evaluation of central slices only (Additional Study 1).

Model	Sensitivity	Specificity	Precision	Accuracy	AUC
VGG16	76.7 ± 1.52	63.3 ± 4.71	67.6 ± 3.34	70.0 ± 2.84	0.75 ± 0.02
VGG19	70.0 ± 4.16	80.0 ± 1.56	77.8 ± 2.05	75.0 ± 2.36	0.78 ± 0.01
ResNet50	73.3 ± 3.16	76.7 ± 2.74	75.9 ± 1.39	75.0 ± 0.80	0.83 ± 0.01
DenseNet121	73.3 ± 1.56	80.0 ± 1.56	78.6 ± 1.27	76.7 ± 0.80	0.82 ± 0.01
DenseNet169	73.3 ± 2.74	76.7 ± 0.00	75.9 ± 0.69	75.0 ± 1.39	0.77 ± 0.01
DenseNet201	66.7 ± 3.11	83.3 ± 0.00	80.0 ± 0.71	75.0 ± 1.56	0.82 ± 0.02

Table 5. Classification results without data augmentation (Additional Study 2).

Model	Sensitivity	Specificity	Precision	Accuracy	AUC
VGG16	66.7 ± 3.11	76.7 ± 4.15	74.1 ± 3.98	71.7 ± 2.81	0.75 ± 0.03
VGG19	63.3 ± 4.16	66.7 ± 6.27	65.5 ± 5.26	65.0 ± 4.08	0.70 ± 0.03
ResNet50	60.0 ± 5.43	83.3 ± 4.16	78.3 ± 2.11	71.7 ± 0.75	0.81 ± 0.01
DenseNet121	63.3 ± 1.56	70.0 ± 6.86	67.9 ± 6.19	66.7 ± 3.60	0.72 ± 0.04
DenseNet169	70.0 ± 2.69	76.7 ± 0.00	75.0 ± 0.73	73.3 ± 1.35	0.77 ± 0.02
DenseNet201	63.3 ± 4.16	83.3 ± 1.60	79.2 ± 2.50	73.3 ± 3.37	0.84 ± 0.02

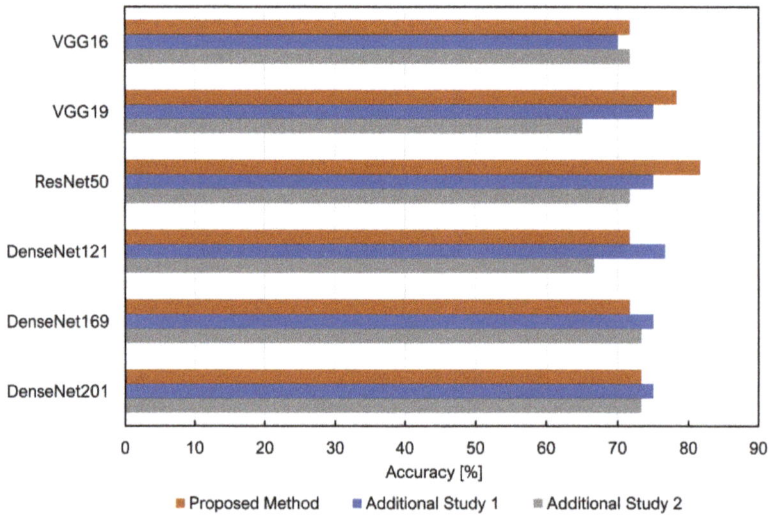

Figure 6. Comparison of proposed method and additional study.

The images that were correctly classified by ResNet50 are shown in Figure 7, and those that were incorrectly classified are shown in Figure 8.

Figure 9 shows the saliency map output when ResNet50 correctly classifies a case, and Figure 10 shows the heatmap output when ResNet50 incorrectly classifies a case. Note that the presented case is the same patient as the one presented in Figures 7 and 8.

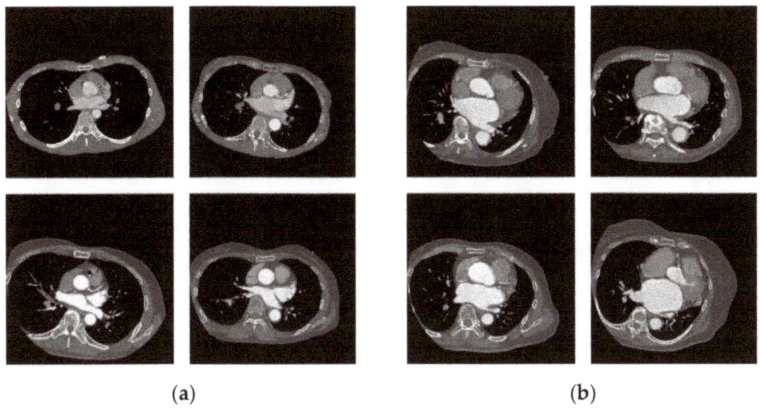

Figure 7. Correctly classified cases. (a) PAF; (b) LSAF.

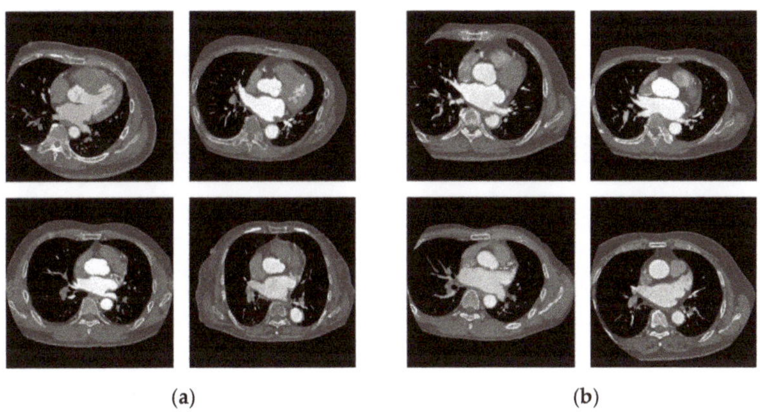

Figure 8. Incorrectly classified cases. (a) PAF; (b) LSAF.

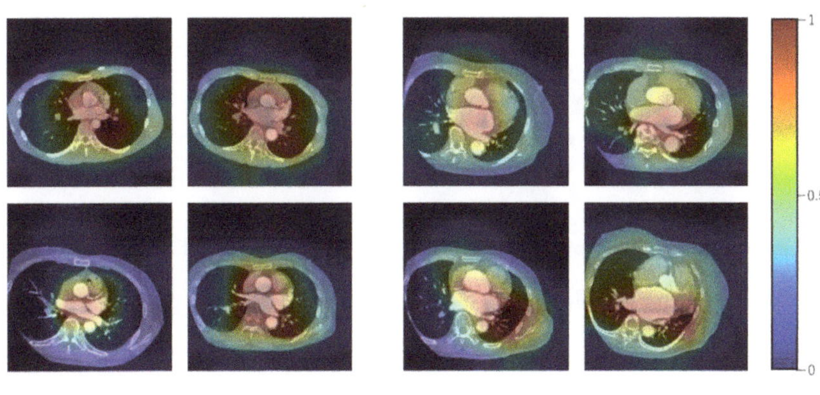

Figure 9. Saliency maps of correctly classified cases. (a) PAF; (b) LSAF.

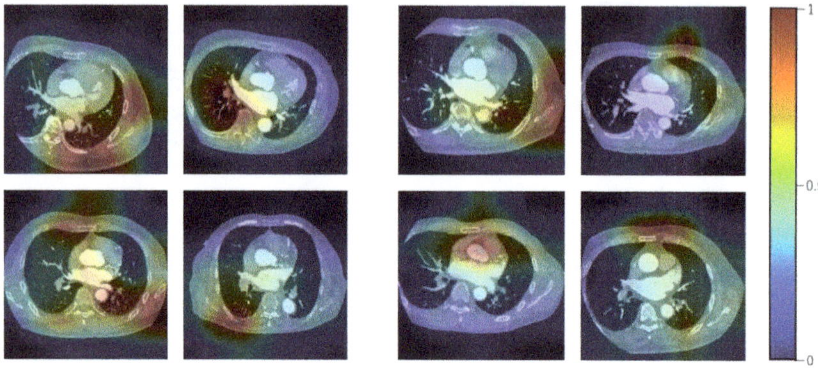

(a) (b)

Figure 10. Saliency maps of incorrectly classified cases. (**a**) PAF; (**b**) LSAF.

3.2. Classification Results by Physicians

Table 6 shows the number (%) of responses to each of the following questions: (1) years of experience as a physician, (2) specialty, and (3) number of catheter ablation therapies performed per year. In Case (2), all 18 physicians specialized in cardiovascular medicine.

Table 6. Survey results on years of experience as a physician and areas of specialization.

Experience (years)	Responses (%)	Specialty	Responses (%)
5–10	3 (16.7)	cardiovascular	18 (100)
11–15	4 (22.2)		
16–20	7 (38.9)		
21–25	2 (11.1)		
26–30	1 (5.6)		
31–35	1 (5.6)		
Total	18 (100)	Total	18 (100)

Six physicians responded to question (3), the number of catheter ablation therapy performed in a year. The results are summarized in Table 7.

Table 7. Survey results of the number of catheter ablation therapies performed in a year.

Number of Treatments (Cases)	Responses (%)
1–50	2 (33.3)
51–100	2 (33.3)
101–150	1 (16.7)
151–200	1 (16.7)
Total	6 (100)

Nine physicians responded to the question about (4) whether preoperative CT images could predict the efficacy of catheter ablation therapy. Of these, eight physicians answered that preoperative contrast-enhanced CT could predict the efficacy of catheter ablation therapy.

Figure 11 shows the percentage of correct answers for the 20 cases used in the questionnaire classified by ResNet50, the percentage of correct answers for 18 physicians, and the average percentage for all physicians. In addition, Figure 12 shows the ROC of the physicians' classification results, and Table 8 shows details of the physicians' classification accuracy and AUC. The mean accuracy was 73.6% and the median was 75%. The mean

AUC was 0.802. The 20 cases used to evaluate ResNet50 were the same as those used in the survey of physicians, and the overall correct response rate for physicians was widely distributed, ranging from 55% to 90%; however, the average correct response rate was 73.6%, which was slightly lower than that of ResNet50.

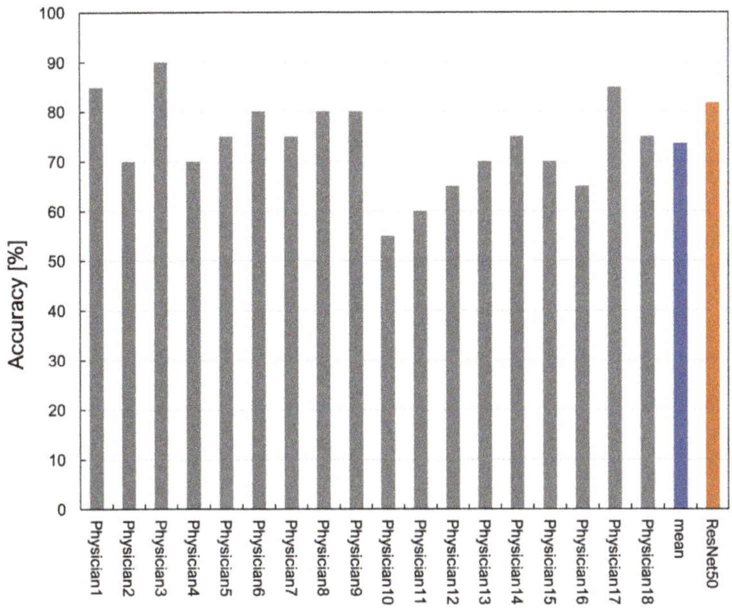

Figure 11. Physicians' classification results and comparison between CNN models.

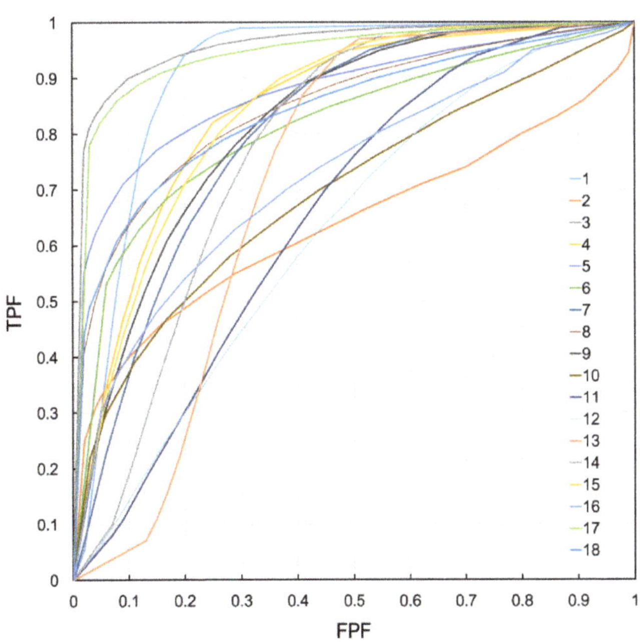

Figure 12. ROC curves of physicians.

Table 8. Physicians' classification results.

Physician	Accuracy(%)	AUC	Physician	Accuracy(%)	AUC
1	85.0	0.895	10	55.0	0.690
2	70.0	0.640	11	60.0	0.670
3	90.0	0.955	12	65.0	0.675
4	70.0	0.820	13	70.0	0.770
5	75.0	0.865	14	75.0	0.780
6	80.0	0.825	15	70.0	0.800
7	75.0	0.825	16	65.0	0.740
8	80.0	0.830	17	85.0	0.945
9	80.0	0.885	18	55.0	0.825

The respondents had diverse opinions based on their judgments. Generally, LSAF is characterized by left atrial enlargement, roundness of the left atrium, coronary artery calcification, left auricular enlargement, poor contrast, auricular thrombus closure, uneven contrast density, retraction of the comb muscle, atrial wall thickening, and fibrosis of the atrial septum. The most common finding of persistent atrial fibrillation is enlargement of the left atrium.

4. Discussion

4.1. Comparison of CNN Models

In this study, six CNN models were evaluated on their performance in classifying the AF types. ResNet50 performed the best in terms of overall accuracy, followed by VGG19. The reason these CNN outperformed DenseNet121, 169, and 201 could be that the number of layers in the network was shallow, which made it possible to extract features in a localized region. The long-term persistence of AF results in structural remodeling, such as left atrial shape changes and auricular enlargement, also affected the results. Therefore, ResNet50 and VGG19 should focus on these localized areas for classification purposes. The best overall correct response rate for ResNet50 was achieved because ResNet50 is optimized using a residual function and performs batch normalization for each residual block. We hypothesize that this resulted in stable learning without the gradient vanishing problem.

In addition, Figure 6 shows a comparison of the classification correctness rate between the proposed method and Additional Studies 1 and 2. In most cases, the proposed method performs better than Additional Studies 1 and 2. The reason for the better accuracy rate than that of Additional Study 1 is that the proposed method uses a total of five slices (located 5 mm above and below) centered on the slice with the most enlarged left atrium for training; therefore, it is possible to analyze information in the body axis direction, in addition to the slice direction, and classification is more accurate than when only one slice is used for evaluation. The reason for the higher rate of correct answers compared to Additional Study 2 is thought to be that the data augmentation increased the number of pseudo-variations because of the various body inclinations and CT values due to the contrast agent and was able to respond to the effects on the image caused during imaging. Furthermore, data augmentation increased the number of images used for training by a factor of nine; therefore, it was assumed that efficient training was possible.

4.2. Insights from Saliency Map in CNN Classifications

Score-CAM was used to output a color map showing the pixels contributing to the CNN classification results. In the heatmap output for the correct classification in Figure 8, the left atrium and pulmonary veins tended to attract more CNN attention. In addition, when attention was focused on structures other than the heart, which was often seen in the heatmap output when the patient was incorrectly classified, as shown in Figure 10, there was a tendency toward incorrect classification. Focusing on the left atrium, cases of PAF were misclassified with findings of major LSAF, including an enlarged left atrium, the loss of comb-like muscular structures, and large rounded anterior and posterior structural left atria. In the cases of LSAF, there was also a tendency to misclassify cases in which the left atrium was not enlarged, especially when the anteroposterior diameter of the left atrium was short. Based on these findings, CNN classification focuses on the shape and surrounding structures of the left atrium and is considered a valid classification for the findings of LSAF.

4.3. Comparison with Physician's Results

In response to the physician's description of the basis for judgment, enlargement of the left atrium is a feature of LSAF in many cases. In the correctly classified cases shown in Figure 7, (a) the PAF has a small, flat left atrial structure, whereas (b) the LSAF has a large, rounded left atrial structure in the front and back. The CNN model is expected to classify patients using the same criteria as physicians because the heatmap also shows that the left atrium area attracts more attention. The cases in which the CNN model and averaged results of the physicians' responses differed are shown in Figure 13. Case (a) involved LSAF, but the left atrium was relatively small (left), and there was no loss of the pectinate muscle structure (right). The CNN model can classify these cases. However, it was misclassified, even when the typical findings of LSAF in the size of the left atrium were observed, as shown in (b). The possible reason is that by using the entire CT image as the input image, information other than the left atrial region may have led to misclassification. This problem could be improved by increasing the variation with more training data and narrowing the field of view to the left atrial region alone.

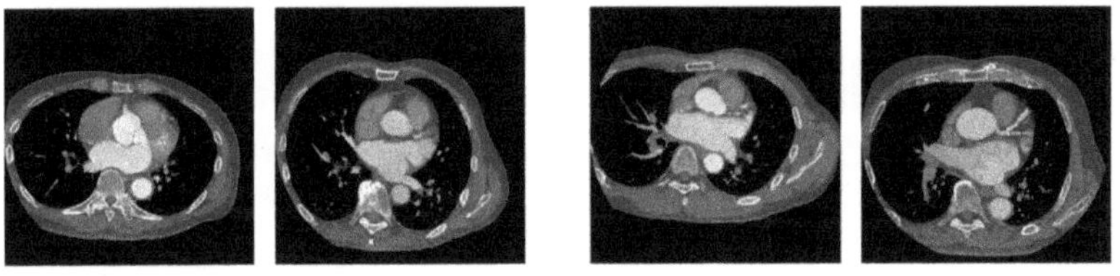

(a) (b)

Figure 13. LSAF cases with different results between physicians and the proposed method. (**a**) Correctly classified only by CNN model; (**b**) correctly classified only by physician.

4.4. Comparison with Previous Studies

The results of this study showed a higher accuracy than those of the study by Ortigosa et al. using ECG (classification accuracy rate 77.1%) [10]. Furthermore, the method of this study has the advantage of being able to classify the pathology of AF using the assessment of structural remodeling of the left atrium, even when other diseases that affect the ECG waveform are present at the same time. AF is usually detected using an ECG, but we think that the limitation of using an ECG is that the time of detection of an attack is considered to be the moment of the first appearance of the attack. The advantage of this study using contrast CT images is that it allows for an objective evaluation of the state of the atrium regardless of the type of disease. We think that by evaluating the stress on the atrial muscle when atrial fibrillation is first discovered and confirming long-term findings, it will be possible to get closer to starting treatment at an earlier stage.

4.5. Practical Applications in Clinical Settings

We hypothesize that by using deep learning to classify AF types from CT images, this study will facilitate a standardized assessment of structural remodeling of the left atrium, which was originally determined subjectively by physicians, thereby reducing subjective bias. By integrating these systems into clinical workflows, it will become possible to evaluate the strain on the atrial muscle at the initial detection of AF. Additionally, if signs of long-term persistence are confirmed, early treatment can be initiated. This approach could potentially reduce unnecessary catheter ablation procedures, allow for more tailored treatment recommendations, and decrease healthcare costs. Furthermore, computational resources and processing time need to be discussed for practical application. Although model training requires substantial hardware resources and prolonged processing time (2–5 h), we believe that once the model is trained, the prediction process can be completed in under one minute, making it sufficiently feasible for clinical use because of the reduced hardware requirements for inference.

4.6. Limitation of This Study

There are two limitations of this study. The first is that it is a small and single-facility dataset. Furthermore, potential confounding factors, such as patient comorbidities, are not discussed. When the number of data is increased and external validation is performed in the future, comorbidities should be included in the analysis and evaluated. In addition, contrast-enhanced CT provides a clearer image of the left atrium than simple CT, but patients who cannot use contrast media and variations in contrast media and image quality among facilities remain a challenge. We hypothesize that this challenge can be resolved by using simple CT images or by preparing a dataset that includes images taken at other facilities and performing data augmentation, as in this study. The second limitation is that the classification does not include persistent AF, which we think does not allow for continuous evaluation. The definition of the duration of persistent AF ranges from 7 days to less than 1 year, making it difficult to accurately identify it through the assessment of left atrial geometry. Therefore, persistent atrial fibrillation was excluded from classification in this study and classified as paroxysmal and long-standing persistent; these cases have predominantly different results in ablation therapy and can be evaluated for structural remodeling based on imaging features. In the future, it is necessary to develop a method to evaluate AF types continuously by adding cases of persistent AF. The use of left atrial volume, dynamic modality information, additional machine learning models, and natural language processing models is also possible and will be explored.

5. Conclusions

Catheter ablation therapy is a treatment for AF; however, its efficacy is not well established due to the high recurrence rate in patients with PAF. In this study, we attempted to classify AF types using a convolutional neural network based on features obtained from contrast-enhanced CT images. As a result of the classification, ResNet50, which is a CNN model, showed the best performance in terms of the overall correct response rate and AUC value. The output of the heatmap and the survey of physicians' judgment criteria indicated that many patients tend to focus on the shape of the left atrium in both classifications, suggesting that this method can classify AF types more accurately than physicians in a manner similar to the physicians' judgment criteria. In the future, we plan to address the challenges of this study, such as using plain CT images, preparing a dataset that includes images from other facilities, and conducting continuous evaluations that include persistent AF. Furthermore, once these issues are resolved, this study can potentially be applied in predicting the efficacy of catheter ablation therapy. A future direction is to predict the efficacy of catheter ablation therapy in patients with atrial fibrillation based on contrast-enhanced CT images with the goal of providing quality information for patients to choose their treatment options.

Author Contributions: Conceptualization, H.K. and A.T.; formal analysis, H.K. and A.T.; methodology, H.K. and A.T.; data curation, T.O. and Y.S.; software, H.K. and A.T.; writing—original draft preparation, H.K. and A.T.; writing—review and editing, T.O., Y.S., E.W., and H.F. All authors have read and agreed to the published version of the manuscript.

Funding: This research received no external funding.

Institutional Review Board Statement: This study was approved by the Ethical Review Committee of Fujita Health University (HM22-095) and was carried out in accordance with the World Medical Association's Declaration of Helsinki.

Informed Consent Statement: Informed consent was obtained in the form of an opt-out at Fujita Health University Bantane Hospital, and all data were anonymized.

Data Availability Statement: The source code and additional information used to support the findings of this study are available from the corresponding author upon request.

Conflicts of Interest: The authors declare no conflicts of interest.

References

1. Morillo, C.A.; Banerjee, A.; Perel, P.; Wood, D.; Jouven, X. Atrial fibrillation: The current epidemic. *J. Geriatr. Cardiol.* **2017**, *14*, 195–203. Available online: https://www.ncbi.nlm.nih.gov/pmc/articles/PMC5460066 (accessed on 9 December 2023). [PubMed]
2. Kirchhof, P.; Benussi, S.; Kotecha, D.; Ahlsson, A.; Atar, D.; Casadei, B.; Castella, M.; Diener, H.-C.; Heidbuchel, H.; Hendriks, J.; et al. 2016 ESC guidelines for the management of atrial fibrillation developed in collaboration with EACTS. *Eur. Heart J.* **2016**, *37*, 2893–2962. [CrossRef] [PubMed]
3. Developed with the special contribution of the European Heart Rhythm Association (EHRA); Endorsed by the European Association for Cardio-Thoracic Surgery (EACTS); Camm, A.J.; Kirchhof, P.; Lip, G.Y.; Schotten, U.; Savelieva, I.; Ernst, S.; Van Gelder, I.C.; Al-Attar, N.; et al. Guidelines for the management of atrial fibrillation: The Task Force for the Management of Atrial Fibrillation of the European Society of Cardiology (ESC). *Eur. Heart J.* **2010**, *31*, 2369–2429. [CrossRef]
4. Nogami, A.; Kurita, T.; Abe, H.; Ando, K.; Ishikawa, T.; Imai, K.; Usui, A.; Okishige, K.; Kusano, K.; Kumagai, K.; et al. 2018 Revised Guidelines for Non-Pharmacologic Treatment of Arrhythmia. *Circ. J.* **2021**, *85*, 1692–1700. [CrossRef] [PubMed]
5. Sultan, A.; Lüker, J.; Andresen, D.; Kuck, K.H.; Hoffmann, E.; Brachmann, J.; Hochadel, M.; Willems, S.; Eckardt, L.; Lewalter, T.; et al. Predictors of Atrial Fibrillation Recurrence after Catheter Ablation: Data from the German Ablation Registry. *Sci. Rep.* **2017**, *7*, 16678. [CrossRef] [PubMed]
6. Njoku, A.; Kannabhiran, M.; Arora, R.; Reddy, P.; Gopinathannair, R.; Lakkireddy, D.; Dominic, P. Left atrial volume predicts atrial fibrillation recurrence after radiofrequency ablation: A meta-analysis. *EP Eur.* **2018**, *20*, 33–42. [CrossRef] [PubMed]
7. Zhou, X.; Nakamura, K.; Sahara, N.; Takagi, T.; Toyoda, Y.; Enomoto, Y.; Hara, H.; Noro, M.; Sugi, K.; Moroi, M.; et al. Deep Learning-Based Recurrence Prediction of Atrial Fibrillation After Catheter Ablation. *Circ. J.* **2022**, *86*, 299–308. [CrossRef] [PubMed]
8. Kim, J.Y.; Kim, Y.; Oh, G.-H.; Choi, Y.; Hwang, Y.; Kim, T.-S.; Kim, S.-H.; Kim, J.-H.; Jang, S.-W.; Oh, Y.-S.; et al. A deep learning model to predict recurrence of atrial fibrillation after pulmonary vein isolation. *Int. J. Arrhythmia* **2020**, *21*, 19. [CrossRef]
9. McGann, C.; Akoum, N.; Patel, A.; Kholmovski, E.; Revelo, P.; Damal, K.; Wilson, B.; Cates, J.; Harrison, A.; Ranjan, R.; et al. Atrial Fibrillation Ablation Outcome Is Predicted by Left Atrial Remodeling on MRI. *Circ. Arrhythmia Electrophysiol.* **2014**, *7*, 23–30. [CrossRef] [PubMed]
10. Ortigosa, N.; Cano, Ó.; Ayala, G.; Galbis, A.; Fernández, C. Atrial fibrillation subtypes classification using the General Fourier-family Transform. *Med. Eng. Phys.* **2014**, *36*, 554–560. [CrossRef] [PubMed]
11. Alcaraz, R.; Sandberg, F.; Sörnmo, L.; Rieta, J.J. Classification of Paroxysmal and Persistent Atrial Fibrillation in Ambulatory ECG Recordings. *IEEE Trans. Biomed. Eng.* **2011**, *58*, 1441–1449. [CrossRef] [PubMed]
12. Fujita, H. AI-based computer-aided diagnosis (AI-CAD): The latest review to read first. *Radiol. Phys. Technol.* **2020**, *13*, 6–19. [CrossRef] [PubMed]
13. Suman, G.; Panda, A.; Korfiatis, P.; Goenka, A.H. Convolutional neural network for the detection of pancreatic cancer on CT scans. *Lancet Digit. Health* **2020**, *2*, 453. [CrossRef] [PubMed]
14. Xiang, L.; Wang, Q.; Nie, D.; Zhang, L.; Jin, X.; Qiao, Y.; Shen, D. Deep embedding convolutional neural network for synthesizing CT image from T1-Weighted MR image. *Med. Image Anal.* **2018**, *47*, 31–44. [CrossRef] [PubMed]
15. Teramoto, A.; Fujita, H.; Yamamuro, O.; Tamaki, T. Automated detection of pulmonary nodules in PET/CT images: Ensemble false-positive reduction using a convolutional neural network technique. *Med. Phys.* **2016**, *43*, 2821–2827. [CrossRef] [PubMed]
16. Wang, Q.; Shen, F.; Shen, L.; Huang, J.; Sheng, W. Lung Nodule Detection in CT Images Using a Raw Patch-Based Convolutional Neural Network. *J. Digit. Imaging* **2019**, *32*, 971–979. [CrossRef] [PubMed]
17. Liu, C.; Cao, Y.; Alcantara, M.; Liu, B.; Brunette, M.; Peinado, J.; Curioso, W. TX-CNN: Detecting tuberculosis in chest X-ray images using convolutional neural network. In Proceedings of the 2017 IEEE International Conference on Image Processing (ICIP), Beijing, China, 17–20 September 2017; Volume 23, pp. 14–18.
18. Rohini, A.; Praveen, C.; Mathivanan, S.K.; Muthukumaran, V.; Mallik, S.; Alqahtani, M.S.; Al-Rasheed, A.; Soufiene, B.O. Multimodal hybrid convolutional neural network based brain tumor grade classification. *BMC Bioinform.* **2023**, *24*, 382. [CrossRef] [PubMed]
19. Shorten, C.; Khoshgoftaar, T.M. A survey on image data augmentation for deep learning. *J. Big Data* **2019**, *6*, 60. [CrossRef]
20. Simonyan, K.; Zisserman, A. Very Deep Convolutional Networks for Large-Scale Image Recognition. In Proceedings of the 3rd International Conference on Learning Representations (ICLR), San Diego, CA, USA, 7–9 May 2015; pp. 11–14.
21. He, K.; Zhang, X.; Ren, S.; Sun, J. Deep Residual Learning for Image Recognition. In Proceedings of the 2016 IEEE Conference on Computer Vision and Pattern Recognition (CVPR), Las Vegas, NV, USA, 27–30 June 2016; pp. 770–778.

22. Huang, G.; Liu, Z.; Van Der Maaten, L.; Weinberger, K.Q. Densely Connected Convolutional Networks. In Proceedings of the 2017 IEEE Conference on Computer Vision and Pattern Recognition (CVPR), Honolulu, HI, USA, 21–26 July 2017; pp. 2261–2269.
23. Wang, H.; Wang, Z.; Du, M.; Yang, F.; Zhang, Z.; Ding, S.; Mardziel, P.; Hu, X. Score-CAM:Score-Weighted Visual Explanations for Convolutional Neural Networks. In Proceedings of the IEEE Computer Society Conference on Computer Vision and Pattern Recognition Workshops, Seattle, WA, USA, 14–19 June 2020; pp. 111–119.

computers MDPI

Article

Modified Multiresolution Convolutional Neural Network for Quasi-Periodic Noise Reduction in Phase Shifting Profilometry for 3D Reconstruction

Osmar Antonio Espinosa-Bernal *, Jesús Carlos Pedraza-Ortega *, Marco Antonio Aceves-Fernandez, Juan Manuel Ramos-Arreguín, Saul Tovar-Arriaga and Efrén Gorrostieta-Hurtado

Facultad de Ingeniería, Universidad Autónoma de Querétaro, Querétaro 76010, Mexico; marco.aceves@uaq.mx (M.A.A.-F.); jsistdig@yahoo.com.mx (J.M.R.-A.); saul.tovar@uaq.mx (S.T.-A.); efrengorrostieta@gmail.com (E.G.-H.)

* Correspondence: oespinosa07@alumnos.uaq.mx (O.A.E.-B.); caryoko@yahoo.com (J.C.P.-O.)

Abstract: Fringe profilometry is a method that obtains the 3D information of objects by projecting a pattern of fringes. The three-step technique uses only three images to acquire the 3D information from an object, and many studies have been conducted to improve this technique. However, there is a problem that is inherent to this technique, and that is the quasi-periodic noise that appears due to this technique and considerably affects the final 3D object reconstructed. Many studies have been carried out to tackle this problem to obtain a 3D object close to the original one. The application of deep learning in many areas of research presents a great opportunity to to reduce or eliminate the quasi-periodic noise that affects images. Therefore, a model of convolutional neural network along with four different patterns of frequencies projected in the three-step technique is researched in this work. The inferences produced by models trained with different frequencies are compared with the original ones both qualitatively and quantitatively.

Keywords: quasi-periodic noise; frequency; convolutional neural network; 3D object; computer vision; fringe profilometry; synthetic objects

1. Introduction

The fringe projection is one method without contact that permits to measure heights from objects to generate 3D objects, and it is considered one of the most reliable for this aim [1–3].

The acquisition of 3D information is very essential in many areas, e.g., computer vision [4–6], industrial applications [7–9], optics [10,11], and biomedical applications [12–14], among others [15]. However, this method presents an inconvenience in the final 3D reconstruction due to the quasi-periodic noise [16–20] that is produced during the acquisition of images at the stage of phase unwrapping [21,22]. This stage of phase unwrapping recovers the 3D information from the image capture depending on the number of images. In this work, we apply the three-step technique [1,17], and therefore three images are required. This quasi-periodic or Moire noise, as is also known, has the particularity of affecting the shape of the 3D object [8,23–25], as it is shown in Figure 1, and it depends on the frequency of the pattern employed in the projection. This number of frequencies affects the way the noise appears in the images, as it is shown below in Figures 1 and 2.

The reduction or elimination in periodic or quasi-periodic noise, known as Moire noise, began as soon as the first digital images could be obtained; however, it was not until it was analyzed in terms of how much noise was produced that research began on ways to attenuate or eliminate it from the images. Once the noise on the images was detected and analyzed, it was found that it is formed in a repetitive pattern and in different ways. Many studies have been conducted to reduce or eliminate such quasi-periodic noise, some processing the image in its spatial domain [18], others in its frequency domain [17]. In recent studies, thanks to the advances in artificial intelligence, specifically in the field of deep learning, images can be processed for different tasks, including image reduction or restoration. Convolutional neural networks are networks composed of neurons and are part of deep learning. They are composed of many layers of stacked neurons. These networks are designed to process an image by convolution, which is a technique that infers a pixel by calculating an average from information of neighboring pixels [26].

When all pixels of an image are completely processed, a complete image is produced by a model that is trained for this specific task. Many tasks are carried out with convolutional neural networks, such as classification [27,28], segmentation [29,30], restoration [31,32], object detection [33,34], among other tasks [35–39].

In this work, we propose a convolutional neural network to restore images affected by quasi-periodic noise in the process of 3D reconstruction by using the technique of fringe projection in three steps. The trained model will act as an image pre-processor by reducing the repetitive pattern present in the affected images, whose pattern appears like horizontal fringes that affect the surface of an object, improving the speed of this stage and obtaining an accurate 3D object. The convolutional neural network is based on the same architecture proposed by Sun [40], namely the multiresolution convolutional neural network, for the reduction in Moire patterns in digital images whose parameters will be described below. Section 3 will describe the results and Section 4 will present the conclusions.

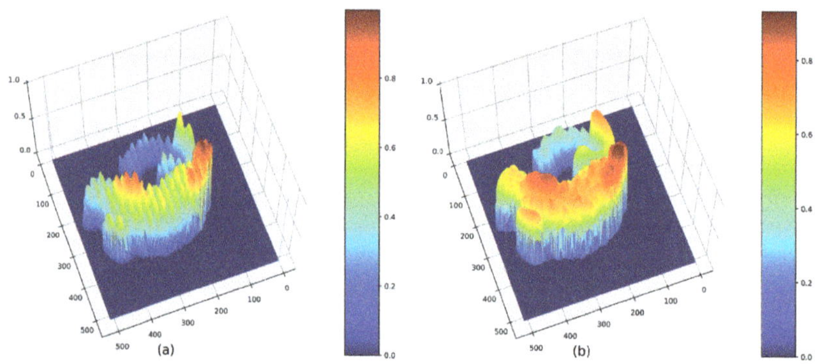

Figure 1. Three-dimensional reconstruction of an object, (**a**) affected by quasi-periodic noise, and (**b**) original object. The image shows the deformation of the surface caused by the noise present in images acquired by the fringe projection in three steps.

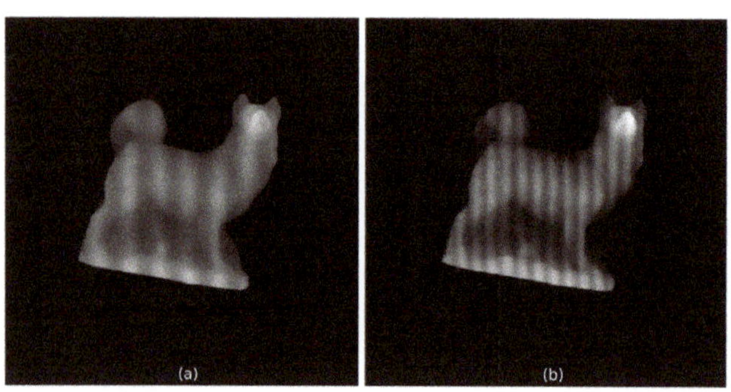

Figure 2. *Cont.*

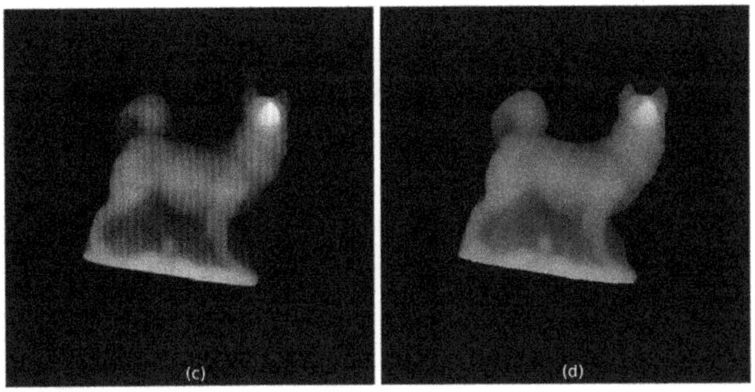

Figure 2. Images from the database with quasi-periodic noise at different frequencies: (**a**) quasi-periodic noise at 4 frequencies, (**b**) quasi-periodic noise at 8 frequencies, (**c**) quasi-periodic noise at 16 frequencies, (**d**) quasi-periodic noise at 32 frequencies.

2. Materials and Methods

The software Blender (https://www.blender.org/) emulates a 3-step fringe profilometry system and the 3D object models used for generating the database were acquired from platform Turbosquid and were free to use. Here, 75 different 3D models were used, and in Figure 3 some examples of these models are shown.

In the simulated system, a lamp is used to project the fringes over objects; then, pictures are acquired with four different patterns. For capturing the images, a camera with a focal length setting of 28 mm [41] was selected and the size of the captured images was 512 × 512 pixels. With the simulation system, a database of 1350 images with different objects at different positions was generated, but as four frequencies were applied to the pattern projected over the object, the total images were 5400. Each scene was composed of 16 different pictures plus 12 more that correspond to the references −3 for each different pattern projected shared by every scene. Figure 4 shows a complete set of all pictures of a single scene that conform to the generated database [17,41].

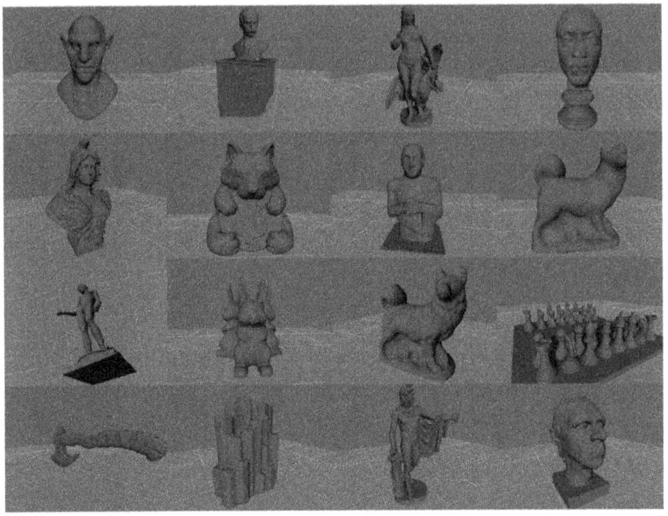

Figure 3. Three-dimensional models acquired from platform Turbosquid.

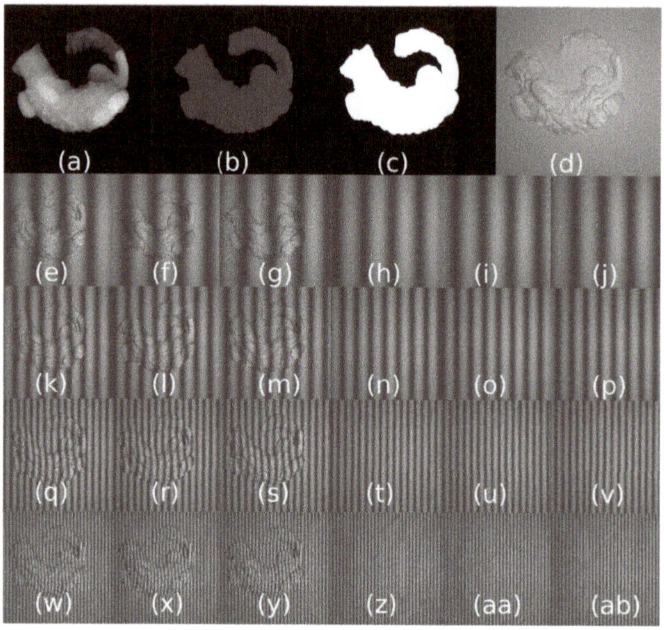

Figure 4. Set of images obtained from a single scene with a 3D model. (**a**) Ground-truth, (**b**) original 3D model, (**c**) region of interest, (**d**) 3D model with background, (**e–g**) images with object with 120° shifting pattern projected composed of 4 frequencies, (**h–j**) reference images with a 4-frequency composite pattern, (**k–m**) images with object with 120° shifting pattern projected composed of 8 frequencies, (**n–p**) reference images with a 8-frequency composite pattern, (**q–s**) images with object with 120° shifting pattern projected composed of 16 frequencies, (**t–v**) reference images with a 16-frequency composite pattern, (**w–y**) images with object with 120° shifting pattern projected composed of 32 frequencies, (**z,aa,ab**) reference images with a 32-frequency composite pattern.

Figure 2 shows a single picture affected by four different patterns of quasi-periodic noise, and the process to obtain such images is shown in Figure 5.

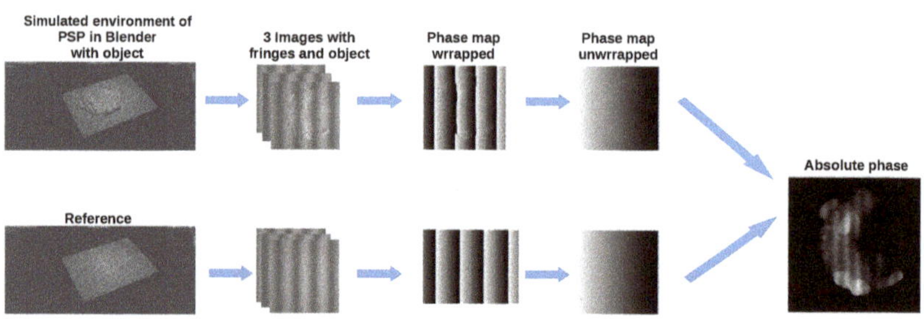

Figure 5. The methodology used to generate a database of images with quasi-periodic noise.

All images were obtained using a laptop with NVIDIA GeForce RTX 3060 graphic card with 6 Gb of memory RAM, 16 Gb of memory RAM, and an I7-10750H processor @2.60 GHz. The images for training were 90% of 1050 images, for validation 10% of 1050 images, and 300 additional images were used for the test set. All this was only used to train a model with one single frequency, which was either 4, 8, 16, or 32. For the training of a model with multiple frequencies, were combined images with all four frequencies, adding up to a total of 4200 images, 90% for the training set, 10% for the validation set, and 1200 images affected with the four different patterns for the test set. Figure 6 shows some images with quasi-periodic noise at different frequencies and their respective targets generated by Blender.

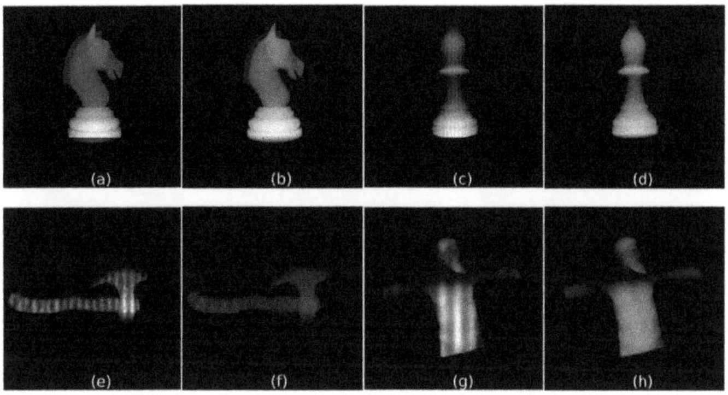

Figure 6. Images from database created with Blender software: (**a**,**c**,**e**,**g**) images affected with quasi-periodic noise at different frequencies, (**b**,**d**,**f**,**h**) ground-truth image.

The database of images generated with Blender includes three images of different 3D models with a pattern of 4 different frequencies and shifting 120° degrees. Applying a phase unwrapping algorithm (in this case, the PEARLS algorithm [21]) to obtain an absolute phase image, results in the generation of an image with noise known as quasi-periodic noise or Moire noise, as shown in Figure 2. Such noise is inherent in the technique of 3-step fringe profilometry to obtain the heights of an object from images using a single camera and affects the final 3D object reconstructed by altering its shape and losing 3D information.

When the stage to obtain the absolute phase of images pre-processed with the PEARLS algorithm is finished, the images are used to generate a database. The algorithm called PEARLS (Phase Estimation using Adaptive Regularization based on Local Smoothing) is described in the following pseudocode:

1. Each pixel (x, y) in $h \in H$
   (a) The zero-order phase $\tilde{\varphi}_h(x, y)$ estimate is calculated;
   (b) Adaptive window size is applied to estimates $\tilde{\varphi}_h(x, y)$ to properly select a window size $h^+(x, y)$;
   (c) Compute first-order phase estimates with adaptive window size;
   (d) end.
2. Unwrap the phase $\varphi_{\tilde{h}^+}$ using one of the procedures developed for noise-free data.

For further information, see [21].

The database is then used as the source for training a CNN to learn to reduce or eliminate the quasi-periodic noise present in images that are affected by such noise. Finally, the trained model is used in the stage of pre-processing to generate a 3D object as a filter of noise. The process of the methodology to generate the images to train a model to reduce the noise in images is shown in Figure 5.

Once the database of images is obtained, a convolutional neural network based on Multiresolution-CNN proposed by Sun [40] is applied. The proposed model was modified to have 9 layers after the down-sampling and up-sampling operation with 3×3 kernel and 64 channels which were completely convolutional, contrary to the original one that had 5 layers in this stage of the architecture. In addition to this change, a layer as input and output of grayscale images or one channel was added as well. Figure 7 shows the architecture developed and implemented.

The original Multiresolution-CNN model was developed to reduce the Moire noise in color and white and black images. Therefore, the proposed model was modified to be trained with images that contain both quasi-periodic and Moire noise and reduce such noise. The trained model to reduce such noise was finally used as part of pre-processing images to generate a 3D object, improving the speed and the quality of the 3D objects generated. The novelty of this paper relies on the proposal of a modified multiresolution CNN in order to reduce the quasi-periodic noise on phase shifting profilometry at four different frequencies to generate a more reliable 3D reconstruction of an object.

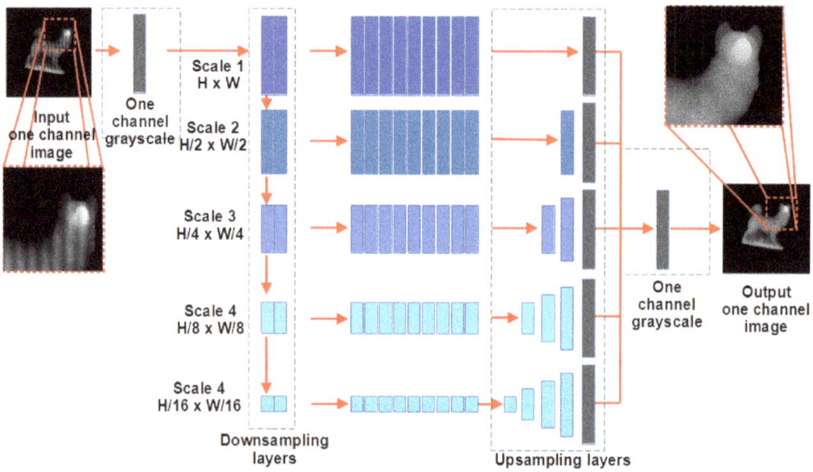

Figure 7. The architecture of convolutional neural network model developed and implemented.

The model was trained using a set of 1050 grayscale images with a size of 549 × 540 but adjusted to a size of 512 × 512 before feeding the model, and five experiments were carried out, one for every frequency present in the images. The last experiment was carried out using the set of images of every frequency gathered in one set of 4200 images. The projected frequency patterns were 4, 8, 16, and 32 fringes. Every experiment was performed using the optimizer Adam() [42,43] and the MSELoss() function [44] to calculate the training and validation loss. Internally, the algorithm took 10% of images randomly to be used as validation set in every training.

The fringe profilometry method allows for obtaining information on object heights through images. Therefore, a large number of images with a wide variety of shapes, surfaces, and contours are required to remove this specific noise. Although there are techniques to augment data and give them variety during the training of models for noise reduction and image restoration, this first approximation was carried out without data augmentation. This is performed in order to observe the results obtained and make the corresponding improvements. However, since this is a specific noise to be reduced, we leave some training techniques for future work. For now, we just add a large variety of objects to have a model trained with enough data to generalize to the greatest number of possible scenarios or objects to reduce or restore noise in images affected by quasi-periodic noise.

The selection of the neural network architecture is based on a previously published article, wherein a comparative study between three different architectures was carried out and the most appropriate neural network for this purpose was selected using performance criteria [23].

2.1. Optimizer and Loss Function

The optimizer Adam() has the advantage of requiring little memory, and it is computationally efficient and has an adaptive estimation to calculate moments of first and second order.

$$m_t = \beta_1 m_{t-1} + (1 - \beta_1) g_t \tag{1}$$

$$v_t = \beta_2 v_{t-1} + (1 - \beta_2) g_t^2, \tag{2}$$

g_t evaluates the gradient in a timestep t, m_t calculates the average of moving, v_t is the squared gradient, and β_1 and β_2 calculate the decay rates for every moment estimates.

Equation (3) calculates the MSELoss() function

$$l(x,y) = L = \{l_1,\ldots,l_N\}^T, l_n = (x_n - y_n)^2, \quad (3)$$

the batch-size is represented by N, x, and y which represent the dimensions that form a matrix of a given size with n elements [42,43].

2.2. IMMSE

The inverse mean square error (IMMSE) is a metric used to evaluate the quality of reconstructed images by comparing the original image with the generated image. The IMMSE formula is based on the calculation of the mean square error (MSE), but is applied in an inverse manner [45]. This equation is shown below

$$IMSSE = \frac{1}{mn}\sum_{i=1}^{m}\sum_{i=j}^{n}(I(i,j) - K(i,j))^2 \quad (4)$$

where I is the original image, K is the processed image, m number of rows, n number of cols, and $K(i,j)$ is the value of the corresponding pixel in the reconstructed image. The IMMSE provides a measure of how similar the two images are, where higher values indicate better quality.

2.3. PSNR (Peak Signal-to-Noise Ratio)

Peak Signal-to-Noise Ratio (PSNR) is a widely used metric to assess the quality of compressed or reconstructed images. PSNR measures the ratio of the maximum power of a signal (the original image) to the noise that affects the quality of its representation (the reconstructed image) [45,46]. It is defined as follows:

$$PSNR(f,g) = 10log_{10}(255^2/MSE(f,g)) \quad (5)$$

where

$$MSE(f,g) = \frac{1}{MN}\sum_{i=1}^{M}\sum_{j=1}^{N}(f_{ij} - g_{i,j})^2 \quad (6)$$

A higher PSNR indicates that the reconstructed image is more similar to the original, i.e., it has less noise. Typical PSNR values for high-quality images are in the range of 30–50 dB.

3. Results

The results were obtained by experimenting with different parameters and the parameters proposed by the author of the model, which were based on the model proposed in [40]. These parameters are summarized in Table 1.

In addition to the parameters shown in Table 1, 50 epochs were set and, if the obtained model had a better validation loss, it was saved as the best, but if a bad validation loss was obtained, the model was penalized. After training the model, the results obtained after every epoch were charted to show the evolution of the training and validation loss and were scaled for a better appreciation of the loss. The graphs of the evolution of every training are shown in Figure 8.

Figure 8 shows the training and validation loss of every model trained. The evolution of training and validation loss shows a constant decline, which is consistent and shows that the model is effectively "learning", and it is also observed that the learning is performed rapidly and at the end the rate of learning is very low.

The time of learning and the training and validation loss are shown in Table 2.

Table 1. Parameters used during network training for comparison, trained with images affected by quasi-periodic noise at four different patterns (4, 8, 16, and 32 frequencies), as seen in Figure 2.

Parameter	Pattern 1 (Number of Fringes 4)	Pattern 2 (Number of Fringes 8)	Pattern 3 (Number of Fringes 16)	Pattern 4 (Number of Fringes 32)	Pattern 5 (Multifrequency Pattern)
Batch size	4	4	4	4	4
Initials weights	Gaussian random (average = 0.0, standard deviation = 0.01)	Gaussian random (average = 0.0, standard deviation = 0.01)	Gaussian random (average = 0.0, standard deviation = 0.01)	Gaussian random (average = 0.0, standard deviation = 0.01)	Gaussian random (average = 0.0, standard deviation = 0.01)
Bias	0.0	0.0	0.0	0.0	0.0
Learning rate	0.007	0.007	0.007	0.007	0.007
Optimizer	Adam()	Adam()	Adam()	Adam()	Adam()
Training loss	MSELoss()	MSELoss()	MSELoss()	MSELoss()	MSELoss()
Validation loss	MSELoss()	MSELoss()	MSELoss()	MSELoss()	MSELoss()
Test planing (train, val)	90%, 10%	90%, 10%	90%, 10%	90%, 10%	90%, 10%
Images size (Width, Height)	512 × 512 pixels	512 × 512 pixels	512 × 512 pixels	512 × 512 pixels	512 × 512 pixels
Set train images	1050	1050	1050	1050	4200
Set validation images	105	105	105	105	420
Set test images	300	300	300	300	300

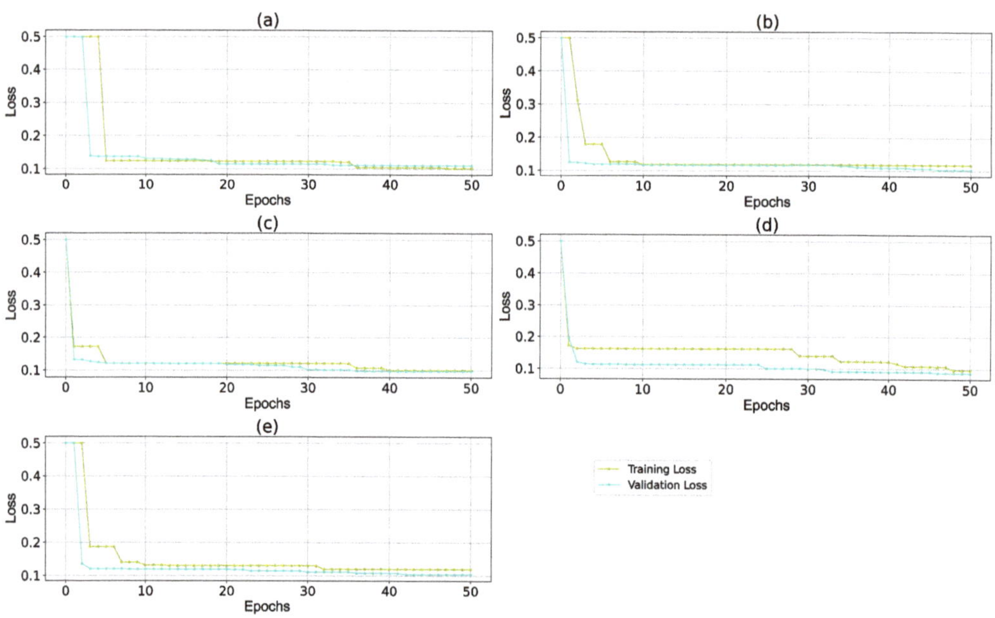

Figure 8. Evolution of training and validation loss. Models train with noisy images affected by different frequencies due to different patterns projected. (**a**) Images with 4 frequencies, (**b**) images with 8 frequencies, (**c**) images with 16 frequencies (**d**) images with 32 frequencies, and (**e**) images with multifrequencies (4, 8, 16, and 32).

Table 2. Time employed to perform each training and training and validation loss reached during network training for comparison using images with four different patterns (4, 8, 16, and 32 frequencies), as seen in Figure 2.

	Pattern 1 (Number of Fringes 4)	Pattern 2 (Number of Fringes 8)	Pattern 3 (Number of Fringes 16)	Pattern 4 (Number of Fringes 32)	Pattern 5 (Multifrequency Pattern)
Training loss	0.10275	0.11939	0.09801	0.08825	0.12041
Validation loss	0.11187	0.10390	0.10042	0.09749	0.10443
Training time (HH:MM:SS)	0:59:37	1:08:49	0:58:12	1:00:16	5:20:22

According to the data obtained after performing the training of the models, these trainings took around one hour to complete, while the training with the set that contains all the images with the four frequencies lasted a bove five hours because its set contained more than 4000 images. The training and validation loss reached values equal to or below 0.1, indicating a constant learning by the trained models.

3.1. Inferences Obtained from Images Affected with Quasi-Periodic Noise of 4 Frequencies

The inferences obtained from images affected by quasi-periodic noise composed of four frequencies using all the trained models are shown in Figure 9, and the 3D reconstructions are shown in Figure 10.

The profiles obtained from these inferences, the ground-truth image, and the original image affected by quasi-periodic noise of four frequencies are compared and are charted in Figure 11. The heights are normalized from 0.0 to 1.0 and the x-axis represents pixels.

The error between the inferences made by the models trained and the ground-truth image is identified using the PSNR, SSIM, IMMSE, and the MSE Profile between the inference and the ground-truth image. The measures obtained for the images affected by quasi-periodic noise of four frequencies are summarized in Table 3.

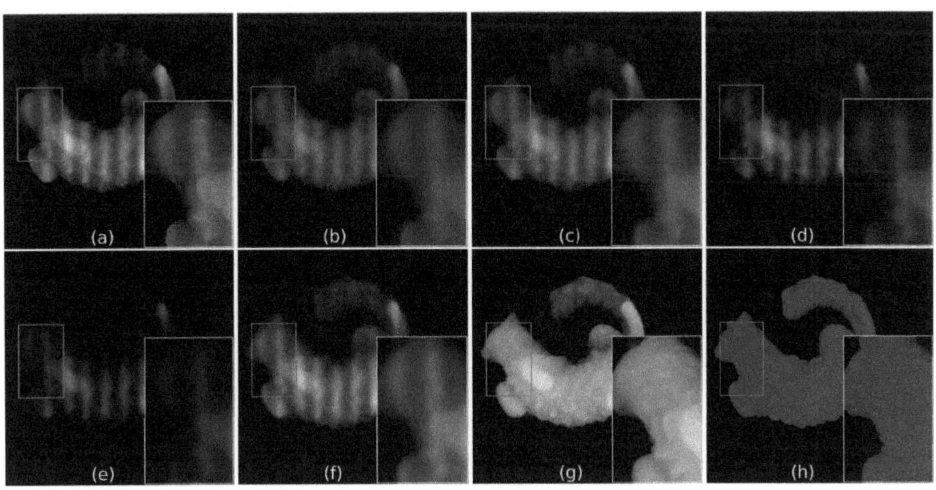

Figure 9. Two-dimensional representation of an object Cat. (**a**) Image with quasi-periodic noise produced by projection of a four-frequency pattern, inference obtained with models trained with (**b**) four frequencies, (**c**) 8 frequencies, (**d**) 16 frequencies, (**e**) 32 frequencies, and (**f**) Multifrequencies. (**g**) ground-truth image, and (**h**) original object.

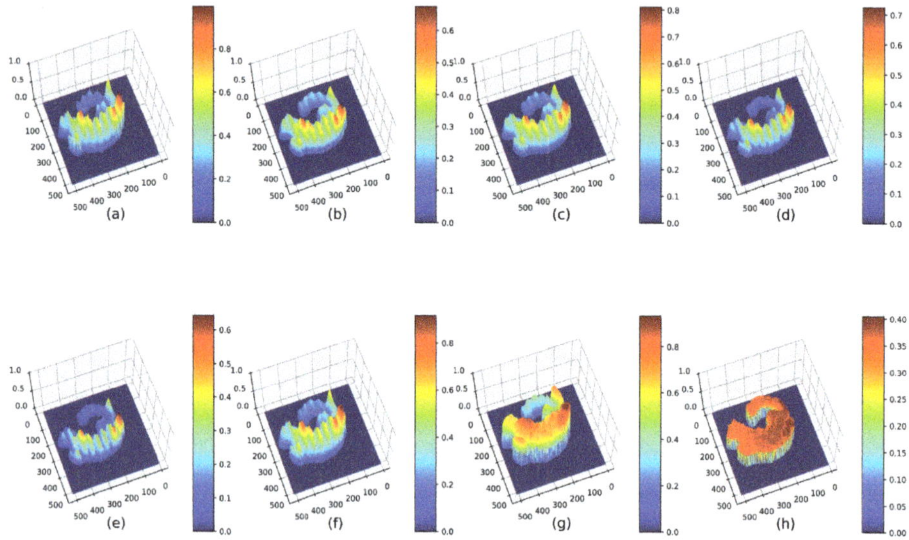

Figure 10. Three-dimensional representation of an object Cat. (**a**) Image with quasi-periodic noise produced by projection of a four-frequency pattern, inference obtained with models trained with (**b**) four frequencies, (**c**) 8 frequencies, (**d**) 16 frequencies, (**e**) 32 frequencies, and (**f**) Multifrequencies. (**g**) ground-truth image, and (**h**) original object.

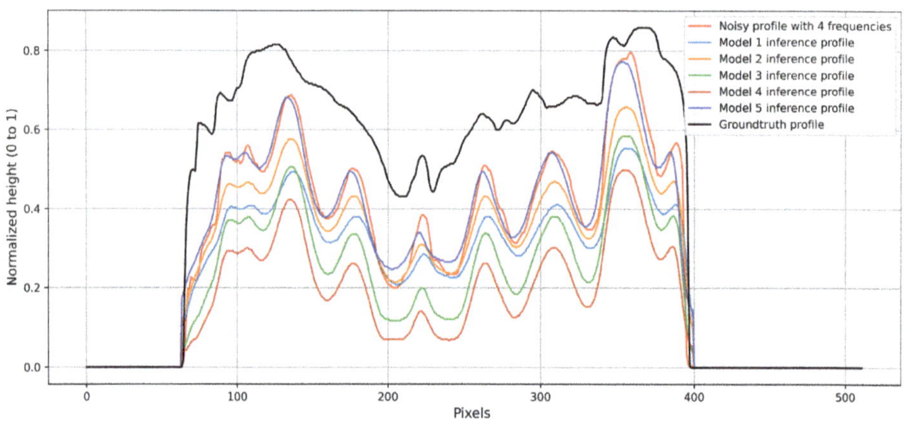

Figure 11. Profile comparison of 3D objects.

Table 3. Measures obtained with model trained with images affected by noise of four frequencies.

Inference	IMMSE	SSIM	PSNR	MSE (Profile)
1	0.022	0.871	64.676	0.064
2	0.017	0.879	65.767	0.048
3	0.033	0.828	62.900	0.089
4	0.046	0.793	61.547	0.124
5	0.012	0.873	67.263	0.034

3.2. *Inferences Obtained from Images Affected with Quasi-Periodic Noise of 8 Frequencies*

The inferences obtained from images affected by quasi-periodic noise composed of 8 frequencies using all the trained models are shown in Figure 12, and the 3D reconstructions are shown in Figure 13.

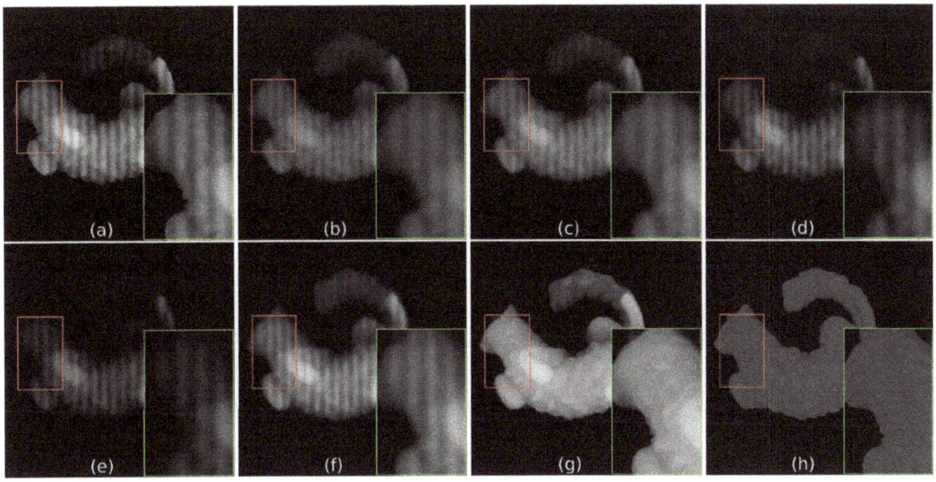

Figure 12. Two-dimensional representation of an object Cat. (**a**) Image with quasi-periodic noise produced by projection of an 8-frequency pattern, inference obtained with models trained with (**b**) four frequencies, (**c**) 8 frequencies, (**d**) 16 frequencies, (**e**) 32 frequencies, and (**f**) Multifrequencies. (**g**) ground-truth image, and (**h**) original object.

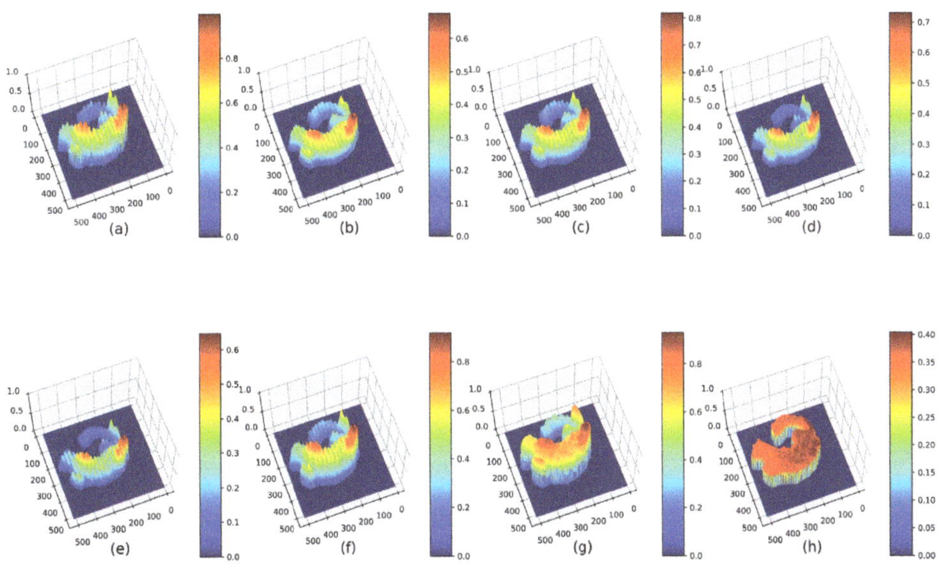

Figure 13. Three-dimensional representation of an object Cat. (**a**) Image with quasi-periodic noise produced by projection of an 8-frequency pattern, inference obtained with models trained with (**b**) four frequencies, (**c**) 8 frequencies, (**d**) 16 frequencies, (**e**) 32 frequencies, and (**f**) Multifrequencies. (**g**) ground-truth image, and (**h**) original object.

The profiles obtained from these inferences, the ground-truth image, and the original image affected by quasi-periodic noise of eight frequencies are compared and are charted in Figure 14. The heights are normalized from 0.0 to 1.0 and the x-axis represents pixels.

The error between the inferences made by the models trained and the ground-truth image is identified using the PSNR, SSIM, IMMSE, and the MSE Profile between the inference and the ground-truth image. The measures obtained in images affected by quasi-periodic noise of eight frequencies are summarized in Table 4.

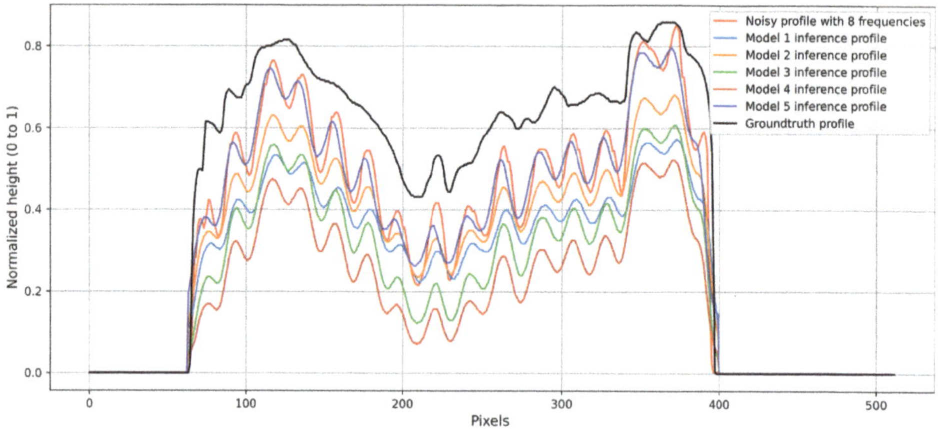

Figure 14. Profile comparison of 3D objects.

Table 4. Measures obtained with model trained with images affected by noise of 8 frequencies.

Inference	IMMSE	SSIM	PSNR	MSE (Profile)
1	0.017	0.882	65.838	0.048
2	0.012	0.889	67.488	0.031
3	0.025	0.846	64.224	0.063
4	0.036	0.813	62.561	0.095
5	0.007	0.878	69.646	0.018

3.3. *Inferences Obtained from IMAGES Affected with Quasi-Periodic Noise of 16 Frequencies*

The inferences obtained from images affected by quasi-periodic noise composed of 16 frequencies using all the trained models are shown in Figure 15, and the 3D reconstructions are shown in Figure 16.

The profiles obtained from these inferences, the ground-truth image, and the original image affected by quasi-periodic noise of 16 frequencies are compared and are charted in Figure 17. The heights are normalized from 0.0 to 1.0 and the x-axis represents pixels.

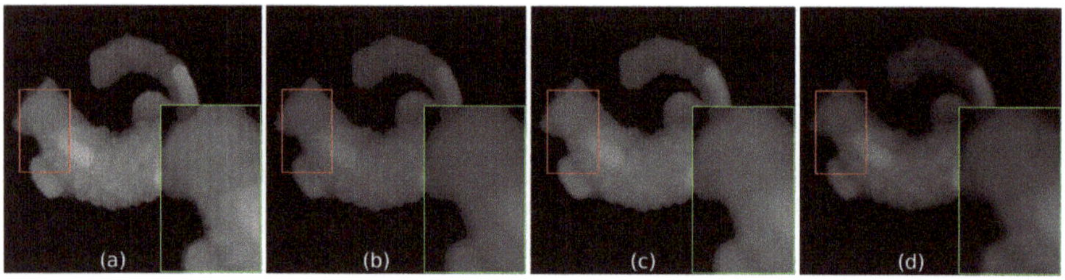

Figure 15. *Cont.*

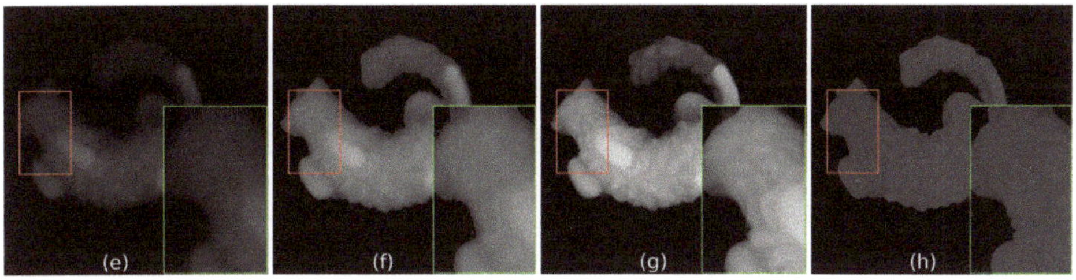

Figure 15. Two-dimensional representation of an object Cat. (**a**) Image with quasi-periodic noise produced by projection of a 16-frequency pattern, inference obtained with models trained with (**b**) four frequencies, (**c**) 8 frequencies, (**d**) 16 frequencies, (**e**) 32 frequencies, and (**f**) Multifrequencies. (**g**) ground-truth image, and (**h**) original object.

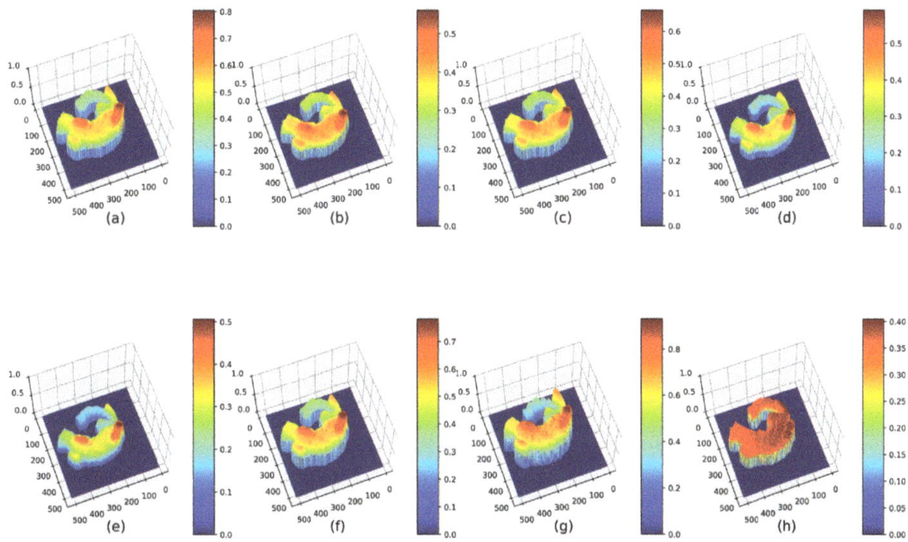

Figure 16. Three-dimensional representation of an object Cat. (**a**) Image with quasi-periodic noise produced by projection of a 16-frequency pattern, inference obtained with models trained with (**b**) four frequencies, (**c**) 8 frequencies, (**d**) 16 frequencies, (**e**) 32 frequencies, and (**f**) Multifrequencies. (**g**) ground-truth image, and (**h**) original object.

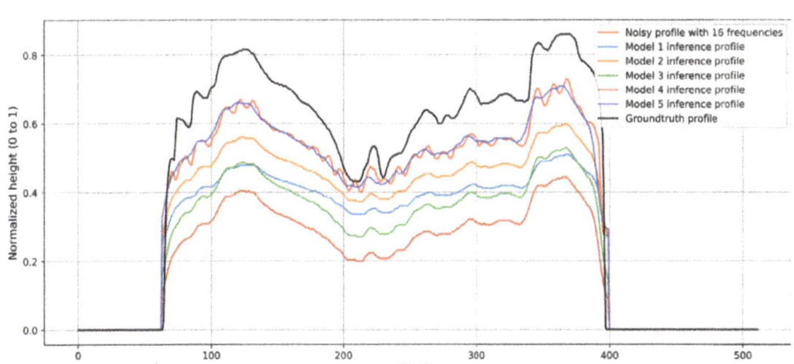

Figure 17. Profile comparison of 3D objects.

The error between the inferences made by the models trained and the ground-truth image is identified using the PSNR, SSIM, IMMSE, and the MSE Profile between the inference and the ground-truth image. The measures obtained in images affected by quasi-periodic noise of 16 frequencies are summarized in Table 5.

Table 5. Measures obtained with model trained with images affected by noise of 16 frequencies.

Inference	IMMSE	SSIM	PSNR	MSE (Profile)
1	0.014	0.886	66.517	0.043
2	0.009	0.903	68.549	0.025
3	0.017	0.897	65.771	0.050
4	0.028	0.872	63.609	0.082
5	0.005	0.914	71.465	0.011

3.4. Inferences Obtained from Images Affected with Quasi-Periodic Noise of 32 Frequencies

The inferences obtained from images affected by quasi-periodic noise composed of 32 frequencies using all the trained models are shown in Figure 18, and the 3D reconstructions are shown in Figure 19.

The profiles obtained from these inferences, the ground-truth image, and the original image affected by quasi-periodic noise of 32 frequencies are compared and are charted in Figure 20. The heights are normalized from 0.0 to 1.0 and the x-axis represents pixels.

The error between the inferences made by the models trained and the ground-truth image is identified using the PSNR, SSIM, IMMSE, and the MSE Profile between the inference and the ground-truth image. The measures obtained in images affected by quasi-periodic noise of 32 frequencies are summarized in Table 6.

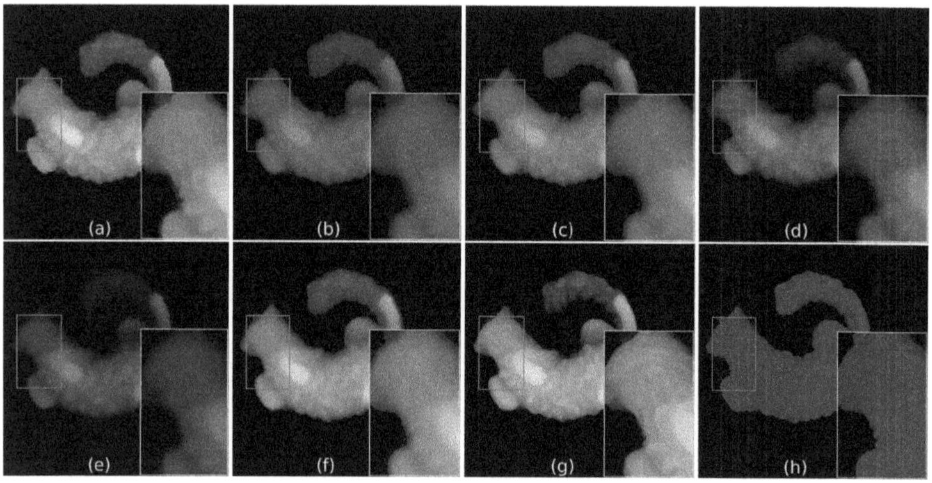

Figure 18. Two-dimensional representation of an object Cat. (**a**) Image with quasi-periodic noise produced by projection of a 32-frequency pattern, inference obtained with models trained with (**b**) four frequencies, (**c**) 8 frequencies, (**d**) 16 frequencies, (**e**) 32 frequencies, and (**f**) Multifrequencies. (**g**) ground-truth image, and (**h**) original object.

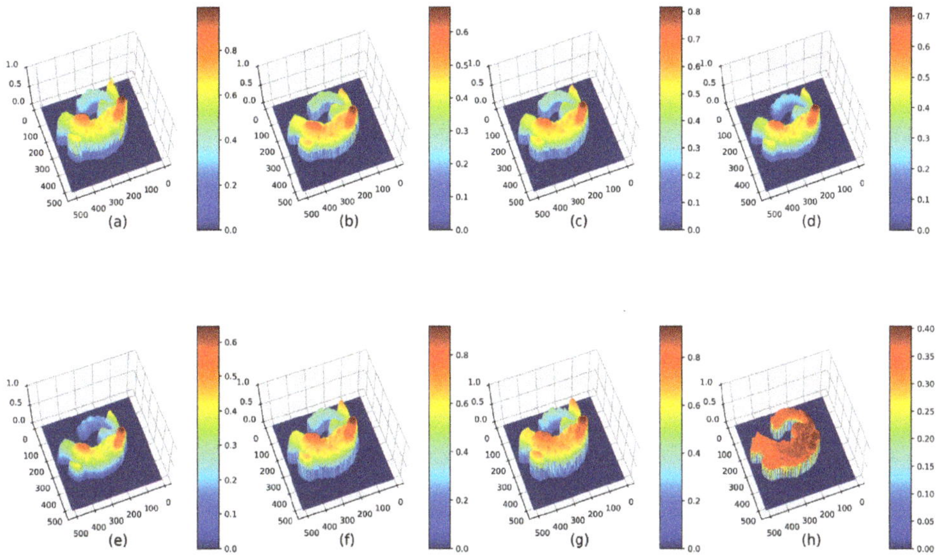

Figure 19. Three-dimensional representation of an object Cat. (**a**) Image with quasi-periodic noise produced by projection of a 32-frequency pattern, inference obtained with models trained with (**b**) four frequencies, (**c**) 8 frequencies, (**d**) 16 frequencies, (**e**) 32 frequencies, and (**f**) Multifrequencies. (**g**) ground-truth image, and (**h**) original object.

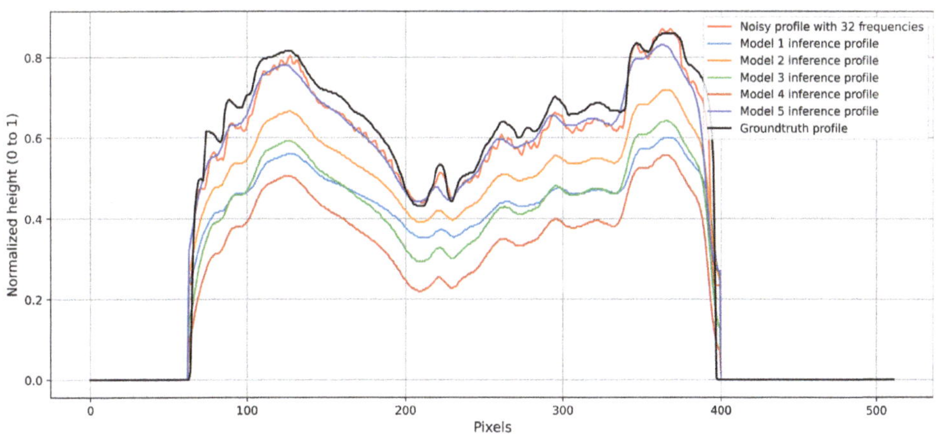

Figure 20. Profile comparison of 3D objects.

Table 6. Measures obtained with model trained with images affected by noise of 32 frequencies.

Inference	IMMSE	SSIM	PSNR	MSE (Profile)
1	0.010	0.905	68.307	0.027
2	0.005	0.923	71.543	0.011
3	0.010	0.922	68.098	0.028
4	0.019	0.901	65.273	0.054
5	0.002	0.927	75.116	0.002

4. Discussion

The inferences obtained from each trained model with a different set of images affected with quasi-periodic noise of different frequencies show, in every case, a better performance when the model is trained with a set that contains images affected with different frequencies instead of using only a set of images with one frequency. Although an image affected with quasi-periodic noise of only four frequencies appears to show a better similarity with the ground-truth image, preserving better details of the object, it is difficult for the trained models to obtain a better inference in quantitative terms. This is observed in the metrics shown in the Tables 3–6. In quantitative terms, in the four inferences performed with 4, 8, 16, and 32 fringes, the IMMSE value is reduced in each inference compared to the original model. In addition, it is observed that the inferences with model 5, which was trained with multiple frequencies, presented a better performance in the SSIM, PSNR, and MSE (Profile) metrics, compared to models 1 to 4.

At first glance at the images with quasi-periodic noise, it can be seen that those that are affected by a lower frequency of such noise lose fewer details of the 3D object. However, as the number of fringe frequencies in the projected patterns increases, this quasi-periodic noise decreases, but only in size. It therefore merges and blends with the details of the 3D object, making it almost impossible to determine what is noise and what is part of the 3D information. Another effect shown by using a low fringe frequency in the projected patterns is that the final height of the object inferred by the model better preserves the original height of the object. This is clearly appreciated in the images that compare the profiles at each frequency of the projected pattern analyzed, where the inferences represented as model 3 (fringe pattern with 16 frequencies) and model 4 (fringe pattern with 16 frequencies) are always lower in normalized height.

It is expected that training using images affected by noise of the same frequency may adequately restore images with similar noise present; however, it was found that performance improved when using images affected by other frequencies. Therefore, training was carried out wherein all the images affected by different frequencies were put together, achieving better results. Although better results were obtained by generalizing the training data more by combining affected images with different frequencies, another limitation was the number of images. By increasing the number of images in the database, it may be possible to further improve the results obtained.

Generating data using Blender allows us to obtain data in a way that is very similar to real data. On the one hand, extensive methodologies must be followed, such as calibration of cameras and objects that do not have restrictions of any kind, while synthetic data save us time and can be used freely. Since models tend to mimic real-world objects, it is possible to use them to represent even people or people's faces roughly, but without the inconvenience of having to obtain them from real people. Furthermore, one can include images of objects captured from the real world, and carry out the 3D reconstruction process at the testing stage.

These results show the difficulty of eliminating the quasi-periodic noise that affects this particular fringe profilometry method for 3D reconstruction, even when trying with different frequencies. Trying different frequencies was found out that the speed of acquisition of image by fringe profilometry of 3-step, while less the frequency pattern projected is faster than with a high frequency. The next research will aim to improve the inferences obtained by either increasing the number of images in the training set or trying other models of convolutional neural networks or networks known as GAN.

5. Conclusions

The experiments performed using a set of images affected with quasi-periodic noise of four different frequencies show how these frequencies affect the 3D object reconstructed and the results obtained when an inference is generated after training a CNN model with these images. Quantitative results show better performance when the model is trained with a set of images that contains, in this case, a quasi-periodic noise pattern of four different frequencies showing that images affected with a higher frequency are the ones that obtain a better result and visually show greater similarity with the ground-truth image.

On the other hand, using a model trained to reduce noise in images obtained in PSP increases the speed of image pre-processing to obtain a 3D object. Trying different frequencies to produce images with different kinds of noise helps to create a high variety of such noise in datasets to train models of CNNs, generating good results both quantitatively and qualitatively.

Author Contributions: Conceptualization, O.A.E.-B., J.C.P.-O., M.A.A.-F., S.T.-A., J.M.R.-A., and E.G.-H.; methodology, O.A.E.-B.; software, O.A.E.-B.; validation, J.C.P.-O.; formal analysis, J.C.P.-O.; investigation, O.A.E.-B.; data curation, O.A.E.-B.; writing—original draft preparation, O.A.E.-B.; writing—review and editing, J.C.P.-O., M.A.A.-F., S.T.-A., J.M.R.-A., and E.G.-H.; supervision, J.C.P.-O., M.A.A.-F., S.T.-A., J.M.R.-A., and E.G.-H. All authors have read and agreed to the published version of the manuscript.

Funding: This research received no external funding.

Institutional Review Board Statement: Not applicable.

Informed Consent Statement: Not applicable.

Data Availability Statement: The data presented in this study are available upon request from the corresponding author.

Acknowledgments: This work was supported in part by the Consejo Nacional de Humanidades, Ciencias y Tecnologías (CONAHCYT), México, in the Postgraduate Faculty of Engineering by the Universidad Autonoma de Querétaro, under Grant CVU 1099050. We also would like to thank FONDO PARA EL FORTALECIMIENTO DE LA INVESTIGACIÓN, VINCULACIÓN Y EXTENSIÓN (FONFIVE-UAQ 2024) for the support of this research.

Conflicts of Interest: The authors declare no conflicts of interest.

Abbreviations

The following abbreviations are used in this manuscript:

CNN	Convolutional Neural Network
MSE	Media Square Error
PEARLS	Phase Estimation using Adaptive Regularization based on Local Smothing

References

1. Gorthi, S.S.; Rastogi, P. Fringe projection techniques: Whither we are? *Opt. Lasers Eng.* **2010**, *48*, 133–140. [CrossRef]
2. Feng, S.; Zuo, C.; Zhang, L.; Tao, T.; Hu, Y.; Yin, W.; Qian, J.; Chen, Q. Calibration of fringe projection pro-filometry: A comparative review. *Opt. Lasers Eng.* **2021**, *143*, 106622. [CrossRef]
3. Hu, Y.; Chen, Q.; Feng, S.; Zuo, C. Microscopic fringe projection profilometry: A review. *Opt. Lasers Eng.* **2020**, *135*, 106192. [CrossRef]
4. Frank Chen, G.M.; Mumin, S. Overview of three-dimensional shape measurement using optical methods. *Opt. Eng.* **2000**, *39*, 10–21.
5. Huang, L.; Idir, M.; Zuo, C.; Asundi, A. Review of phase measuring deflectometry. *Opt. Lasers Eng.* **2018**, *107*, 247–257. [CrossRef]
6. Chen, C.; Gao, N.; Wang, X.; Zhang, Z.; Gao, F.; Jiang, X. Generic exponential fringe model for alleviating phase error in phase measuring profilometry. *Opt. Lasers Eng.* **2018**, *110*, 179–185. [CrossRef]
7. Land, W.S., II; Zhang, B.; Ziegert, J.; Davies, A. In-situ metrology system for laser powder bed fusion additive process. *Procedia Manuf.* **2015**, *1*, 393–403. [CrossRef]
8. Li, B.; Xu, Z.; Gao, F.; Cao, Y.; Dong, Q. 3D reconstruction of high reflective welding surface based on binocular structured light stereo vision. *Machines* **2022**, *10*, 159. [CrossRef]
9. Sun, B.; Zheng, G.; Zhang, X.; Bai, L. Research on aero-engine blade surface detection based on three datum points integrating algorithm. *AIP Adv.* **2020**, *10*, 075305. [CrossRef]
10. Qian, J.; Feng, S.; Tao, T.; Hu, Y.; Liu, K.; Wu, S.; Chen, Q.; Zuo, C. High-resolution real-time 360 3d model reconstruction of a handheld object with fringe projection profilometry. *Opt. Lett.* **2019**, *44*, 5751–5754. [CrossRef]
11. Song, K.; Hu, S.; Wen, X.; Yan, Y. Fast 3D shape measurement using Fourier transform profilometry without phase unwrapping. *Opt. Lasers Eng.* **2016**, *84*, 74–81. [CrossRef]
12. Jiang, C.; Jia, S.; Xu, Y.; Bao, Q.; Dong, J.; Lian, Q. The application of multi-frequency fringe projection profilometry on the measurement of biological tissues. *Biomed. Mater. Eng.* **2015**, *26*, S395–S403. [CrossRef] [PubMed]

13. Chatterjee, A.; Dhanotia, J.; Bhatia, V.; Prakash, S. Non-destructive 3D profiling of orthopaedic titanium bone plate using fringe projection profilometry and Fourier transform analysis. In Proceedings of the 2017 6th International Conference on Computer Applications In Electrical Engineering-Recent Advances (CERA), Roorkee, India, 5–7 October 2017; pp. 389–392.
14. Chatterjee, A.; Singh, P.; Bhatia, V.; Prakash, S. Ear biometrics recognition using laser biospeckled fringe projection profilometry. *Opt. Laser Technol.* **2019**, *112*, 368–378. [CrossRef]
15. Xing, H.Z.; Zhang, Q.B.; Braithwaite, C.H.; Pan, B.; Zhao, J. High-speed photography and digital optical measurement techniques for geomaterials: Fundamentals and applications. *Rock Mech. Rock Eng.* **2017**, *50*, 1611–1659. [CrossRef]
16. Aizenberg, I.N.; Butakoff, C. Frequency domain medianlike filter for periodic and quasi-periodic noise removal. *Image Process. Algorithms Syst.* **2002**, *4667*, 181–191.
17. Espinosa-Bernal, O.A.; Pedraza-Ortega, J.C.; Aceves-Fernández, M.A.; Martínez-Suárez, V.M.; Tovar-Arriaga, S. Adaptive Based Frequency Domain Filter for Periodic Noise Reduction in Images Acquired by Projection Fringes. In *International Congress of Telematics and Computing*; Springer International Publishing: Cham, Switzerland, 2022; pp. 18–32.
18. Aizenberg, I.; Butakoff, C. A windowed Gaussian notch filter for quasi-periodic noise removal. *Image Vis. Comput.* **2008**, *26*, 1347–1353. [CrossRef]
19. López-Torres, C.V.; Salazar Colores, S.; Kells, K.; Pedraza-Ortega, J.C.; Ramos-Arreguin, J.M. Improving 3D reconstruction accuracy in wavelet transform profilometry by reducing shadow effects. *IET Image Process.* **2020**, *14*, 310–317. [CrossRef]
20. Wang, J.; Yang, Y. Phase extraction accuracy comparison based on multi-frequency phase-shifting method in fringe projection profilometry. *Measurement* **2022**, *199*, 111525. [CrossRef]
21. Bioucas-Dias, J.; Katkovnik, V.; Astola, J.; Egiazarian, K. Absolute phase estimation: Adaptive local denoising and global unwrapping. *Appl. Opt.* **2008**, *47*, 5358–5369. [CrossRef]
22. Bioucas-Dias, J.M.; Valadao, G. Phase unwrapping via graph cuts. *IEEE Trans. Image Process.* **2007**, *16*, 698–709. [CrossRef]
23. Espinosa-Bernal, O.A.; Pedraza-Ortega, J.C.; Aceves-Fernandez, M.A.; Martínez-Suárez, V.M.; Tovar-Arriaga, S.; Ramos-Arreguín, J.M.; Gorrostieta-Hurtado, E. Quasi/Periodic Noise Reduction in Images Using Modified Multiresolution-Convolutional Neural Networks for 3D Object Reconstructions and Comparison with Other Convolutional Neural Network Models. *Computers* **2024**, *13*, 145. [CrossRef]
24. Qian, J.; Feng, S.; Tao, T.; Hu, Y.; Li, Y.; Chen, Q.; Zuo, C. Deep-learning-enabled geometric constraints and phase unwrapping for single-shot absolute 3D shape measurement. *APL Photonics* **2020**, *5*, 046105. [CrossRef]
25. Alvarado Escoto, L.A.; Ortega, J.C.P.; Ramos Arreguin, J.M.; Gorrostieta Hurtado, E.; Tovar Arriaga, S. The effect of bilateral filtering in 3D reconstruction using PSP. In *Telematics and Computing, Proceedings of the 9th International Congress, WITCOM 2020, Puerto Vallarta, Mexico, 2–6 November 2020*; Proceedings 9; Springer International Publishing: Cham, Switzerland, 2020; pp. 268–280.
26. Chollet, F. *Deep Learning with Python*; Manning Publications: Shelter Island, NY, USA, 2020.
27. Dhiman, P.; Kaur, A.; Balasaraswathi, V.R.; Gulzar, Y.; Alwan, A.A.; Hamid, Y. Image acquisition, preprocessing and classification of citrus fruit diseases: A systematic literature review. *Sustainability* **2023**, *15*, 9643. [CrossRef]
28. Alkhatib, M.Q.; Al-Saad, M.; Aburaed, N.; Almansoori, S.; Zabalza, J.; Marshall, S.; Al-Ahmad, H. Tri-CNN: A three branch model for hyperspectral image classification. *Remote Sens.* **2023**, *15*, 316. [CrossRef]
29. Yuan, F.; Zhang, Z.; Fang, Z. An effective CNN and Transformer complementary network for medical image segmentation. *Pattern Recognit.* **2023**, *136*, 109228. [CrossRef]
30. Nasreen, G.; Haneef, K.; Tamoor, M.; Irshad, A. A comparative study of state-of-the-art skin image segmentation techniques with CNN. *Multimed. Tools Appl.* **2023**, *82*, 10921–10942. [CrossRef]
31. Ali, A.M.; Benjdira, B.; Koubaa, A.; El-Shafai, W.; Khan, Z.; Boulila, W. Vision transformers in image restoration: A survey. *Sensors* **2023**, *23*, 2385. [CrossRef]
32. Wang, Q.; Li, Z.; Zhang, S.; Chi, N.; Dai, Q. A versatile Wavelet-Enhanced CNN-Transformer for improved fluorescence microscopy image restoration. *Neural Netw.* **2024**, *170*, 227–241. [CrossRef]
33. Shah, A.; Shah, M.; Pandya, A.; Sushra, R.; Sushra, R.; Mehta, M.; Patel, K.; Patel, K. A comprehensive study on skin cancer detection using artificial neural network (ANN) and convolutional neural net-work (CNN). *Clin. eHealth* **2023**, *6*, 76-84. [CrossRef]
34. Jakubec, M.; Lieskovská, E.; Bučko, B.; Zábovská, K. Comparison of CNN-based models for pothole detection in real-world adverse conditions: Overview and evaluation. *Appl. Sci.* **2023**, *13*, 5810. [CrossRef]
35. Dash, A.; Ye, J.; Wang, G. A review of generative adversarial networks (GANs) and its applications in a wide variety of disciplines: From medical to remote sensing. *IEEE Access* **2024**, *12*, 18330–18357. [CrossRef]
36. Chakraborty, T.; KS, U.R.; Naik, S.M.; Panja, M.; Manvitha, B. Ten years of generative adversarial nets (GANs): A survey of the state-of-the-art. *Mach. Learn. Sci. Technol.* **2024**, *5*, 011001. [CrossRef]
37. Ahmad, Z.; Jaffri, Z.U.A.; Chen, M.; Bao, S. Understanding GANs: Fundamentals, variants, training challenges, applications, and open problems. *Multimed. Tools Appl.* **2024**, 1–77. [CrossRef]
38. Dunmore, A.; Jang-Jaccard, J.; Sabrina, F.; Kwak, J. A comprehensive survey of generative adver-sarial networks (GANs) in cybersecurity intrusion detection. *IEEE Access* **2023**, *11*, 76071–76094 [CrossRef]
39. Chen, C.; Wu, Y.; Dai, Q.; Zhou, H.Y.; Xu, M.; Yang, S.; Han, X.; Yu, Y. A survey on graph neural networks and graph transformers in computer vision: A task-oriented perspective. *IEEE Trans. Pattern Anal. Mach. Intell.* **2024**, *46*, 10297–10318. [CrossRef]

40. Sun, Y.; Yu, Y.; Wang, W. Moiré photo restoration using multiresolution convolutional neural networks. *IEEE Trans. Image Process.* **2018**, *27*, 4160–4172. [CrossRef]
41. Martínez-Suárez, V.M.; Pedraza-Ortega, J.C.; Salazar-Colores, S.; Espinosa-Bernal, O.A.; Ra-mos-Arreguin, J.M. Environment emulation in 3d graphics software for fringe projection profilometry. In *International Congress of Telematics and Computing*; Springer International Publishing: Cham, Switzerland, 2022; pp. 122–138.
42. Haji, S.H.; Abdulazeez, A.M.; Darrell, T. Comparison of optimization techniques based on gradient descent algorithm: A review. *PalArch's J. Archaeol. Egypt/Egyptol.* **2021**, *18*, 2715–2743.
43. Kingma, D.P.; Ba, J. Adam: A method for stochastic optimization. *arXiv* **2014**, arXiv:1412.6980.
44. Jiang, J.; Bao, S.; Shi, W.; Wei, Z. Improved traffic sign recognition algorithm based on YOLO v3 algorithm. *J. Comput. Appl.* **2020**, *40*, 2472.
45. Martinez-Carranza, J.; Falaggis, K.; Kozacki, T. Fast and accurate phase-unwrapping algorithm based on the transport of intensity equation. *Appl. Opt.* **2017**, *56*, 7079–7088. [CrossRef]
46. Hore, A.; Ziou, D. Image quality metrics: PSNR vs. SSIM. In Proceedings of the 2010 20th International Conference on Pattern Recognition, Istanbul, Turkey, 23–26 August 2010; pp. 2366–2369.

computers

MDPI

Article

Empowering Communication: A Deep Learning Framework for Arabic Sign Language Recognition with an Attention Mechanism

R. S. Abdul Ameer, M. A. Ahmed *, Z. T. Al-Qaysi, M. M. Salih and Moceheb Lazam Shuwandy

Department of Computer Science, Faculty of Computers & Mathematics, Tikrit University, Tikrit 34001, Iraq; rafalsaleh@tu.edu.iq (R.S.A.A.); ziadoontareq@tu.edu.iq (Z.T.A.-Q.); mahmaher1989@gmail.com (M.M.S.); moceheb@tu.edu.iq (M.L.S.)

* Correspondence: mohamed.aktham@tu.edu.iq

Abstract: This article emphasises the urgent need for appropriate communication tools for communities of people who are deaf or hard-of-hearing, with a specific emphasis on Arabic Sign Language (ArSL). In this study, we use long short-term memory (LSTM) models in conjunction with MediaPipe to reduce the barriers to effective communication and social integration for deaf communities. The model design incorporates LSTM units and an attention mechanism to handle the input sequences of extracted keypoints from recorded gestures. The attention layer selectively directs its focus toward relevant segments of the input sequence, whereas the LSTM layer handles temporal relationships and encodes the sequential data. A comprehensive dataset comprised of fifty frequently used words and numbers in ArSL was collected for developing the recognition model. This dataset comprises many instances of gestures recorded by five volunteers. The results of the experiment support the effectiveness of the proposed approach, as the model achieved accuracies of more than 85% (individual volunteers) and 83% (combined data). The high level of precision emphasises the potential of artificial intelligence-powered translation software to improve effective communication for people with hearing impairments and to enable them to interact with the larger community more easily.

Keywords: deaf communication; sign language recognition; dynamic hand gestures; deep learning; LSTM networks; attention mechanism; MediaPipe framework; human–computer interaction; multimodal integration; assistive technology

1. Introduction

People with hearing loss and speech impairments are deprived of effective contact with the rest of the community. According to the statistics of the International Federation of the Deaf and the World Health Organisation (WHO), more than 5% of people around the world are deaf and have severe difficulties communicating with those without hearing impairments, which means approximately 360 million people. Deaf individuals use another method to communicate instead of speech called sign language (SL) [1]. SL facilitates communication between the deaf community and people who are either deaf or nondisabled. SL is a visual communication system that encompasses both manual elements, such as hand gestures, and nonmanual elements, such as facial emotions and body movements [2]. SL is a complicated style of communication based mostly on hand gestures. These gestures are formed by different components, such as hand shape, hand motion, hand location, palm orientation, the movement of the lips, facial expressions, and points of contact between the hands or between the hands and other parts of the body, to express words, letters, and numbers.

Many sign languages exist in the deaf community, roughly one per country, which vary as much as spoken languages [3], e.g., Arabic Sign Language (ArSL), American Sign Language (ASL), British Sign Language (BSL), Australian Sign Language (Auslan), French Sign Language (LSF), Japanese Sign Language (JSL), Chinese Sign Language (CSL), German

Sign Language (DGS), Spanish Sign Language (LSE), Italian Sign Language (LIS), Brazilian Sign Language (LIBRAS), and Indian Sign Language, among others. Sign languages vary in lexicon, grammar, phonology, gesture form, and nonmanual elements, as do alphabets and words. Each language has its own unique features and regional variations, which reflect the diverse cultural and linguistic backgrounds of deaf communities worldwide. This diversity adds another difficulty, which is the lack of a unified sign language that serves universally as a vital means of communication and cultural expression for deaf individuals. Therefore, translating SL is indeed a necessary solution to bridge communication gaps between deaf and hearing individuals [4,5]. The development of automatic sign language translation systems reduces the reliance on human interpreters, lowers communication barriers, and promotes social inclusion in the deaf community. Hand gesture recognition is essential for automatic sign language translation systems. Researchers are increasingly interested in hand gesture recognition to solve communication challenges for deaf individuals, along with advances in gesture-controlled gadgets, gaming, and assistive technology [6].

Sign language recognition (SLR) systems focus on recognising and understanding sign language gestures and translating them into text or speech [7,8]. SLR systems typically involve artificial intelligence techniques to recognise and interpret the movements and forms of hands, fingers, and other relevant body parts used in SL. Several studies on sign language recognition (SLR) have attempted to bridge the communication gap between deaf and hearing individuals by eliminating the need for interpreters. However, sign language recognition systems have several obstacles, including a low accuracy, complex movements, a lack of large and full datasets containing various signals, and the models' inability to analyse them appropriately. Additionally, there are distinct indicators for each language [4,9,10].

This study proposes a deep learning (DL)-based model that leverages MediaPipe alongside RNN models to address the issues of dynamic sign language recognition. MediaPipe generates keypoints from hands and faces to detect position, form, and orientation, while LSTM models recognise dynamic gesture movements. Additionally, we introduce a new Arabic Sign Language dataset that focuses on dynamic gestures, as existing datasets predominantly feature static gestures in ArSL. In contrast, sensor-based solutions such as glove usage are expensive and impractical for everyday use due to power requirements and user annoyance. As a result, we abandoned this approach in favour of a more cost-effective approach involving the use of smartphone cameras to acquire data. The contributions of this study can be summarised as follows:

1. The DArSL50 dataset is a large-scale dataset comprised of 50 dynamic gestures in Arabic Sign Language (ArSL), including words and numbers, resulting in a total of 7500 video samples. This extensive dataset addresses the lack of sufficient data for dynamic gestures in ArSL and supports the development and evaluation of robust sign language recognition systems.
2. The proposed model leverages long short-term memory (LSTM) units with an attention mechanism combined with MediaPipe for keypoint extraction. This architecture effectively handles the temporal dynamics of gestures and focuses on relevant segments of input sequences.
3. The model's performance was evaluated in the following two scenarios: individual volunteer data and combined data from multiple volunteers. This dual evaluation approach ensures that the model is tested for its ability to generalise across different individuals and in different signing styles.
4. The proposed framework is validated for real-time performance.

The rest of this paper is organised as follows. Section 2 describes the methodology of the proposed ArSL recognition system and includes details about the DArSL 50 dataset. The experimental results are reported in Section 3, while an explanation of the results is presented in Section 4. Section 6 concludes the discussion and outlines future research directions.

The following two categories of sign language recognition systems can be distinguished according to the method used for data collection in the academic literature: sensor-based and vision-based [11], as shown in Figure 1.

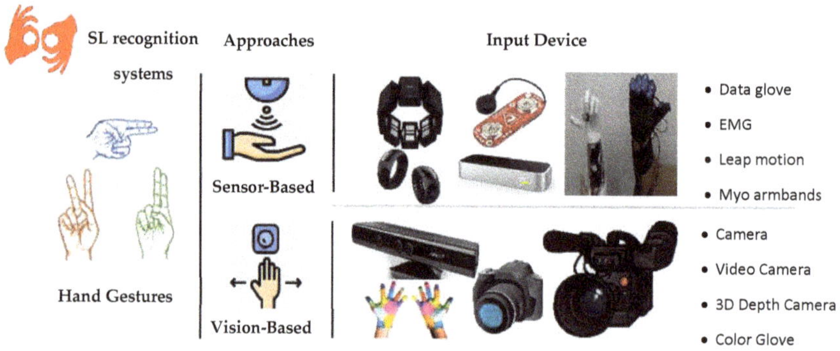

Figure 1. Sign language recognition approaches.

In the sensor-based method, sensors and equipment are used to collect the position, hand motion, wrist orientation, and velocity. Flex sensors, for instance, are used to measure finger movements. The inertial measurement unit (IMU) measures the acceleration of the fingers using a gyroscope and an accelerometer. The IMU is also used to detect wrist orientation. Wi-Fi and radar detect variations in the intensity of communications in the air using electromagnetic indicators. Electromyography (EMG) identifies finger mobility by measuring the electrical pulse in human muscles and then decreasing the biosignal. Other devices include haptic, mechanical, electromagnetic, ultrasonic, and flex sensors [12]. Sensor-based systems have an important advantage over vision-based systems, since gloves can rapidly communicate data to computers [13]. The device-based sensors (Microsoft Kinect sensor, Leap Motion Controller, and electronic gloves) can directly extract features without preprocessing, which means that the device-based sensors can minimise the time needed to prepare sign language datasets, data can be obtained directly, and a good accuracy rate can be achieved in comparison with vision-based devices [14]. Figure 2 demonstrates the primary phases of the SL gesture data collection and detection utilising the sensor-based system. The sensor-based approach has the issue of requiring the end-user to have a physical connection to the computer, making it unsuitable. Furthermore, it is expensive due to the use of sensitive gloves [13]. Despite the accuracy of the data that may be obtained from these devices, whether they wear gloves or are coupled to a computer, gadgets such as a Leap Motion or Microsoft Kinect device remain unpleasant [14].

Another option is the vision-based approach, which involves using a video camera to capture hand gestures. This gesture-detection solution combines appearance information with a 3D hand model. Key gesture capture technology in a vision-based technique was developed in Ref. [13]. Body markers such as colourful gloves, wristbands, and LED lights were used in this study, as well as active light projection systems that make use of the Kinect: Manufactured by Microsoft Corporation, Redmond, WA, USA. and Leap Motion Controller (LMC): Manufactured by Ultraleap Inc., San Francisco, CA, USA). A single camera might be employed with a smartphone camera, a webcam, or a video camera, as well as stereo cameras, which deliver rich information by using numerous monocular cameras. The primary benefit of employing a camera is that it removes the need for sensors in sensory gloves, lowering the system's manufacturing costs. Cameras are fairly inexpensive, and most laptops employ a high-specification camera due to the blurring effect of a webcam [13]. A simplified representation of the camera vision-based method for extracting and detecting hand movements is shown in Figure 3.

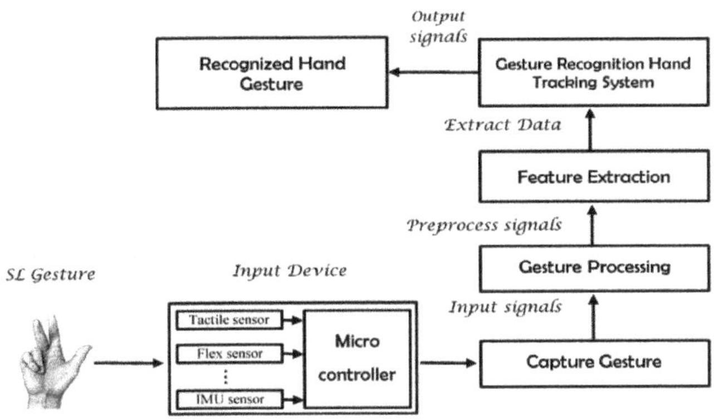

Figure 2. The main phases of recognising the SL gesture data using a sensor-based system [13].

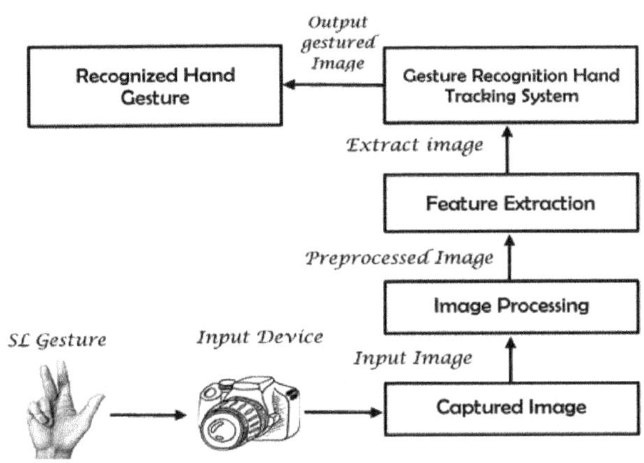

Figure 3. The procedure of vision-based sign language recognition [13].

In the literature, many SLR systems use traditional machine learning algorithms to classify the features of images to recognise SL gestures. In addition, the former uses traditional image segmentation algorithms to segment hand shapes from sign language images or the video frames of sign language video and then uses a machine-learning approach (such as SVM, HMM, or the k-NN algorithm). Using traditional machine learning algorithms has disadvantages related to handicraft features, which have a limited representational capability. It is difficult to extract representative semantic information from complex material, and step-by-step gesture recognition performs poorly in real-time. Other researchers have used deep neural networks to detect and recognise the gestures of SL. Deep neural network models such as CNNs, RNNs, GRUs, long short-term memory (LSTM), and bidirectional long short-term memory (LSTM) networks are used to address the issue of frame dependency in sign movement. These models employ an object-detection neural network to learn the video frame's features, allowing it to find the hand while also classifying the movements. Compared to traditional image processing and machine learning algorithms, deep neural network-based target detection networks frequently achieve a higher accuracy and recognition speed, as well as better real-time performance, and have become the mainstream method of dynamic target detection. The advantage of deep learning is its ability to automatically learn data representations directly from raw inputs. Deep learning models can autonomously extract features and patterns from complex datasets without the need for manual feature engineering [15].

SLR studies can also be divided into static sign language recognition and dynamic sign language recognition. The former performs gesture recognition by judging the hand posture, and it does not contain dynamic information. The latter contains hand movements and performs gesture recognition based on the video sequence, which is essentially a classification problem. Dynamic sign language recognition is much more difficult to implement than static sign language recognition, but it is more meaningful and valuable.

The following presents a review of SLR studies, including methods and datasets. In Ref. [16], a recognition system was utilised as a communication tool between those who are hearing-challenged and others who are not. This work describes the first automatic Arabic Sign Language (ArSL) recognition system using hidden Markov models (HMMs). A vast number of samples were utilised to identify 30 isolated terms from the standard Arabic Sign Language. The recognition accuracy of the system was between 90.6 and 98.1%. In Ref. [17], ArSL was based on the hidden Markov model (HMM). They collected a large dataset to detect 20 isolated phrases from the genuine recordings of deaf persons in various clothing and skin hues, and they obtained a recognition rate of approximately 82.22%. In Ref. [18], the authors presented an ArSL recognition system. The scope of this study includes the identification of static and dynamic word gestures. This study provides an innovative approach for dealing with posture fluctuations in 3D object identification. This approach generates picture features using a pulse-coupled neural network (PCNN) from two separate viewing angles. The proposed approach achieved a 96% recognition accuracy. Ref. [19] provided an automated visual SLRS that converted solitary Arabic word signals to text. The proposed system consisted of the following four basic stages: hand segmentation, tracking, feature extraction, and classification. A dataset of 30 isolated words used in the everyday school lives of hearing-challenged students was created to evaluate the proposed method, with 83% of the words having varied occlusion conditions. The experimental findings showed that the proposed system had a 97% identification rate in the signer-independent mode. Ref. [20] presented a framework for the field of Arabic Sign Language recognition. A feature extractor with deep behaviour was utilised to address the tiny intricacies of Arabic Sign Language. A 3D convolutional neural network (CNN) was utilised to detect 25 motions from the Arabic Sign Language vocabulary. The recognition system was used to obtain data from depth maps using two cameras. The system obtained a 98% accuracy for the observed data, but the for fresh data, the average accuracy was 85%. The results might be enhanced by including more data from various signers. In Ref. [21], a computational mechanism was described that allowed an intelligent translator to recognise the separate dynamic motions of ArSL. The authors utilised ArSL's 100-sign vocabulary and 1500 video clips to represent these signs. These signs included static signs such as alphabets, numbers ranging from 1 to 10, and dynamic words. Experiments were carried out on our own ArSL dataset, and the matching between ArSL and Arabic text was evaluated using Euclidian distance. The suggested way to automatically find and translate single dynamic ArSL gestures was tested and found to work well and correctly. The test findings revealed that the proposed system can detect signs with a 95.8% accuracy. In Ref. [4], the authors generated a video-based Arabic Sign Language dataset with 20 signs generated by 72 signers and suggested a deep learning architecture based on CNN and RNN models. The authors separated the data preprocessing into three stages. In the first stage, the proportions of each frame decreased to reach a lower total complexity. In the second stage, they sent the result to a code that subtracted every two consecutive frames to determine the motion between them. Finally, in the third stage, the attributes of each class were merged to produce 30 frames, with each unified frame combining 3 frames. The goal of stage three was to decrease the duplication while not losing any information. The primary idea behind the proposed architecture was to train two distinct CNNs independently for feature extraction, then concatenate the output into a single vector and transmit it to an RNN for classification. The proposed model scored 98% and 92% on the validation and testing subsets of the specified dataset, respectively. Furthermore, they attained promising accuracies of 93.40% and 98.80% on the top one and top five rankings of the UFC-101 dataset, respectively. The study by Ref. [22] provides a computer application for translating Iraqi Sign Language into Arabic (text). The translation process began with the capture of videos to create the dataset (41 words). The proposed system then employed a convolutional neural network (CNN) to categorise the sign language based on its attributes to infer the meaning of the signs. The proposed system's section that translates the sign language into Arabic text had an accuracy rate of 99% for the sign words.

Research on Arabic Sign Language recognition lacks common datasets available for researchers. Despite the publication of two volumes of "A Unified Arabic Sign Language Dictionary" in 2008, researchers in this field continue to face a lack of large-scale datasets. As such, each researcher needed to create a sufficiently large dataset to develop the ArSL recognition systems. Therefore, this study endeavoured to create a comprehensive dataset that was explicitly tailored for Arabic Sign Language recognition. Subsequently, this dataset serves as the foundation for the development of an accurate Arabic Sign Language recognition system capable of recognising the dynamic gestures inherent in ArSL.

2. Materials and Methods

The suggested system for recognising dynamic hand gestures uses keypoints that have been extracted. It is a neural network model that is constructed for learning from one sequence to another. Figure 4 depicts the primary phases of the proposed framework for recognising the dynamic gestures of Arab Sign Language.

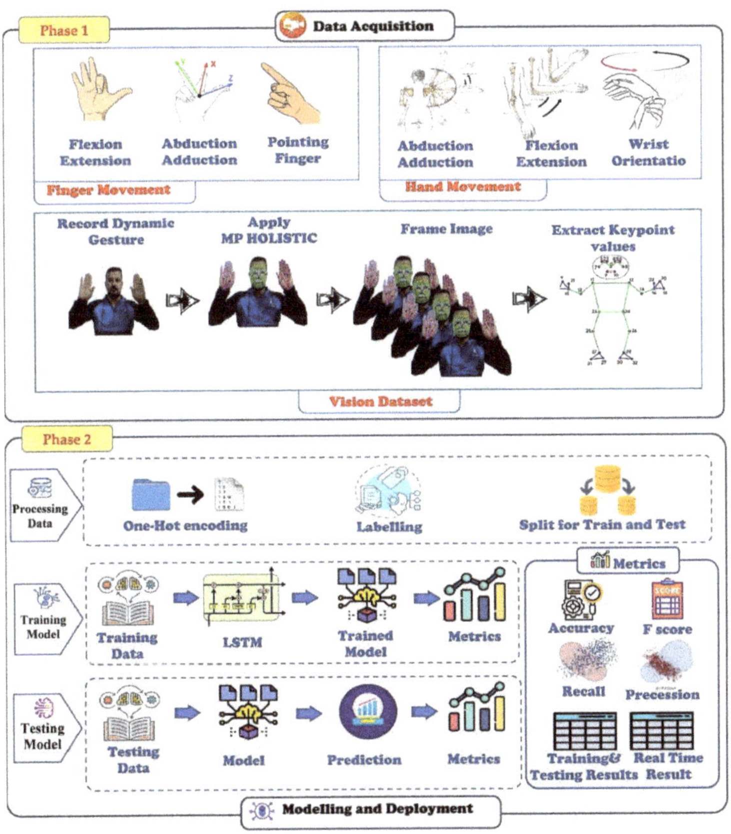

Figure 4. The proposed sign language recognition framework for dynamic Arabic gestures.

The model architecture incorporates both long short-term memory (LSTM) units and an attention mechanism. The model received a series of extracted keypoints from recorded gestures that indicate hand spatial configurations in a frame. The LSTM layer is responsible for processing the input sequence, identifying the temporal dependencies, and encoding the sequential information in its output sequence. The LSTM output sequence was also improved with an attention layer that allows the model to focus on different parts of the input sequence based on how relevant they are to the task at hand. The incorporation of this attention mechanism enhanced the ability of the model to recognise significant temporal patterns and spatial configurations within the sequences of gestures. Ultimately, the output layer generates a probability distribution over the potential classes of hand gestures, enabling the model to categorise the input sequences into predetermined gesture categories.

Anaconda Navigator (Anaconda3) and the free Jupyter Notebook Version 6.4.3 environment service were used to create the framework software package for the selected models. By utilising the Open-Source Computer Vision Library (OpenCV) Version 4.5.3, a specialised photo and video processing library that enables a wide range of tasks, including image analysis, facial recognition, and the identification of sign language gestures, along with the Mediapipe library, which extracts information from multimedia and which is the main tool for tracking motion and video analysis, the MP-holistic model was put into action along with some drawing functions. A dataset was recorded and gathered in which the volunteer represented all of the gestures by recording 30 videos of 30 frames each. The next stage was the conversion of frameworks from BGR to RGB colour coordination, because MediaPipe prefers RGB and Open CV coordination prefers BGR colour coordination. For the application of an activated model in each framework and the extraction of keypoint values, we created subvolumes under a major folder to store video clips for each class, where a separate folder was created for each class and each video under this volume, and these data were the data used to train the learning model to classify these classes. The dataset was collected and recorded using a webcam, and analysed using the MediaPipe model. The volunteer had to follow the criteria, which will be mentioned later, and then perform them. The key values discovered from the multimedia library's total model were extracted and stored for training. Then, we started the pretreatment phase, which involved labelling each class. A label was used to convert the correct name into a binary representation. For example, in our search for 50 classes of (0–49), Class 1 will become [0, 1, 0] and Class 2 will become [1, 0, 0]. A sequential neural network model comprising LSTM layers and fully linked layers was constructed for the classification. The training approach involved utilising data and the "Adam" algorithm to optimise the weight parameters, while the "categorical_crossentropy" function was employed to compute the loss during training. The term "categorical accuracy" refers to the correctness of the categorisation and served as a metric for evaluating the model's performance. The subsequent step involved saving the model, which could then be employed to recover the model and make predictions or to conduct the training. The last phase involved evaluating and using the confusion matrix, accuracy, and classification energy.

2.1. Dataset

In recent years, there has been tremendous development in the field of deep learning algorithms in artificial intelligence (AI). The success of AI applications depends on the quality and quantity of training and testing data. To improve AI systems, vast datasets must be collected and used. As far as we are aware, there is a lack of sufficient datasets for dynamic signals in Arabic Sign Language, which impedes the progress of recognition systems. Thus, it is crucial to create a large-scale dataset for dynamic signals in Arabic Sign Language. Accordingly, we created a DArSL50 dataset with a wide range of Arabic Sign Language dynamic motions. The DArSL50 dataset is comprised of 50 Arabic gestures representing 44 words and 6 digits. Each gesture was recorded by five participants. We selected signs from two dictionaries, "قاموس لغة الاشارة للاطفال الصم" (Sign Language Dictionary for Deaf Children) and "قاموس الاشاري العربي" (The Arabic Sign Language Dictionary for the Deaf).

Figure 5 displays a segment of the sign language database, which includes 50 dynamic signals in the Arabic Sign Language (ArSL) database. Five volunteers recorded each sign, with each participant performing each sign 30 times. Hence, the aggregate number of videos reached 7500, which was calculated by multiplying 50 by 5 and then by 30. The Video Capture function in OpenCV enabled the collection of data, which were then saved in NumPy format for further analysis.

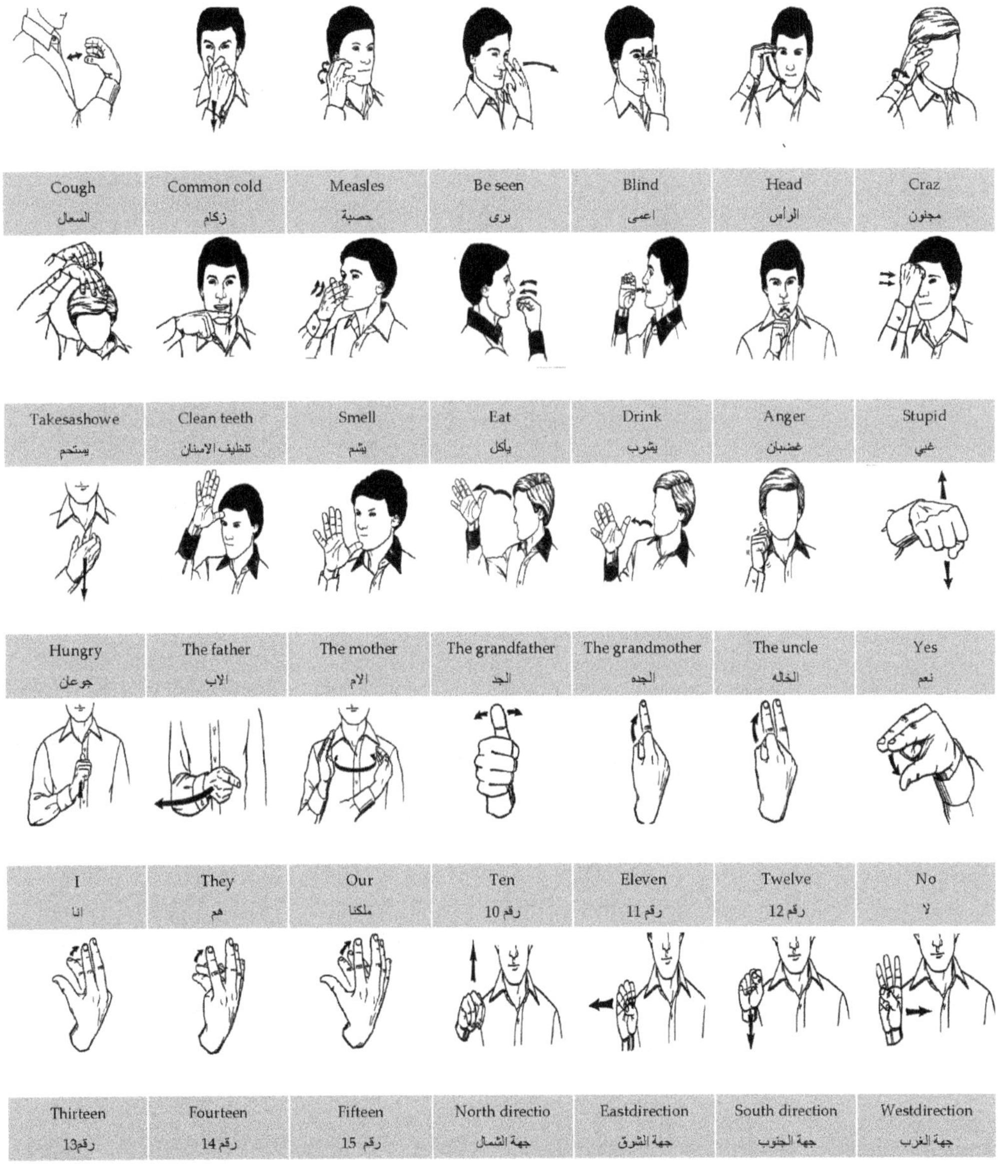

Figure 5. Images from the ArSL Words and Numbers dataset, which includes the lexicon for sign language for children that are deaf and the Arabic Sign Language Dictionary.

To collect the dataset, a series of processes were carried out. Initially, a collaboration was formed with the Deaf Centre, ensuring access to resources and specialised knowledge in Arabic Sign Language. Two dictionaries were examined to understand the signs. This study focused on 50 frequently used words and numbers, with a particular emphasis on those that may be expressed using only the right hand for the sake of simplicity. A group of volunteers was enlisted to imitate the signs, with each sign being replicated 30 times to capture variations. Data collection involved recording videos using a laptop camera, while the OpenCV program analysed the video clips by extracting important characteristics and preparing the data for additional analysis. This meticulous approach resulted in the creation of a complete and representative dataset for the study of ArSL signs. Volunteers of diverse demographics participated without limitations, ensuring inclusivity and diversity within the dataset. In addition, it is important to guarantee that the volunteer's body and all of their movements fit within the camera frame. A consistent and unchanging background setting should be ensured, with a particular emphasis on capturing volunteers' hands and faces. A robust camera tripod was used to generate crisp and dependable video recordings. In addition, it is advisable to establish the duration and frame count of the clip before recording, and to strive for a resolution of 640 × 480 or greater to achieve the best possible quality.

2.2. Feature Extraction Using MediaPipe

Google created MediaPipe, an open-source framework that allows developers to build multimodal (video, audio, and time-series data) cross-platform applied ML pipelines. MediaPipe contains a wide range of human body identification and tracking algorithms that were trained using Google's massive and diverse dataset. As the skeleton of the nodes and edges, or landmarks, they track keypoints on different parts of the body. All of the coordinated points are three-dimensionally normalised. Models built by Google developers using TensorFlow lite facilitate the flow of information that is easily adaptable and modifiable via graphs [23]. Sign language is based on hand gestures and stance estimation, yet the recognition of dynamic gestures and faces presents several challenges as a result of the continual movement. The challenges involved recognising the hands and establishing their form and orientation. MediaPipe was used to address these issues. It extracts the keypoints for the three dimensions of X, Y, and Z for both hands and estimates the postures for each frame. The pose estimation approach was used to forecast and track the hand's position relative to the body. The output of the MediaPipe architecture was a list of keypoints for hand and posture estimation. MediaPipe extracted 21 keypoints for each hand [24], as shown in Figure 6. The keypoints were determined in three dimensions, X, Y, and Z, for each hand. Therefore, the number of extracted keypoints for the hands is determined as follows [25]:

$$\text{keypoints in hand} \times \text{Three dimensions} \times \text{No. of hands} = (21 \times 3 \times 2) = 126 \text{ keypoints.}$$

For the pose estimation, MediaPipe extracted 33 keypoints [26], as shown in Figure 7. They were calculated in three dimensions (X, Y, and Z), in addition to the visibility. The visibility value indicates whether a point is visible or concealed (occluded by another body component) in a frame. Thus, the total number of keypoints extracted from the pose estimate is computed as follows [27]:

$$\text{keypoints in pose} \times (\text{Three dimensions} + \text{Visibility}) = (33 \times (3 + 1)) = 132 \text{ keypoints.}$$

For the face, MediaPipe extracted 468 keypoints [28], as shown in Figure 8. Lines linking landmarks define the contours around the face, eyes, lips, and brows, while dots symbolise the 468 landmarks. They were computed in three dimensions (X, Y, and Z). Thus, the number of retrieved keypoints from the face is computed as follows:

$$\text{Key points in face} \times \text{Three dimensions} = (468 \times 3) = 1404 \text{ keypoints.}$$

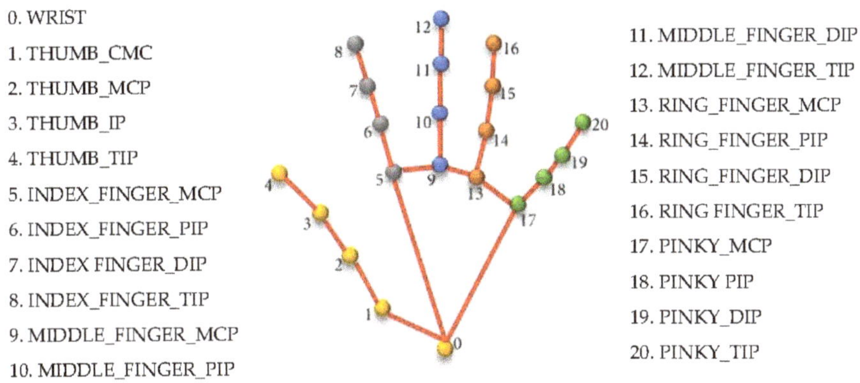

Figure 6. A total of 21 keypoints for the hand.

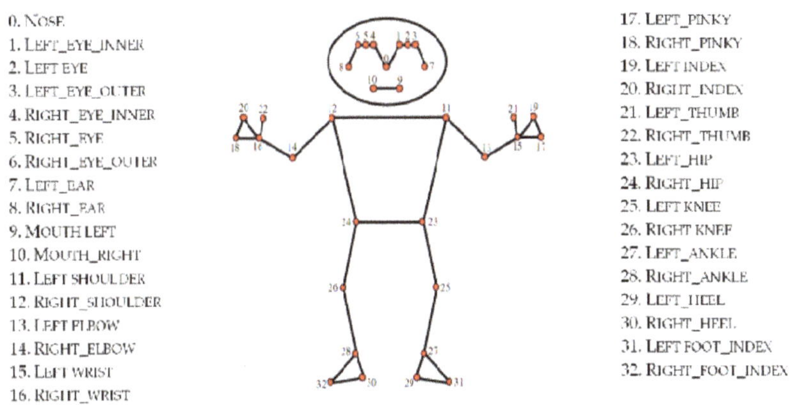

Figure 7. A total of 33 keypoints for the pose.

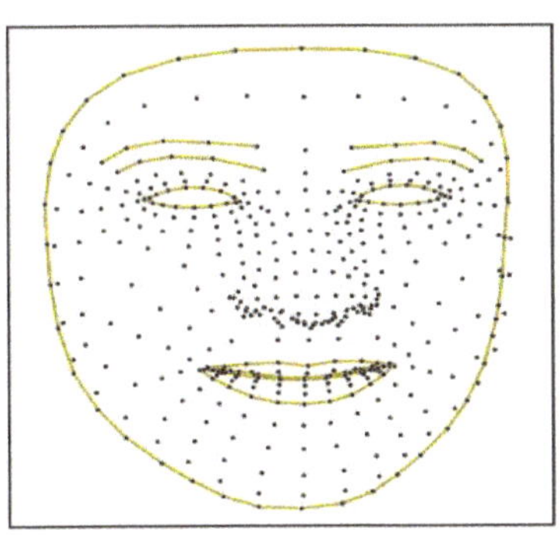

Figure 8. A total of 468 keypoints for the face.

The total number of keypoints for each frame was determined by summing the number of keypoints in the hands, the pose, and the face. This calculation resulted in a total of 1662 keypoints. Figure 9 displays the keypoints retrieved from a sample of frames.

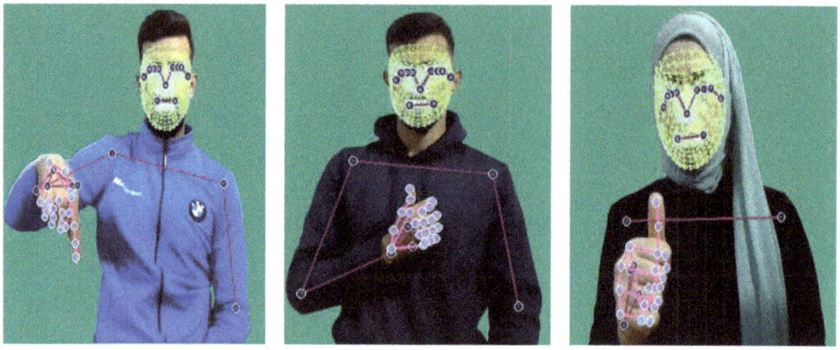

Figure 9. Keypoints that were extracted from a sample of frames.

2.3. Model

To process the dynamic gestures, data were represented as a series of frames, with each frame containing a collection of values representing the features of the hand posture in that frame. A recurrent neural network, specifically long short-term memory (LSTM), was used to process the resulting set of frames. LSTM is a well-known tool for encoding time series by extracting latent sign language expressions [29]. The model used in this study combines LSTM units with an attention mechanism. The model structure comprises the following three primary layers: an LSTM layer, an attention mechanism layer, and an output layer. The LSTM layer consists of 64 units, which contribute the most parameters to the model because of its recurring nature and the related parameters for each unit. The attention mechanism layer introduces a limited number of parameters, consisting of 10 units that govern the attention weights. The output layer, which is responsible for predicting the hand gesture classes, has a set of parameters that are dictated by the size of the context vector generated by the attention mechanism and the number of classes that need to be predicted. In total, the model consists of 89,771 parameters, with the LSTM layer accounting for the largest proportion. This architecture was specifically designed to efficiently handle sequential data, exploit temporal relationships, and dynamically prioritise essential sections of the input sequence, ultimately facilitating precise hand motion detection. The choice of the optimal parameter was pivotal for building these layers. Table 1 displays the utilised model parameters. During the use of the model, the parameters of each layer can be modified by picking values from Table 1 in preparation for the training phase.

Table 1. Model layer parameters.

Parameters	Value
Model	LSTM
Number of Nodes	64
Input Shape	(timesteps, 1662)
Attention Units	10
Activation	'softmax'
Optimiser	'adam'
Epochs	40

The choice of 64 hidden units and the specific activation function (ReLU) was based on preliminary experiments and established practices in similar research domains. An LSTM model with 64 hidden nodes was used to balance the model complexity and computational performance. We wanted a model that could learn complex data patterns without overfitting, which may occur with large networks. Experiments showed that 10 attention units offered enough attentional concentration without too much of a processing burden. We used 'SoftMax' for the activation function because it is common for classification tasks, especially multiclass problems. The LSTM model underwent training for a total of 40 epochs, with early stopping based on validation loss to prevent overfitting. The models' inputs include the sequence length and total number of keypoints. The sequence length is the number of frames contained in each clip. The total number of keypoints was 1662. At this point, the model is ready to accept the dataset and begin the training phase using the sequence of keypoints collected. Thus, the sign movement was examined and a hand gesture label could be used. As a result, DArSL-50 could be accurately detected.

2.4. Experiments

This research collected data from five participants, resulting in two separate scenarios. The first scenario involved creating the model by using the data from each volunteer separately. In the second scenario, the data gathered from the volunteers were combined, and then the suggested model was implemented. In Scenario 1, the dataset comprised data from five volunteers, with each volunteer contributing 1500 data points. For the training set, 1125 data points were selected, representing 75% of the total data, ensuring a comprehensive representation of the variability within the dataset. The remaining 375 data points were allocated to the testing set, representing 25% of the total data. This subset was reserved for evaluating the performance and generalizability of the trained models, as shown in Table 2.

Table 2. Data size, training set, and test set for each volunteer.

Number of Volunteers	Dataset Size	Train	Test	Size Test
One volunteer	1500	1125	375	0.25

In Scenario 2, four datasets were generated by combining the volunteer data. Data-I was composed of data collected from two volunteers, resulting in 3000 data points. Subsequently, Data-II, Data-III, and Data-V were formed by merging the data from three, four, and five volunteers, resulting in dataset sizes of 4500, 6000, and 7500 data points, respectively. To evaluate the proposed model, the dataset was partitioned into training and testing sets using a split ratio of 75–25 respectively. As a result, the training set consisted of 3375, 4500, and 5625 data points, while the testing set contained 1125, 1500, and 1875 data points for the datasets with three, four, and five volunteers, respectively, as shown in Table 3.

Table 3. Data size, training set, and test set for Scenario 2.

Dataset	Number of Volunteers	Dataset Size	Train Size	Test Size
Data-I	Two volunteers	3000	2250	750
Data-II	Three volunteers	4500	3375	1125
Data-III	Four volunteers	6000	4500	1500
Data-IV	Five volunteers	7500	5625	1875

The objective of integrating the dataset with data from numerous individuals was to improve the reliability and applicability of the trained models across a wide variety of signers and signing styles. By integrating the data from several individuals, the models were enhanced to effectively manage variances in gestures and signing styles, resulting in enhanced performance in real-world applications. This training and testing technique allowed for a thorough assessment and validation of the models, ensuring their dependability and efficacy in different settings and populations.

2.5. Evaluation Metrics

Evaluation metrics, such as the accuracy, precision, recall, and F1 score, are commonly used to evaluate the performance of classification models. These metrics provide crucial information about how well the model is doing and where it may require improvement.

Accuracy is the most commonly used simple metric for classification. It represents the ratio of the number of correctly classified predictions to the total number of predictions. A high level of accuracy indicates that the model is making correct predictions overall. The accuracy was calculated using Equation (1), as follows:

$$Accuracy = \frac{TP + TN}{TP + FP + TN + FN} \tag{1}$$

Precision measures the proportion of true positive predictions among all positive predictions.

Interpretation: A high precision indicates that, when the model predicts a positive class, it is likely to be correct. The precision is calculated using Equation (2), as follows:

$$Precision = \frac{TP}{TP + FP} \tag{2}$$

Recall measures the proportion of true positive predictions among all actual positive instances.

Interpretation: A high recall indicates that the model can identify most of the positive instances. The recall is calculated using Equation (3), as follows:

$$Recall = \frac{TP}{TP + FN} \tag{3}$$

The F1 score is the harmonic mean of the precision and recall, providing a balanced measure between the two metrics. The F1 score considers both the precision and recall, making it suitable for imbalanced datasets where one class dominates. The F1 score is calculated using Equation (4), as follows:

$$F1 - Score = \frac{(2 \times \ Precision \ \times \ Recall \ )}{(\ Precision \ + \ Recall \ )} \tag{4}$$

where:

The number of true positives (*TPs*) is the number of positive class samples correctly classified by a model. True negatives (*TNs*) are the number of negative class samples correctly classified by a model. False positives (*FPs*) are the number of negative class samples that were predicted (incorrectly) to be of the positive class by the model. False negatives (*FNs*) are the number of positive class samples that were predicted (incorrectly) to be of the negative class by the model. The classification report provides the accuracy, recall, and F1 score for each class, as well as the overall metrics. The assessment measures were used to determine how well the trained models performed on the testing datasets. This showed how well, accurately, and consistently they could recognise Arabic Sign Language gestures.

3. Results

The studies were carried out on a PC with an Intel(R) Core (TM) i7-10750H CPU operating at a base frequency of 2.60 GHz, which has 12 cores and 16,384 MB of RAM. The framework was developed using the Python programming language. The source code for this study may be accessed at the following URL: https://drive.google.com/file/d/1FcXudNQqXb_IzehsdMWb0tSBplcq-8LJ/view?usp=sharing (accessed on 10 June 2024). The dataset was gathered by a team of five volunteers, including a total of 50 distinct categories. Every participant captured recordings for the dataset consisting of 50 classes, and the outcomes were examined using the DArSL50 dataset. The DArSL50 dataset was divided randomly, with 75% used for training and 25% used for testing in the experiment. The performance criteria, such as the accuracy, precision, recall, and F1 score, were assessed under different situations to evaluate the functioning of the suggested system. In the first scenario, we evaluated the classification model with a dataset that included five participants' recordings; each participant provided 1500 data points. A training set was created from 1125 data points (representing 75% of the total), and a testing set was created from 375 data points (representing 25% of the total). Table 4 indicates the performance metrics obtained for each volunteer in Scenario 1.

Table 4. Results for Scenario 1.

Volunteer	Accuracy	Precision	Recall	F1 Score
Volunteer1	0.82	0.84	0.81	0.80
Volunteer2	0.83	0.83	0.83	0.82
Volunteer3	0.85	0.86	0.85	0.83
Volunteer4	0.83	0.84	0.85	0.83
Volunteer5	0.84	0.84	0.83	0.82

The data presented in Table 4 indicate that the third volunteer achieved the highest accuracy, approximately 85%, while the first volunteer achieved the lowest accuracy, approximately 82%. Nevertheless, the dataset's accuracy ratio for all volunteers was highly similar, indicating a highly effective discrimination mechanism for each individual. The results of Scenario 1 provide valuable insights into the model's efficacy in categorising hand movements using the given dataset. Through the evaluation of parameters such as accuracy, precision, recall, and the F1 score, we can determine the model's ability to generalise across various volunteers and accurately recognise gestures. The model's high accuracy, precision, recall, and F1 score demonstrate its effectiveness in recognising hand gestures from varied recordings. This indicates that the model is resilient and generalisable across multiple volunteers and signing styles. Table 5 shows the findings of Scenario 2, which included experiments to recognise dynamic hand gestures for four datasets. These datasets represent a combination of volunteer data.

Table 5. The proposed framework results for Scenario 2.

Dataset	Accuracy	Precision	Recall	F1 Score
Data-I	0.83	0.83	0.83	0.82
Data-II	0.82	0.83	0.83	0.82
Data-III	0.80	0.82	0.80	0.80
Data-IV	0.80	0.82	0.80	0.80

The results presented in Table 5 indicate that the highest level of accuracy, reaching 83%, was achieved by Data-I, which represents the combined data of two participants. However, Data-III and Data-IV achieved the minimum accuracy, which was approximately 80%. The accuracy of the four experiments varied between 83% and 80%, which is near and relevant in terms of the precision and recall. The F1 score, a metric that combines precision and recall using the harmonic mean, provides a well-balanced evaluation of the models' overall performance, with scores ranging from 0.82 to 0.80. By analysing Table 5, it is clear that the best accuracy ever achieved after the merger of volunteers is almost very close to the accuracy of the merger of the five volunteers, which suggests that the system is good with discrimination and has a strong impact, depending on the multiple people and the magnitude of the dataset. Overall, the models had good precision and recall scores, indicating that they could make accurate predictions and successfully detect positive events. These results show that the trained models are effective at recognising Arabic Sign Language. Compared to Data-IV, Table 6 shows the performance metrics (precision, recall, and the F1 score) for recognising 50 different types of ArSL gestures. Every row represents a particular class, and the metrics indicate the model's performance in accurately differentiating between gestures of that class.

Table 6. Results for the scenarios with classification reports for each class of Scenario 5.

Class Label	Dynamic Arabic Gesture	English Meaning	Precision	Recall	F1 Score
0	سعال	Cough	0.71	0.75	0.73
1	زكام	Common cold	0.84	0.82	0.83
2	حصبة	Measles	0.88	0.93	0.90
3	يرى	Be seen	0.73	0.84	0.78
4	اعمى	Blind	0.83	0.67	0.74
5	الرأس	Head	0.97	0.92	0.94
6	يستحم	Takes a shower	1.00	0.97	0.99
7	فرشاة اسنان	Cleaning teeth	0.79	0.98	0.87
8	يشم	Smell	0.86	0.65	0.68
9	يأكل	Eat	0.69	0.81	0.75
10	يشرب	Drink	0.76	0.77	0.76
11	غضبان	Anger	0.97	0.92	0.95
12	جوعان	Hungry	0.97	0.85	0.90
13	ابو	The father	0.97	0.88	0.92
14	ام	The mother	0.90	0.72	0.80
15	جد	The grandfather	0.86	1.00	0.92
16	جدة	The grandmother	0.91	0.94	0.93
17	خالة	The uncle	0.96	0.72	0.83
18	انا	I	0.87	0.84	0.85
19	هم	They	0.92	0.77	0.84
20	ملكنا	Our	0.92	0.87	0.89
21	10رقم	Ten number	0.71	0.75	0.73
22	11رقم	Eleven number	0.81	0.65	0.65
23	12رقم	Twelve number	0.65	0.65	0.67
24	13رقم	Thirteen number	0.65	0.67	0.65
25	14رقم	Fourteen number	0.65	0.68	0.65

Table 6. *Cont.*

Class Label	Dynamic Arabic Gesture	English Meaning	Precision	Recall	F1 Score
26	15رقم	Fifteen number	0.65	0.65	0.66
27	جهة الشمال	North direction	0.68	0.94	0.79
28	جهة الشرق	East direction	0.94	0.72	0.82
29	جهة الجنوب	South direction	0.84	0.65	0.71
30	جهة الغرب	West direction	0.79	0.89	0.84
31	نعم	Yes	0.68	0.83	0.75
32	لا	No	0.74	0.89	0.81
33	يفهم	Understand	0.67	0.88	0.74
34	غبي	Stupid	0.83	0.88	0.85
35	مجنون	Crazy	0.90	0.74	0.81
36	مع السلامة	Goodbye	0.94	1.00	0.97
37	مهم	Important	0.79	0.76	0.77
38	نمو	To grow	1.00	0.98	0.99
39	(صمت)اسكت	Shut up (silence)	0.88	0.88	0.88
40	(الان)حالا	Immediately (now)	0.71	0.89	0.79
41	(دمعة)حزين	Sad (tear)	0.97	0.91	0.94
42	حضور	Presence (coming)	0.95	0.97	0.96
43	ذهاب	To go	1.00	0.91	0.95
44	اهلا	Hello (congratulations)	0.96	0.69	0.80
45	توقف	To stop	0.88	0.94	0.91
46	امانة	Honesty	0.92	0.70	0.71
47	اعطى	To give	0.74	0.94	0.83
48	(قضى على)اهلك	To destroy	0.69	0.88	0.77
49	تخلص من	To get rid of	0.91	0.91	0.91

Table 6 presents a comprehensive analysis of the performance metrics of the model for each class in the classification report. Some classes demonstrate exceptional performance, as seen by their high precision, recall, and F1 score levels. For instance, the classes "Takes a shower", "Our", "The grandfather", and "Understand" exhibit high scores in all measures, indicating that the model accurately recognises these actions. However, specific classes exhibit disparities in performance indicators. For example, the "Blind" class exhibits relatively high precision but lower recall and F1 scores, suggesting that the model can accurately detect certain instances of this gesture but may fail to detect certain actual occurrences.

Classes such as "Common cold", "Measles", and "Stupid" consistently and effectively display strong recognition abilities across all parameters, indicating their robustness in gesture recognition. Conversely, classes such as "North direction", "East direction", and "To grow" display different performance metrics, with higher precision but lower recall values. This suggests that the model might have difficulty in accurately identifying all occurrences of these gestures. Based on the categorisation report results, we discovered that classes 11, 12, 13, and 14 (equivalent to classes 23, 24, 25, and 26, respectively) performed relatively poorly compared to the other classes. This is due to the nature of the movement in these classes, where the distinction between individual movements may be unclear. For example, the movement could be a slight hand gesture with no substantial variations in motion, or the difference between one movement and another may not be obvious enough, making classification more difficult for these classes. High values of accuracy, precision, recall, and the F1 score indicate successful model performance, while lower values may signify areas for improvement in the model's predictive capabilities.

To evaluate the system performance in real-time sign language detection, measurements were made concerning the reading error rate at the first stage. Algorithm 1 presents the approach used to measure the system performance metrics. Each letter was tested individually with five participants, and 40 iterations were applied to each letter to determine the frequency of the recognition. Consequently, the performance of the proposed system can be assessed by calculating the recognition accuracy of each gesture, followed by the total accuracy of the entire system, as shown in Algorithm 1. Errors in the results may be categorised as either "misclassification" (incorrect recognition) or "gesture not recognised" (not detection). The accuracy and error rates are determined using the equations provided below:

$$\text{Accuracy\%} = \frac{\text{detected right}}{\text{Num.of itration}} \times 100 \tag{5}$$

$$\text{Wrong recognise\%} = \frac{\text{detected wrong}}{\text{Num.of itration}} \times 100 \tag{6}$$

$$\text{Not detected\%} = \frac{\text{not detected}}{\text{Num.of itration}} \times 100 \tag{7}$$

Algorithm 1 Inference procedures for real-time sign language detection.

```
Input: D—new data                    {perform dynamic gesture}
Output: M real-time sign language detection model performance metrics
Initialise I ← 0, D ← 0, Z ← 0, E ← 0 {Initialise counts}
while I < 40 do
    gesture ← CaptureGesture()       {Capture the gesture}
    if RecogniseGesture(gesture) == DesiredGesture then
        D ← D + 1                    {Increment correct detection count}
        Display("Gesture is found")
    else
        if gesture == "No detection", then
            Z ← Z + 1                {Increment no detection count}
            Display("Gesture is not recognised")
        else
            E ← E + 1                {Increment misclassification count}
            Display("Misclassification: Wrong recognition")
        end if
    end if
    I ← I + 1                        {Increment iteration count}
end while
Display("Total Correct Detections: " + D)
Display("Total Misclassifications: " + E)
Display("Total Nondetections: " + Z)
Display("Total Iterations: " + I)
```

The real-time results are summarised in Table 7, which shows the accuracy, error of incorrect recognition, and error of not detecting each sign. The real-time performance analysis of dynamic Arabic gesture recognition reveals high accuracy for gestures such as "مع السلامة" (Goodbye) and "فرشاة اسنان" (Cleaning teeth), indicating the model's proficiency with distinct patterns. However, lower accuracy and higher error rates in gestures such as "اعمى" (Blind) and " يشم" (Smell) suggest difficulties in distinguishing these gestures, highlighting areas for improvement.

Table 7. The Real-Time Performance Result.

Class Label	Dynamic Arabic Gesture	English Meaning	Accuracy (%)	Err of Wrong Detected (%)	Err of Not Detected (%)
0	سعال	Cough	75	17	8
1	زكام	Common cold	82	11	7
2	حصبة	Measles	93	7	0
3	يرى	Be seen	84	0	16
4	اعمى	Blind	72	12	16
5	الرأس	Head	92	2	6
6	يستحم	Takes a shower	97	0	3
7	فرشاة اسنان	Cleaning teeth	98	0	2
8	يشم	Smell	75	5	20
9	يأكل	Eat	81	10	9
10	يشرب	Drink	77	16	7
11	غضبان	Anger	92	3	5
12	جوعان	Hungry	85	3	12
13	ابو	The father	88	3	9
14	ام	The mother	72	10	18
15	جد	The grandfather	100	0	0
16	جدة	The grandmother	94	0	6
17	خالة	The uncle	72	8	20
18	انا	I	84	13	3
19	هم	They	77	8	15
20	ملكنا	Our	87	0	13
21	رقم10	Ten number	75	20	5
22	رقم11	Eleven number	65	22	13

Table 7. *Cont.*

Class Label	Dynamic Arabic Gesture	English Meaning	Accuracy (%)	Err of Wrong Detected (%)	Err of Not Detected (%)
23	رقم12	Twelve number	65	25	10
24	رقم13	Thirteen number	67	26	7
25	رقم14	Fourteen number	68	28	4
26	رقم15	Fifteen number	65	15	20
27	جهة الشمال	North direction	94	3	3
28	جهة الشرق	East direction	72	6	22
29	جهة الجنوب	South direction	75	6	19
30	جهة الغرب	West direction	89	2	9
31	نعم	Yes	83	8	9
32	لا	No	89	4	7
33	يفهم	Understand	88	0	12
34	غبي	Stupid	88	3	9
35	مجنون	Crazy	74	0	26
36	مع السلامة	Goodbye	100	0	0
37	مهم	Important	76	11	13
38	نمو	To grow	98	0	2
39	(صمت)اسكت	Shut up (silence)	88	6	6
40	(الان)حالا	Immediately (now)	89	0	11
41	(دمعة)حزين	Sad (tear)	91	3	6
42	حضور	Presence (coming)	97	0	3
43	ذهاب	To go	91	0	9
44	اهلا	Hello (congratulations)	85	11	4

The results presented in Table 7 evaluate the real-time recognition proficiency of dynamic Arabic gestures, which achieved an overall accuracy rate of 83.5%. The accuracy of dynamic Arabic gestures indicates a generally high performance for many gestures, such as "مع السلامة" (Goodbye) and "فرشاة اسنان" (Cleaning teeth), with a 100% and 98% accuracy, respectively, and minimal errors. This reflects the model's effectiveness in recognising distinct gestures. Conversely, gestures such as "يشم" (Smell) and "اعمى" (Blind) achieved a moderate accuracy, with significant errors not detected (20% and 16%). Numeric gestures, particularly "رقم11"

(Eleven number) and "رقم12" (Twelve number), provide lower accuracy and higher error rates, suggesting challenges in distinguishing similar visual patterns. Figure 10 shows examples of complex signs that achieved low accuracy due to similarity problems.

Number 11: The hand is contracted and facing upwards, with the thumb extended. The hand moves from the wrist to the right and left.

Number 12: The hand is contracted and facing upwards, with the index finger extended.

Number 13: The hand is contracted and facing upwards, with the index and middle fingers extended.

Number 14: The hand is contracted and facing upwards, with the index, middle, and ring fingers extended, while the thumb is joined to the palm.

Number 15: The hand is contracted and facing upwards, with all fingers extended.

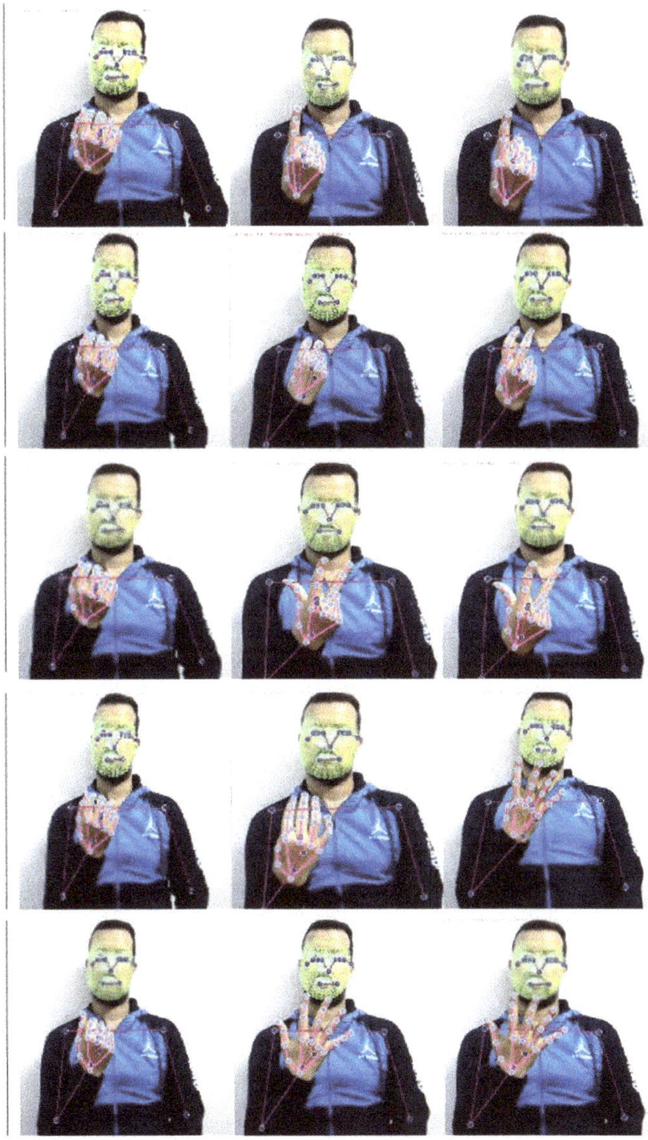

Figure 10. The similarity between the signs in ArSL.

4. Discussion

The evaluation of the model performance through the comparison of "macro-" and "weighted" averages offers useful insights into how the distribution of classes affects the accuracy of categorisation. While "macro-averages" provide a simple average over all classes, "weighted" averages take into consideration class imbalance by assigning weights to the average based on the number of instances in each class. Our investigation revealed that both types of averages showed similar patterns across different circumstances, indicating the continuous impact of class distribution on the model results. Analysing the outcomes of every scenario clarifies the connection between the model performance, volunteer contributions, and dataset size. The best accuracy and F1 score were obtained in Scenario 1, when each volunteer provided 1500 data points, demonstrating the potency of the individual volunteer datasets. We observed a modest decline in the accuracy and F1 score in Scenario 2, as the dataset size rose with the merged data from several participants. Larger datasets may have advantages, but adding a variety of volunteer contributions could complicate things and impair the model performance according to this tendency. Additional analysis of the classification report offers valuable information about the specific difficulties faced by the model in distinct categories. Classes 10, 11, 12, and 13 demonstrated worse precision, recall, and F1 scores than did the other classes, suggesting challenges in successfully recognising these gestures. This difference highlights the significance of analysing metrics relevant to each class to discover areas where the model may need more refinement or training data augmentation to enhance its performance.

Several factors contribute to these classes' inferior performance. First, the nature of the movements within these classes may provide complexity that is difficult to fully determine. For example, these movements may include subtle gestures or minor differences between different signs, making it difficult for the model to distinguish between them efficiently. Furthermore, the classification model may have problems catching the intricacies of these movements, particularly if they include small fluctuations or sophisticated hand movements that are difficult to identify precisely. Moreover, the minimal size and diversity of the dataset for these classes may have contributed to the poor performance. A larger and more diversified dataset would give the model a broader set of instances, improving its capacity to generalise and identify these complex movements. To summarise, while the model's overall performance is acceptable, further modification and augmentation of the dataset, as well as the model architecture, are required to enhance the classification accuracy for these hard classes. This highlights the need for ongoing research and development efforts in the field of sign language recognition to solve these unique issues while also improving the accessibility and effectiveness of sign language recognition technology. The observed influence of an increasing dataset size emphasises the need for data augmentation and the establishment of larger, more diverse datasets in sign language recognition research. As part of the study's objectives, the goal was to create a comprehensive dataset exclusively for Arabic Sign Language recognition. By expanding the dataset, the model can be trained on a broader collection of instances, boosting its capacity to generalise and reliably identify sign language movements, especially in difficult categories. This is consistent with the overall goal of improving the accessibility and effectiveness of sign language recognition systems, ultimately leading to greater inclusivity and accessibility for people with hearing impairments.

5. A Comparison with Previous Studies

This study focused on the recognition of dynamic gestures performed with a single hand captured using a single camera setup. The primary goal was to recognise isolated dynamic words and dynamic numbers expressed through sign language gestures. The data collection process involved recording sessions where individuals performed these gestures in front of the camera, ensuring that the dataset captured a diverse range of hand movements and expressions, and by limiting the scope to dynamic gestures performed with one hand. Table 8 provides a comparison with prior studies that align with our objectives.

Table 8. Comparison with similar ArSL recognition systems.

Aspect	Proposed Work	Study [4]	Study [23]	Study [17]
Model Used	Long short-term memory (LSTM) with an attention mechanism	Convolutional neural network (CNN)	Convolutional neural network (CNN)	Hidden Markov models (HMMs)
Dataset Size	7500	7200	390	4045
Number of gestures	50 (30 simple, 20 complex)	20 (simple signs)	30 (simple signs)	30 (simple signs)
Gestures	Words and numbers	Words	Words	Words
Balanced data	YES	NO	NO	NO
Preprocessing	No need to convert the frames into greyscale	Convert the frames into greyscale	Convert the frames into greyscale	Convert the frames into greyscale
Feature Extraction Method	MediaPipe framework for hand and body keypoints	An adaptive threshold and adding a unique factor to each class	Two convolution layers with 32 and 64 parameters	Discrete cosine transform (DCT)
Best Accuracy	85% (individual volunteers), 83% (combined data)	92%	99.7%	90.6%
Real-World Applicability	Verified	Not verified	Not verified	Not verified

The dataset size in the proposed work is also significantly larger, at 7500 samples, compared to 7200 in Ref. [4], 390 in Ref. [23], and 4045 in Ref. [17]. A larger dataset contributes to better model generalizability and robustness, ensuring that the model performs well on diverse and unseen data. Moreover, the proposed framework handles 50 gestures, including both simple and complex signs, whereas the other studies focus primarily on simple signs (20 in Ref. [4], 30 in Ref. [23] and Ref. [17]). This broader range of gestures, which includes words and numbers, demonstrates the versatility and applicability of the proposed model for more comprehensive sign language recognition tasks. The data used in the proposed framework are balanced, ensuring that the model is trained on an equal representation of all gesture classes, reducing bias and improving the overall performance. In contrast, the datasets in Refs. [4,17,23] are not balanced, which could lead to skewed results favouring more frequent classes. For data collection, the proposed framework uses recorded videos with keypoint extraction using MediaPipe, a state-of-the-art framework for extracting hand and body keypoints. This method captures more detailed motion data than do the simpler approaches used in other studies, such as the smartphone videos in Ref. [4] and OpenPose version 1.4 in Ref. [17]. In terms of preprocessing, the proposed framework simplifies the process by not converting frames to greyscale, preserving more information from the original videos.

The MediaPipe feature extraction method used in the proposed framework is more advanced than methods, such as adaptive thresholding, convolution layers, and discrete cosine transform (DCT), which have been used in other studies. The proposed framework might not be as accurate as those used in other studies, but it is a strong and flexible solution for sign language recognition because it can better handle complex gestures, has a larger and more balanced dataset, uses advanced data collection and preprocessing methods, and can evaluate performance in real-time.

6. Conclusions

In this study, we attempted to meet the pressing need for effective communication tools for the deaf community by developing a model that can recognise dynamic hand gestures from video recordings. This was accomplished by combining the attention mechanism with LSTM units developed on a new ArSL dataset, namely, the DArSL50_Dataset. Keypoints were extracted from videos in the DArSL50 dataset using the MediaPipe framework. Subsequently, the features were fed into the proposed LSTM model to detect gestures. The results of our method were encouraging, with an average performance of 80–85%. The proposed model architecture demonstrated robustness in classifying hand motions despite variances in signing styles and recording conditions. The attention mechanism enhanced the framework's ability to recognise spatial arrangements and temporal relationships in sign language gestures by selectively focusing on key parts of the input sequences. Our research indicates that our method has considerable promise in enabling smooth communication between deaf and hearing populations. Future research could investigate other model architectures, such as Bi-LSTM, one-dimensional convolutional neural networks, convolutional recurrent neural networks, and transformer models. Additionally, there is potential for the creation of a large-scale dataset encompassing a variety of sign language gestures. Augmentation techniques could also be investigated to further enrich the dataset and improve the model's ability to generalise across various signing styles.

Author Contributions: R.S.A.A.: Conceptualization, Methodology, Writing—Original Draft; M.A.A.: Supervision, Methodology, Project Administration, Writing—Review & Editing; Z.T.A.-Q.: Data Curation, Software, Formal Analysis; M.M.S.: Validation, Investigation, Visualization; M.L.S.: Resources, Writing—Review & Editing. All authors have read and agreed to the published version of the manuscript.

Funding: No funding was received for this study.

Data Availability Statement: The source code for this study may be accessed at the following URL: https://drive.google.com/file/d/1FcXudNQqXb_IzehsdMWb0tSBplcq-8LJ/view?usp=sharing (accessed on 10 June 2024).

Conflicts of Interest: The authors declare no conflict of interest.

References

1. Ahmed, A.M.; Alez, R.A.; Taha, M.; Tharwat, G. Automatic translation of Arabic sign to Arabic text (ATASAT) system. *J. Comput. Sci. Inf. Technol.* **2016**, *6*, 109–122.
2. Ahmed, M.A.; Zaidan, B.; Zaidan, A.; Salih, M.M.; Al-Qaysi, Z.; Alamoodi, A. Based on wearable sensory device in 3D-printed humanoid: A new real-time sign language recognition system. *Measurement* **2021**, *168*, 108431. [CrossRef]
3. Alrubayi, A.; Ahmed, M.; Zaidan, A.; Albahri, A.; Zaidan, B.; Albahri, O.; Alamoodi, A.; Alazab, M. A pattern recognition model for static gestures in malaysian sign language based on machine learning techniques. *Comput. Electr. Eng.* **2021**, *95*, 107383. [CrossRef]
4. Balaha, M.M.; El-Kady, S.; Balaha, H.M.; Salama, M.; Emad, E.; Hassan, M.; Saafan, M.M. A vision-based deep learning approach for independent-users Arabic sign language interpretation. *Multimedia Tools Appl.* **2023**, *82*, 6807–6826. [CrossRef]
5. Tharwat, A.; Gaber, T.; Hassanien, A.E.; Shahin, M.K.; Refaat, B. Sift-based arabic sign language recognition system. In *Afro-European Conference for Industrial Advancement: Proceedings of the First International Afro-European Conference for Industrial Advancement AECIA 2014*; Springer: Berlin/Heidelberg, Germany, 2015.
6. Abdul, W.; Alsulaiman, M.; Amin, S.U.; Faisal, M.; Muhammad, G.; Albogamy, F.R.; Bencherif, M.A.; Ghaleb, H. Intelligent real-time Arabic sign language classification using attention-based inception and BiLSTM. *Comput. Electr. Eng.* **2021**, *95*, 107395. [CrossRef]
7. Suharjito; Anderson, R.; Wiryana, F.; Ariesta, M.C.; Kusuma, G.P. Sign language recognition application systems for deaf-mute people: A review based on input-process-output. *Procedia Comput. Sci.* **2017**, *116*, 441–448. [CrossRef]
8. Al-Saidi, M.; Ballagi, Á.; Hassen, O.A.; Saad, S.M. Cognitive Classifier of Hand Gesture Images for Automated Sign Language Recognition: Soft Robot Assistance Based on Neutrosophic Markov Chain Paradigm. *Computers* **2024**, *13*, 106. [CrossRef]
9. Samaan, G.H.; Wadie, A.R.; Attia, A.K.; Asaad, A.M.; Kamel, A.E.; Slim, S.O.; Abdallah, M.S.; Cho, Y.-I. MediaPipe's landmarks with RNN for dynamic sign language recognition. *Electronics* **2022**, *11*, 3228. [CrossRef]
10. Almasre, M.A.; Al-Nuaim, H. Comparison of four SVM classifiers used with depth sensors to recognize arabic sign language words. *Computers* **2017**, *6*, 20. [CrossRef]
11. Al-Shamayleh, A.S.; Ahmad, R.; Jomhari, N.; Abushariah, M.A.M. Automatic Arabic sign language recognition: A review, taxonomy, open challenges, research roadmap and future directions. *Malays. J. Comput. Sci.* **2020**, *33*, 306–343. [CrossRef]
12. Cheok, M.J.; Omar, Z.; Jaward, M.H. A review of hand gesture and sign language recognition techniques. *Int. J. Mach. Learn. Cybern.* **2019**, *10*, 131–153. [CrossRef]

13. Ahmed, M.A.; Zaidan, B.B.; Zaidan, A.A.; Salih, M.M.; Bin Lakulu, M.M. A review on systems-based sensory gloves for sign language recognition state of the art between 2007 and 2017. *Sensors* **2018**, *18*, 2208. [CrossRef]
14. Mohammed, R.; Kadhem, S. A review on arabic sign language translator systems. In *Journal of Physics: Conference Series*; IOP Publishing: Bristol, UK, 2021.
15. Jiang, X.; Satapathy, S.C.; Yang, L.; Wang, S.-H.; Zhang, Y.-D. A survey on artificial intelligence in chinese sign language recognition. *Arab. J. Sci. Eng.* **2020**, *45*, 9859–9894. [CrossRef]
16. Al-Rousan, M.; Assaleh, K.; Tala'a, A. Video-based signer-independent Arabic sign language recognition using hidden Markov models. *Appl. Soft Comput.* **2009**, *9*, 990–999. [CrossRef]
17. Youssif, A.A.; AAboutabl, E.; Ali, H.H. Arabic sign language (arsl) recognition system using hmm. *Int. J. Adv. Comput. Sci. Appl.* **2011**, *2*, 45–51.
18. Elons, A.S.; Abull-Ela, M.; Tolba, M. A proposed PCNN features quality optimization technique for pose-invariant 3D Arabic sign language recognition. *Appl. Soft Comput.* **2013**, *13*, 1646–1660. [CrossRef]
19. Ibrahim, N.B.; Selim, M.M.; Zayed, H.H. An automatic Arabic sign language recognition system (ArSLRS). *J. King Saud Univ. -Comput. Inf. Sci.* **2018**, *30*, 470–477. [CrossRef]
20. ElBadawy, M.; Elons, A.S.; Shedeed, H.A.; Tolba, M.F. Arabic sign language recognition with 3d convolutional neural networks. In Proceedings of the 2017 Eighth International Conference on Intelligent Computing and Information Systems (ICICIS), Cairo, Egypt, 5–7 December 2017; IEEE: Piscataway, NJ, USA, 2017.
21. Ahmed, A.M.; Alez, R.A.; Tharwat, G.; Taha, M.; Belgacem, B.; Al Moustafa, A.M.; Ghribi, W. Arabic sign language translator. *J. Comput. Sci.* **2019**, *15*, 1522–1537. [CrossRef]
22. Mohammed, R.; Kadhem, S.M. Iraqi sign language translator system using deep learning. *Al-Salam J. Eng. Technol.* **2023**, *2*, 109–116. [CrossRef]
23. Halder, A.; Tayade, A. Real-time vernacular sign language recognition using mediapipe and machine learning. *J. Homepage* **2021**, *2582*, 7421.
24. Zhang, F.; Bazarevsky, V.; Vakunov, A.; Tkachenka, A.; Sung, G.; Chang, C.L.; Grundmann, M. Mediapipe hands: On-device real-time hand tracking. *arXiv* **2020**, arXiv:2006.10214.
25. Wu, T.-L.; Senda, T. Pen Spinning Hand Movement Analysis Using MediaPipe Hands. *arXiv* **2021**, arXiv:2108.10716.
26. Bazarevsky, V.; Grishchenko, I.; Raveendran, K. BlazePose: On-device Real-time Body Pose tracking. *arXiv* **2020**, arXiv:2006.10204.
27. Chen, K.-Y.; Shin, J.; Hasan, A.M.; Liaw, J.-J.; Yuichi, O.; Tomioka, Y. Fitness Movement Types and Completeness Detection Using a Transfer-Learning-Based Deep Neural Network. *Sensors* **2022**, *22*, 5700. [CrossRef]
28. Kartynnik, Y.; Ablavatski, A.; Grishchenko, I.; Grundmann, M. Real-time facial surface geometry from monocular video on mobile GPUs. *arXiv* **2019**, arXiv:1907.06724.
29. Alnahhas, A.; Alkhatib, B.; Al-Boukaee, N.; Alhakim, N.; Alzabibi, O.; Ajalyakeen, N. Enhancing the recognition of Arabic sign language by using deep learning and leap motion controller. *Int. J. Sci. Technol. Res.* **2020**, *9*, 1865–1870.

computers

MDPI

Article

Enhancing Brain Segmentation in MRI through Integration of Hidden Markov Random Field Model and Whale Optimization Algorithm

Abdelaziz Daoudi [1,*] and Saïd Mahmoudi [2,*]

[1] Department of Computer Science, Faculty of Exact Sciences, Tahri Mohammed University, Bechar 08000, Algeria
[2] ILIA Department, Faculty of Engineering, University of Mons, 7000 Mons, Belgium
* Correspondence: daoudi.abdelaziz@univ-bechar.dz (A.D.); said.mahmoudi@umons.ac.be (S.M.)

Abstract: The automatic delineation and segmentation of the brain tissues from Magnetic Resonance Images (MRIs) is a great challenge in the medical context. The difficulty of this task arises out of the similar visual appearance of neighboring brain structures in MR images. In this study, we present an automatic approach for robust and accurate brain tissue boundary outlining in MR images. This algorithm is proposed for the tissue classification of MR brain images into White Matter (WM), Gray Matter (GM) and Cerebrospinal Fluid (CSF). The proposed segmentation process combines two algorithms, the Hidden Markov Random Field (HMRF) model and the Whale Optimization Algorithm (WOA), to enhance the treatment accuracy. In addition, we use the Whale Optimization Algorithm (WOA) to optimize the performance of the segmentation method. The experimental results from a dataset of brain MR images show the superiority of our proposed method, referred to HMRF-WOA, as compared to other reported approaches. The HMRF-WOA is evaluated on multiple MRI contrasts, including both simulated and real MR brain images. The well-known Dice coefficient (DC) and Jaccard coefficient (JC) were used as similarity metrics. The results show that, in many cases, our proposed method approaches the perfect segmentation with a Dice coefficient and Jaccard coefficient above 0.9.

Keywords: brain tissue segmentation; HMRF method; WOA; classification

1. Introduction

In the human body, the most complex organ is the brain. It is responsible for coordinating and controlling many bodily activities and every process that regulates the body. Alzheimer's disease, epilepsy, encephalitis, meningitis, and brain abscesses and tumors are different forms of brain disease [1].

In recent years, the manual examination and interpretation of images obtained from various imaging modalities such as Radiography, Magnetic Resonance Imaging (MRI), and Computed Tomography (CT) have become challenging and intensive processes. This underscores the fact that that automatic image analysis by several operations is a necessity [2–4]. MRI brain segmentation helps in detecting brain diseases, analyzing brain changes, identifying pathological areas, and measuring and visualizing the anatomical structures of the brain. Furthermore, brain segmentation is a difficult task due to the homogeneities and correlations of image intensity among brain tissues. Nevertheless, many research methodologies have been proposed for brain tissue MR image segmentation. For example, Qaiser Mahmood et al. [5] present a fully automatic unsupervised segmentation algorithm called BAMS, where a combination of the Bayesian method and Adaptive Mean-Shift (BAMS) are applied to real multimodal MR images to segment brain tissues into four regions: White Matter (WM), Gray Matter (GM), Cerebrospinal Fluid (CSF), and background. In the last step, the authors used the voxel-weighted kmeans clustering algorithm to merge the homogeneous regions obtained in the previous steps.

In another work, Henri A. Vrooman et al. [6] proposed a brain segmentation process based on an automatically trained kNN classifier. This kNN classification method incorporates voxel intensities from a T1-weighted MRI scan and a FLAIR sequence scan. In [7], the authors introduced a hybrid approach based on techniques for brain MRI segmentation. The method utilizes the Gabor transform for computing features of brain MRI. Subsequently, these features are subjected to classification using various classifiers, including Incremental Supervised Neural Network, K-NN, Probabilistic Neural Network (PNN), and Support Vector Machine (SVM). A drawback of these approaches [5–7] is that they may give poor tissue classifications in the presence of noise, and that they are computationally expensive.

In recent years, there has been more research in the field of brain tumor MR image segmentation. For example, the study of Jalab H A et al. [8] presented and evaluated a novel convolutional neural autoencoder designed for brain tumor segmentation using semantic segmentation principles. The evaluation was conducted on a dataset consisting of 3064 T1-weighted Contrast-Enhanced Magnetic Resonance Images. In [9], Hasan AM et al. used three techniques to precisely pinpoint the area of pathological tissues in volumetric MRI brain scans: the first one is a three-dimensional active contour model without boundaries, the second one is a multi-layer perceptron neural network adopted as a classifier, and the third one is a bounding box-based genetic algorithm. The most important limitations that make brain tumor segmentation [8,9] a challenging task are the varieties of the shape and intensity of tumors, along with the probability of inhomogeneity within tumorous tissue.

The Hidden Markov Random Field Model is a segmentation algorithm popularly used in image segmentation, such as by Ahmadvand et al. [10], Jianhua et al. [11], Shah Saurabh [12], and Mingsheng Chen [13]. A combination of fuzzy clustering and the MRF model was presented by Mingsheng Chen et al., where the Fuzzy C-Means (FCM) algorithm was combined with the MRF model to filter the effect of noise and to increase the integrity of segmented regions. An additional work using the HMRF model for segmenting brain tissue was presented by Alansary et al. [14], in which the authors proposed the unsupervised learning of different brain structures from T1-weighted MR brain images, by using the Maximum A posteriori Probability (MAP) estimate with a joint Markov–Gibbs Random Field Model (MGRF). In [15], the authors proposed the optimization of the MRFM by using the Broyden–Fletcher–Goldfarb–Shanno algorithm to segment brain tissues. In [16], a generalization of the HMRF model with the Expectation Maximization (EM) method was applied and tested on brain MRI data. These hybrid methods are used to significantly decrease computational time in comparison to classical MRF. However, they often lack accurate segmentation of MRI brain tissue.

Some other studies used a Fuzzy C-Means algorithm to improve the segmentation accuracy of brain images. For example, in [17], the authors used an improved multi-view FCM with an adaptive learning mechanism to segment brain images.

In some references, brain segmentation methods based on deep learning techniques have been proposed in brain segmentation, such as by Zhao L et al. [18], Brudfors Mikael et al. [19], and Bento M [20]. For example, Lee B et al. [21] introduced a non-overlapping patch-wise U-net architecture to remedy the drawbacks of the conventional U-Net with greater retention of local information. On the other hand, Renukadevi [22] et al. proposed a medical image classification with a Histogram and Time–Frequency Differential Deep Learning method using brain Magnetic Resonance Imaging. First, a supervised training method was applied by an intensity-oriented Histogram to prepare the feature extraction step. Then, time and frequency factors were applied to the pre-processed features to obtain a set of features. These features are used in the Differential Deep Learning process. The main drawback of these approaches is their expensive computational cost, as the training process needs to be repeated multiple times. Other researchers have used hybrid approaches combining deep learning with fuzzy logic to segment MRI brain tumors. For example, in [23], the authors propose a novel approach combining fuzzy logic-based edge detection and U-Net CNN classification for brain tumor detection. This work demonstrates superior performance in identifying meningioma and non-meningioma brain images, outperforming existing methods in terms of performance metrics. But the analysis provided in this work lacks a detailed analysis of the drawbacks associated with the fuzzy logic-based edge detection or U-Net CNN classification methods used for the brain tumor detection process.

Among the optimization algorithms that have appeared in the 1980s used in images segmentation, we can cite metaheuristics methods. In the study proposed in [24], a biologically inspired ant colony algorithm was proposed to optimize the thresholding technique for MR brain image segmentation, but the thresholding methods faced some limitations that decreased the overall accuracy of the segmentation method. On the other hand, Thuy Xuan Pham et al. [25] presented an optimization method that combines metaheuristic methods (cuckoo search and particle swarm optimization algorithms) and an HMRF model to provide brain tissue segmentation. The authors of this work applied their model to both simulated and real MR images. This method is limited by its tendency to increase computational complexity due to the problem of selecting an appropriate value for the parameter β, as well as the running time for both the ICS and IPSO algorithms.

On the other hand, many techniques have been proposed suggested to aid in detecting brain lesions and diseases. The authors in [26] have proposed a pre-trained U-Net encoder–decoder system to extract ischemic stroke lesions (ISLs), using image processing techniques on brain MRI slices from the ISLES2015 database. This study achieved high Jaccard, Dice, and accuracy values on a dataset of 500 images. However, the main limitation of this approach is that the number of test images may not fully represent the variability in ischemic stroke lesions and increasing the training dataset size may introduce biases or artifacts in the segmentation process. Ramya, J et al. [27] present a novel method for Alzheimer's disease classification using MRI data. This method focuses on image processing techniques such as 2D Adaptive Bilateral Filtering, the ECLAHE algorithm for image enhancement, and feature extraction using GLCM and PCA. The paper lacks comparisons with other advanced classification techniques, and the proposed method presents high computational complexity. Rangaraju et al. [28] introduce a novel deep learning-based method for automated Alzheimer's disease detection using 3D brain MRI data, where the authors used a Patch Convolutional Neural Network and Octave convolution for feature identification and spatial redundancy reduction. The limitation of this method is that the accuracy metric may not be adequate for evaluating the model's efficacy if the dataset has an uneven distribution of classes.

In this proposal, our concern is to solve the problem of segmenting brain MR images into three tissues: GM, WM, and CSF, without apparent disease. To attain this objective, the whale optimization algorithm (WOA) is employed to optimize the HMRF model, offering an automated segmentation tool for brain MR images. Then, the proposed method performance evaluation is achieved on ground truth images from the BrainWeb and Internet Brain Segmentation Repository (IBSR) databases, using the Dice coefficient metric (DC) and the Jaccard coefficient (JC).

The overall contributions of this paper are as follows:

- A new optimization method applied to MRI image segmentation.
- A novel technique using the combination of HMRF and the WOA is proposed.
- The proposed method improves the accuracy of segmenting brain images into three tissues: GM, WM, and CSF.
- This manuscript primarily focuses on brain tissue segmentation to aid experts and radiologists.

The efficacy of the HMRF-WOA is tested on six datasets with various parameters collected from BrainWeb and the IBSR. The experimental results demonstrate remarkable performance when segmenting different types of homogeneous and heterogeneous tissues. By employing this architecture, our aim is to achieve improved accuracy, efficiency, and reliability compared to existing state-of-the-art models.

This paper is organized as follows: In Sections 2 and 3, we give a detailed explanation of the HMRF model and Whale Optimization Algorithm. The algorithm design (HMRF-WOA) is presented in Section 4, followed by the experimental results and discussions in Section 5, and the conclusion in the last section.

2. Hidden Markov Random Field Model

The Hidden Markov Random Field model is a stochastic process whose state sequence can be indirectly deduced from observations. The MRF includes a set of random variables. Let y be the observed image (i.e., the image for segmentation) and x the hidden image (i.e., the resulting segmented image). Both images (y and x) are formed of L sites or positions set; we note these sites as $S = \{s_1, s_2 \ldots, s_L\}$.

So, we consider that $y = \{y_1, y_2, \ldots, y_L\}$ is the image to be segmented, where y_s is one of the pixel values and $x = \{x_1, x_2, \ldots, x_L\}$ is the resulting segmented image, where x_s is one of the pixel classes. We consider $Ey = \{0 \ldots 255\}$ and $Ex = \{1 \ldots K\}$ to be the gray-level intensity space and the discrete space, respectively, where K denotes the number of homogeneous zones in the image. In classification methods, pixels are organized based on these gray levels. The random variables $Y = (y_1 \ldots, y_L)$ and $X = (x_1, \ldots, x_L)$ adopt their values from Ey and Ex, respectively.

We propose to use the HMRF model to segment the image y by searching for the optimal realization x* of X by maximizing the posteriori probability value $P[X = x/Y = y]$.

$$x^* = argmax\{P[X = x/Y = y]\}, x \in E_x \tag{1}$$

which is written by the law of Bayes:

$$P(X = x \ / \ Y = y) = \frac{P(Y = y \ / \ X = x) \, .P(X = x)}{P(Y = y)} \tag{2}$$

where $P(Y = y/X = x)$ indicates the probability distribution of $Y = y$; given that $X = x$ has occurred, it is called likelihood. $P(X = x)$ is the preliminary probability of $X = x$ based on prior knowledge. The denominator $P(Y = y)$ is the probability of $Y = y$ occurring; it is called the evidence.

For each site, we associated a descriptor which represents a gray level. Any family V(s) possessing the following properties was labelled as a neighborhood system:

- Where $s \notin V(s)$ ⇔, a site is not a neighborhood to itself.
- Where $s \in V(t)$ ⇔ $t \in V(s)$, the neighborhood relationship is symmetrical.

The most frequently used neighborhoods are either the four or the eight nearest neighbors: they are referred to as the first- and second-order neighborhoods, respectively. The neighborhood relationship between sites is the clique $c \in C$. (C represents the set of all potential cliques.)

A Random Field X is identical to a Gibbs distribution (Hammersley–Clifford theorem) [29] if the joined probability distribution is:

$$P(X = x) = W^{-1} \, exp(-H(X = x)) \tag{3}$$

where $W^{-1} = \sum_x \exp(-H(X = x))$ is a normalization function, also called the partition function, and H is a nearly constant energy which decomposes into the sum of potential U_c functions associated with cliques $c \in C$.

$$H(X = x) = \textstyle\sum_{c \, \in \, C} U(X_C) \tag{4}$$

Equation (3) becomes:

$$P(X = x) = \frac{exp(U(X_C))}{\sum_{c \, \in \, C} exp(U(X_C \,))} \tag{5}$$

In the image space, we take the second-order neighborhood system as the interactions system between pixels (i.e., 8 neighbors of each pixel), so we have 8 cliques for each pixel. A pair of neighboring pixels (i, j), defined as a clique potential, is used as a factor in the energy function $U(X_c)$ of the Potts model [30]. In this Potts model, the energy function is generally based on the interactions between neighboring pixels, and the formula for this energy function for image segmentation using this Potts model is written as:

$$U_c(x_i, x_j) = \beta(1 - V(x_i, x_j)) \tag{6}$$

where i and j are indices of the neighboring pixels.

β is a weight associated with the pair of neighboring pixels (a constant).

x_i, x_j are the classes assigned to pixels i, j, respectively.

$V(x_i, x_j)$ is a function which equals 1 if the two pixels of the clique belong to the same class and 0 otherwise.

$$V(x_i, x_j) = \begin{cases} 1 & if \quad x_i = x_j \\ 0 & if \quad x_i \neq x_j \end{cases} \tag{7}$$

The fundamental assumption of the HMRF model is that for any configuration x of X, the random variables Y are conditionally independent, and the distribution of the pixels follows the normal law, i.e., there is an independence between classes, and the field of observations can be modeled by the following function:

$$P(Y = y \;/\; X = x) = \prod\nolimits_{s \in S} P(Y_s = y_s \;/ X_s = x_s) \tag{8}$$

Given that $P(Y_s = y_s \;/ X_s = x_s)$ follows the Gaussian distribution, it can be written as:

$$P(Y_s = y_s \;/ X_s = x_s) = \frac{1}{\sqrt{2\pi\sigma_{x_s}^2}} \exp\left[\frac{-(y_s - \mu_{x_s})^2}{2\sigma_{x_s}^2}\right] \tag{9}$$

where μ_{x_s} is the mean and σ_{x_s} is the standard deviation.

According to Equations (8) and (9), we obtain:

$$P(Y = y \;/\; X = x) = \prod\nolimits_{s \in S} \frac{1}{\sqrt{2\pi\sigma_{x_s}^2}} \exp\left[\frac{-(y_s - \mu_{x_s})^2}{2\sigma_{x_s}^2}\right]$$

With

$$\frac{1}{\sqrt{2\pi\sigma_{x_s}^2}} = \exp\left(ln\left(\frac{1}{\sqrt{2\pi\sigma_{x_s}^2}}\right)\right) \quad and \quad \ln\left(\frac{1}{\sqrt{2\pi\sigma_{x_s}^2}}\right) = -\ln\left(\sqrt{2\pi\sigma_{x_s}^2}\right)$$

Then, we obtain

$$P(Y = y \;/\; X = x) = \prod\nolimits_{s \in S} \left(\exp\left(-\ln\left(\sqrt{2\pi\sigma_{x_s}^2}\right)\right).\exp\left[\frac{-(y_s - \mu_{x_s})^2}{2\sigma_{x_s}^2}\right]\right)$$

$$P(Y = y \;/\; X = x) = \prod_{s \in S} \exp\left(-\ln\left(\sqrt{2\pi\sigma_{x_s}^2}\right) - \frac{(y_s - \mu_{x_s})^2}{2\sigma_{x_s}^2}\right)$$

$$P(Y = y \;/\; X = x) = \exp\left[-\left[\sum\nolimits_{s \in S}\left[\ln\left(\sqrt{2\pi\sigma_{x_s}^2}\right) + \frac{(y_s - \mu_{x_s})^2}{2\sigma_{x_s}^2}\right]\right]\right]$$

We come back to Bayes' law in Equation (2), with $P(Y = y)$ being the constant value C, and obtain:

$$P(X = x\ /\ Y = y) = \frac{1}{C}\exp\left[-\left[\sum_{s\in S}\left[\ln\left(\sqrt{2\pi\sigma_{x_s}^2}\right) + \frac{(y_s - \mu_{x_s})^2}{2\sigma_{x_s}^2}\right]\right]\right].\exp\left[\beta\sum_{c\in C}[1 - V(x_i, x_j)]\right]$$

$$P(X = x\ /\ Y = y) = C'.\exp\left[-\left[\sum_{s\in S}\left[\ln\left(\sqrt{2\pi\sigma_{x_s}^2}\right) + \frac{(y_s - \mu_{x_s})^2}{2\sigma_{x_s}^2}\right]\right]\right].\exp\left[\beta\sum_{c\in C}[1 - V(x_i, x_j)]\right]$$

$$P(X = x\ /\ Y = y) = C'.\exp\left[-\left[\sum\nolimits_{s\in S}\left[\ln\left(\sqrt{2\pi\sigma_{x_s}^2}\right) + \frac{(y_s - \mu_{x_s})^2}{2\sigma_{x_s}^2}\right]\right] + \beta\sum\nolimits_{c\in C}[1 - V(x_i, x_j)]\right]$$

$$\begin{cases} P(X = x\ /\ Y = y) = C'.\exp(-\varphi(x,y)) \\ \varphi(x,y) = \sum\limits_{s\in S}\left[\ln\left(\sqrt{2\pi\sigma_{x_s}^2}\right) + \frac{(y_s-\mu_{x_s})^2}{2\sigma_{x_s}^2}\right] + \beta\sum\limits_{c\in C}[1 - V(x_i, x_j)] \end{cases}$$

where C' is a positive constant and β is used to control the size of homogeneous regions and the interaction between their sites. μ_{x_i}, σ_{x_i} are the mean and standard deviation of the class x_i, respectively (i.e., the ith region $\Omega_i = \{s\ /\ x_s = i\}$ in the image). Then, μ_{x_i}, σ_{x_i} are described as follows:

$$\begin{cases} \mu_i = \frac{1}{|\Omega_i|}\sum_{s\in\Omega_i} y_s \\ \sigma_i = \sqrt{\frac{1}{|\Omega_i|}\sum_{s\in\Omega_i}(y_s - \mu_i)} \end{cases} \quad (10)$$

Once we know all the parameters of the HMRF model, we can perform the segmentation itself, i.e., find the value to maximize the probability $P(X = x/Y = y)$, which is equivalent in this context to minimize $\varphi(x, y)$ such that $x^* = \text{argmin}\ \{\ \varphi(x, y)\}$.

To seek a given pixel class x_s, we can consider an approximation of the exact segmentation using optimization techniques. Furthermore, we can obtain the optimal segmentation $x^*(x_1, \ldots x_s \ldots x_L)$ through $\mu^*\ (\mu_1, \ldots \mu_i, \ldots, \mu_k)$ by classifying y_s into the same category of the nearest mean μ_i of μ (i.e., $x_s = i$ if the nearest mean of y_s is μ_i). We seek μ^* instead of x^* and the optimal means value μ^* as follows:

$$\mu^* = \text{argmin}\{\varphi(\mu)\} \quad (11)$$

where $\varphi(\mu)$ is defined as:

$$\varphi(\mu) = \sum\nolimits_{s\in S}\left[\ln\left(\sqrt{2\pi\sigma_{x_s}^2}\right) + \frac{(y_s - \mu_{x_s})^2}{2\sigma_{x_s}^2}\right] + \beta\sum\nolimits_{c\in C}[1 - V(x_i, x_j)] \quad (12)$$

This objective function (Equation (12)) is simply a formula that can be applied in the optimization process. Accordingly, in the section below, we will define the optimization method applied in this work.

3. Whale Optimization Algorithm

The Whale Optimization Algorithm is among the latest bio-inspired optimization algorithms. It is proposed for optimizing numerical problems [31]. Humpback whales are among the largest and oldest animals in the world; they are highly intelligent animals that feel emotion and never sleep [32–34]. This algorithm emulates the intelligent foraging behavior of this animal. This hunting comportment is called the bubble net feeding method and is an exclusive method of hunting that can only be observed in humpback whales.

In recent years, a large number of works in the literature have applied the WOA for optimization in several fields, such as [35–39]. In order to perform optimization, including the exploitation and exploration phases, the mathematical model is explained below. For more details, please refer to [31,40].

Step 1: Encircling Prey phase

When the prey's location is identifiable, humpback whales start to circle their prey. Then, the humpback whales create bubble nets to catch their prey. $X_i^t = \left(x_{i,1}^t \cdots x_{N,D}^t\right)$ denotes the place of the ith whale at time t (iteration value), with i ∈ [1...N], where N represents the whale population and *D* is the dimensions of the problem. In the search zone, the whales consider the target prey or prey in the close vicinity as the optimal solution; during this phase, other whales seek to come closer to the best search agent and update their position using Equation (13).

$$D = |C.X^*(t) - X_i(t)| \tag{13}$$

$$X_i(t+1) = X^*(t) - A.D \tag{14}$$

where *t* indicates the present iteration, the parameter $X_i(t)$ denotes the position of each individual i at the tth iteration, $X^*(t)$ signifies the optimal global position at the tth iteration, and | | is the absolute value. Equations (15) and (16) are used to define the factor vectors *A* and C, respectively:

$$A = 2ar - a \tag{15}$$

$$C = 2r \tag{16}$$

$$a = 2.\left(1 - \frac{t}{T_{max}}\right) \tag{17}$$

The parameter (a) linearly declines over the course of the iteration from 2 to 0, and r is a random value in [0, 1].

Step 2: Bubble-Net Attacking Method (Exploitation Phase)

Two mechanisms are designed to mathematically model the predation behavior of humpback whales, which can be described as follows:

1. Shrinking encircling mechanism: According to Equation (15), the decrease in the value of A depends on the decrease in the value of the control parameter a. Note that the search agent approaches the current optimal solution when the value of the random variable A is set in the range [−1, 1].
2. Spiral updating position: To capture food, humpback whales take a spiral-shaped path around their prey. Equations (18) and (19) are used to reproduce the helix-shaped movement of humpback whales and to calculate the distance between the whale and the prey, respectively:

$$X_i(t+1) = D'.\, e^{bl}.\cos(2\pi.l) + X^*(t) \tag{18}$$

$$D' = |X^*(t) - X_i(t)| \tag{19}$$

where D' is the distance between the whale and prey (the best solution obtained so far), *b* is a constant that defines the logarithmic shape, and *l* is a random value in [−1, 1]. During the iterations of the algorithm, the movement behavior of humpback whales is either shrinking encircling or spiral movement. For this behavior, assuming a probability of 50%, the mathematical model can be described as follows:

$$X_i(t+1) = \begin{cases} X^*(t) - A.D & if \quad p < 0.5 \\ D'.\, e^{bl}.\cos(2\pi.l) + X^*(t) & if \quad p \geq 0.5 \end{cases} \tag{20}$$

where *p* is an arbitrary value in [0, 1].

Step 3: Search for Prey (Exploration Phase)

In the exploration phase, the search is performed randomly. First, one of the whales' populations is selected randomly to allow the global search, then according to this randomly chosen population the position of the search is updated. In this phase, it is necessary to use the random values of the parameter A higher than 1 or lower than -1 to obligate the search agent to move far away from a reference whale. The model's equations are expressed as follows:

$$D = |C.X_{rand} - X \ | \tag{21}$$

$$X_i(t+1) = X_{rand} - A.D \tag{22}$$

where X_{rand} represents a random position vector chosen from the available whales in the population.

As mentioned earlier, the Whale Optimization Algorithm (WOA) is one of the latest swarm-based algorithms and it showed high performance when addressing various optimization problems, such as an analysis of medical image segmentation [41] and optimization tasks [42]. Recently, the WOA gained significant attention from researchers due to its ability to be quickly implemented and its requirement of only a few parameters to fine-tune [43]. The simplicity of this method and its success in solving some optimization problems attracted our attention to employ it to address MRI brain segmentation problems.

The WOA depends on the initial values of the population obtained by a set of random solutions. First, the WOA takes the initial values randomly, whereas, during iterations, the search agents optimize their positions accorded by the randomly selected search agent or based on the current optimal solution. The current solution is calculated according to the fitness function values as the optimal solution. To apply this algorithm and track its steps, a new hybrid method was proposed to solve the optimization issues called HMRF-WOA, a proposed hybrid algorithm that links the steps of the WOA with the HMRF model. The HMRF-WOA is depicted in the next section.

4. HMRF and Whale Optimization Algorithm (HMRF-WOA)

This section explains the connection between the Hidden Markov Random Field Model and the Whale Optimization Algorithm. As discussed in Section 2, MRF is one of the most effective methods for achieving image segmentation of images using the maximum a posterior (MAP) criterion. However, due to some problems such as noise, overlapping regions, and low contrast in medical images, MRF seems to be inadequate. Moreover, in order to accurately identify the class of a given pixel, we can consider an approximation of the exact segmentation using optimization techniques. In addition, to seek a given pixel class, we can consider an approximation of the exact segmentation using optimization techniques. For these reasons, we employed WOA as an optimizing tool to aid in segmenting MR brain images. WOA is utilized to define the optimal class of pixel in brain MR images.

Therefore, by combining MRF- and WOA-based methods, we can leverage the advantages of both techniques to significantly improve the accuracy of segmentation and also to address issues related to low contrast in MRI images. Additionally, we can achieve optimal segmentation by considering the mean and standard deviation of each class. So, pixels are classified into the same category as the nearest mean, and during the algorithm iterations, the best solution is selected based on the fitness function values (Equation (12)) referenced in Section 2. This objective function serves to quantify the proximity of a solution to the optimal solution.

Moreover, the brain tissue segmentation problem can be solved by the HMRF-WOA method, where the objective function given in Equation (12) can converge or close in on the optimal solution. The HMRF-WOA initiates using a random value of the populations with predefined search elements $(X_1 \ldots X_i \ldots X_n)$, and each one has a set of predefined value of the initial locations $X_i = (X_{i1}, \ldots X_{ij} \ldots X_{ik})$. Through the iterations of the algorithm, we calculated, for each search agent i, the new position by the fitness function, obtaining a set of positions for all populations and conserving the best set of positions.

Let $\mu_i(t) = (\mu_{i1}(t), \ldots, \mu_{ij}(t), \ldots, \mu_{ik}(t))$ be the best location visited by the search agent i until the time t calculated by the fitness function, which allows us to define its own resulting segmented image $x_i(t) = (x_{i1}(t),...,x_{is}(t),...,x_{iM}(t))$ by using its location $\mu_i(t)$, where $x_{is}(t) = j$, on the condition that the mean $\mu_{ij}(t)$ is nearest to y_s. After identifying the optimal search element by its best position μ_i, other search elements will adjust their positions towards the best search element. Consequently, the best position obtained by the population thus far is $\mu = (\mu_1, \ldots, \mu_i, \ldots \mu_k)$.

Our proposed segmentation method of brain MRIs by the HMRF-WOA has the following main steps (Algorithm 1).

Algorithm 1: The main steps of our proposed segmentation method of brain MRIs by the HMRF-WOA.

Input: Initialize randomly a population X_i

1. Initialization of the search elements (agents X_i) and i = 1, 2. . .n.
2. For each element i, compute the fitness value by Equation (12).
3. X* designed the best search element.
4. Do while (t $\leq$ number of iterations) is true.
5. For each i in the population of the search agents
6. These parameters (a, A, C, l, and p) are updated.
7. If ($p < 0.5$)
8. If (| A | < 1)
9. The current search agent's position is updated by Equation (14)
10. Else if (i.e., | A | $\geq$ 1)
11. A random search agent (Xrand) is selected.
12. The current search agent's position is updated by Equation (22).
13. End if
14. Else if (i.e., $p \geq 0.5$)
15. The current search agent's position is updated by Equation (18).
16. End if
17. End for
18. Check that if any search agent exceeds the boundaries of the search space and make the correction.
19. Recompute the fitness value of all the population (each search agent) by Equation (12).
20. Getting better solution, update X*.
21. Increment the iteration (t).
22. End while

Output: The optimal solution is X*.

5. Experimental Results

In this part of the manuscript, we will explain the segmentation method results in detail. Our proposed method is a hybrid algorithm that links the HMRF model and the WOA metaheuristic algorithm, called HMRF-WOA, and our goal is to classify each pixel of the brain tissues into four categories: WM, GM, CSF, and background. To obtain this result, firstly, we applied the median filter to reduce noise with a structure of [3 $\times$ 3] and to improve the segmentation results to achieve a high quality. Then, we started our proposed HMRF-WOA process to research each region in the image and obtain its optimal mean intensity.

One of the most successful research approaches is acquiring appropriate data for testing the proposed methods, which often presents a major challenge for researchers, especially in studies related to the human body. BrainWeb provides a valuable resource for the research community by offering a set of realistic simulated brain MR image volumes (Simulated Brain Database, SBD) with reference data (ground truth). These databases are particularly suitable for brain tissue research. For this reason, we have chosen these datasets as they offer a sufficient amount of data for brain image segmentation and are highly appropriate for our purpose.

5.1. Datasets

In this experimental phase, we chose two datasets of the MR images, including both T1-weighted simulated and real 2D MRI brain images. The Simulated Brain Database (SBD) was downloaded from the BrainWeb database [44], which can be accessed at this link (https://brainweb.bic.mni.mcgill.ca/brainweb/), accessed on 20 October 2022. On the one hand, we have five BrainWeb databases with different input image parameters. Table 1 below contains all these parameters.

Table 1. The parameters of the databases used in the proposed method.

Databases	Types	Dimensions	Noises (%)	INU * (%)	Voxels (mm)
1	Brainweb	181 × 217 × 181	0	0	1 × 1 × 1
2	Brainweb	181 × 217 × 181	3	20	1 × 1 × 1
3	Brainweb	181 × 217 × 181	5	20	1 × 1 × 1
4	Brainweb	181 × 217 × 181	7	20	1 × 1 × 1
5	Brainweb	181 × 217 × 181	9	40	1 × 1 × 1
6	IBSR	256 × 256 × 63	-	-	1 × 3 × 1

* Intensity non-uniformity = INU.

On the other hand, the real MR images with T1-weighted modality, known as the Internet Brain Segmentation Repository (IBSR), were collected from the 20 normal MR brain datasets, which are available at (https://www.nitrc.org/projects/ibsr/), accessed on 20 October 2022, where the input image parameters were dimensions = 256 × 256 × 63 and voxels = 1 × 3 × 1 mm. In totality, six datasets with various parameters were considered as input data to apply our algorithm.

5.2. Performance Measures

With the purpose of interpreting the HMRF-WOA's performance, this manuscript uses two measures which are most often used in the evaluation of medical volume segmentation: the Dice coefficient metric (DC) [45] and the Jaccard coefficient (JC) [46].

5.2.1. Dice Coefficient (Dice)

This is a metric based on overlap that directly evaluates the similarity between a segmented image and a ground truth image. If the value of DC equals or is close to 1, this indicates the best performance of the method.

$$Dice = \frac{2.\ area\ of\ overlap}{total\ area} = \frac{2.TP}{2.TP + FP + FN} \quad (23)$$

5.2.2. Jaccard Coefficient (JC)

JC is an evaluation index that summarizes the area of overlap between two groups of binary segmentations. This metric is defined as the ratio of intersection over union of the ground truth image and the resulting segmented image. A higher result of this metric signifies a better result. The JC index is defined as follows:

$$JC = \frac{area\ of\ overlap}{area\ of\ union} = \frac{TP}{TP + FP + FN} \quad (24)$$

where TP, FP, and FN are the true positive, the false positive, and the false negative, respectively.

Furthermore, the parameter called β in the fitness function (Equation (12)) can influence the performance of the algorithm. In this case, it is necessary to fix the coefficient β when the weights present a part of the energy of the model. We chose $\beta = 1$ in this work. Table 1 defines the different databases used in our proposed method.

5.3. Discussion

The accuracy of any segmentation method depends on several factors, including the choice of the proposed technique, and a number of its parameters, such as the dataset, number of regions to be segmented or classified, the number of iterations, and the workstation configuration. Within this framework, we have achieved superior segmentation results compared to other methods (see Tables 2–4). This is due to the use of prior knowledge.

Table 2. Mean DC values of the simulated MR brain images (BrainWeb).

Tissue	Method	Database 1	Database 2	Database 3	Database 4	Database 5
GM	HMRF-WOA	0.982	0.974	0.953	0.955	0.935
	HMRF-BFGS	0.973	0.942	0.918	NA *	NA *
	MV-FCM	0.885	0.876	0.866	0.854	0.836
	Amiri et al. [47]	0.975	0.960	0.930	0.925	0.895
	AWSFCM	NA *	0.895	0.836	0.809	NA *
	WMT-FCM	NA *	0.9508	0.9219	0.8818	NA *
WM	HMRF-WOA	0.997	0.990	0.986	0.986	0.976
	HMRF-BFGS	0.991	0.969	0.951	NA *	NA *
	IMV-FCM	0.952	0.950	0.938	0.929	0.918
	Amiri et al. [47]	0.960	0.950	0.920	0.920	0.880
	AWSFCM	NA *	0.865	0.836	0.813	NA *
	WMT-FCM	NA *	0.9729	0.9550	0.9306	NA *
CSF	HMRF-WOA	0.979	0.977	0.951	0.952	0.968
	HMRF-BFGS	0.960	0.939	0.919	NA *	NA *
	IMV-FCM	0.850	0.844	0.837	0.870	0.813
	Amiri et al. [47]	0.970	0.960	0.940	0.930	0.925
	AWSFCM	NA *	0.692	0.672	0.658	NA *
	WMT-FCM	NA *	0.9628	0.9424	0.9090	NA *

* The performance of the method for this tissue was not reported.

Table 3. Mean JC values of simulated MR brain images from BrainWeb.

Tissue	Method	Database 1	Database 2	Database 3	Database 4	Database 5
GM	HMRF-WOA	0.966	0.944	0.925	0.916	0.879
	HMRF-BFGS	NA *	NA *	NA *	NA *	NA *
	IMV-FCM	0.797	0.781	0.765	0.753	0.722
	Amiri et al. [47]	0.959	0.920	0.880	0.860	0.820
	AWSFCM	NA *	0.787	0.742	0.726	NA *
WM	HMRF-WOA	0.995	0.987	0.977	0.973	0.953
	HMRF-BFGS	NA *	NA *	NA *	NA *	NA *
	IMV-FCM	0.904	0.892	0.877	0.858	0.835
	Amiri et al. [47]	0.925	0.915	0.870	0.850	0.800
	AWSFCM	NA *	0.760	0.743	0.721	NA *

Table 3. *Cont.*

Tissue	Method	Database 1	Database 2	Database 3	Database 4	Database 5
CSF	HMRF-WOA	0.961	0.949	0.927	0.914	0.939
	HMRF-BFGS	NA *	NA *	NA *	NA *	NA *
	IMV-FCM	0.707	0.679	0.670	0.675	0.718
	Amiri et al. [47]	0.925	0.920	0.920	0.885	0.860
	AWSFCM	NA *	0.520	0.516	0.485	NA *

* The performance of the method for this tissue was not reported.

Table 4. Mean DICE coefficient values of MR brain images from the IBSR.

Tissue	Method	Mean Dice
GM	HMRF-WOA	0.916
	hMRF-BFGS	0.859
	PLA-SOM	0.780
	Amiri et al. [47]	0.863
	Gardens2	0.740
	KPSFCM	0.80
WM	HMRF-WOA	0.856
	hMRF-BFGS	0.855
	PLA-SOM	0.740
	Amiri et al. [47]	0.814
	Gardens2	0.720
	KPSFCM	0.81
CSF	HMRF-WOA	0.459
	hMRF-BFGS	0.381
	PLA-SOM	0.230
	Amiri et al. [47]	0.423
	Gardens2	0.230
	KPSFCM	0.31

As mentioned before, the images of the first five datasets in Table 3 were used to evaluate the performance of the HMRF-WOA. Figures 1–5 show some slices of a T1-weighted image (slices: 84, 95, 105, 108, 120). These brain images correspond to the slices under different types of conditions, such as database type, dimension image, noise level, intensity non-uniformity level, and slice thickness (mm). In Table 1, rows 1 to 5 summarize the parameters of Figures 1–5, respectively. Figure 6 represents the ground truth segmentation of slices 84, 95, 105, 108, and 120. In this figure, each column contains the three tissues, GM, WM, and CSF, of each slice. Figures 7–11 show the segmentation results, where the four tissues (BG, GM, WM, and CSF) are shown with different colors. The yellow, red, and green colors represent the segmented regions of GM, WM, and CSF, respectively. As we can also see from these figures, the resulting segmented images in Figures 7–11 are almost close to the initial images in Figures 1–5.

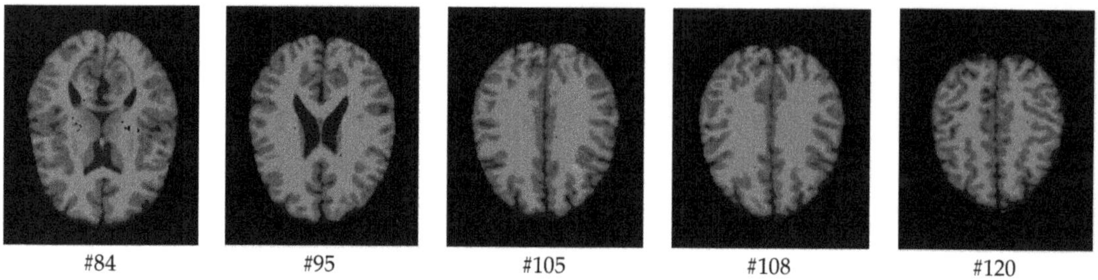

Figure 1. Slices with Noise = 0%, INU = 0% of database 1.

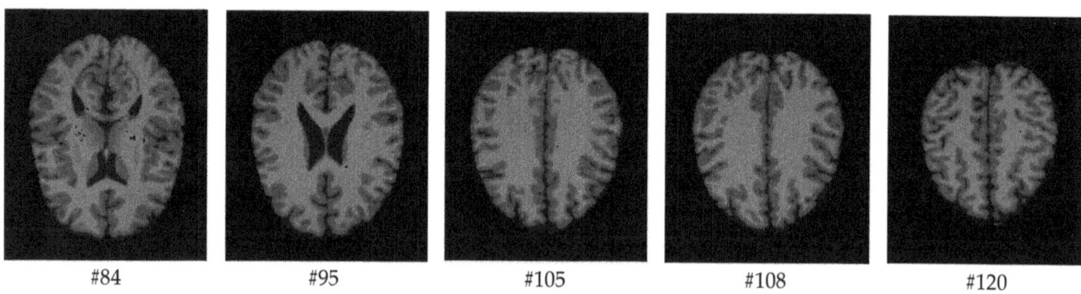

Figure 2. Slices with Noise = 3%, INU = 20% of database 2.

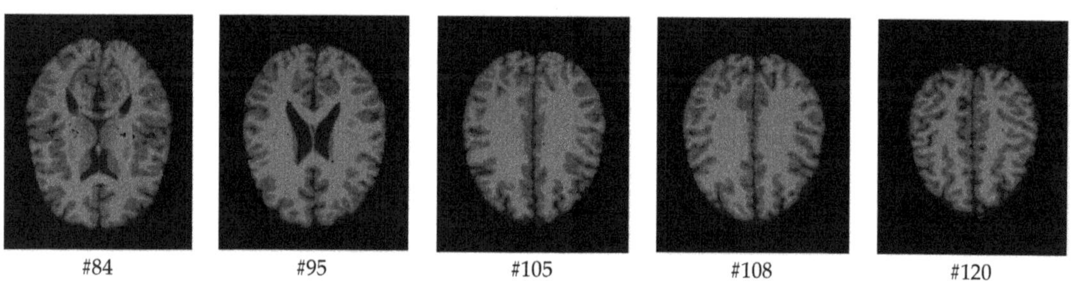

Figure 3. Slices with Noise = 5%, INU = 20% of database 3.

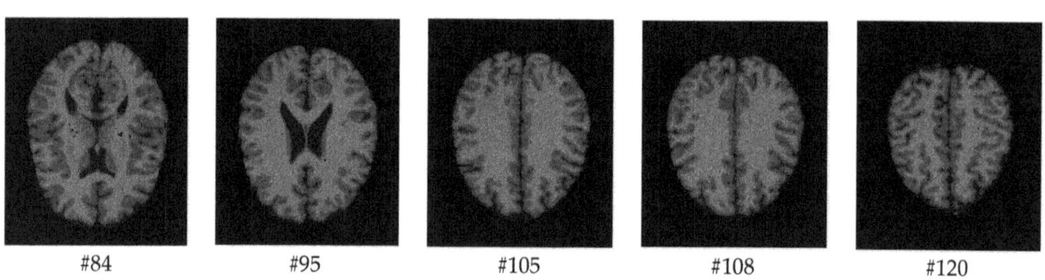

Figure 4. Slices with Noise = 7%, INU = 20% of database 4.

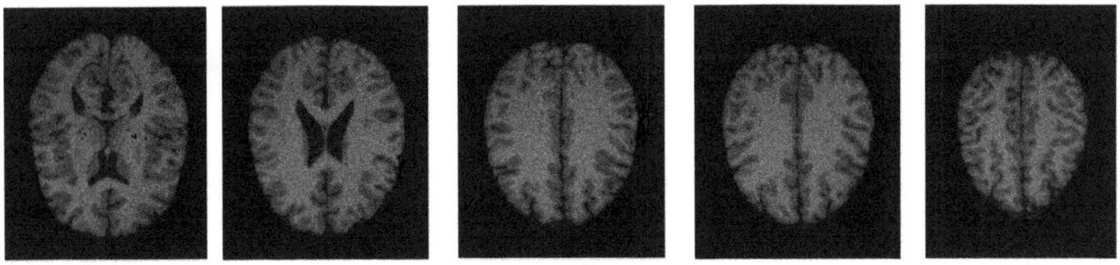

#84 #95 #105 #108 #120

Figure 5. Slices with Noise = 9%, INU = 40% of database 5.

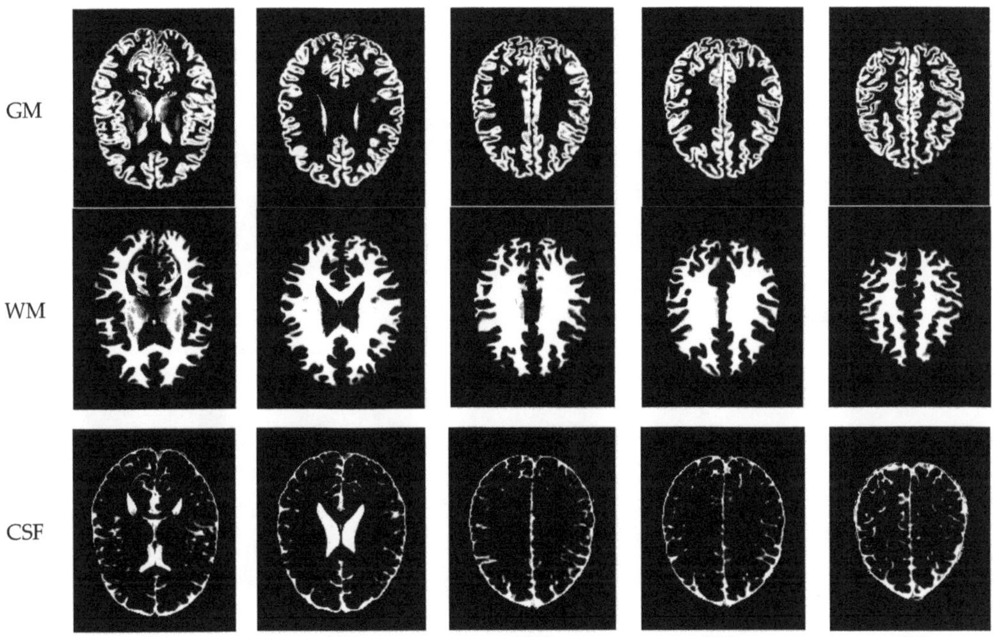

#84 #95 #105 #108 #120

Figure 6. Ground truth segmentation of the GM, WM, and CSF tissues.

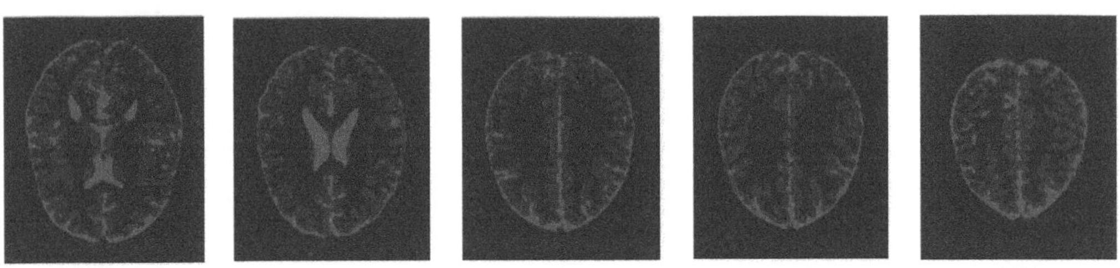

#84 #95 #105 #108 #120

Figure 7. Segmentation results of the slices illustrated in Figure 1.

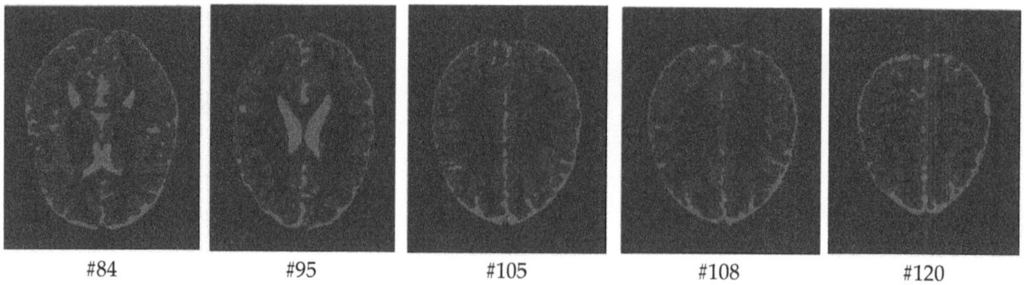

Figure 8. Segmentation results of the images illustrated in Figure 2.

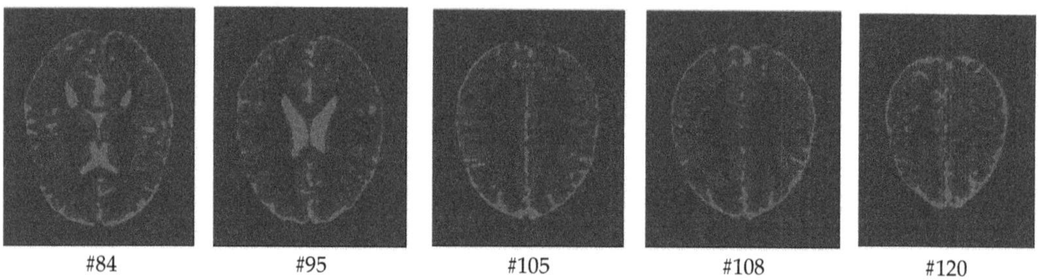

Figure 9. Segmentation results of the images illustrated in Figure 3.

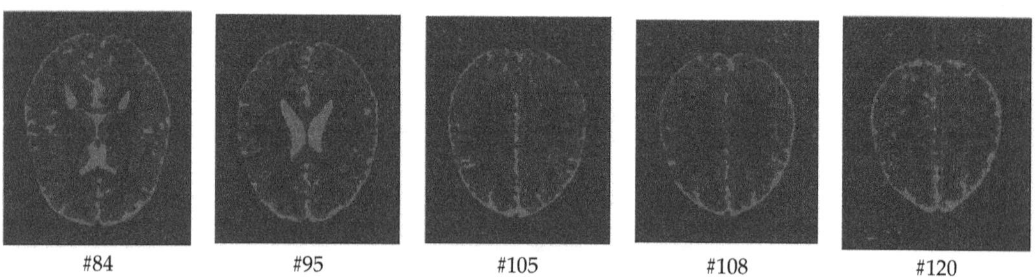

Figure 10. Segmentation results of the images illustrated in Figure 4.

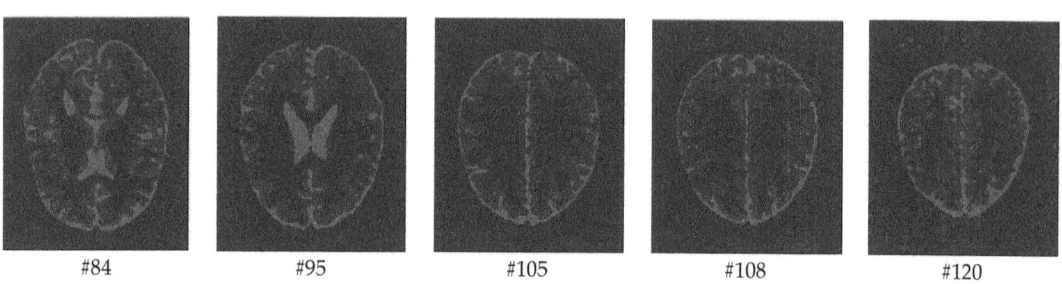

Figure 11. Segmentation results of the images illustrated in Figure 5.

Hence, we have demonstrated the high performance of our method, despite existing artifacts on the MR brain images. To evaluate the performances of the HMRF-WOA more clearly, two criteria were used to compare the similarities between the manual (GT) and automatic segmentations: DC and AC, which are described in the previous section.

The results are summarized in Tables 2 and 3. Moreover, Figures 12–17 illustrate the comparison of the DC and JC coefficients between five approaches: HMRF-BFGS, IMV-FCM, Amiri et al. [47], AWSFCM [48], WMT-FCM [49], and HMRF-WOA. According to these figures, the test results show that the present approach brings satisfactory results compared with the literature methods for all brain tissues.

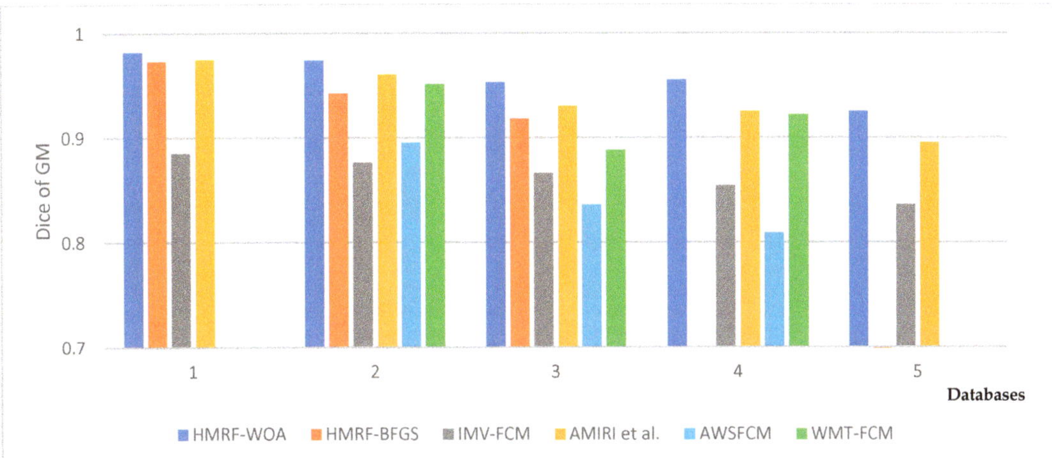

Figure 12. Dice coefficient of GM (BrainWeb dataset) for each algorithm [47].

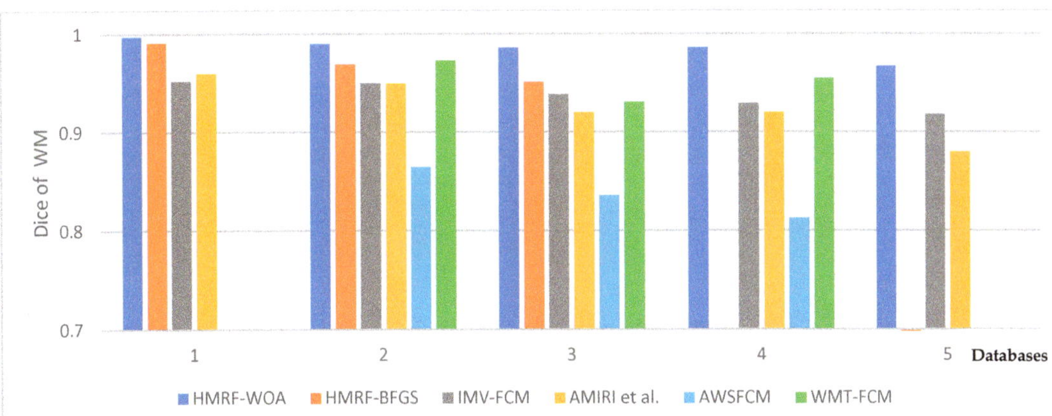

Figure 13. Dice coefficient of WM (BrainWeb dataset) for each algorithm [47].

With regard to the T1-weighted MRI brain datasets, the performance of the HMRF-WOA was evaluated for 20 normal subjects. Figure 18 shows some slices of one subject (slices 20, 28, 32, 35, and 39); Figure 18a presents the initial slices images, (b) represents the ground truth segmentation, and (c) shows the HMRF-WOA segmentation results.

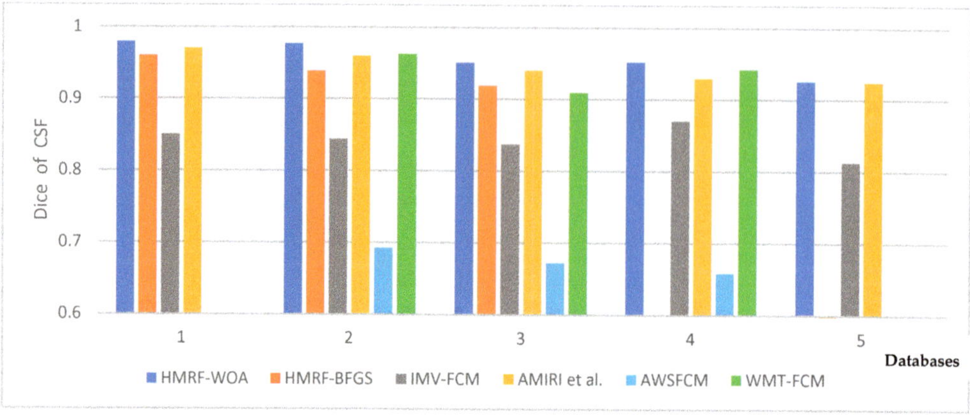

Figure 14. Dice coefficient of CSF (BrainWeb dataset) for each algorithm [47].

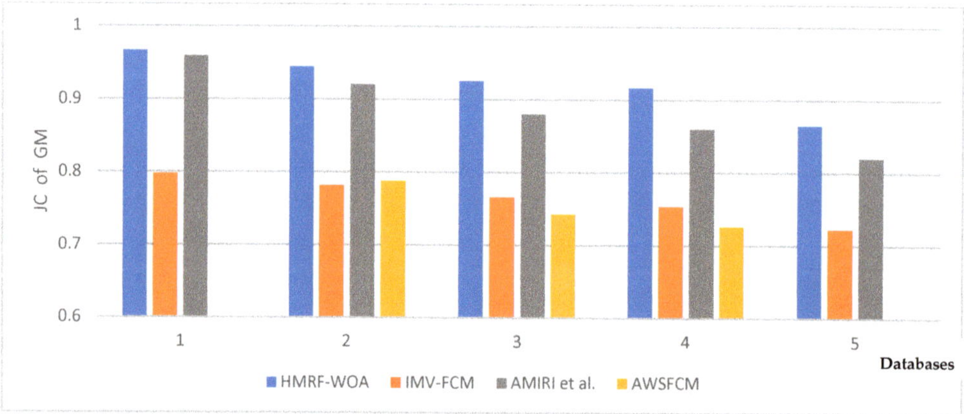

Figure 15. Jaccard coefficient of GM (BrainWeb dataset) for each algorithm [47].

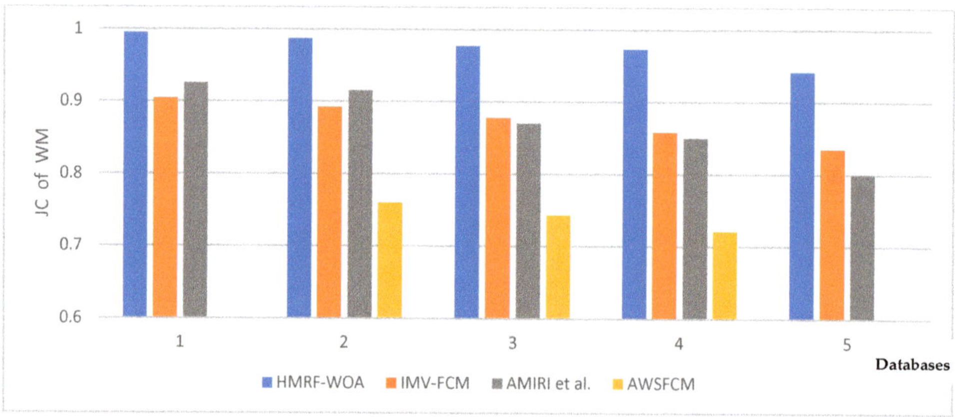

Figure 16. Jaccard coefficient of WM (BrainWeb dataset) for each algorithm [47].

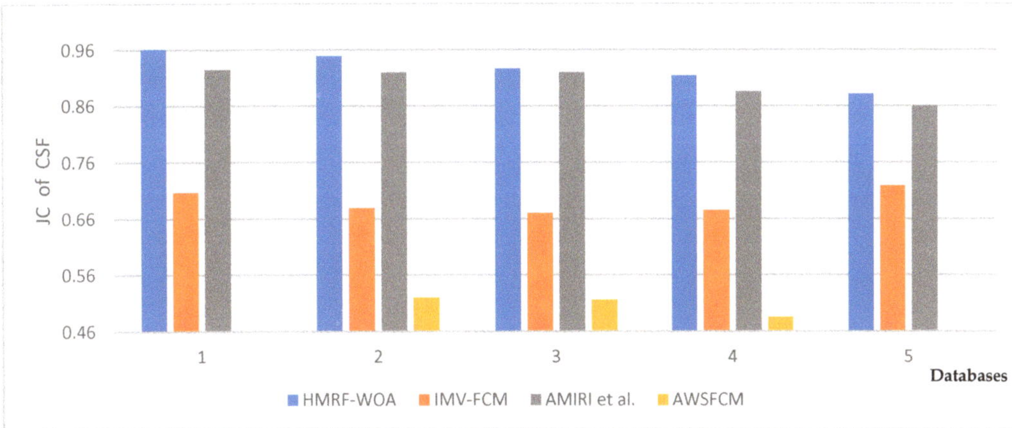

Figure 17. Jaccard coefficient of CSF (BrainWeb dataset) for each algorithm [47].

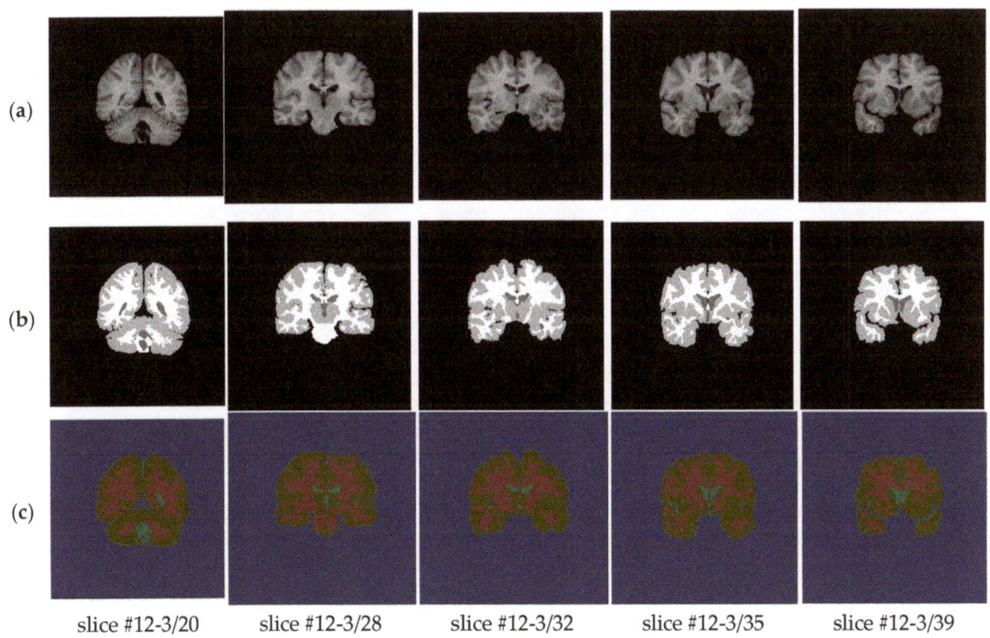

Figure 18. Segmentation results of IBSR dataset: (**a**)—initial images; (**b**)—ground truth images; (**c**)—segmentation results.

Table 4 below illustrates the Mean DC values of the MR brain images from the IBSR obtained by our proposed method (HMRF-WOA) and the literature methods. In this assessment, we have added other approaches, such as PLA-SOM [50], Gardens2 [51], andKPSFCM [52], for GM, WM, and CSF segmentation. All the comparative methods shown in this table use the same database images. So, this comparison shows that the HMRF-WOA performed significantly better than the other methods.

The graphical presentation of the mean DC index for the three tissues (CSF, WM, and GM) between our proposed method and the literature methods is shown in Figure 19. This comparison shows that the average DC index of the GM and CSF segmentations is strongly improved in the IBSR dataset. On the other hand, the average DC indexes of the WM segmentations between our method and hMRF-BFGS suggests that the improvement is slight.

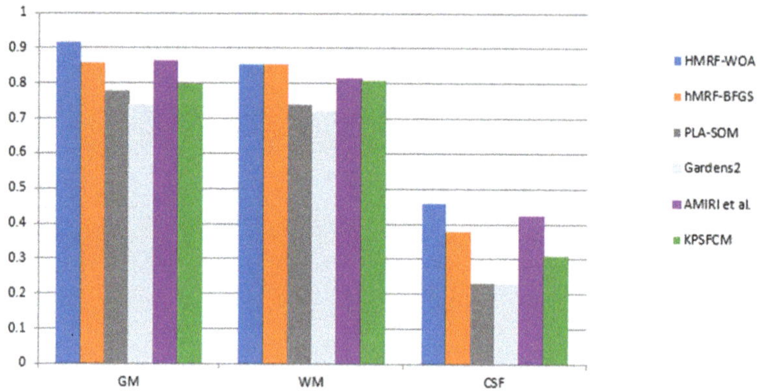

Figure 19. Mean DC of brain tissues in IBSR dataset [47].

As shown, these analyses confirmed the accuracy and the robustness of our automatic method. In addition, the proposed method, called HMRF-WOA, outperforms the literature methods used for our comparison.

The qualitative analysis provides a visual representation of the segmentation approaches. The visual comparison of the resulting images using the HMRF-WOA appears to be more similar to the reference image (ground truth), where Figures 1–5 show the GM, WM, and CSF tissue regions of the reference image with higher values of noise levels (3, 5, 7, and 9%) and intensity non-uniformity levels (20, 40%), whereas Figures 7–11 show the subject images obtained using the proposed technique. However, this result shows that with higher values of noise and intensity non-uniformity, the algorithm, with its hyperparameters, is able to segment the tissue regions correctly.

Moreover, Figure 18 illustrates the segmentation results of the proposed algorithm using MR brain images from the IBSR database. Figure 18a presents the slices of the original brain image; Figure 18b is the ground truth slice images; and Figure 18c shows the segmented brain MR images using the HMRF-WOA approach on the sample image of one subject. GM is shown in yellow, WM in red, CSF in green, and the background in blue.

Therefore, these analyses confirmed the accuracy and the robustness of our automatic method. In most cases, we achieved acceptable results using these brain datasets.

In this framework, the HMRF-WOA incorporates three hyperparameters:

1. The weight β associated with the pair of neighboring pixels is a positive constant that controls the size of homogeneous regions. Also, increasing the value of the β parameter e can increase the contribution of the neighboring sites in the estimation of the class of a given pixel. So, we chose $\beta = 1$ as we obtained a good performance for the segmentation method using this value.
2. The whale population size parameter represents the total number of whales used in the WOA to optimize the MRI image segmentation. We have tested three values of this parameter (10, 20, and 30). Using 20 search agents gave the best accuracy result and a good computational cost compared to other values.
3. The number of iterations represents the number of loops used to evaluate the HMRF-WOA process. We tested values ranging between 5 and 40 iterations. The best result was obtained with 20 iterations.

The choice of these parameters shows its effect on the performance of the HMRF-WOA.

Computational Complexity Analysis

Computing time serves as a crucial measure for justifying the computational effectiveness of any method. Our proposed approach with these hyperparameters showed a good efficiency and a better performance compared to other segmentation methods. However, a notable drawback of this method is its computational complexity. A critical limitation arises from the selection of hyperparameters, where the balance between computational cost and accurate results must be carefully considered. Another limitation is that we have not tested the algorithm's performance to evaluate its generalizability on other MRI types or imaging modalities.

In addition to this, the computational complexity of the algorithm is computed as follows:

1. Initializing the whale population is $O(N)$, where N is the size of the population.
2. Computing the fitness value of the initial population is $O(N)$.
3. Obtaining the best solution is $O(N^2)$.
4. Iteration, updating whale population, and evaluating fitness are $O(2N)$.
5. Iteration and obtaining the best solution are $O(N^2)$.

Therefore, the total time complexity of HMRF-WOA is:

$$O(2N) + O\,(N^2) + maxiter\,(O\,(2N) + O(N^2)) == (maxiter + 1)\,(O\,(N^2 + 2N))$$

where *maxiter* is the maximum number of iterations used as the termination criteria for the algorithm.

6. Conclusions

Efficient methods of segmentation and classification are some of the most challenging tasks for physicians and radiologists. The automation of these methods thus occupies a major proportion of research in the domain of medical imaging.

The motive of medical image processing for handling human organs is to precisely segment or classify the tissue regions to make operations easier.

In this study, a novel combination of the HMRF model and a whale optimization algorithm (WOA) are applied to segment the images of two well-known brain datasets: BrainWeb and IBSR. We conclude that our HMRF-WOA outperforms all the other methods or techniques compared in this study, where the assessment results of the segmented tissues as illustrated in all the figures indicate that the HMRF-WOA can precisely segment the brain tissues at different noise levels, despite the presence of the intense inhomogeneity in the input images. Overall, comparing the proposed method with the results of other techniques shows that the method can yield an acceptable result for GM, WM, and CSF segmentation. The results are summarized in Tables 2 and 3.

This increased robustness and accuracy of our HMRF-WOA optimization method-based MRI brain segmentation technique will hopefully help the application of MR image segmentation techniques, such as measuring the anatomical structures measurement of the brain, surgical planning, and image-guided interventions.

In the future, we would like to hybridize the WOA method with other techniques to show their main benefits and to achieve higher performances in the treatment process.

Author Contributions: Conceptualization, A.D.; Methodology, A.D.; Software, A.D.; Validation, A.D.; Supervision, S.M. All authors have read and agreed to the published version of the manuscript.

Funding: This research received no external funding.

Institutional Review Board Statement: Not applicable.

Data Availability Statement: All data were contained in the main text.

Conflicts of Interest: The authors declare no conflict of interest.

References

1. Falaq, N.; Yasir, S. Human brain disorders: A Review. *Open Biol. J.* **2020**, *8*, 6–21. [CrossRef]
2. Catalina, T.G.; Geers, A.J.; Peters, J.; Weese, J.; Pinto, K.; Karim, R.; Ammar, M.; Daoudi, A.; Margeta, J.; Sandoval, Z.; et al. Benchmark for Algorithms Segmenting the left atrium from 3D CT and MRI datasets. *IEEE Trans. Med. Imaging* **2015**, *34*, 1460–1473. [CrossRef] [PubMed]
3. Abdelaziz, D.; Said, M.; Chikh, M. Automatic segmentation of the left atrium on CT images. In *Statistical Atlases and Computational Models of the Heart. Imaging and Modelling Challenges. STACOM 2013*; Springer: Berlin/Heidelberg, Germany, 2014; Volume 8330, pp. 14–23. [CrossRef]
4. Abdelaziz, D.; Said, M.; Chikh, M. Automatic Segmentation of the Right Ventricle by Active Shape Model and a Distance Transform. *JMIHI J. Med. Imaging Health Inform.* **2015**, *5*, 27–35. [CrossRef]
5. Qaiser, M.; Alipoor, M.; Chodorowski, A.; Mehnert, A.; Persson, M. Multimodal MR Brain segmentation using Bayesian based Adaptive Mean-Shift. *MIDAS J.* **2013**. [CrossRef]
6. Henri, A.V.; Fedde, V.; Wiro, J. Auto knn: Brain tissue segmentation using automatically trained k-nearest-neighbor classification. *MIDAS J.* **2011**. [CrossRef]
7. Fiaz, M.; Ali, K.; Rehman, A.; Gul, M.J.; Jung, S.K. Brain MRI Segmentation using rule-based hybrid approach. *arXiv* **2019**, arXiv:1902.04207. [CrossRef]
8. Jalab, H.A.; Hasan, A.M. Magnetic resonance imaging segmentation techniques of brain tumors: A Review. *Arch. Neurosci.* **2019**, *6*, e84920. [CrossRef]
9. Hasan, A.M.; Meziane, F.; Aspin, R.; Jalab, H. Segmentation of Brain Tumors in MRI Images using three-dimensional active contour without edge. *Symmetry* **2016**, *8*, 132. [CrossRef]
10. Ahmadvand, A.; Yousefi, S.; Manzuri, M. A novel markov random field model based on region adjacency graph for T1 magnetic resonance imaging brain segmentation. *IJIST Int. J. Imaging Syst. Technol.* **2017**, *27*, 78–88. [CrossRef]
11. Jianhua, S.; Lei, Y. Brain tissue segmentation via non-local fuzzy c-means clustering combined with markov random field. *MBE Math. Biosci. Eng.* **2021**, *19*, 1891–1908. [CrossRef]
12. Shah, S.A.; Chauhan, N.C. An automated approach for segmentation of Brain MR Images using gaussian mixture model based Hidden Markov Random Field with Expectation Maximization. *BJHMR Br. J. Healthc. Med. Res.* **2015**, *2*, 57. [CrossRef]
13. Chen, M.; Yan, Q.; Qin, M. A segmentation of brain MRI images utilizing intensity and contextual information by Markov random field. *Comput. Assist. Surg.* **2017**, *22*, 200–211. [CrossRef] [PubMed]
14. Alansary, A.; Soliman, A.; Khalifa, F.; Elnakib, A.; Mostapha, M.; Nitzken, M.; Casanova, M.; El-Baz, A. MAP Based framework for segmentation of MR Brain Images based on visual appearance and prior shape. *MIDAS J.* **2014**. [CrossRef]
15. Elhachemi, G.; Samy, A.; Dominique, M.; Ramdane, M. Hidden markov random field model and broyden fletcher goldfarb shanno algorithm for brain image segmentation. *JETAI J. Exp. Theor. Artif. Intell.* **2017**, *30*, 415–427. [CrossRef]
16. Castillo, D.; Peis, I.; Martínez, F.; Segovia, F.; Górriz, J.; Ramírez, J.; Salas, D. A Heavy tailed expectation maximization hidden markov random field model with applications to segmentation of MRI. *Front. Neurosci.* **2017**, *11*, 66. [CrossRef]
17. Hua, L.; Gu, Y.; Gu, X.; Xue, J.; Ni, T. A novel brain MR image segmentation method using an improved multi view fuzzy c-means clustering algorithm. *Front. Neurosci.* **2021**, *15*, 662674. [CrossRef]
18. Zhao, L.; Asis-Cruz, J.D.; Feng, X.; Wu, Y.; Kapse, K.; Largent, A.; Quistorff, J.; Lopez, C.; Wu, D.; Qing, K.; et al. Automated 3D fetal brain segmentation using an optimized deep learning approach. *AJNR Am. J. Neuroradiol.* **2022**, *43*, 448–454. [CrossRef]
19. Brudfors, M.; Balbastre, Y.; Ashburner, J.; Rees, G.; Nachev, P.; Ourselin, S.; Cardoso, M.J. An MRF Unet product of experts for image segmentation. In Proceedings of the Machine Learning Research, Proceedings of the Fourth Conference on Medical Imaging with Deep Learning, Lübeck, Germany, 7–9 July 2021; ML Research Press: Westminster, UK, 2021; Volume 143, pp. 48–59.
20. Bento, M.; Fantini, I.; Park, J.; Rittner, L.; Frayne, R. Deep learning in large and multi site structural brain MR imaging datasets. *Front. Neuroinform.* **2022**, *15*, 805669. [CrossRef] [PubMed]
21. Lee, B.; Yamanak, K.; Nagaraj, M.; Muhammad, A.; Choi, J. Automatic segmentation of brain MRI using a novel patch-wise U net deep architecture. *PLoS ONE* **2022**, *17*, e0264231. [CrossRef]
22. Renukadevi, T.; Saraswathi, K.; Prabu, P.; Venkatachalam, K. Brain image classification using time frequency extraction with histogram intensity similarity. *CSSE Comput. Syst. Sci. Eng.* **2022**, *41*, 645–660. [CrossRef]
23. Maqsood, S.; Damasevicius, R.; Shah, F.M. An Efficient Approach for the Detection of Brain Tumor Using Fuzzy Logic and U-NET CNN Classification. In *Computational Science and Its Applications—ICCSA*; Lecture Notes in Computer Science; Springer: Cham, Switzerland, 2021; pp. 105–118. [CrossRef]
24. Khorram, B.; Yazdi, M. A New optimized thresholding method using ant colony algorithm for MR brain image segmentation. *J. Digit. Imaging* **2019**, *32*, 162–174. [CrossRef] [PubMed]
25. Thuy, X.; Patrick, S.; Hamouche, O. Segmentation of MR Brain images through Hidden Markov Random Field and hybrid metaheuristic algorithm. *IEEE Trans. Image Process.* **2020**, *29*, 6507–6522. [CrossRef] [PubMed]
26. Kadry, S.; Damaševičius, R.; Taniar, D.; Rajinikanth, V.; Lawal, I.A. U-Net Supported Segmentation of Ischemic-Stroke-Lesion from Brain MRI Slices. In Proceedings of the Seventh International Conference on Bio Signals, Images, and Instrumentation (ICBSII), Chennai, India, 25–27 March 2021; pp. 1–5. [CrossRef]

27. Ramya, J.; Maheswari, B.U.; Rajakumar, M.P.; Sonia, R. Alzheimer's Disease Segmentation and Classification on MRI Brain Images Using Enhanced Expectation Maximization Adaptive Histogram (EEM-AH) and Machine Learning. *Inf. Technol. Control.* **2022**, *51*, 786–800. [CrossRef]
28. Rangaraju, B.; Chinnadurai, T.; Natarajan, S.; Raja, V. Dual Attention Aware Octave Convolution Network for Early-Stage Alzheimer's Disease Detection. *Inf. Technol. Control.* **2024**, *53*, 302–316. [CrossRef]
29. Clifford, P.; Hammersley, J. *Markov Fields on Finite Graphs and Lattices*; University of Oxford: Oxford, UK, 1971.
30. Potts, R. Some generalized order-disorder transformations. *Math. Proc. Camb. Philos. Soc.* **1952**, *48*, 106–109. [CrossRef]
31. Mirjalili, S.; Lewi, A. The whale optimization algorithm. *AES Adv. Eng. Softw.* **2016**, *95*, 51–67. [CrossRef]
32. Goldbogen, J.; Friedlaender, A.; Calambokidis, J.; McKenna, M.; Malene, S.; Nowacek, D. Integrative approaches to the study of baleen whale diving behavior, feeding performance, and foraging ecology. *BioScience* **2013**, *63*, 90–100. [CrossRef]
33. Hof, P.; Gucht, E. Structure of the cerebral cortex of the humpback whale, megaptera novaeangliae (Cetacea, Mysticeti, Balaenopteridae). *Anat. Rec.* **2007**, *290*, 1–31. [CrossRef] [PubMed]
34. Watkins, W.; Schevill, W.E. Aerial Observation of feeding behavior in four baleen whales: Balaena glacialis, balaenoptera borealis, Megaptera novaeangliae, and Balaenoptera physalus. *J. Mammal.* **1979**, *60*, 155–163. [CrossRef]
35. Nasiri, J.; Khiyabani, F.M.; Yoshise, A. A whale optimization algorithm (WOA) approach for clustering. *CMS Cogent Math. Stat.* **2018**, *5*, 1483565. [CrossRef]
36. Yue, Y.; You, H.; Wang, S.; Cao, L. Improved whale optimization algorithm and its application in heterogeneous wireless sensor networks. *IJDSN Int. J. Distrib. Sens. Netw.* **2021**, *17*. [CrossRef]
37. Mohammed, A.K.; Suhaib, A.A.; Zakariya, Y.A. Improving whale optimization algorithm for feature selection with a time-varying transfer function. *NACO Numer. Algebra Control Optim.* **2021**, *11*, 87–98. [CrossRef]
38. Zhihong, Y.; Shuqian, W.; Bin, L.; Xinde, L. Application of whale Optimization Algorithm in Optimal Allocation of Water Resources. *E3S Web Conf.* **2018**, *53*, 04019. [CrossRef]
39. Reddy, P.; Reddy, V.; Manohar, T. Whale optimization algorithm for optimal sizing of renewable resources for loss reduction in distribution systems. *Renewables* **2017**, *4*, 3. [CrossRef]
40. Nadimi, S.; Zamani, H.; Asghari, V.Z.; Mirjalili, S. A Systematic Review of the Whale Optimization Algorithm: Theoretical Foundation, Improvements, and Hybridizations. *Arch. Comput. Methods* **2023**, *30*, 4113–4159. [CrossRef] [PubMed]
41. Mostafa, A.; Hassanien, A.E.; Houseni, M.; Hefny, H. Liver segmentation in MRI images based on whale optimization algorithm. *Multimed. Tools Appl.* **2017**, *76*, 24931–24954. [CrossRef]
42. Kaur, R.; Khehra, B.S. Modified Whale Optimisation Algorithm and minimum CROSS entropy-based segmentation of CT Liver image. *J. Pharm. Negat. Results* **2023**, *14*, 2908–2931.
43. Chakraborty, S.; Saha, A.K.; Nama, S.; Debnath, S. COVID-19 X-ray image segmentation by modified whale optimization algorithm with population reduction. *Comput. Biol. Med.* **2021**, *139*, 104984. [CrossRef] [PubMed]
44. Kwan, R.; Evans, A.; Pike, G. MRI simulation-based evaluation of image-processing and classification methods. *IEEE Trans. Med. Imaging* **1999**, *18*, 1085–1097. [CrossRef] [PubMed]
45. Dice, L. Measures of the Amount of Ecologic Association between Species. *Ecology* **1945**, *26*, 297–302. [CrossRef]
46. Jaccard, P. The Distribution of the Flora of the Alpine Zone. *New Phytol.* **1912**, *11*, 37–50. [CrossRef]
47. Amiri, S.; Movahedi, M.; Kazemi, K.; Parsaei, H. 3D cerebral MR image segmentation using multiple-classifier system. *Med. Biol. Eng. Comput.* **2017**, *55*, 353–364. [CrossRef] [PubMed]
48. Mishro, P.; Agrawal, S.; Panda, R.; Abraham, A. A Novel Type-2 Fuzzy C-Means Clustering for Brain MR Image Segmentation. *IEEE Trans. Cybern.* **2021**, *51*, 3901–3912. [CrossRef] [PubMed]
49. Yunlan, Z.; Zhiyong, H.; Hangjun, C.; Fang, X.; Man, L.; Mengyao, W.; Daming, S. Segmentation of Brain Tissues from MRI Images Using Multitask Fuzzy Clustering Algorithm. *JHE J. Health Eng.* **2023**, 4387134. [CrossRef] [PubMed]
50. Jonas, G.B.; Pilar, G. Pseudo Label Assisted Self-Organizing Maps for Brain Tissue Segmentation in Magnetic Resonance Imaging. *JDI J. Digit. Imaging* **2022**, *35*, 180–192. [CrossRef] [PubMed]
51. Jonas, G.B.; Pilar, G. Segmentation of MRI brain scans using spatial constraints and 3D features. *Med. Biol. Eng. Comput.* **2020**, *58*, 3101–3112. [CrossRef]
52. Padmanaban, S.; Thiruvenkadam, K.; Karuppanagounder, S.; Rangasami, R. A Rapid Knowledge Based Partial Supervision Fuzzy C Means for Brain Tissue Segmentation with CUDA Enabled GPU Machine. *IJIST Int. J. Imaging Syst. Technol.* **2019**, *29*, 547–560. [CrossRef]

computers

Article

Computer Vision Approach in Monitoring for Illicit and Copyrighted Objects in Digital Manufacturing

Ihar Volkau [1,*], Sergei Krasovskii [1], Abdul Mujeeb [1] and Helen Balinsky [2,*]

[1] HP–NTU Digital Manufacturing Corporate Lab, Nanyang Technological University, Singapore 637460, Singapore; krasovskii.sergei.gen@gmail.com (S.K.); amujeeb@ntu.edu.sg (A.M.)
[2] Workforce Solutions, HP Inc., Bristol BS1 6NP, UK
* Correspondence: volkau.ihar@ntu.edu.sg (I.V.); helen.balinsky@hp.com (H.B.)

Abstract: We propose a monitoring system for detecting illicit and copyrighted objects in digital manufacturing (DM). Our system is based on extracting and analyzing high-dimensional data from blueprints of three-dimensional (3D) objects. We aim to protect the legal interests of DM service providers, who may receive requests for 3D printing from external sources, such as emails or uploads. Such requests may contain blueprints of objects that are illegal, restricted, or otherwise controlled in the country of operation or protected by copyright. Without a reliable way to identify such objects, the service provider may unknowingly violate the laws and regulations and face legal consequences. Therefore, we propose a multi-layer system that automatically detects and flags such objects before the 3D printing process begins. We present efficient computer vision algorithms for object analysis and scalable system architecture for data storage and processing and explain the rationale behind the suggested system architecture.

Keywords: computer vision; high-dimensional data; digital manufacturing; illicit object; copyright object; illegal printing

1. Introduction

Almost any new technology, along with creating new possibilities, gives rise to immediate attempts to misuse it. For example, the introduction of color printers enabled attempts to print counterfeit currency [1], forge official documents, and so on. It was difficult to conduct counterfeit investigations for illegal activities using color printing, and almost impossible to find the person or people who performed it and the printer itself. As a cybersecurity measure that facilitates the search for the offender, some color laser printer manufacturers started including tracking information as part of the printout [2]. A similar problem emerged in additive manufacturing, or 3D printing, a technology that enables the creation of physical objects from digital blueprints. However, these blueprints can be stolen or tampered with. In addition to illegal 3D printing of counterfeits, another cybersecurity challenge relates to producing 3D-printed weapons, explosives, etc. [3,4]. For example, ghost guns are almost impossible to trace [5], and workshops conducting their manufacturing are discovered mainly by chance [6].

There is an emerging need to detect the printing of objects (hereafter called controlled objects or COs) that potentially infringe on laws, authorship rights, legal or other constraints. We suggest detecting such objects before the 3D printing process begins to avoid legal consequences for manufacturers. We cannot control digital manufacturing at illegal workshops. Still, our approach could help "to keep honest people honest", e.g., online 3D printing digital manufacturers (like Shapeways.com) with large volumes of customers uploading parts for 3D printing. Our approach can prevent the printing of COs and alleviate the accompanying legal and other challenges for an unsuspecting manufacturer. We could help to mitigate the risk to business owners of accidentally manufacturing something forbidden.

This paper proposes a monitoring system for detecting illicit and copyrighted objects in digital manufacturing (DM). Our system is based on extracting and analyzing high-dimensional data from blueprints of three-dimensional objects and can automatically detect and flag such objects before the 3D printing process begins. The system employs efficient computer vision algorithms for object analysis and scalable system architecture for data storage and processing.

The paper is organized as follows: Section 2 discusses the legal issues of DM. Section 3 states the goals and objectives of our work and contains related prior art. Section 4 includes a description of the main parts of our system. Section 5 discusses the results, performance issues, and possible future directions. Section 6 finalizes the article.

2. Legal Framework for Digital Manufacturing and Physical Control at IP Protection

Three-dimensional printing allows the production of a wide variety of objects, ranging from children's toys to weapons, bringing new opportunities and security challenges. In [7], the cybersecurity implications of additive manufacturing are described, and serious concerns have been raised about the security of storage, transmission, and execution of 3D models in digital networks and systems. The International Conference on 3D-Printed Firearms [8] addressed the latest challenges law enforcement faces in tackling the digital manufacturing threat. The Peace Research Institute Frankfurt (PRIF) 2017 report [9] describes the potential of this new technology and analyzes its possible risks concerning the proliferation of small arms, major weapons systems, and even weapons of mass destruction.

Besides the printing of dangerous objects, there are concerns about the 3D printing of counterfeit products, which could be a severe copyright issue [10]. Printing 3D objects without permission is illegal if the original design is protected under copyright law [11,12]. If a 3D model is protected by copyright, copyright holders can use technical protection measures to safeguard patented property. Circumvention of such protection measures is expressly prohibited by the World Intellectual Property Organization (WIPO) [13].

Several theoretical approaches for IP protection in 3D printing have been proposed, in addition to legal measures and prohibitions. In [14], for example, it is offered to tag an object and its associated 3D printing file with a unique identifier to track usage. However, an engineering solution for the implementation was not provided. Similarly, partnering with sharing platforms that make 3D files public can help limit unauthorized use. In [15], proposals were made to incorporate blockchain into the 3D printing process, providing creators with an additional layer of legal protection with copyright information and a watermark. To reduce the illegal use of 3D printers, ref. [16] proposed a method for extrusion manufacturing to trace the origin of printed objects. When a 3D printer has an extruder that pushes the building material through, the hot end of the extruder melts the material and places it on the print platform to create the model. Each extruder's hot end has unique properties, affecting how the 3D model is built. These thermodynamic properties can be used to identify a particular extruder and, therefore, a 3D printer model as unique as a human fingerprint or "ThermoTag". Thus, the model's buyer can be traced for using the printer to make an illegal copy.

The existing solutions for IP protection in 3D printing to combat 3D-printed counterfeiting and forgery are mainly focused on controlling the original production. For example, embedding NFC tags and QR codes in genuine products helps consumers validate their authenticity [17,18]. In [19], it was proposed to use specially placed nanorods in the final product, which do not affect the integrity of the material but could be a compliance "watermark" to distinguish it from a counterfeit, the same way as the watermark is applied to detect fraudulently printed documents.

The control of original production cannot decrease the production of counterfeits using 3D custom printing, which remains and will be the main issue. Along with the violation of trademarks, patents, and other intellectual rights, illegally printed parts could result in severe or even fatal consequences, e.g., due to incorrect materials being utilized or substandard production [20].

3. Problem Statement and the Related Works

Our starting point was to analyze the following situation: There is a 3D printing facility (automated or semi-automated) which receives requests for 3D printing. There is a chance to receive an order to print a controlled object. To avoid legal consequences [4,5], detecting such objects before the 3D printing process begins is recommended. Nowadays, manufactured objects without official permission or license can only be discovered by human inspection, and this process is prone to errors. To the best of our knowledge, currently, there are no existing supporting technical systems, and the enforcement of law mainly relies on the legal bodies' operational activities and information from the public. The introduction of automated tools could be an initial step, allowing at least primary automated law enforcement for 3D printing.

Hereafter, we propose the concept of an automated system for pre-scanning COs in 3D printing, along with the algorithms for the extraction and analysis of high-dimensional data from blueprints of 3D objects. In general, all printable 3D objects can be considered either technical or decorative. The structure and extent of the technical objects are considered fixed. Otherwise, its functionality will be compromised. Currently, we do not consider cases when the specific technical part could be heavily modified aesthetically without changing functionality, nor is there the possibility of including large-scale features that can be easily removed in post-processing.

At first glance, restricting unauthorized objects from printing boils down to checking if two 3D objects represented by blueprints are the same or different. The existing methods for 3D-object matching can be categorized into three groups: shape-based, view-based, and hybrid [21].

3.1. Shape-Based Methods

In the shape-based category, features are extracted from 3D shape representations (such as polygons, voxels, graphs, etc.) and later used for similarity measurement. The descriptor of the shape is found using some algorithm that characterizes the geometric properties of the object. Statistical descriptors employ histograms to encapsulate the distributions of shape features. While they are efficient and quick to compute, their ability to discriminate is limited, as they do not adequately capture the local characteristics of the object's shape. In this category of methods, we mention the following descriptors:

- A 3D shape spectrum descriptor [22] is related to the first and second principal curvature along the object's surface.
- A D2 descriptor [23,24] takes samples of distances between two points on the model's surface and then creates a distance distribution histogram that serves as the model's shape descriptor.
- A descriptor [25] compares the similarity of two 3D objects by generating distance histograms and determining the appropriate alignment of the two objects.
- A graph-based approach [26] utilizes hierarchical structures to represent 3D objects, accompanied by graph-matching techniques.
- A spherical function-based descriptor [27] suggests using a volumetric representation of the Gaussian Euclidean Distance Transform for a 3D object, expressed by the norms of spherical harmonic frequencies.

3.2. View-Based Methods

View-based methods are becoming increasingly popular due to the progress in 2D-3D reconstruction. The primary concept in visual representation for 3D model retrieval involves initially converting the 3D model into a 2D projection image. Subsequently, various image processing techniques are employed to extract diverse features from this image [28]. For example:

- Ansary et al. [29] selected optimal 2D views of a 3D model and created K-mean clustering of views. Then, the similarity between pairwise 3D objects was measured by applying Bayesian models.

- Wang et al. [30] solved the retrieval problem using group sparse coding. The query object was constructed again by the view sets of each shape; then, the restoration error was considered the similarity measurement for retrieval.
- In [31], it was proposed to project a 3D object to a 2D space and use multi-views. These view-based methods combine a trainable system with 2D projection attributes adopted by the Convolutional Neural Networks (CNNs).
- Ref. [32] introduced a 3D shape descriptor known as the spherical trace transform, which generalizes the 2D trace transform. This approach involves calculating a range of 2D features for a collection of planes that intersect the volume of a 3D model.

3.3. Hybrid Methods

The hybrid methods involve fusing various 3D shape features to improve retrieval accuracy [33]. According to [34], a 3D shape representation incorporating more shape features tends to excel in retrieving more relevant models. In a study by Papadakis et al. [35], a novel hybrid 3D model shape descriptor called PANORAMA was introduced. PANORAMA relies on a set of panoramic views of a 3D model. This approach involves projecting an object onto three perpendicular cylinders and, for each projection, calculating the corresponding 2D Discrete Fourier Transform and 2D Discrete Wavelet Transform.

4. System Architecture

The lack of a universally accepted and consistently effective solution is evident from the multitude of methods available. One of the main requirements for an industrial system is stable, error-free work, and one of the ways to improve reliability is by combining existing approaches and using them in the ensemble.

For a real-life proof of concept system, besides comparing two 3D objects, many other issues should be considered, such as:

- How to store COs securely without unauthorized leakage of their blueprints.
- How to represent the objects in the database of controlled objects.
- How to evaluate objects-in-question quickly and provide a fast search of this information to keep up with 3D printing operations.

We need to address three problems:

1. How to describe controlled objects in a compact way that is good for comparison and storage: Confidentiality Preserving Descriptors (CPDs) should be used for object feature representation. Even if a descriptor of a CO is leaked, it cannot be used to manufacture COs.
2. How to keep a Database of Controlled Objects (DCO) containing the descriptions of the controlled objects: this database should be maintained by the authorities, who decide which objects should be controlled.
3. How to compare an object to be manufactured (an object-under-analysis, OUA) to controlled objects from the DCO in rapid, reliable, and efficient ways.

4.1. Storing of Controlled Objects

The decision of what is forbidden and what should be considered controlled objects should be decided by some authority. It might depend on the country and local laws, and local authorities and enforcement organizations should maintain this information.

The information about forbidden and controlled objects (e.g., in airport security) can be kept today in the following forms:

- Human knowledge (a border control officer can recognize a forbidden item).
- Databases of 2D photographs for camera/video recognition.
- In a neural network (NN) for photo/video recognition. This NN should first be trained on many cases to extract the patterns typical for the specific class (classes) of objects to recognize.

These forms cannot be directly utilized for our 3D recognition project. For example, human knowledge cannot be embedded into a device for automation and checks before manufacturing. Two-dimensional photos do not show the internal architecture, so non-functional replicas of the controlled object (for example, a 3D-printed foam gun for hobbyists for play) could be identified as a CO. The usage of a NN could be questionable as sometimes there is only one sample of a controlled object. It does not represent any class, so extracting common patterns from this unique object is pointless.

Both the visual appearance and the object's internal structure should be analyzed to make an informed decision. Furthermore, we do not like to constrain the CO's geometry. COs may have the following: (a) complex geometry with embedded surfaces and structures (this is a unique feature of 3D printers (3DPs) when several objects can be printed at the same time, and some objects may be embedded into others, e.g., a sphere in a hollow cube); (b) a topology with holes and many fine-grain details; and (c) various curvatures with/without edges at the surface, etc.

To date, there are no 3D DCOs or prohibited blueprints in the public domain. If such databases existed, they would be an excellent source for illegal manufacturing and would encourage a proliferation of illicit items, for example, ghost guns. An open-access DCO would substantially increase the scope of attack, so a real DCO (with guns, explosives, etc.) could be created only by relevant government agencies and supervisory authorities and be securely kept out of public access. This consideration sets high-security requirements for a DCO, as the DCO itself would be a target for attacks to extract COs.

One more consideration relates to the question of where to keep the DCO. We assume there should be a centralized DCO, and we propose keeping the local copy of this DCO at the edge (at the printing facility) and keeping both options to perform validation locally at the facility, or as part of a cloud service.

Each edge device subscribes to a centralized DCO (in the cloud) and fetches the latest updates on controlled objects, creating a local DCO copy in-device. The gains from this could be the following:

- Local validation provides performance benefits; large 3D design files do not need to be uploaded through the Internet.
- A deployment model where designs are pre-validated by a cloud service is possible, assuming design owners are ready to get their designs pre-approved from authority services. In some cases, in-device validation could be beneficial as it limits design exposure service. To ensure the confidentiality of designs-to-be-produced, there may be a requirement not to move the blueprint out of the 3D printer to protect intellectual rights and provide secure printing operations.
- Additive manufacturing factories (or devices) could be operating offline.
- A DCO will store information about 3D objects in the form of CPDs.

4.2. Confidentiality Preserving Descriptors: Describing CO

At the system core, there are CPDs—a set of "fingerprints" for 3D objects.

The concept behind CPDs is as follows:

- Each of these descriptors describes a distinctive feature of 3D objects. It could [36–38] be the number of holes in the object, volume of the object, area of the surface, volume of the convex hull, surface- or boundary-based centroid, center of mass, principal axes, convexity, aspect ratios, sphericity, mean radius, ellipsoidal variance, EGI [39], spherical harmonic coefficients [27], etc. Multiple CPDs are used as an ensemble to facilitate rapid object identification.
- Three-dimensional objects are encoded by their feature vector. Each object's CPDs contain essential information about the shape of the 3D object in a compressed and low-dimensionality form, sufficient for object identification.
- Descriptors must be lossy and nonreversible, making the restoration of original blueprints from CPDs impossible even if the 3DP device is breached and fully disassembled.

- Descriptors need to be computationally light/fast for in-device processing. We assume $k = 10^2$–10^3 physical objects per 3DP job, so using object-per-object comparison will require k times the number of controlled objects for comparisons. This processing should not create a "bottleneck" for the primary 3D printing process by demanding too many resources.
- At least some descriptors should be able to capture the internal structure of the 3D object, not only the appearance.
- Descriptors could be efficiently stored in the DCO and allow effective comparison of descriptors.
- As objects in the 3DP job may be rotated for better packing of objects in the printing volume, the descriptors should either provide the same output when the 3D objects are rotated and translated or the most efficient method to compare the descriptors of the rotated and translated objects should be known.

4.3. Identification Process

The objective of the identification process is to analyze the object in a 3D printing (3DP) job as being a CO before printing. CPDs are computed for each object in a 3DP job (for each OUA) and compared to CPDs of controlled objects from the DCO before allowing manufacturing to commence. This identification process should be time- and resource-efficient and include the analysis of the internal structure of the 3D object, not only the surface.

One possible option during the analysis is that the CO in the 3DP job may be rotated and translated for better packing of objects in the printing volume. Assuming that the technical OUA has an established and (almost) unchangeable geometry, its mesh could still be modified to change the number of vertices/triangles (and keep the original geometry and topology) in the blueprint. Such a modification is one of the simplest methods to make the object misidentified if the recognition of the object is based on the number of vertices and triangles of the original blueprint.

We assume that most objects to be printed at the facility are non-controlled. This brings us to a two-level architecture, where at the first level we would like to identify the non-controlled objects as fast as possible and leave only the suspicious objects to be controlled. We use more time-consuming but high-accuracy approaches at the second level to check if the object is a CO.

The error of the first type (the allowed object is considered controllable) will annoy the customer of the 3D printer as the legitimate order will be rejected. This event will likely negatively affect customer satisfaction and future usage of the manufacturing facility. The error of the second type (the controlled object is considered as allowed) could cause severe consequences for the facility owner/operator for breaking the law. For example, per Singapore law, the operator of the printing facility is responsible for printing illegal objects [4].

The proposed two-layer system can be considered a two-factor authentication (2FA) system, where the printable object is checked and authenticated by distinctively different methods at each stage.

This 2FA system is a cascade of classifiers:

- The decision making about object identification is performed as a cascade of classifiers, i.e., in a hierarchical manner.
- The probability of encountering a CO is low, so we must filter out non-COs quickly and efficiently.
- We start from low-complexity discriminative algorithms to reject the object as being a CO as fast as possible (e.g., it is too small, too "square", has no holes, etc.).
- Then, at later stages, we progress to complex, computationally expensive, and accurate determination algorithms.
- All objects (models) from a 3D print job should pass through a hierarchy of classifiers (it could be imagined as a set of sieves with smaller and smaller chances to make an

inaccurate decision due to being more computationally expensive at each consequent level); refer to Figure 1.

- We aim to identify (eliminate) most objects by the least computationally expensive classifier.
- Ideally, it is expected that identification aims for 100% accuracy within an acceptable time.
- Different methods have different complexity and accuracy (usually, the more complex the approach, the longer the calculations and the better the final accuracy).
- Some models could take a long time to process to reach high-accuracy results.
- The acceptable level of object identification accuracy may depend on the object type. We might need to weigh the importance of correctly identifying the object against the time spent on decision making and the type of the object itself.

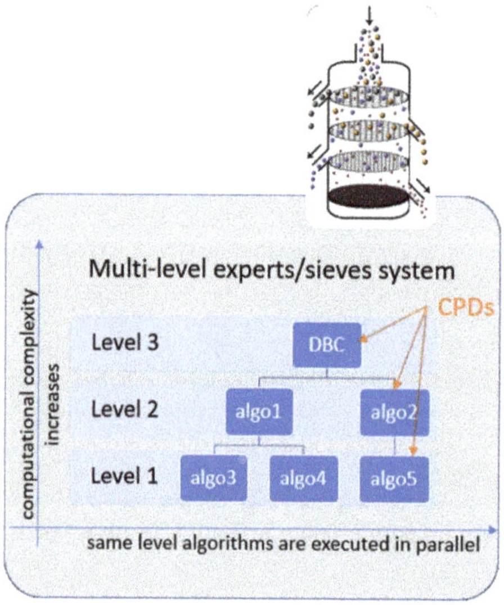

Figure 1. The sieve system is used to identify a CO in a 3DP job.

The method of object identification should be immune to:

- Rotation in R^3 (any degree) and translation (as objects in a 3D printing job could be moved to be better packed in the printing volume).
- Remeshing of 3D object mesh.

Many descriptors for the first layer can be found in [36–38]. We can apply these descriptors according to a decrease in complexity (and an increase in speed) and calculate some descriptors in parallel. The calculation and comparison of different descriptors can be separated into several levels (Figure 1).

We can choose all the descriptors available to perform the object's comparison. However, there is a more advanced way. In [40], different sets of descriptors were analyzed for their usage for object "fingerprinting" and for their efficacy and efficiency. A small set of four descriptors was found to describe and compare 3D objects efficiently. These descriptors are also efficient for information retrieval from the big database of 3D objects. One of the sets of the champion CPDs consists of the convex hull area of the 3D object, convex hull volume, modified extended gaussian image (which is the energy of the spherical harmonics corresponding to the extended gaussian image [39,41] of the 3D object), and the central moment of inertia of the surface of the object calculated relative to the centroid of the 3D object [40]. These CPDs were chosen based on their computational simplicity and the power of feature extraction, and their efficacy is the same as for the much more comprehensive set of descriptors.

The specialized algorithm called Discriminative Base Comparison (DBC) was used for the second layer. Following Kazhdan's [27] approach, it cuts the 3D object into concentric spheres (shells) and then finds the intersection of the object by each shell. A sequence of spherical harmonic coefficients represents the resulting indicator function for each shell, and then the corresponding energies for each degree and shell are calculated. The valuable property of energies is that an energy is not changed by any rotation in R^3 around the center of mass (or centroid) and does not depend on the object's translation.

In a concentric manner, shell-by-shell and degree-by-degree, the energies of the spherical coefficients are compared for the OUA and COs from the DCO. If a correspondence is found, the object similar to the CO is identified. DBC is a non-iterative and non-gradient method of searching for similarity.

The computational complexity of this method is much higher than the complexity for calculations of the simple descriptors at the first layer of the process. That is why the OUA is first tested by fast and simple descriptors, which provide quick rejection of non-similar objects, and only after passing this sieving-out do we apply the more complex check. Let us recall that most of the objects in the 3DP job are assumed to be non-controllable, so the first layer efficiently identifies and rejects non-COs, leaving only the cases where extra investigation is required.

The overall workflow is depicted in Figure 2. The OUA is represented in the form of a set of descriptors and is compared with the descriptors of the COs from the DCO using the sieve system (Figure 1).

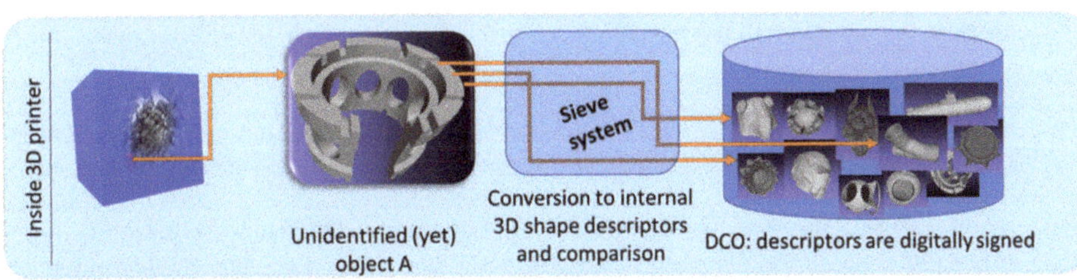

Figure 2. The overall workflow.

5. Results and Discussion

The current developed proof of concept demonstrates its functionality and verifies a principal concept of usage of CPDs for object "fingerprinting" and identification (Figure 3). We also developed an initial prototype that allows for the visualization of how the system will function; there is a working interactive model that gives an idea of the functionality, design, navigation, and layout (Figure 3).

To test the software for the identification of COs, we used several standard internet datasets that contain 3D polygonal models collected from the World Wide Web:

- The ShapeNet dataset (The Princeton Shape Benchmark (PSB), Version 1) [42].
- The Engineering Shape Benchmark (ESB, Purdue University) dataset [43].
- Princeton ModelNet40 [44].
- Free downloadable models from different Internet websites.

All in all, we collected more than 14,000 models and placed them in the database. These 3D objects represented potential objects of interest with unique features.

Our approach was tested in the following way: We took every object from the database (considered as our DCO), then randomly rotated, translated, and re-meshed them, and then performed a database search using our two-layer approach. The first layer checked the correspondence of features of two objects; if the objects are scaled versions of each other, they will be considered as non-matching (as they have, for example, different volumes).

In case we needed to identify the scaled objects as matching, then before the analysis, we additionally needed to scale the objects to the same standard size.

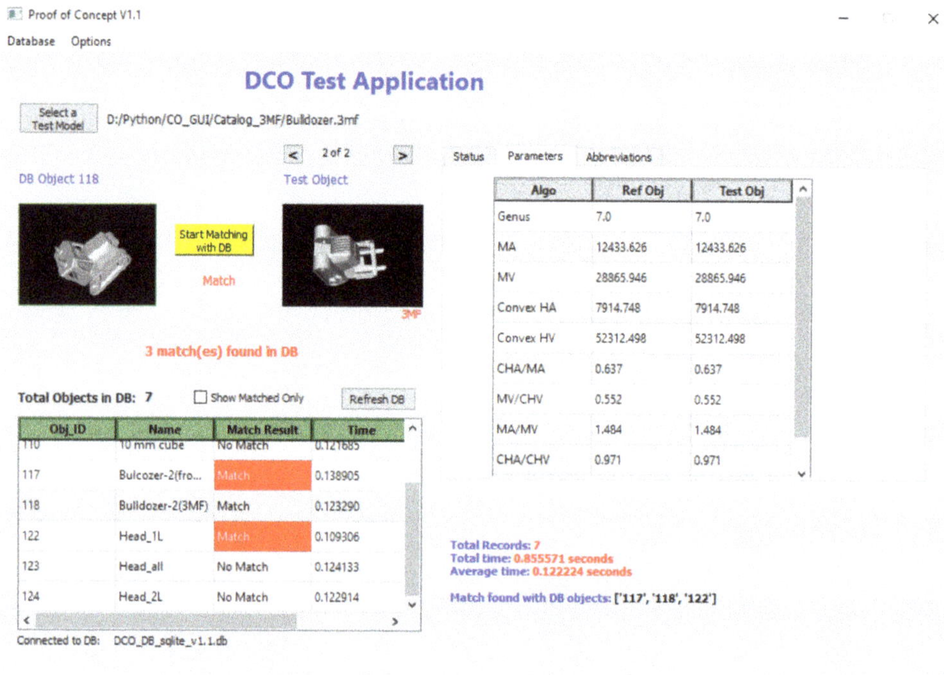

Figure 3. Application interface for comparison of object-under-printing against the DCO objects.

The result showed that, using the architecture suggested and the CPDs described, it was possible in all cases (100% accuracy, 0% false positive/false negative) to successfully identify the models from the database. These identified models could comprise duplicates or mirror images of the OUA, or objects found in the database that possess a slight variation of the surface of the OUA.

The second experiment conducted to check our method used the ESB [34,43] as a DCO. The set of 3D models input to check against the DCO included transformed and re-meshed models from ModelNet40 [44] (a set of unprotected objects) and ESB (protected objects). Our descriptor-based approach correctly identified whether the input model was contained in the DCO with 100% accuracy; shifted, rotated, and mirrored objects, and objects with minor modifications were identified correctly.

The ultimate validation of the proposed method of CO identification could be accomplished by using a real DCO (with guns, explosives, etc.) To our knowledge, there is no existing open-access database of controlled (prohibited) blueprints, and even keeping a controlled blueprint on a computer without official permission is a criminal offense in some countries, including, for example, Singapore. The existence of such a database would be a significant security threat, and the creation and maintenance of such a DCO should be developed only by relevant government agencies and supervisory authorities. Hence, real-life experiments could be conducted only after the appearance of such a DCO and only by the appointed people.

The system proposed is not a panacea, and expecting the same 100% accuracy in a real-life situation would be really naive. Currently, it can only identify technical objects with (almost) unchangeable geometry. The objects' scaling, rotation, translation, and remeshing do not affect the identification results. This system would mainly help when attempting to print a known controlled object without significant modification. By analogy, in Internet cyberattacks where people try to use a vulnerability discovered by some pioneer hacker, we hope that most attackers (people who would try to print COs) would use the blueprints found on the Internet without modifications.

We see a rapid adoption of 3D printing technology for manufacturing illegal or counterfeit objects. Wikipedia provides a list of 3D-printed weapons and parts [45] which consists of 50 individual designs printed in metal and plastic. For comparison, only five to six designs were available two years ago. As a result, laws and regulations were rapidly introduced to prohibit/restrict 3D printing, identify legally guilty parties, and introduce penalties. Finding people/organizations illegally printing counterfeit objects and proving that the objects were illegally printed will be an enforcement nightmare for patent holders and relevant law enforcement authorities. Incorporating constraints in 3D printing will allow manufacturers to satisfy current and future legal requirements and enable programmable control for printing unauthorized/copyrighted 3D objects.

Zero-day attacks and different (from those considered above) types of attempts to print COs should be addressed when these new attacks are detected. This is the same never-ending attack and defense game we see for viruses and antiviruses.

One of the types of attacks presently challenging to detect involves modifying the surface of a 3D object in a way that does not impact its functionality but alters the object's shape. Establishing local surface correspondences with the CO could shield them from this attack, and the authors are currently working on this idea. This approach requires time to develop to make it practical (to work in real time and to be accurate and robust under possible modifications).

5.1. Efficiency of Search in a Big Database of Controlled Objects

A potential bottleneck could appear for efficient data retrieval from a big database (~1 M controlled objects and more). A set of CPDs represents each object; hence, for the fast retrieval of an object from a database, we need to find a "good" subset of CPDs to discriminate the database objects efficiently. Next, we need to index and filter the database using the subset of CPDs found. If the database is modified (the number of records is growing), the "good" set of descriptors for fast retrieval might also change. It poses the question: how do you find a quick and efficient method of information retrieval for a database of, say, 1 million or 1 billion records?

The distribution of object features in a database appears to have colossal information "inertia". The distribution does not change a lot when the database grows. It is the same concept as for public opinion surveys: there is no need to ask everyone, and there is a need to choose a representative subset. Statistically representative results for a database of up to 1 million records require a sample size of fewer than 400 records to be analyzed (with a 95% confidence level and 5% margin of error). We conducted experimental checks of the claim as it sounds counterintuitive and found that the statistical approach (unlike intuition) is correct. We can, therefore, discover optimal filtering for a big database based on samples from this database.

5.2. Possible Future Directions

There are a lot of interesting future continuations for this project. For example:

- Making the identification of a CO possible even if no blueprint for this CO is available. This could be done by scanning the object and representing it as a point cloud.
- Identifying a CO even if an intentional change in the design (to escape detection) is made. We assume that this design change does not affect the object's functionality.
- Verifying that the blueprint object was not modified during printing (parts of the blueprint should not be changed during manufacturing due to a malicious attack).
- Performing modeling of attacks and countering attacks.

- Incorporating ML/DL techniques to detect similarity to the class of COs even if we have a limited number (or even one only) of class representatives (e.g., the object looks like a known CO) using one-shot learning.

6. Conclusions

There is a clear need for new solutions in intellectual property protection and the production of controlled objects in the emerging world of 3D printing. In this world, the proliferation of 3D manufacturing of fake spare parts and real weapons is the upcoming reality.

Preventing counterfeiting and printing of controlled objects promises to be a growth market (the same as 3D additive manufacturing) with several clearly defined stakeholders. The incorporation of constraints before the 3D printing process starts might benefit:

- Patents, copyrights, and trademarks holders;
- Three-dimensional manufacturers (this could help address current and future regulatory challenges for the production of COs);
- Law enforcement organizations (to tighten controls for high-risk items).

We have proposed a system architecture for the fast, efficient, and secure identification of whether a design-to-be-produced inside a 3D printing system is a controlled object. The computer vision algorithms developed analyze the features of 3D objects in multi-dimensional space. This project is currently in the process of building a prototype. Pre-screening software could indemnify a 3D printer owner from liability related to the unintentional printing of a controlled object. This technology could help protect manufacturers and rights owners from unscrupulous customers and insider threats (e.g., "after-hours manufacturing", (un)intentional oversight, etc.).

Copyright/trademark holders could protect their intellectual rights, e.g., by subscribing to a service that prevents (prohibits) the reproduction of protected objects through 3D printing at additive manufacturing facilities.

Author Contributions: Conceptualization, I.V. and H.B.; investigation, methodology, writing original draft, review & editing, I.V., S.K., A.M. and H.B.; project administration, I.V. and H.B.; data curation, formal analysis, software, validation, I.V., S.K. and A.M.; supervision, funding acquisition, H.B. All authors have read and agreed to the published version of the manuscript.

Funding: This study is supported under the RIE2020 Industry Alignment Fund—Industry Collaboration Projects (IAF-ICP) Funding Initiative, as well as by cash and in-kind contributions from industry partner HP Inc. through the HP-NTU Digital Manufacturing Corporate Lab.

Data Availability Statement: The open access data [42–44] were used.

Acknowledgments: This study is supported under the RIE2020 Industry Alignment Fund—Industry Collaboration Projects (IAF-ICP) Funding Initiative, as well as by cash and in-kind contributions from industry partner HP Inc. through the HP-NTU Digital Manufacturing Corporate Lab.

Conflicts of Interest: The authors declare that this study received funding from HP Inc. The funder was not involved in the study design, collection, analysis, interpretation of data, the writing of this article or the decision to submit it for publication. In addition, author Helen Balinsky is employed by HP Inc. The remaining authors declare that the research was conducted in the absence of any commercial or financial relationships that could be construed as a potential conflict of interest.

References

1. HP Helps U.S. Clamp Down on Counterfeiting. Imaging Expertise Used to Deter Digital Fakes. Available online: https://www.hpl.hp.com/news/2003/july_sept/counterfeit.html (accessed on 31 October 2023).
2. Secret Code in Colour Printers Lets Government Track You. Available online: https://www.eff.org/press/archives/2005/10/16 (accessed on 31 October 2023).
3. When 3D Printing Gets into the Wrong Hands. Available online: https://www.forbes.com/sites/zurich/2016/05/06/when-3d-printing-gets-into-the-wrong-hands/ (accessed on 31 October 2023).

4. Elangovan, N. Parliament Enacts New Law to Keep 3D-Printed Guns off the Streets, Better Regulate Weapons. Available online: https://www.todayonline.com/singapore/parliament-enacts-new-law-keep-3d-printed-guns-streets-better-regulate-weapons (accessed on 31 October 2023).
5. Fact Sheet: The Biden Administration Cracks Down on Ghost Guns, Ensures that ATF Has the Leadership it Needs to Enforce Our Gun Laws. Available online: https://www.whitehouse.gov/briefing-room/statements-releases/2022/04/11/fact-sheet-the-biden-administration-cracks-down-on-ghost-guns-ensures-that-atf-has-the-leadership-it-needs-to-enforce-our-gun-laws/ (accessed on 31 October 2023).
6. Spain Dismantles Workshop Making 3D-Printed Weapons. Available online: https://www.bbc.com/news/world-europe-56798743 (accessed on 31 October 2023).
7. Bridges, S.M.; Keiser, K.; Sissom, N.; Graves, S.J. Cyber security for additive manufacturing. In Proceedings of the 10th Annual Cyber and Information Security Research Conference (CISR'15), Oak Ridge, TN, USA, 7–9 April 2015.
8. Printing Insecurity: Tackling the Threat of 3D Printed Guns in Europe. Available online: https://www.europol.europa.eu/media-press/newsroom/news/printing-insecurity-tackling-threat-of-3d-printed-guns-in-europe (accessed on 31 October 2023).
9. Fey, M. *3D Printing and International Security: Risks and Challenges of an Emerging Technology*; Report No. 144; Peace Research Institute Frankfurt: Frankfurt am Main, Germany, 2017.
10. Ebrahim, T. 3D Printing: Digital Infringement & Digital Regulation. *Northwest. J. Technol. Intellect. Prop.* **2016**, *14*, 2.
11. U.S. Code. Title 17. Ch. 1. § 102—Subject Matter of Copyright: In General. Available online: https://www.law.cornell.edu/uscode/text/17/102 (accessed on 31 October 2023).
12. Ogburu-Ogbonnay, H. 3D Printing as a Copyright Infringement, JIPEL Blog 2016–2017. Available online: https://blog.jipel.law.nyu.edu/2017/03/3d-printing-as-a-copyright-infringement/ (accessed on 31 October 2023).
13. WIPO Copyright Treaty (Adopted in Geneva on December 20, 1996), WIPO IP Portal. Available online: https://wipolex.wipo.int/en/text/295166 (accessed on 31 October 2023).
14. Malaty, E.; Rostama, G. 3D printing and IP law. *WIPO Mag.* **2017**, *1*, 6.
15. Blockchain to Play a Key Part in Ensuring Copyright Laws Can Be Used for 3D Printing. Available online: https://news-archive.exeter.ac.uk/homepage/title_908509_en.html (accessed on 31 October 2023).
16. Gao, Y.; Wang, W.; Jin, Y.; Zhou, C.; Xu, W.; Jin, Z. ThermoTag: A hidden ID of 3D printers for fingerprinting and watermarking. *IEEE Trans. Inf. Forensics Secur.* **2021**, *16*, 2805–2820. [CrossRef]
17. 3D-Printed Counterfeits on the Rise: How to Protect Your Brand. Available online: https://www.nanomatrixsecure.com/3d-printed-counterfeits-on-the-rise-how-to-protect-your-brand/ (accessed on 31 October 2023).
18. Roche, S. The New World of 3D Printing... and Counterfeiting. Available online: https://www.linkedin.com/pulse/new-world-3d-printing-counterfeiting-sebastien-roche (accessed on 31 October 2023).
19. O'Heir, J. Protecting a New World of 3D-Printed Products, the American Society of Mechanical Engineers. Available online: https://www.asme.org/topics-resources/content/protecting-new-world-3dprinted-products (accessed on 31 October 2023).
20. Counterfeit Product Alert: How to Identify Counterfeit BMW Group Vehicle Parts. Available online: https://www.thecounterfeitreport.com/product/599/BMW-Group-Vehicle-Parts.html (accessed on 31 October 2023).
21. Zhuang, T.; Zhang, X.; Hou, Z.; Zuo, W.; Liu, Y. A novel 3D CAD model retrieval method based on vertices classification and weights combination optimization. *Math. Probl. Eng.* **2017**, *2017*, 6049750. [CrossRef]
22. Zaharia, T.; Petreux, F. 3D shape-based retrieval within the mpeg-7 framework. In Proceedings of the SPIE Conference on Nonlinear Image Processing and Pattern Analysis XII, San Jose, CA, USA, 30–31 July 2001; pp. 133–145.
23. Osada, R.; Funkhouser, T.A.; Chazelle, B.; Bobkin, D.B. Shape distribution. *ACM Trans. Graph.* **2002**, *21*, 807–832. [CrossRef]
24. Shih, J.-L.; Lee, C.-H.; Wang, J.T. 3D object retrieval system based on grid D2. *Electron. Lett.* **2005**, *41*, 179–181. [CrossRef]
25. Novotni, M.; Klein, R. A geometric approach to 3D object comparison. In Proceedings of the International Conference on Shape Modeling and Applications, Genoa, Italy, 7–11 May 2001; pp. 167–175.
26. Zhang, J.; Siddiqi, K.; Macrini, D.; Shokoufandeh, A.; Dickinson, S. Retrieving articulated 3-d models using medial surfaces and their graph spectra. In Proceedings of the Energy Minimization Methods in Computer Vision and Pattern Recognition: 5th International Workshop, EMMCVPR 2005, St. Augustine, FL, USA, 9–11 November 2005.
27. Kazhdan, M.; Funkhouser, T.; Rusinkiewicz, S. Rotation invariant spherical harmonic representation of 3D shape descriptors. In Proceedings of the 2003 Eurographics/ACM SIGGRAPH Symposium on Geometry Processing (SGP '03), Aachen, Germany, 23–25 June 2003; pp. 156–164.
28. Gao, Y.; Dai, Q. View-based 3D object retrieval: Challenges and approaches. *IEEE Multimed.* **2014**, *21*, 52–57. [CrossRef]
29. Ansary, T.F.; Daoudi, M.; Vandeborre, J. Bayesian 3D search engine using adaptive views clustering. *IEEE Trans. Multimed.* **2007**, *9*, 78–88. [CrossRef]
30. Wang, X.; Nie, W. 3D model retrieval with weighted locality constrained group sparse coding. *Neurocomputing* **2015**, *151*, 620–625. [CrossRef]
31. Hoang, L.; Lee, S.-H.; Kwon, K.-R. A deep learning method for 3D object classification and retrieval using the global point signature plus and deep wide residual network. *Sensors* **2021**, *21*, 2644. [CrossRef] [PubMed]
32. Zarpalas, D.; Daras, P.; Axenopoulos, A.; Tzovaras, D.; Strintzis, M.G. 3D model search and retrieval using the spherical trace transform. *EURASIP J. Adv. Signal Process.* **2006**, *2007*, 23912. [CrossRef]

33. Daras, P.; Axenopoulos, A.; Litos, G. Investigating the effects of multiple factors towards more accurate 3-D object retrieval. *IEEE Trans. Multimed.* **2012**, *14*, 374–388. [CrossRef]
34. Jayanti, S.; Kalyanaraman, Y.; Iyer, N.; Ramani, K. Developing an engineering shape benchmark for CAD models. *Comput.-Aided Des.* **2006**, *38*, 939–953. [CrossRef]
35. Papadakis, P.; Pratikakis, I.; Theoharis, T.; Perantonis, S. Panorama: A 3D shape descriptor based on panoramic views for unsupervised 3d object retrieval. *Int. J. Comput. Vis.* **2010**, *89*, 177–192. [CrossRef]
36. Peura, M.; Iivarinen, J. Efficiency of simple shape descriptors. In Proceedings of the 3rd International Workshop on Visual Form (IWVF3), Capri, Italy, 28–30 May 1997; pp. 443–451.
37. Wäldchen, J.; Mäder, P. Plant species identification using computer vision techniques: A systematic literature review. *Arch. Comput. Methods Eng.* **2008**, *25*, 507–543. [CrossRef] [PubMed]
38. Sonka, M.; Hlaváč, V.; Boyle, R.D. *Image Processing, Analysis and Machine Vision*, 4th ed.; Springer: New York, NY, USA, 1993.
39. Kang, S.B.; Horn, P.K. Extended Gaussian image (EGI). In *Computer Vision*; Ikeuchi, K., Ed.; Springer: Cham, Switzerland, 2021; pp. 420–424.
40. Volkau, I.; Krasovskii, S.; Mujeeb, A.; Balinsky, H. Whether 3D object is copyright protected? Controlled object identification in additive manufacturing. In Proceedings of the IEEE 22nd International Conference on Cyberworlds (CW2023), Sousse, Tunisia, 3–5 October 2023.
41. Horn, B.K.P. *Robot Vision*; The MIT Press: Cambridge, MA, USA, 1986.
42. Shilane, P.; Min, P.; Kazhdan, M.; Funkhouser, T. Princeton Shape Benchmark. Available online: https://shape.cs.princeton.edu/benchmark/benchmark.pdf (accessed on 15 May 2023).
43. Engineering Shape Benchmark (ESB, Purdue University). Available online: https://engineering.purdue.edu/cdesign/wp/downloads/ (accessed on 31 October 2023).
44. Wu, Z.; Song, S.; Khosla, A.; Yu, F.; Zhang, L.; Tang, X.; Xiao, J. 3D ShapeNets: A Deep Representation for Volumetric Shapes. In Proceedings of the IEEE Conference on Computer Vision and Pattern Recognition (CVPR 2015), Boston, MA, USA, 7–12 June 2015; pp. 1912–1920.
45. List of 3D Printed Weapons and Parts. Available online: https://en.wikipedia.org/wiki/List_of_3D_printed_weapons_and_parts (accessed on 31 October 2023).

computers

MDPI

Review

The YOLO Framework: A Comprehensive Review of Evolution, Applications, and Benchmarks in Object Detection

Momina Liaqat Ali [1] and Zhou Zhang [2,*]

[1] Department of Computer Science, Middle Tennessee State University, 1301 E Main St., Murfreesboro, TN 37132, USA; ma2mp@mtmail.mtsu.edu
[2] Farmingdale State College, State University of New York, 2350 NY-110, Farmingdale, NY 11735, USA
* Correspondence: zhangz@farmingdale.edu

Abstract: This paper provides a comprehensive review of the YOLO (You Only Look Once) framework up to its latest version, YOLO 11. As a state-of-the-art model for object detection, YOLO has revolutionized the field by achieving an optimal balance between speed and accuracy. The review traces the evolution of YOLO variants, highlighting key architectural improvements, performance benchmarks, and applications in domains such as healthcare, autonomous vehicles, and robotics. It also evaluates the framework's strengths and limitations in practical scenarios, addressing challenges like small object detection, environmental variability, and computational constraints. By synthesizing findings from recent research, this work identifies critical gaps in the literature and outlines future directions to enhance YOLO's adaptability, robustness, and integration into emerging technologies. This review provides researchers and practitioners with valuable insights to drive innovation in object detection and related applications.

Keywords: YOLO; single stage detection; YOLOv10; YOLOv11; performance evaluation; deep neural network; real-time object detection

1. Introduction

Object detection, a core task in computer vision, has seen remarkable advancements in recent years due to the ongoing development of more efficient and accurate algorithms [1,2]. One of the most significant breakthroughs in this field is the You Only Look Once (YOLO) framework, a pioneering one-stage object detection algorithm that has drawn widespread attention for its ability to achieve real-time detection with high precision [3,4]. YOLO's approach simultaneously predicting bounding boxes and class probabilities in a single forward pass sets it apart from traditional multi-stage detection methods [5–7]. This capability makes YOLO exceptionally well-suited for applications requiring rapid decision-making, such as autonomous driving, medical diagnostics, and surveillance systems [8,9]. The evolution of object detection methods has paved the way for YOLO, offering a novel solution to the longstanding challenge of balancing speed and accuracy in detection tasks [10,11]. Its real-time performance, coupled with its flexibility across a wide range of domains, has cemented YOLO as a leading algorithm in both academic research and practical applications. As object detection continues to evolve, a deeper understanding of YOLO's architecture and its extensive applicability becomes increasingly important, particularly as newer versions introduce significant architectural improvements and optimizations [12].

This review provides a comprehensive exploration of the YOLO framework, beginning with an overview of the historical development of object detection algorithms, leading to the emergence of YOLO [13]. The subsequent sections delve into the technical details of YOLO's architecture, focusing on its core components, the backbone, neck, and head, and how these elements work in unison to optimize the detection process. By examining these components, we highlight the key innovations that enable YOLO to outperform many of its counterparts in real-time detection scenarios. A central theme of this review is the versatility of YOLO across diverse application domains. From detecting COVID-19 in X-ray images to enhancing road safety under adverse weather conditions [14], YOLO has demonstrated its ability to address complex challenges across fields such as medical imaging, autonomous vehicles, and agriculture. In each of these domains, YOLO's ability to process high-resolution images quickly and accurately has driven substantial improvements in detection efficiency and accuracy.

Throughout this review, we address several key research questions, including the major applications of YOLO, its performance compared to other object detection algorithms, and the specific advantages and limitations of its various versions. We also consider the ethical implications of using YOLO in sensitive applications, particularly regarding privacy concerns, dataset biases, and broader societal impacts. As YOLO continues to be deployed in applications such as surveillance and law enforcement, these ethical considerations become increasingly critical to responsible AI development. Therefore, this review synthesizes insights from various domains to provide a holistic understanding of the YOLO framework's contributions to the field of object detection. By highlighting both the strengths and limitations of YOLO, this paper offers a foundation for future research directions, particularly in optimizing YOLO for emerging challenges in the ever-evolving landscape of computer vision.

This paper is structured to provide a holistic understanding of the YOLO framework, beginning with an overview of its fundamental architecture and evolutionary advancements. It then delves into a benchmark-based evaluation of various YOLO versions, offering critical insights into their performance across diverse datasets and scenarios. The discussion extends to YOLO's extensive applications across multiple domains, such as healthcare, autonomous systems, agriculture, and industrial automation, highlighting its transformative impact in real-world settings. Finally, the paper addresses ethical considerations associated with YOLO's deployment, including privacy concerns, societal implications, and the need for responsible use. This comprehensive approach aims to provide readers with a well-rounded perspective on the technical capabilities, practical applications, and ethical dimensions of YOLO, serving as a valuable resource for researchers, practitioners, and policymakers alike.

2. Literature Search Strategy

Conducting a comprehensive literature review of the YOLO framework requires a systematic and methodologically rigorous approach. This study employed a well-structured strategy to navigate the extensive and multidisciplinary body of literature on YOLO, ensuring a thorough and representative selection of the most relevant and impactful studies.

2.1. Search Methodology

To ensure an exhaustive review, we focused on reputable and high-impact sources such as IEEE Xplore, SpringerLink, and key conference proceedings, including CVPR, ICCV, and ECCV. In addition, we utilized search engines like Google Scholar and academic databases, leveraging Boolean search operators to construct detailed queries with phrases such as "object detection", "YOLO", "deep learning", and "neural networks". This approach allowed us to capture the latest research and most significant papers across disciplines related to computer vision and machine learning.

The search covered an array of top-tier publications, including but not limited to the following:

- *IEEE Transactions on Pattern Analysis and Machine Intelligence (TPAMI);*
- *Computer Vision and Image Understanding (CVIU);*
- *Journal of Machine Learning Research (JMLR);*
- *International Journal of Computer Vision (IJCV);*
- *Journal of Artificial Intelligence Research (JAIR).*

The search results yielded an initial pool of 53,200 articles. To manage this large collection, a two-step screening process was applied:

1. Title Screening: The titles were reviewed to eliminate papers not directly related to YOLO or object detection methodologies.
2. Abstract Screening: Abstracts were thoroughly examined to assess the relevance of each article in terms of its focus on YOLO's architectural innovations, applications, or comparative analysis.

2.2. Selection Criteria

We applied stringent inclusion and exclusion criteria to refine the literature pool:

- Inclusion Criteria:
    - Studies providing in-depth analysis of YOLO architecture and methodologies.
    - High-impact and widely cited papers.
    - Research papers offering empirical results from YOLO-based applications in various domains.
    - Articles that address both the strengths and limitations of YOLO.
- Exclusion Criteria:
    - Articles that merely mention YOLO without exploring its methodologies or applications.
    - Research papers lacking substantive contributions to the development or application.
    - Duplicate or redundant publications across multiple conferences or journals.

This process refined the literature pool to 135 articles, which were selected for a full-text review. The chosen articles span a wide range of topics, including YOLO's architectural developments, training and optimization strategies, and its application across diverse domains such as medical imaging, autonomous vehicles, and agriculture.

2.3. Coding and Classification

The selected articles were further categorized based on specific features of the YOLO framework. Each article was coded according to the following dimensions:

- *Architectural Innovations:* Backbone, neck, and head components, and innovations across YOLO versions (e.g., YOLOv3, YOLOv4, YOLOv5, YOLOv9).
- *Training Strategies:* Data augmentation, transfer learning, and optimization techniques.
- *Performance Metrics:* Evaluation metrics such as mAP (mean Average Precision), FPS (Frames Per Second), and computational cost (FLOPs).
- *Applications:* Medical imaging, autonomous driving, agriculture, industrial applications, and more.

Table 1 provides a detailed breakdown of the different versions of YOLO, their architectural innovations, and methodological approaches. For each version, we analyzed training strategies, loss functions, post-processing techniques, and optimization methods. This systematic classification allows for a nuanced understanding of YOLO's progression and its practical applications.

Table 1. YOLO framework version and research methodologies.

YOLO Version	Architectural Innovations	Training Strategies	Optimization Techniques
YOLOv1	Simplified CNN backbone, basic bounding box prediction	Geometric transformations, hue jitter	Stochastic gradient descent, non-maximum suppression (NMS)
YOLOv2	DarkNet-19 backbone, K-means clustering for anchor box refinement	Fine-tuning, pre-trained weights	SGD with momentum, hyperparameter tuning, Adam optimizer

Table 1. *Cont.*

YOLO Version	Architectural Innovations	Training Strategies	Optimization Techniques
YOLOv3	DarkNet-53, multi-scale detection, residual connections	Mix-up, data augmentation, noise	Non-maximum suppression, thresholding, multi-scale object detection
YOLOv4	CSPDarkNet-53, PANet, mosaic data augmentation	Transfer learning, knowledge distillation	Generalized IoU, focal loss, dynamic quantization
YOLOv5	CSPNet, dynamic anchor refinement, lightweight architecture	Mosaic, CutMix, early stopping	Post-training quantization, filter pruning, low-rank approximation
YOLOv6	PANet, CSPDarkNet53	Adversarial training, domain-specific augmentation	IoU loss, confidence thresholding, multi-scale fusion
YOLOv7	EfficientRep backbone, dynamic label assignment	Fine-tuning, adversarial patch detection	NAS, quantization, gradient clipping
YOLOv8	Path Aggregation Network, Dynamic Kernel Attention	Adversarial training, data augmentation	Momentum and Adam optimizer, post-training quantization
YOLOv9	Multi-level auxiliary feature extraction	Fine-tuning, domain-specific augmentation	GELAN module, deep supervision for resource-constrained systems
YOLOv10	Lightweight classification head and separate spatial and channel transformations	NMS free training, dual label assignment	Distinct spatial and channel transformations to increase overall efficiency during down sampling stage
YOLOV11	Introduced C3k2 block in backbone and used C2PSA to enhance spatial attention	Fine-tuning, mix-up, augmentation, adaptive gradient clipping	Quantization, stochastic gradient descent (SGD)

3. Single-Stage Object Detectors

3.1. Understanding Single-Stage Detectors in Object Detection: Concepts, Architecture, and Applications

Single-stage object detectors represent a class of models designed to detect objects in an image through a single forward pass of the neural network [15]. Unlike two-stage detectors, which involve separate steps for region proposal and object classification, single-stage detectors perform both tasks simultaneously, streamlining the detection process [16]. This approach has gained popularity due to its simplicity, computational efficiency, and real-time processing capabilities, making it particularly well suited for applications that demand quick inference, such as autonomous vehicles and surveillance systems [17].

A typical single-stage detector directly predicts object class probabilities and bounding boxes without the need for a region proposal network (RPN) [18]. Several key concepts define single-stage object detectors:

1. Unified Architecture: These detectors employ a unified neural network architecture that predicts bounding boxes and class probabilities simultaneously, eliminating the need for a separate region proposal phase [19].
2. Anchor Boxes or Default Boxes: To accommodate varying object scales and aspect ratios, single-stage detectors use anchor boxes (also referred to as default boxes) [20]. These predefined boxes allow the network to make adjustments to better fit objects of different shapes and sizes.
3. Regression and Classification Head: Single-stage detectors consist of two main components: a regression head for predicting bounding box coordinates and a classification head for determining object classes. Both heads operate on the feature maps extracted from the input image [15].

4. Loss Function: The model's training objective involves minimizing a combination of three losses: localization loss (for accurate bounding box predictions), confidence loss (for object presence or absence), and classification loss (for class label accuracy) [21].
5. Non-Maximum Suppression (NMS): After predicting multiple bounding boxes, non-maximum suppression is applied to filter out low-confidence and overlapping predictions. This ensures that only the most confident and non-redundant bounding boxes are retained [22,23].
6. Efficiency and Real-time Processing: One of the primary advantages of single-stage detectors is their computational efficiency, making them suitable for real-time processing. The absence of a separate region proposal step reduces computational overhead, allowing for rapid detection [24].
7. Applications: Single-stage detectors find applications in various domains, including autonomous vehicles, surveillance, robotics, and object recognition in images and videos. Their speed and simplicity make them particularly well-suited for scenarios where real-time detection is crucial. These applications are supported by numerous studies that highlight the efficiency and effectiveness of single-stage detectors in dynamic environments, especially in autonomous driving and pedestrian detection scenarios [25–28]. The effectiveness of single-stage detectors in surveillance systems enables continuous monitoring and quick response, which is essential for security applications [29]. In robotics, these detectors assist in real-time object recognition, facilitating navigation and interaction with the environment [30]. Therefore, the versatility and performance of single-stage detectors have made them a critical component in various modern technology applications.

These characteristics make single-stage detectors a critical tool in object detection, providing a balance between speed and accuracy while supporting a wide range of real-world applications. The flowchart of a single-stage detector's operation is depicted in Figure 1 in which there are convolutional layers of different scales followed by FC layers.

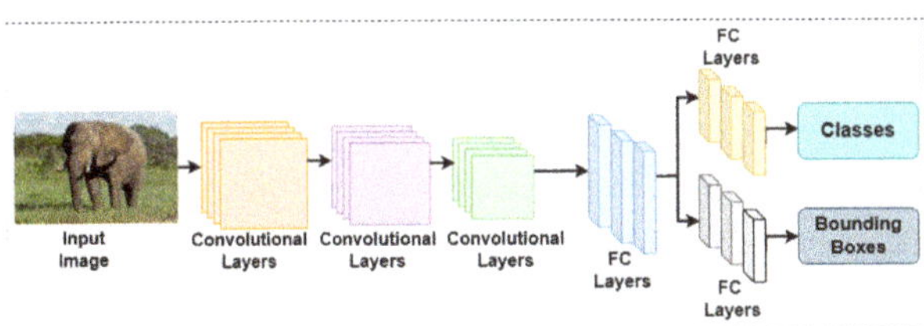

Figure 1. Overview of single-stage detectors.

3.2. *Typical Single-Stage Object Detectors*

Several single-stage detectors have been developed over the years, each with unique innovations and optimizations. Below is an overview of key single-stage detectors, their architectures, and contributions to the field of object detection.

3.2.1. SSD (Single Shot Detectors)

Introduced by Liu et al. in 2016 [31], the Single Shot MultiBox Detector (SSD) leverages a Convolutional Neural Network (CNN) as its backbone for feature extraction. SSD utilizes multiple layers from the base network to generate multi-scale feature maps, allowing it to detect objects at various scales. For each feature map scale, the SSD assigns anchor boxes with different aspect ratios and sizes, simultaneously predicting object class scores and bounding box offsets. After predictions are made, non-maximum suppression is applied to remove duplicate bounding boxes and retain the most confident detections. The overall architecture of an SSD is illustrated in Figure 2. The architecture of an SSD is a combination of convolutional layers that form the backbone and then the SSD head, which performs detection, and the head is composed of a few convolutional layers.

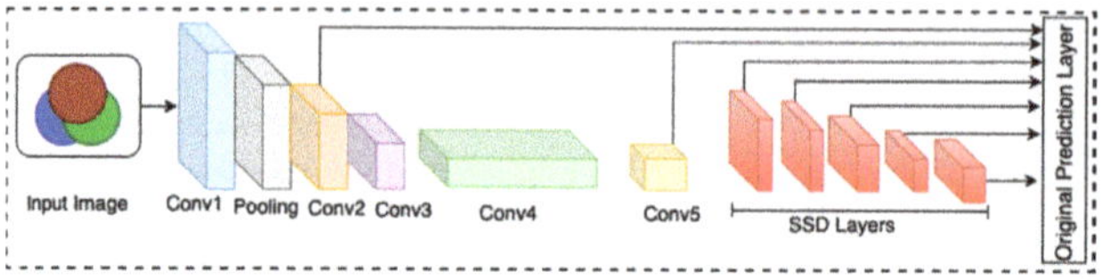

Figure 2. Flow diagram of SSD architecture.

3.2.2. DenseBox

DenseBox [32], developed by Huang et al., integrates object localization and classification within a single framework. Unlike other models that rely on sparse anchor boxes, DenseBox densely predicts bounding boxes across the entire image, improving localization accuracy. The model employs a deep CNN for feature extraction, followed by non-maximum suppression to refine object detections. DenseBox's dense prediction mechanism allows for enhanced performance in detecting small and closely packed objects Figure 3 shows the detailed architecture of DenseBox. The whole architecture consists of 16 convolutional layers, the initial 12 layers of which are used VGG19 for initialization.

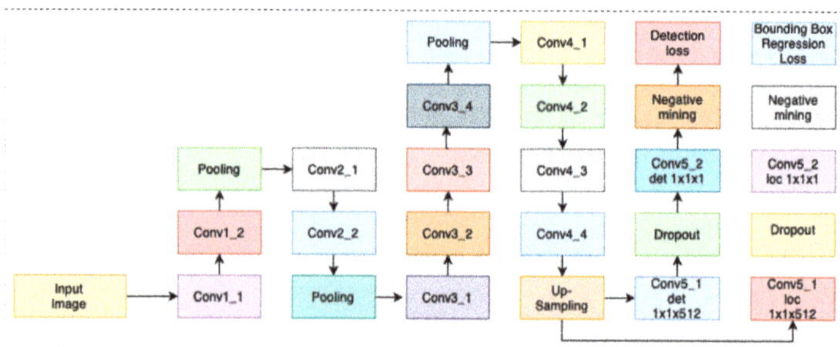

Figure 3. Detailed architecture of DenseBox.

3.2.3. RetinaNet

RetinaNet [33], introduced by Lin et al., addresses the issue of class imbalance commonly found in object detection tasks. The architecture incorporates a Feature Pyramid Network (FPN) for multi-scale feature extraction and employs a novel focal loss function to give higher priority to harder-to-detect objects during training. This loss function helps mitigate the imbalance between foreground and background classes, making RetinaNet particularly effective in scenarios with sparse object occurrences. The workflow of RetinaNet is shown in Figure 4. From the figure below, it can be seen that RetinaNet uses both top-down and bottom-up approaches to extract features at different scales and this technique helps in obtaining enriched feature space.

3.2.4. RFB Net

The RFB Net (RefineNet with Anchor Boxes) [34], developed by Niu and Zhang, builds upon the basic RefineNet architecture. RFB Net introduces anchor boxes of varying sizes and aspect ratios to improve detection performance, particularly for small objects. This model applies a series of refinement stages that iteratively enhance both localization accuracy and classification confidence. The architecture of RFB Net is shown in Figure 5. A significant difference between the RFB net and SSD is that RFB net uses VGG as a backbone; otherwise, it is architecturally close to SSD.

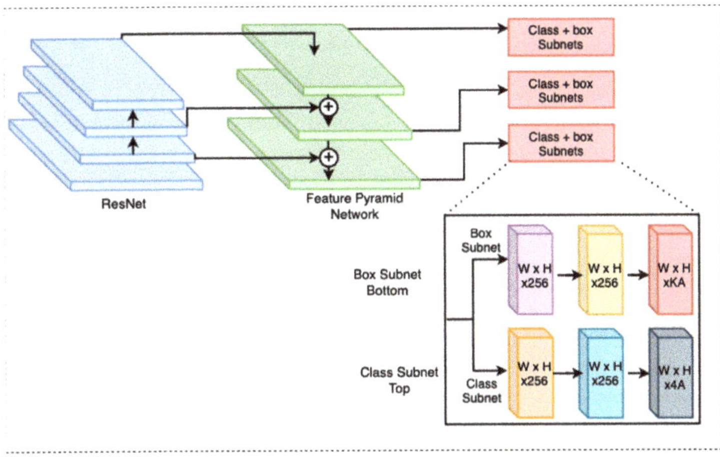

Figure 4. Detailed workflow of RetinaNet.

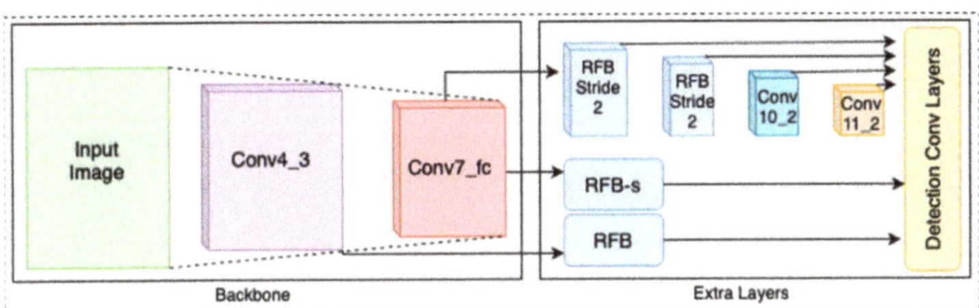

Figure 5. The workflow diagram of RFB Net.

3.2.5. Efficient Det

EfficientDet [35], proposed by Tan and Le, introduces a compound scaling approach to simultaneously increase network depth, width, and resolution while maintaining computational efficiency. EfficientDet uses a BiFPN (Bidirectional Feature Pyramid Network) for efficient multi-scale feature fusion, balancing model size and performance. This design achieves state-of-the-art object detection results with reduced computational complexity, making it ideal for resource-constrained applications. The architecture of EfficientDet is shown in Figure 6. EfficientDet uses EfficientNet as its backbone architecture and uses repeated layers of Bidirectional Feature Pyramid Network (BiFPN) in the neck part.

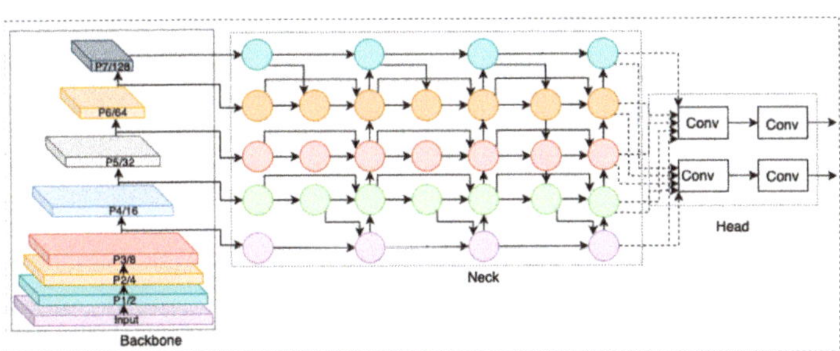

Figure 6. The architectural overview of EfficientDet.

3.2.6. YOLO

The YOLO framework, pioneered by Joseph Redmon, revolutionized real-time object detection by introducing a grid-based approach to predict bounding boxes and class probabilities simultaneously [36]. This innovative design facilitates a highly efficient detection process, making YOLO particularly suitable for applications needing real-time performance.

Since its inception, the YOLO architecture has undergone continuous evolution, with each version from YOLOv1 through to the latest YOLOv9 introducing enhancements in accuracy, speed, and efficiency [37]. Significant advancements include the introduction of anchor boxes, which improve the model's ability to detect objects of varying shapes and sizes, as well as new loss functions aimed at optimizing performance. Additionally, each YOLO iteration features optimized backbones that contribute to faster processing times and better detection capabilities.

The evolution of the YOLO framework from 2015 to 2023 showcases the iterative enhancements made in response to emerging challenges in object detection [38]. Each revision has made strides in minimizing latency while maximizing detection accuracy central goals in the continuing development of real-time object detection technologies Figure 7. illustrates the timeline of YOLO's evolution from 2015 to 2023.

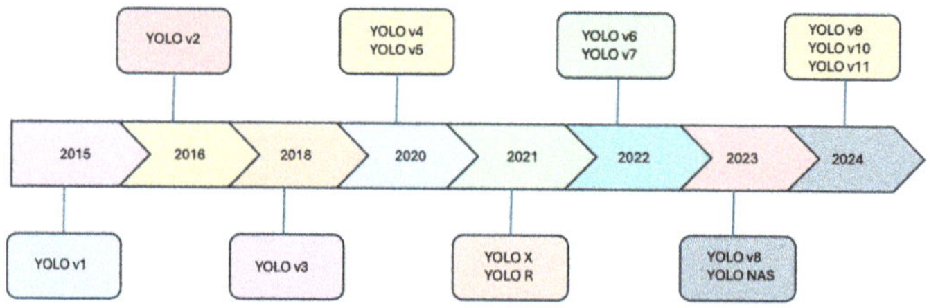

Figure 7. Timeline of YOLO models starting from 2015 to 2023.

To quickly and accurately identify objects, YOLO divides an image into a grid and predicts both bounding boxes and class probabilities simultaneously. Bounding box coordinates and class probabilities are generated by convolutional layers, following feature extraction by a deep Convolutional Neural Network (CNN). YOLO improves the detection of objects at varying sizes using anchor boxes at multiple scales. The final detections are refined using Non-Maximum Suppression (NMS), which filters out redundant and low-confidence predictions, making YOLO a highly efficient and reliable method for object detection.

Each YOLO variant introduces distinct innovations aimed at optimizing both speed and accuracy. For example, YOLOv4 and YOLOv5 integrated advanced backbones and loss functions such as Complete Intersection over Union (CIoU) to improve object localization.

The basic loss function for the YOLO model introduced by Redmon et al. [39] is presented in equation below:

$$
\begin{aligned}
&\lambda_{coord} \sum_{i=0}^{S^2} \sum_{j=0}^{B} 1_{ij}^{obj} \left[(x_i - \hat{x}_i)^2 + (y_i - \hat{y}_i)^2 \right] \\
&+\lambda_{coord} \sum_{i=0}^{S^2} \sum_{j=0}^{B} 1_{ij}^{obj} \left[(\sqrt{w_i} - \sqrt{\hat{w}_i})^2 + \left(\sqrt{h_i} - \sqrt{\hat{h}_i} \right)^2 \right] \\
&+\sum_{i=0}^{S^2} \sum_{j=0}^{B} 1_{ij}^{obj} (C_i - \hat{C}_i)^2 \\
&+\lambda_{noobj} \sum_{i=0}^{S^2} \sum_{j=0}^{B} 1_{ij}^{noobj} (C_i - \hat{C}_i)^2 \\
&+\sum_{i=0}^{S^2} 1_i^{obj} \sum_{c \in classes} (p_i(c) - \hat{p}_i(c))^2
\end{aligned}
$$

where 1_i^{obj} is used to check if there is an object in cell i while 1_{ij}^{obj} is used to tell that the *jth* bounding box in cell i is responsible for making that prediction. In this basic YOLO loss function, we can see that only the classification error and bounding box coordinate error are penalized. Table 2 below provides an overview of the loss functions used across YOLO variants, highlighting their contributions to classification and bounding box regression.

Table 2. Overview of loss function in YOLO variants.

Model	Bounding Box Regression	Classification
YOLOv1	Mean Squared Error (MSE)	Binary Cross Entropy (BCE)
YOLOv2	Sum Squared Error	BCE
YOLOv3	GIoU/DIoU	Cross Entropy (CE)
YOLOv4	CIoU	BCE/Focal Loss
YOLOv5	CIoU	Focal Loss
YOLOv6	CIoU/DFL	VariFocal Loss
YOLOv7	CIoU	BCE
YOLOv8	CIoU/DFL	CE
YOLOv9	L1 Loss	BCE
YOLOv10	Coordinate loss and confidence loss	Cross Entropy (CE)
YOLOv11	IoU based loss	BCE/Focal Loss + CIoU

Note: Mean Squared Error (MSE), Generalized Intersection over Union (GIoU), Distance based Intersection over Union (DIoU), Binary Cross Entropy (BCE), Cross Entropy (CE), Complete Intersection over Union (CIoU), Distributed Focal Loss (DFL).

3.3. The YOLO Architecture: Backbone, Neck, and Head

The three primary components of the YOLO architecture backbone, neck, and head undergo significant modifications across its variants to enhance performance:

- *Backbone*: Responsible for extracting features from input data [40], the backbone is typically a CNN pre-trained on large datasets such as ImageNet. Common backbones in YOLO variants include ResNet50, ResNet101, and CSPDarkNet53.
- *Neck*: The neck further processes and refines the feature maps generated by the backbone. It often employs techniques like Feature Pyramid Networks (FPN) and Spatial Attention Modules (SAM) [41] to improve feature representation.
- *Head*: The head processes fused features from the neck to predict bounding boxes and class probabilities. YOLO's head typically uses multi-scale anchor boxes, ensuring effective detection of objects at different scales [42].

Table 3 provides a comparison of the strengths and weaknesses of various YOLO variants, showcasing the tradeoffs between speed, accuracy, and complexity.

Table 3. Strengths and weakness comparisons of YOLO variants.

Model	Strengths	Weaknesses
YOLOv1	Fast performance, real-time detection	Lower accuracy compared to two-stage detectors
YOLOv2	Better performance with anchor boxes	Still suffers from accuracy issues
YOLOv3	Improved accuracy with Darknet-53 backbone	Increased complexity, slower than earlier versions
YOLOv4	Adaptable with various heads and backbones	Less user-friendly
YOLOv5	Faster training and more accurate than YOLOv3	Less adaptable than YOLOv4
YOLOv6	Fewer computations and parameters	Less research and resource availability
YOLOv7	Accuracy and speed improvements over YOLOv6	Higher complexity, risk of overfitting
YOLOv8	Lighter and faster compared to YOLOv7	Case-specific optimizations
YOLO-NAS	Good balance of accuracy and speed	Less widely adopted
YOLOv9	Reduced model size, ideal for real-time applications	Focuses too much on specific objects, ignoring the rest

4. Investigation, Evaluation with Benchmark

YOLO's real-time detection capabilities and versatility have revolutionized object detection across numerous domains. In cultural heritage, YOLO is employed to detect and classify artifacts in archaeological studies, aiding in the preservation of cultural history and restoration of structural defects in heritage sites [43,44]. In environmental monitoring, YOLO assists in tracking endangered species and identifying deforestation patterns through satellite imagery [45]. In healthcare, YOLO excels in automating critical tasks, such as detecting tumors in medical imaging and monitoring surgical tools during procedures [46]. In autonomous agriculture, YOLO plays a pivotal role in precision farming by identifying pests, diseases, and nutrient deficiencies, thereby enhancing crop yields and optimizing resource efficiency [47]. In industrial automation, YOLO improves defect detection on production lines, ensuring quality control in manufacturing processes [48]. Additionally, YOLO is a powerful tool in surveillance and security, powering facial recognition systems to enable real-time tracking of individuals in sensitive environments such as airports and banks [49]. The application of YOLO is widespread, making it challenging to enumerate all its use cases. Therefore, we have selected a few representative applications with publicly available datasets to conduct an in-depth investigation into the performance of YOLO models. This analysis thoroughly examines the architectures implemented by various researchers and evaluates their corresponding results. YOLO models are particularly popular in real-time applications due to their single-shot detection framework, which enables both speed and efficiency. In our comprehensive comparison study, we examined how YOLO models perform in key domains such as medical imaging, autonomous vehicles, and agriculture. Additionally, we provided an overview of the suitability of these models based on evaluation metrics such as accuracy, speed, and resource efficiency, highlighting their effectiveness across a diverse range of fields.

4.1. Medicine

The YOLO framework has revolutionized medical image analysis with its ability to efficiently and accurately detect, classify, and segment medical images across a range of applications [50]. The core principles behind YOLO's success in medical image analysis can be divided into three main categories: object detection and classification, segmentation and localization, and compression and enhancement. Each of these frameworks offers unique capabilities to address specific challenges in medical imaging.

4.1.1. Object Detection and Classification Frameworks

YOLO's object detection and classification frameworks focus on the accurate identification and categorization of objects within medical images. These applications streamline the detection of key features, abnormalities, and pathologies, reducing the time required for manual analysis and minimizing the risk of human error. By automating object classification, YOLO enables quicker and more precise medical diagnoses.

Breast Cancer Detection in Mammograms: YOLOv3 has been successfully implemented to detect breast abnormalities in mammograms, using fusion models to enhance the accuracy of classification. This model provides reliable detection of early-stage breast cancer, significantly aiding radiologists in making timely and accurate diagnoses [51].

Face Mask Detection in Medical Settings: YOLOv2 has been adapted to detect face masks in hospital and clinical environments, achieving an mAP of 81% [52]. This application was particularly important during the COVID-19 pandemic, ensuring that healthcare facilities maintained proper protective measures [53].

Gallstone Detection and Classification: YOLOv3 has demonstrated high accuracy (92.7%) in detecting and classifying gallstones in CT scans, making it a valuable tool in radiology for diagnosing gallbladder diseases quickly and accurately [54].

Red Lesion Detection in Retinal Images: YOLOv3 has been used to detect red lesions in RGB fundus images, achieving an average precision of 83.3% [55]. This early detection is critical for preventing vision loss in patients suffering from diabetic retinopathy or other retinal diseases [56,57].

4.1.2. Segmentation and Localization Frameworks

Segmentation and localization frameworks extend YOLO's capabilities beyond object detection to identifying specific regions of interest, such as tumors, and delineating their boundaries. This is particularly useful for medical image analysis, where precise localization of pathologies is critical for treatment planning [58].

Ovarian Cancer Segmentation for Real-Time Use: YOLOv5 has been applied for the segmentation of ovarian cancer, providing accurate identification of tumor boundaries [59]. The model's real-time capabilities allow it to be used during surgical procedures, giving doctors valuable information to guide their interventions [60].

Multi-Modality Medical Image Segmentation: YOLOv8, when combined with the Segment Anything Model (SAM), has shown strong results across multiple modalities, including X-ray, ultrasound, and CT scan images [61]. This integration enables more precise segmentation and classification, enhancing the diagnostic capabilities of radiologists and surgeons.

Brain Tumor Localization Using Data Augmentation: YOLOv3, paired with data augmentation techniques like 180° and 90° rotations, has proven effective in brain tumor detection and segmentation. The use of data augmentation strengthens the model's ability to identify tumors in complex orientations, leading to better treatment planning [62,63].

4.1.3. Compression, Enhancement, and Reconstruction Frameworks

YOLO's application in medical image compression and enhancement helps address challenges in transmitting, storing, and reconstructing high-quality medical data. In telemedicine and secure medical data sharing, preserving image fidelity is critical for ensuring accurate diagnoses. YOLO's capabilities in this area provide efficient solutions for compressing medical images without compromising their quality.

Medical Image Compression and Encryption: YOLOv7 has been utilized to compress medical images while maintaining high-quality reconstructions during transmission [64]. In one notable application, liver tumor 3D scans were encrypted and reconstructed with a PSNR of 30.42 and SSIM of 0.94, ensuring that sensitive medical information remains secure and accurate during remote consultations or telemedicine applications [65].

Secure Medical Data Transmission and Image Reconstruction: YOLOv7 has also been applied to enhance the transmission and reconstruction of encrypted medical data, which is especially useful for maintaining data integrity in telemedicine. The chaos and encoding methods used in YOLOv7 ensure that high-quality images are transmitted securely across networks.

Table 4 summarizes various studies in medical research, showcasing the capabilities of different YOLO architectures.

Table 4. Applications of YOLO in medical image analysis.

YOLO Version	Performance Metrics	Observations/Results	Image Domain
YOLO v7 [66]	mAP	Proposed a unique 2D to 3D bounding box adaptation method using NMS for 3D image analysis. Achieved mAP of 82.10%.	Ultrasound Videos
YOLO v3 [67]	F1-Score, Accuracy, Precision, AUC, Recall	Fusion model accurately identified and categorized breast abnormalities in mammograms.	Breast Cancer
YOLO v2 [68]	mAP	Achieved 81% mAP for medical face mask detection.	Face Mask
YOLO v3 [69]	Recall, Precision, Accuracy	Detected and classified gallstones with an average accuracy of 92.7%.	Radiology

Table 4. *Cont.*

YOLO Version	Performance Metrics	Observations/Results	Image Domain
YOLO v8 [70]	Precision, recall, mAP50	Performed comparative analysis of various YOLOv8 variants to perfrom detection and classification using ultrasound images	Ovarian Cancer
YOLO v3 [71]	mAP	Best performance in medical imaging with data augmentation techniques, 180° and 90° rotations.	Brain Tumor
YOLO v3 [72]	Accuracy, Specificity, Sensitivity	Introduced a label-free method for cellular analysis using 2D light scattering and neural networks.	Oncology
YOLO v8 [73]	Dice Score, Precision, Recall, F1-Score	YOLO v8 combined with SAM achieved high scores on X-ray, ultrasound, and CT scan data.	X-Ray, Ultrasound, CT-Scan
YOLOv3 [55]	Average Precision	In the proposed work, they used YOLOv3 to detect red lesion in images and predicts bounding boxes and does classification using logistic regression. They achieved an average precision of 83.3%.	RGB Fundus Images
YOLOv7 [74]	Peak-signal-to-noise-ratio (PSNR), structural similarity index (SSIM)	They did image compression using YOLOv7 while preserving information in the images. They used chaos and encoding to encrypt the input images and performed reconstruction at the receiver. They achieved PSNR of 30.42 and SSIM of 0.94	Liver Tumor 3D scans

4.2. Autonomous Vehicles

The application of YOLO models in the field of autonomous vehicles has proven transformative, particularly for enhancing real-time object detection capabilities [75]. As self-driving technology advances and autonomous vehicles become more prevalent, there is an increasing demand for robust computer vision systems capable of accurately detecting and classifying objects in diverse and often challenging environmental conditions [76]. This capability is essential to ensure the safety and reliability of autonomous driving systems.

4.2.1. Challenges in Real-Time Object Detection for Autonomous Vehicles

One of the primary challenges faced by autonomous vehicles is maintaining accurate object detection under various weather conditions, such as fog, snow, and rain. These adverse conditions can distort images and interfere with navigation, making it difficult for the vehicle to accurately discern critical environmental factors like road signs, pedestrians, and other vehicles. The ultimate objective of integrating YOLO models into autonomous vehicle systems is to develop a reliable detection framework that ensures safe and efficient operation, regardless of external conditions.

YOLO's single-shot detection framework, known for its rapid inference time, makes it particularly well-suited for real-time applications. This is critical for autonomous vehicles, which must make quick decisions in dynamic environments. Moreover, advancements in YOLO's architecture, such as improvements in attention mechanisms, backbone networks, and feature fusion techniques, have further increased its accuracy and speed, allowing it to detect objects of varying sizes even smaller objects like pedestrians and distant vehicles [77].

4.2.2. YOLO's Advancements for Harsh Weather Conditions

Real-time object detection in harsh weather is one of the most critical areas of research in autonomous vehicle systems. Weather conditions like snow, fog, and heavy rain can obscure visibility, making object detection challenging [78]. YOLO's rapid processing capabilities have been enhanced with architectural improvements to handle these conditions effectively. For instance, a study using YOLOv8 applied transfer learning to datasets captured under adverse weather conditions, including fog and snow. The model achieved promising results, with mAP scores of 0.672 and 0.704, demonstrating YOLO's adaptability to real-world challenges and making it a strong candidate for deployment in autonomous driving systems.

4.2.3. Small Object Detection in Autonomous Driving

Detecting small objects at various distances is another significant challenge for autonomous vehicle systems [79]. Small objects, such as pedestrians, cyclists, or road debris, can often be difficult to detect, but they are critical for safe driving. Enhanced versions of YOLO models, particularly YOLOv5, have introduced techniques like structural re-parameterization and the addition of small object detection layers to improve performance. These improvements have been shown to significantly increase the mAP for detecting smaller objects, especially in urban environments where small, fast-moving objects are common.

For example, WOG-YOLO, a variant of YOLOv5, exhibited significant improvements in detecting pedestrians and bikers, increasing the mAP for each by 2.6% and 2.3%, respectively. This focus on small object detection makes YOLO models particularly suitable for urban driving scenarios, where vehicles must detect various obstacles quickly and accurately to ensure safe navigation.

4.2.4. Efficiency and Speed Optimizations for Autonomous Vehicles

In addition to improved accuracy, YOLO models have been optimized for speed and efficiency, making them ideal for edge computing applications in autonomous vehicles, where computational resources are often limited. Lightweight versions of YOLO, such as YOLOv7 and YOLOv5, have incorporated various architectural optimizations such as lightweight backbones, neural architecture search (NAS), and attention mechanisms to improve inference time without sacrificing accuracy.

For instance, YOLOv7 has been enhanced with a hybrid attention mechanism (ACmix) and the Res3Unit backbone, significantly improving its performance, achieving an AP score of 90.8% on road traffic data [80]. These optimizations ensure that YOLO models can deliver real-time performance in dynamic environments, a key requirement for autonomous vehicles operating in various conditions.

4.2.5. YOLO's Performance Across Different Lighting Conditions

Another critical challenge in autonomous vehicle systems is detecting objects under varying lighting conditions, such as nighttime driving. YOLO models, particularly YOLOv8x, have demonstrated strong performance in low-light environments, utilizing advanced feature extraction and segmentation techniques to improve object detection accuracy.

In one study, YOLOv8x outperformed other YOLOv8 variants, achieving precision, recall, and F-score metrics of 0.90, 0.83, and 0.87, respectively, on video data captured during both day and night. This capability ensures that autonomous vehicles can operate safely across different lighting conditions, a vital feature for real-world deployment [81].

Table 5 provides a summary of key studies that highlight YOLO's effectiveness in autonomous vehicle applications. Various YOLO versions, including YOLOv5, YOLOv7, and YOLOv8, have been employed to enhance object detection performance across different datasets and conditions, showcasing YOLO's flexibility and adaptability to the unique challenges of autonomous driving.

Table 5. Application of YOLO in the field of autonomous vehicles.

YOLO Version	Performance Metrics	Observations	Image Domain
YOLOv7 [80]	AP	Proposed modifications including ACmix for hybrid attention, RFLA for feature fusion, and Res3Unit backbone, achieving 89.2% AP.	Road traffic data
YOLOv5 [82]	mAP	Added structural re-parameterization and small object detection layers, achieving 96.1% mAP.	KITTI Dataset (8 classes)

Table 5. *Cont.*

YOLO Version	Performance Metrics	Observations	Image Domain
YOLOv2, YOLOv3 [83]	mAP, Precision, Recall	Complex YOLO outperformed Tiny-YOLO with a mean Average Precision of 0.217.	KITTI Dataset
YOLOv5 [84]	mAP	WOG-YOLO showed improvements in detecting small objects, increasing mAP by 2.6% for pedestrians and 2.3% for bikers.	Self-built dataset
YOLOv5, YOLOv7 [85]	mAP	Evaluated on different activation functions. YOLOv7 with SiLU achieved an mAP of 94%, while YOLOv5 with LeakyReLU reached 88%.	Sandy weather data
YOLOv3 [86]	Accuracy, Recall	The RES-YOLO network improved vehicle detection accuracy and reduced background noise.	Vehicle dataset
YOLOv8 [87]	mAP	Transfer learning applied to hard weather datasets improved object detection, achieving mAP scores of 0.672 and 0.704.	Fog, snow, and hard weather datasets
YOLOv8 [88]	Precision, Recall, F-score	YOLOv8x outperformed other variants, with precision, recall, and F-score of 0.90, 0.83, and 0.87, respectively.	Video road data for day and night
YOLOv8 [89]	Accuracy	A five-stage model using YOLOv8 for detection and Deep Belief Network for classification achieved 95.6% accuracy.	Aerial imagery dataset
YOLOv8, YOLOv7, YOLOv5, YOLOv4 [90]	mAP	YOLOv7 performed the best with mAP50 scores when deployed on edge devices for real-time inference.	Road dataset
YOLOX [91]	mAP	Combined ShuffDet backbone and attention mechanism to achieve 92.20% mAP while reducing parameters by 34%.	KITTI dataset for road traffic
YOLOv4 [92]	mAP, F1-score, Recall	YOLOv4 was trained on a custom dataset for object detection, achieving an mAP of 74.6%, F1-score of 0.70, and recall of 0.81.	Custom vehicle dataset

4.3. Agriculture

YOLO has transformed agricultural practices by enabling fast, accurate detection of crops, pests, and environmental factors affecting crop health. One of its most significant applications is crop monitoring, where YOLO's real-time object detection helps identify issues such as pests, diseases, and nutrient deficiencies early, enabling timely interventions that improve yields. In precision farming, YOLO helps distinguish crops from weeds, allowing selective herbicide application. This reduces chemical usage, lowers costs, and minimizes environmental impact, supporting sustainable agriculture. YOLO's integration with UAVs further enhances its utility, providing large-scale monitoring and detailed insights that would be difficult and time-consuming to gather manually. Beyond crop monitoring, YOLO is applied to tasks such as fire detection, livestock management, and environmental monitoring. By automating these processes, YOLO contributes to efficient farm management and improved resource use.

Table 6 summarizes notable applications of YOLO in agriculture.

Table 6. Application of YOLO in agriculture.

YOLO Version	Performance Metrics	Observations	Image Domain
YOLOv5 [93]	Precision, Recall	UAV-based detection system for forest degradation, effective even in snowy conditions.	UAV imagery of trees
YOLOv5 [94]	Precision, F1-Score, mAP, Recall	DeepForest with YOLO, mAP of 82%, outperformed other models.	Apple trees in UAV RGB images
YOLOv5s, YOLOv5x [95]	IoU, Recall, Precision, mAP	Lightweight YOLOv5s ideal for embedded systems.	RGB forest images

Table 6. *Cont.*

YOLO Version	Performance Metrics	Observations	Image Domain
YOLOv3 [96]	F1-Score	Modified YOLOv3, F1-score of 0.817, used for apple detection.	Apple images from orchards
YOLOv5 [97]	F1-Score, mAP	YOLOv5 ensemble technique for real-time forest fire detection, F1-score of 93%.	FLAME dataset from UAVs
YOLOv3 [98]	IoU	YOLOv3 achieved 91.80% average precision for bird detection.	UAV aerial images
YOLOv4 [99]	mAP	YOLOv4 for cherry ripeness detection, increased mAP by 0.5%.	Cherry ripeness detection
YOLOv8s [100]	mAP	Lightweight YOLOv8s model with mAP of 93.4%, suitable for small devices.	Tomato image data
Ag-YOLO [101]	F1-Score	Ag-YOLO for crop monitoring and spraying, F1-score of 0.9205.	UAV imagery of palm trees

4.3.1. Crop Health Monitoring and UAV Integration

One of the most critical applications of YOLO in agriculture is the continuous monitoring of crop health [102]. With the integration of YOLO models and UAV systems, farmers can now scan large-scale agricultural areas, detecting early signs of pest infestations, diseases, or nutrient deficiencies. This proactive approach helps prevent crop loss and optimize farm productivity.

A noteworthy study employed YOLOv5 integrated into UAVs for detecting forest degradation. The model performed impressively, identifying damaged trees even in challenging conditions such as snow [103]. This advancement has far-reaching implications, allowing farmers and environmental researchers to monitor vast landscapes, particularly in remote or difficult-to-access areas, with unprecedented accuracy and speed [104].

4.3.2. Precision Agriculture and Weed Management

YOLO plays a pivotal role in precision agriculture by facilitating accurate crop and weed differentiation. In precision farming, herbicides can be applied selectively to target weeds without affecting crops [105,106]. This method not only reduces the use of chemicals, lowering the cost of farming, but also minimizes environmental damage, leading to more sustainable agricultural practices.

A modified version of YOLOv3 was deployed to monitor apple orchards, achieving an F1-score of 0.817 [107]. The model utilized DenseNet for improved feature extraction and performed exceptionally well at detecting apples at various developmental stages. This level of precision is invaluable for farmers managing orchards, as it enables better decision-making regarding harvesting and pest control [108].

4.3.3. Real-Time Environmental Monitoring and Fire Detection

YOLO has also been applied to monitor environmental hazards, such as forest fires [109,110]. In a study using an ensemble of YOLOv5 and other detection models like DeepLab and LightYOLO, researchers developed a real-time fire detection system mounted on UAVs. The system outperformed conventional models, achieving an F1-score of 93% and mAP of 85.8%. This real-time capability is crucial in mitigating the spread of fires and protecting valuable forest and agricultural resources [111].

4.3.4. Application in Livestock Management and Other Areas

While YOLO's application in crop monitoring remains a primary focus, it has also been applied to livestock management [112]. UAVs equipped with YOLO models can monitor livestock across large grazing areas, providing real-time updates on animal health and location. This technology is instrumental in reducing the risk of disease outbreaks and improving overall farm management [113].

Furthermore, YOLO's flexibility extends to various agricultural operations. A notable example is Ag-YOLO, a lightweight version of YOLO developed for Intel Neural Compute Stick 2 (NCS2) hardware, which was designed for crop and spray monitoring. Ag-YOLO achieved an F1-score of 0.9205, proving to be an efficient, cost-effective solution for farmers operating in resource-constrained environments [101].

4.4. Industry

In industrial applications, YOLO (You Only Look Once) has become one of the most widely used real-time object detection models due to its high-speed processing and efficient object identification capabilities. The single-stage architecture of YOLO allows it to detect and classify objects in a single pass through the neural network, making it particularly suitable for environments that require rapid decision-making, such as production lines, automated quality control, and anomaly detection. Its adaptability to a wide range of tasks across different industries, from food processing to construction, has made YOLO a versatile tool.

In manufacturing and production, YOLO is used to improve the accuracy and efficiency of automated systems. Whether it's detecting defects in products or monitoring safety in real-time, YOLO contributes to higher-quality outcomes and reduced operational costs [114]. For instance, in food processing, YOLO can be employed to ensure quality control by detecting defects in packaged goods, while in construction, it can help identify safety issues, such as the use of protective gear like helmets [115].

YOLO's implementation in logistics and warehousing has also streamlined processes such as package tracking, inventory management, and equipment monitoring. Robotic systems using YOLO for object detection and identification can automate repetitive tasks, improve safety, and increase production throughput. Despite certain challenges, such as lower accuracy when detecting. Table 7 summarizes various industrial applications of YOLO, showcasing its versatility and effectiveness across different tasks.

Table 7. Applications of YOLO in industry.

YOLO Version	Performance Metrics	Observations	Image Domain
YOLOv5 [116]	mAP	Combined YOLO with transformers to detect small-scale objects and defects. Proposed a bidirectional feature pyramid network, achieving an mAP of 75.2%.	Grayscale imagery of surface defects
YOLOv5 [117]	mAP	PG-YOLO was developed as a lightweight version for edge devices in IoT networks. Improved inference speed without sacrificing accuracy, achieving an mAP of 93.3%.	RGB images of safety-helmet wearing (SHWD)
YOLOv3 [118]	mAP	For detecting weld defects in vehicle wheels, this model achieved an mAP of 98.25% and 84.36% on AP 75 and AP 50, respectively. Environment-specific model.	RGB images of vehicle wheel welding
YOLOv5 [119]	mAP, GFLOPS	ATT-YOLO, inspired by transformers, performed well on surface detection tasks in electronic manufacturing, achieving an mAP of 49.9% with 21.8 GFLOPS.	Laptop surface images
YOLOv3, YOLOv5 [120]	mAP	YOLO models used for process flow tracking in Industry 4.0. Models were applied to datasets with distortions and achieved final mAP scores of 80% (YOLOv3) and 70% (YOLOv5).	Colorful objects in industry setting
YOLO [121]	Precision, Accuracy, mAP	Introduced a deep learning-based system for real-time packaging defect detection. The system achieved 81.8% precision, 82.5% accuracy, and an mAP of 78.6%.	Images of damaged and intact boxes

Table 7. *Cont.*

YOLO Version	Performance Metrics	Observations	Image Domain
YOLOv5s [122]	Precision, Recall, mAP	An upgraded YOLOv5s model used for real-time identification and localization of production line equipment, including robotic arms and AGV carts. Achieved precision of 93.6%, recall of 85.6%, and mAP of 91.8%.	Real-time data from simulated production line
YOLOv5 [123]	mAP	Enhanced YOLOv5 for detecting workpieces on production lines. Improved mAP on COCO dataset by 2.4% and on custom data by 4.2% using ghost bottleneck lightweight deep convolution.	Images of bolts
YOLOD [124]	Average Precision	YOLOD, a unique model addressing uncertainty in object detection, used Gaussian priors in front of YOLOX detection heads. Improved bounding box regression and achieved an AP of 73.9%.	Power line insulator images

4.4.1. Applications of YOLO in Industrial Manufacturing

One of the most impactful uses of YOLO in industry is in manufacturing, where its real-time detection capabilities are leveraged for automated quality control, defect detection, and production optimization. YOLO's speed and accuracy allow manufacturers to identify issues on the production line quickly, reducing downtime and minimizing faulty outputs [125].

Surface Defect Detection: YOLOv5, combined with transformers, was used to detect small defects on surfaces in grayscale imagery, improving detection efficiency. The bidirectional feature pyramid network proposed in this study significantly enhanced the model's ability to identify minor defects, achieving an mAP of 75.2% [126].

Wheel Welding Defect Detection: YOLOv3 was applied to the specific task of detecting weld defects in vehicle wheels, achieving impressive results with mAP scores of 98.25% and 84.36% at different thresholds. While this model was highly effective in its target environment, it was noted that it may not generalize well to other real-time detection tasks without further adaptation [127].

Workpiece Detection and Localization: Another notable application is workpiece detection on production lines, where YOLOv5 was enhanced with lightweight deep convolution layers to improve detection accuracy. The model showed significant improvements, increasing mAP by 2.4% on the COCO dataset and 4.2% on custom industrial datasets [128].

4.4.2. Applications in Automated Quality Control and Safety

YOLO's role in quality control systems is crucial for maintaining the consistency and safety of products in industries like packaging, construction, and electronics. By automatically identifying defects or inconsistencies in real-time, YOLO allows manufacturers to catch problems early in the production process.

Real-Time Packaging Defect Detection: In one study, YOLO was used to develop a deep learning-based system for detecting packaging defects in real-time. The model automatically classified product quality by detecting defects in boxed goods, achieving a precision of 81.8%, accuracy of 82.5%, and mAP of 78.6%. Such systems can be deployed to monitor quality across high-speed production lines, reducing the risk of shipping faulty products to customers [129].

Safety-Helmet Detection in Construction: Safety in construction is another critical area where YOLO has proven its worth. A lightweight version of YOLOv5, known as PG-YOLO, was specifically developed for edge devices in IoT networks, improving inference speed while maintaining accuracy. The model achieved an mAP of 93.3% for detecting workers wearing safety helmets in construction sites, helping ensure compliance with safety regulations [130].

4.4.3. Industrial Robotics and Automation

In logistics and warehouse management, YOLO's ability to detect and identify objects in real-time is a key asset for automating routine tasks, improving both safety and efficiency. YOLO is integrated into robotic systems that handle object detection for sorting, transporting, and monitoring inventory.

Production Line Equipment Monitoring: YOLOv5s was enhanced with a channel attention module, slim-neck, decoupled head, and GSConv lightweight convolution to improve real-time identification and localization of production line equipment, such as robotic arms and AGV carts. This system achieved precision rates of 93.6% and mAP scores of 91.8%, showcasing its effectiveness in automating production line processes [122].

Power Line Insulator Detection: In another study, YOLOD was developed to address uncertainty in object detection by placing Gaussian priors in front of the YOLOX detection heads. This model was applied to power line insulator detection, improving the robustness of object detection by using calculated uncertainty scores to refine bounding box predictions. YOLOD achieved an AP of 73.9% [131].

5. Evolution and Benchmark-Based Discussion

5.1. Evolution

The YOLO family has undergone considerable evolution, with each new iteration addressing specific limitations of its predecessors while introducing innovations that improve its performance in real-time object detection. YOLOv6, YOLOv7, and YOLOv8 represent key advancements in the early evolution of this framework, each contributing significantly to the landscape of object detection in terms of speed, accuracy, and computational efficiency.

YOLOv6: Enhanced Speed and Practicality. YOLOv6 was designed with a focus on speed and practicality, particularly for real-world applications requiring fast and efficient object detection. It introduced modifications in network structure that enabled faster processing while maintaining a decent level of accuracy. YOLOv6 was particularly impactful for lightweight deployment on edge devices, which have limited computing power, making it an attractive option for applications in fields such as surveillance, robotics, and automated inspection systems. However, while YOLOv6 improved efficiency, it faced challenges in complex scenarios involving small or overlapping objects, leading to the need for more advanced versions.

YOLOv7: Improving Accuracy and Feature Extraction. YOLOv7 introduced significant architectural changes that enhanced accuracy and feature extraction capabilities. One of the key advancements in YOLOv7 was the integration of cross-stage partial networks (CSPNet), which improved the model's ability to reuse gradients across different stages, allowing for better feature propagation and reducing the model's overall complexity. This improvement translated into better performance in detecting smaller objects or objects within cluttered environments. YOLOv7 also introduced the concept of extended path aggregation, which helped in merging features from different layers to provide a more detailed and robust representation of the input image. These advancements made YOLOv7 more suitable for applications in industries like medical imaging, autonomous driving, and aerial surveillance, where high accuracy in challenging environments is paramount. However, even with these improvements, YOLOv7 was not immune to the problem of vanishing gradients a common issue in deeper neural networks that leads to poor training outcomes due to the weakening of signal propagation as it moves through multiple layers. This was particularly problematic in cases where high-resolution image data required more sophisticated feature extraction.

YOLOv8: Streamlining for Resource Efficiency. YOLOv8 further refined the architecture, focusing on achieving better resource efficiency without sacrificing accuracy. One of the most notable advancements in YOLOv8 was its ability to scale efficiently across different hardware configurations, making it a flexible tool for both low-power devices and high-performance computing environments. YOLOv8 streamlined the training process and introduced optimizations that improved its ability to generalize across a wide range of object detection tasks. YOLOv8 also enhanced the handling of multi-object detection scenarios, where multiple objects of different sizes and shapes appear in a single frame. Despite these improvements, YOLOv8 faced challenges in deeper architectures, particularly with convergence issues. These issues arose from the model's struggle to balance the computational complexity required for deeper networks with the need for real-time inference. As a result, YOLOv8's performance on complex datasets, especially those involving small, overlapping, or occluded objects, was not always consistent.

Addressing Limitations: The Road to YOLO-NAS and YOLOv9. The limitations observed in YOLOv6 through YOLOv8 such as vanishing gradients and convergence problems were the catalysts for the development of more sophisticated models like YOLO-NAS and YOLOv9. These models aimed to not only enhance speed and accuracy but also tackle the deeper challenges inherent to neural network architectures, such as gradient management and efficient feature extraction.

5.1.1. YOLO-NAS: A Major Turning Point

Before the introduction of YOLOv9 [132], YOLO-NAS [133] developed by Deci AI marked a significant shift in the evolution of the YOLO framework. As object detection models became more widely deployed in real-world applications, there was a growing need for solutions that could balance accuracy with computational efficiency, especially on edge devices that have limited processing power. YOLO-NAS answered this call by incorporating Post-Training Quantization (PTQ), a technique designed to reduce the size and complexity of the model after training [134]. This allowed YOLO-NAS to maintain high levels of accuracy while reducing its computational footprint, making it ideal for resource-constrained environments like mobile devices, embedded systems, and IoT applications.

PTQ enabled YOLO-NAS to deliver minimal latency, which is a crucial factor for real-time object detection, where every millisecond counts. By optimizing the model post-training, PTQ made YOLO-NAS one of the most efficient object detection models for real-time applications, especially in industries where computational resources are scarce, such as autonomous vehicles, robotics, and smart cameras for security systems. The ability to reduce inference time without sacrificing performance positioned YOLO-NAS as a go-to model for developers looking to deploy sophisticated object detection systems on low-power devices.

YOLO-NAS introduced two significant architectural innovations that set it apart from previous models in the YOLO family:

1. Quantization and Sparsity Aware Split-Attention (QSP): The QSP block was designed to enhance the model's ability to handle quantization while still maintaining high accuracy. Quantization often leads to a degradation of model precision because the model is forced to operate with reduced numerical precision (e.g., moving from floating-point to integer operations). QSP mitigated this accuracy drop by using sparsity-aware mechanisms that allowed the model to be more selective in how it used and stored information across different layers. This helped preserve important features, even in a quantized environment.
2. Quantization and Channel-Wise Interactions (QCI): The QCI block further refined the process of quantization by focusing on channel-wise interactions. It enhanced the way features were extracted and processed in the network, ensuring that key information was not lost during the quantization process. By intelligently adjusting how information is passed between channels, QCI ensured that YOLO-NAS could maintain high precision in its predictions, even when the model was reduced to a lightweight architecture. This made it particularly useful for edge applications that require smaller model sizes but cannot afford to lose accuracy.

These innovations were inspired by frameworks like RepVGG and aimed to address the common challenges associated with post-training quantization, specifically the loss of accuracy that typically accompanies such optimization techniques [135]. The combination of QSP and QCI allowed YOLO-NAS to achieve a high level of precision while retaining a small model size, making it an efficient tool for real-time object detection on constrained hardware.

Despite the impressive advancements introduced in YOLO-NAS, the model did face challenges in handling high-complexity image detection tasks. In scenarios where objects were occluded or had intricate patterns, YOLO-NAS struggled to maintain the same level of accuracy as it did in simpler object detection tasks. For example, applications in agriculture, where leaves and crops often occlude one another, or in medical imaging, where subtle variations in texture and shape are critical, highlighted the limitations of YOLO-NAS. The model's performance often dipped when faced with these complex visual environments, underscoring the need for further architectural improvements.

While YOLO-NAS was an excellent solution for resource-efficient detection in straightforward real-time applications, it required additional improvements to handle the nuances of more complex datasets. These limitations laid the groundwork for the development of future models like YOLOv9, which aimed to address these issues through more advanced gradient handling, better feature extraction, and the use of more sophisticated network architectures.

5.1.2. YOLOv9: Groundbreaking Innovations

In response to the challenges encountered by earlier models, YOLOv9 introduced several groundbreaking techniques designed to improve gradient flow, handle error accumulation, and facilitate better convergence during training. These innovations allowed YOLOv9 to extend its applicability to a broader range of real-world object detection tasks.

The key innovations in YOLOv9 include:

1. Programmable Gradient Information (PGI): PGI was designed to tackle the issue of vanishing gradients by enhancing the flow of gradients throughout the model. YOLOv9's PGI ensured smoother backpropagation across multiple prediction branches, significantly improving convergence and overall detection accuracy. PGI is composed of three key components. (a) Main Branch: Responsible for inference tasks. (b) Auxiliary Branch: Manages gradient flow and updates the network parameters. (c) Multi-level Auxiliary Branch: Handles error accumulation and ensures that the gradients propagate effectively across all layers [132]. By addressing gradient backpropagation across complex prediction branches, PGI allowed YOLOv9 to achieve better performance, particularly in detecting multiple objects in challenging environments.
2. Generalized Efficient Layer Aggregation Network (GELAN): The GELAN module was another major innovation in YOLOv9. By drawing from CSPNet [136] and ELAN [137], GELAN provided flexibility in integrating different computational blocks, such as convolutional layers and attention mechanisms. This adaptability allowed YOLOv9 to be fine-tuned for specific detection tasks, from simple object recognition to complex multi-object detection, making it a versatile tool for a wide array of real-time detection applications.
3. Reversible Functions: To ensure information preservation throughout the network, YOLOv9 utilized reversible functions. The formula used for this is: $X = v\zeta\ (r\psi(X))$, $r\psi(X)$ represents the transformation of input data through a reversible function, and $v\zeta$ applies an inverse transformation to recover the original input. These reversible layers allowed YOLOv9 to reconstruct input data perfectly, minimizing information loss during forward and backward passes. The reversible functions allowed for more precise detection and localization of objects, especially in high-dimensional and complex datasets.

5.1.3. Evolution to YOLOv10 and YOLOv11

Following YOLOv9, YOLOv10 and YOLOv11 brought further refinements to the YOLO framework, making significant strides in both speed and accuracy.

YOLOv10 introduced groundbreaking innovations that enhanced performance and efficiency, building on the strengths of its predecessors while pushing the boundaries of real-time object detection. A key advancement in YOLOv10 was the introduction of the C3k2 block, an innovative feature that greatly improved feature aggregation while reducing computational overhead [138]. This allowed YOLOv10 to maintain high accuracy even in resource-constrained environments, making it ideal for deployment on edge devices. Additionally, the model's improved attention mechanisms enabled better detection of small and occluded objects, allowing YOLOv10 to outperform previous versions in tasks such as facemask detection and autonomous vehicle applications. Its ability to balance computational efficiency with detection precision set a new standard, with a final mAP50 of 0.944 in benchmark tests.

YOLOv11 further advanced the framework with the introduction of C2PSA (Cross-Stage Partial with Spatial Attention) blocks, which significantly enhanced spatial awareness by enabling the model to focus more effectively on critical regions within an image [139]. This innovation proved especially beneficial in complex scenarios, such as shellfish monitoring and healthcare applications, where precision and accuracy are crucial. YOLOv11 also featured a restructured backbone with smaller kernel sizes and optimized layers, which improved processing speed without sacrificing performance. The inclusion of Spatial Pyramid Pooling-Fast (SPPF) enabled even faster feature aggregation, solidifying YOLOv11 as the most efficient and accurate YOLO model to date. It achieved a final mAP50 of 0.958 across multiple benchmarks, making YOLOv11 a leading choice for real-time object detection tasks across industries ranging from healthcare to autonomous systems.

5.2. Benchmarks

With the introduction of YOLOv9, the benchmarks for performance have shifted. We conducted a comprehensive evaluation of YOLOv9, YOLO-NAS, YOLOv8, YOLOv10, and YOLOv11 using well-established datasets like Roboflow 100 [140], Object365 [141], and COCO [142]. These datasets offer diverse real-world challenges, allowing us to assess the models' strengths and weaknesses under different conditions.

5.2.1. Benchmark Findings

Our results consistently showed that YOLOv9 outperformed both YOLO-NAS and YOLOv8, particularly in complex image detection tasks where objects are occluded or exhibit detailed patterns. However, with the introduction of YOLOv10 and YOLOv11, the benchmark shifted even further. YOLOv10 introduced new feature aggregation techniques, and YOLOv11's spatial attention mechanisms greatly improved object detection, especially in challenging datasets.

For instance:

- Shellfish Monitoring: In tasks such as shellfish monitoring, which involve complex patterns and occlusions, YOLO-NAS and YOLOv8 struggled to maintain accuracy. While YOLOv9 demonstrated greater adaptability, handling the intricate challenges more effectively, YOLOv10 and YOLOv11 pushed the performance further with their superior spatial attention and feature extraction capabilities. YOLOv11 achieved a final mAP50 of 0.563, the highest among the tested models.
- Medical Image Analysis: On medical image datasets, particularly for tasks such as blood cell detection, YOLOv9 outperformed YOLO-NAS and YOLOv8. However, the architectural advancements in YOLOv10 and YOLOv11 resulted in even better performance, with YOLOv11 achieving an mAP50 of 0.958. This demonstrates its superior capability to detect small and detailed features within cluttered or noisy data, which is critical for applications in medical diagnostics.

These results are summarized in Table 8, highlighting the mAP50 (mean average precision at 50% intersection over union) scores across several datasets.

Table 8. Performance of YOLOv11, YOLOv10, YOLOv9, YOLO-NAS and YOLOv8 on multiple datasets.

Datasets	YOLOv9	YOLO-NAS	YOLOv8	YOLOv10	YOLOv11
Facemask Detection	0.941	0.9199	0.924	0.950	0.962
Shellfish Monitoring	0.534	0.469	0.466	0.542	0.563
Forest Smoke Detection	0.865	0.7811	0.911	0.925	0.945
Human Detection	0.812	0.7145	0.816	0.829	0.854
Pothole Detection	0.78	0.7265	0.745	0.793	0.815
Blood Cell Detection	0.933	0.9041	0.93	0.944	0.958

5.2.2. Performance Insights

Facemask Detection: All models performed well on this dataset, with YOLOv11 dominating, achieving an mAP50 of 0.962. The improved spatial attention mechanisms in YOLOv11 allowed it to detect subtle variations in facemask patterns, making it the best-performing model in this domain. YOLOv10 also showed improvements over YOLOv9, reaching an mAP50 of 0.950.

Shellfish Monitoring: This dataset presented complex challenges with occluded and overlapping objects. Both YOLO-NAS and YOLOv8 struggled, achieving relatively low mAP50 scores of 0.469 and 0.466, respectively. YOLOv9 demonstrated better adaptability with 0.534, while YOLOv10 and YOLOv11 further improved on these results, reaching 0.542 and 0.563, respectively, thanks to their advanced spatial attention mechanisms.

Forest Smoke Detection: YOLOv8 performed particularly well in detecting smoke patterns, achieving an mAP50 of 0.911, while YOLOv9 closely followed with 0.865. However, YOLOv10 and YOLOv11 both improved on this with scores of 0.925 and 0.945, respectively. The improvements in feature extraction and attention mechanisms in YOLOv11 gave it a slight edge over previous versions in detecting subtle smoke patterns.

Human Detection: For human detection, YOLOv9 outperformed YOLO-NAS but was only marginally better than YOLOv8. YOLOv10 reached 0.829, and YOLOv11 achieved the highest mAP50 at 0.854, benefiting from its optimized backbone and better handling of occlusions in complex scenes.

Pothole Detection: YOLOv9 demonstrated superior performance in detecting potholes on road surfaces, achieving an mAP50 of 0.780. However, YOLOv10 and YOLOv11 demonstrated further advancements, reaching 0.793 and 0.815, respectively, making them more reliable for this specific detection task.

Blood Cell Detection: In medical image analysis, YOLOv9 showed great precision with an mAP50 of 0.933. However, YOLOv10 and YOLOv11 set a new standard for this dataset, achieving 0.944 and 0.958, respectively. The enhanced gradient flow and feature extraction capabilities in these models contributed to their superior performance in detecting minute and complex patterns, crucial in medical diagnostics.

5.2.3. Training Considerations: Extended Epochs for Model Optimization

In our benchmark study, the YOLO models (YOLOv9, YOLO-NAS, YOLOv8, YOLOv10, and YOLOv11) were trained for 20 epochs, providing a baseline for performance evaluation. However, it is evident that this limited number of training cycles does not fully tap into the models' potential. Extended training, involving more epochs, would likely result in smoother learning curves and allow the models to achieve even higher levels of accuracy, especially in tasks that involve complex datasets and intricate object patterns.

Extended training is essential for performance improvement across several aspects of object detection models:

1. Refined Feature Extraction: Each epoch allows the model to update and refine its internal feature representations. Models like YOLO-NAS, which are optimized for resource efficiency, benefit from longer training cycles, as this gives the model more op-

portunities to fine-tune its performance on challenging examples like occluded objects or those with non-standard shapes. YOLOv10, with its enhanced feature aggregation blocks, could further refine its detection capabilities with extended epochs, improving accuracy in both resource-constrained environments and complex scenarios.

2. Improved Convergence: While 20 epochs are sufficient for initial insights into performance, convergence when a model reaches its lowest possible error rate often requires more iterations. YOLOv9, YOLOv10, and YOLOv11, featuring more intricate architectures, benefit from prolonged training to reach optimal convergence. Specifically, YOLOv9's use of Programmable Gradient Information (PGI) and Generalized Efficient Layer Aggregation Networks (GELAN) would see further improvements with more epochs, helping the model stabilize gradient flow and improve detection accuracy in environments with occluded or complex objects. YOLOv11, with its C2PSA blocks, would also benefit from more iterations, as this would allow better spatial awareness and feature extraction for difficult detection tasks.
3. Avoiding Overfitting: One concern with prolonged training is overfitting, where the model becomes too tuned to the training data, losing its generalization ability. However, this risk can be mitigated by using early stopping techniques or cross-validation. For models like YOLO-NAS and YOLOv8, incorporating regularization methods such as dropout layers or weight decay would allow them to benefit from extended training epochs without falling prey to overfitting. YOLOv11, with its spatial attention mechanisms, could particularly benefit from extended training, as more iterations would enhance its ability to focus on the most critical regions of the image.
4. Fine-Tuning for Specialized Tasks: In applications like medical imaging, autonomous driving, or industrial automation, where precision is critical, additional training epochs combined with fine-tuning can make a noticeable difference in model performance. YOLOv10, with its enhanced feature aggregation techniques, could greatly benefit from fine-tuning to optimize its performance in specific tasks such as pothole detection or shellfish monitoring. YOLOv11, with its cutting-edge spatial attention blocks, would further improve in complex, specialized tasks like forest smoke detection or health monitoring, where accurate object localization is paramount.
5. Learning Rate Scheduling: As the number of epochs increases, adjusting the learning rate becomes essential. Models like YOLOv9, YOLOv10, and YOLOv11 would benefit from learning rate schedulers that gradually decrease the learning rate during training, ensuring stable convergence and preventing the model from overshooting its optimal parameter values. Adaptive optimization techniques, such as AdamW or RMSProp, could further enhance training performance in extended epochs, particularly in models with complex architectures like YOLOv10 and YOLOv11.

The Specific Impacts on YOLO-NAS, YOLOv9, YOLOv10, and YOLOv11 are as follows:

- YOLO-NAS: Given that YOLO-NAS uses Post-Training Quantization (PTQ), additional epochs would help solidify its quantization strategy, improving performance on both low-resource and high-complexity tasks. The Quantization and Sparsity Aware Split-Attention (QSP) and Quantization and Channel-Wise Interactions (QCI) blocks would benefit from extended training, leading to better feature selection and processing even with quantization. Longer training would also help the model adapt to complex detection tasks that require precision, like health monitoring or industrial automation.
- YOLOv9: YOLOv9's architectural advancements, such as PGI and GELAN, would see improved performance with more training epochs, especially in scenarios involving multiple prediction branches. Extended training would stabilize its gradient flow and error management, improving performance in complex environments like forest smoke detection or medical imaging. Additionally, YOLOv9's reversible functions could further benefit from extended epochs, ensuring that input reconstruction becomes more robust, ultimately enhancing detection precision in real-time applications.

- YOLOv10: As a major advancement over previous versions, YOLOv10 introduced the C3k2 block for more efficient feature aggregation. Extended training would refine its ability to balance computational efficiency and detection precision, particularly for resource-constrained tasks on edge devices. Additional epochs would enable YOLOv10 to improve its performance on specialized tasks like pothole detection and autonomous vehicle applications, achieving better convergence and stability.
- YOLOv11: The most recent and advanced YOLO model, YOLOv11, introduced the Cross-Stage Partial with Spatial Attention (C2PSA) blocks, greatly enhancing spatial awareness. Prolonged training would allow the model to fine-tune these blocks for better detection of small or occluded objects, especially in complex tasks such as shellfish monitoring or industrial safety detection. The use of Spatial Pyramid Pooling-Fast (SPPF) for feature aggregation would also improve with more epochs, enabling YOLOv11 to excel in real-time detection tasks with a final mAP50 score that sets it apart from earlier models.

As we look toward further optimizing the YOLO family models, a comprehensive training regimen that includes extended epochs, dynamic learning rates, and fine-tuning techniques will be crucial in extracting the best performance from these models. Expanding the datasets to include even more diverse real-world scenarios will allow the models to generalize better across different applications, ensuring they maintain top-tier performance in both simple and complex detection tasks.

While our 20-epoch benchmark provided valuable performance insights, longer training cycles combined with the right optimization techniques would likely unlock even greater accuracy and generalization potential for YOLOv9, YOLO-NAS, YOLOv8, YOLOv10, and YOLOv11, particularly in challenging real-time object detection tasks.

5.2.4. Performance Analysis of YOLO Variants on Benchmark Datasets

The mAP50 charts in Figure 8 illustrate how YOLOv11, YOLOv10, YOLOv9, YOLO-NAS, and YOLOv8 perform across a range of benchmark datasets. These plots provide an in-depth comparison of the models over 20 training epochs, offering key insights into how each model handles different detection tasks. The inclusion of YOLOv10 and YOLOv11 further emphasizes the advancements made in real-time object detection, particularly in complex datasets that challenge earlier models. In this study, mAP50 is employed as the primary metric for evaluating and comparing the performance across different YOLO versions. The choice of mAP50 simplifies the benchmarking process by focusing on straightforward detection tasks, providing a consistent and accessible measure of model effectiveness. By setting a fixed IoU threshold of 50%, mAP50 highlights the models' capabilities in identifying objects with acceptable localization accuracy, making it particularly suitable for general-purpose evaluations and less complex detection scenarios. This approach ensures a balanced comparison, especially when dealing with diverse datasets and varying levels of object detection difficulty.

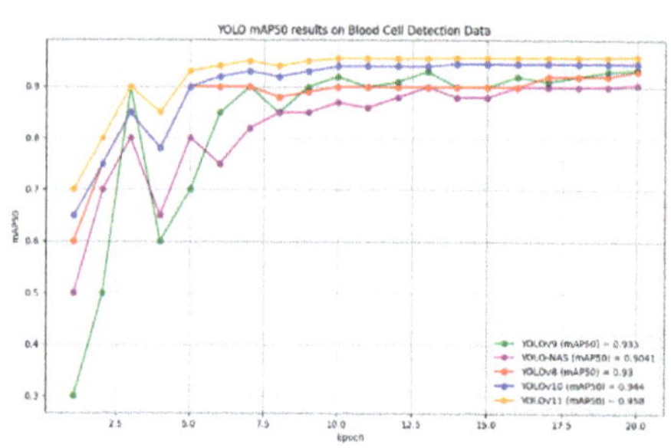

(1)

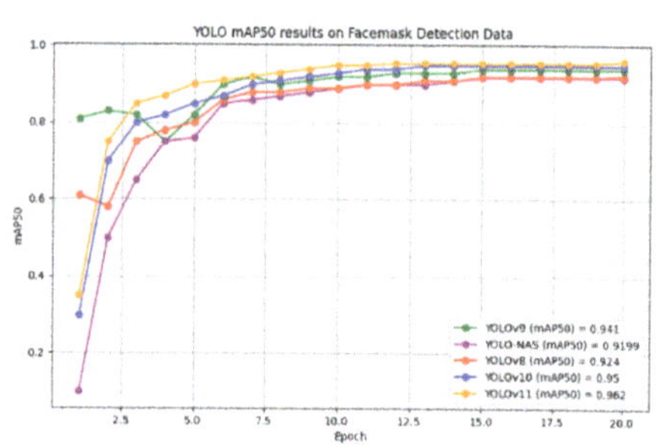

(2)

Figure 8. *Cont.*

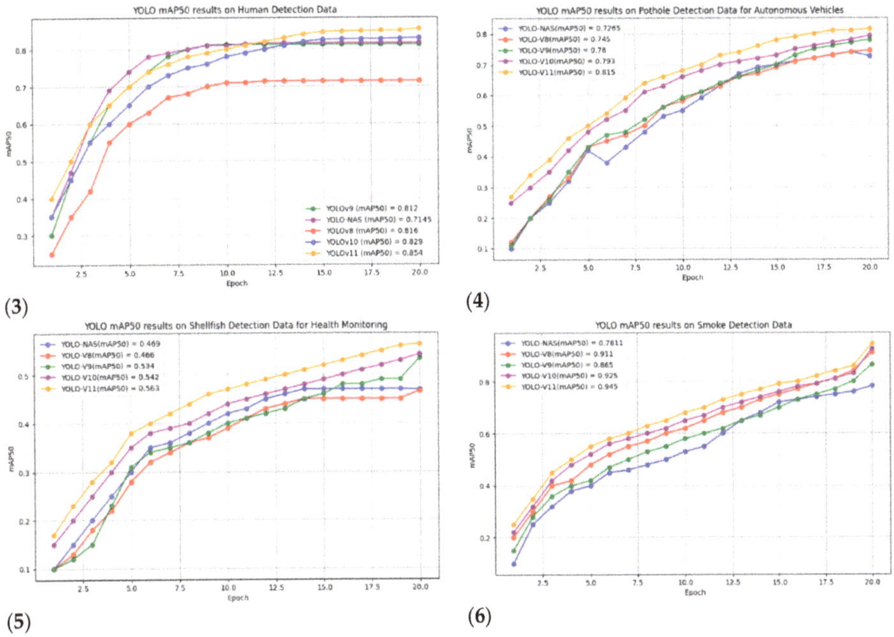

Figure 8. mAP50 plots of YOLO11, YOLO10, YOLOv9. YOLO-NAS and YOLOv8 on benchmark datasets. (**1**) shows the performance of various YOLO models on Blood Cell detection task. (**2**) illustrates the perfoamnce of YOLO models on Face mask detection task. (**3**) Represents the results on human detection problem. (**4**) shows the results on pothole detection task for autonomous vehicles. (**5**) shows the results for shellfish health monitoring task and (**6**) shows results for smoke detection task.

- YOLOv11 and YOLOv10 take the lead: Across almost all benchmarks, YOLOv11 consistently outperforms its predecessors, demonstrating the effectiveness of its C2PSA (Cross-Stage Partial with Spatial Attention) blocks, which allow the model to focus more accurately on important regions within the image. YOLOv10 follows closely behind, benefiting from its C3k2 blocks that optimize feature aggregation and balance computational efficiency with accuracy.
  - Blood cell detection: YOLOv11 achieved the highest mAP50 of 0.958, followed by YOLOv10 at 0.944. Both models surpass YOLOv9 (0.933), YOLO-NAS (0.9041), and YOLOv8 (0.93). The C2PSA and C3k2 blocks in YOLOv11 and YOLOv10 allowed these models to detect intricate patterns, such as those found in medical imaging, more effectively than previous iterations.
  - Facemask detection: YOLOv11 also dominated the facemask detection dataset, achieving a mAP50 of 0.962, compared to YOLOv10's 0.950. This was higher than YOLOv9 (0.941), YOLOv8 (0.924), and YOLO-NAS (0.9199), indicating that the newer models are better suited for precise feature extraction in tasks with clear object boundaries, such as facemask detection.
  - Human Detection: In human detection, YOLOv11 scored a mAP50 of 0.854, with YOLOv10 at 0.829. Although YOLOv9 closely followed at 0.812, YOLOv11 and YOLOv10 demonstrated more stability across the 20 training epochs, thanks to their ability to handle occlusions and dynamic backgrounds.
- Real-Time Applications and Edge Device Suitability

While YOLO-NAS is known for its efficiency in real-time applications, it was outperformed by YOLOv11 and YOLOv10 in tasks requiring more intricate feature extraction.

However, YOLO-NAS's architecture still proves effective for simpler tasks, such as face-mask detection, where it recorded a mAP50 of 0.9199. YOLOv10 and YOLOv11 offer a strong balance between accuracy and computational efficiency, making them suitable for deployment on edge devices that require fast, resource-efficient models.

- Performance on Autonomous Vehicle and Industrial Tasks

In tasks like pothole detection, which are critical for autonomous vehicles, YOLOv11 again led the models with a mAP50 of 0.815, followed by YOLOv10 at 0.793 and YOLOv9 at 0.78. The newer YOLO models consistently improved over time, showing that their architectures are more adaptable to dynamic, real-time environments. This is crucial in applications such as road safety, where detecting subtle features like potholes in various lighting and weather conditions is essential.

- Handling Complex Data: Shellfish and Smoke Detection

Complex datasets, such as shellfish monitoring and smoke detection, present unique challenges due to the overlapping and occluded objects within the images. YOLOv11 stood out in these tasks, with a mAP50 of 0.563 in shellfish monitoring and 0.945 in smoke detection. YOLOv10 also performed well, with scores of 0.542 and 0.925, respectively. In contrast, YOLOv9, YOLO-NAS, and YOLOv8 struggled more with these datasets, particularly in shellfish monitoring, where YOLOv9 only achieved a mAP50 of 0.534, and YOLO-NAS fell behind at 0.469.

In smoke detection, YOLOv8 initially performed better than YOLOv9, with a mAP50 of 0.911 compared to YOLOv9's 0.865. However, YOLOv11 surpassed both models, making it the top performer by the end of the training epochs. YOLO-NAS, while still competitive, recorded a mAP50 of 0.7811, highlighting its limitations in handling more dynamic tasks that require detailed motion analysis and fine-grained object detection.

- Training Epochs: The Importance of Extended Training

As illustrated in the mAP50 charts, extending the training epochs beyond 20 could further enhance the performance of all models, particularly YOLOv10 and YOLOv11. Both models showed a strong upward trajectory throughout the 20 epochs, suggesting that additional training could further improve their ability to handle complex object detection tasks. YOLO-NAS, while designed for efficiency, exhibited earlier flattening in its performance, indicating that its architectural limitations may prevent it from reaching the same level of accuracy in high-complexity tasks.

Therefore, the addition of YOLOv10 and YOLOv11 has shifted the performance standards in real-time object detection. While YOLO-NAS remains a strong candidate for resource-constrained environments, and YOLOv8 continues to deliver adaptable performance, YOLOv11 has emerged as the most versatile and accurate model across a range of challenging datasets. Whether in medical imaging, autonomous driving, or industrial monitoring, YOLOv11's ability to handle complex patterns, occlusions, and dynamic environments makes it the preferred choice for tasks requiring high precision and model stability.

In Table 9, we present the results of testing YOLO variants on a facemask dataset. The objective was to evaluate the performance of older YOLO versions (YOLOv5, YOLOv6, and YOLOv7) to understand their capabilities in handling relatively simple image classification tasks like facemask detection.

Table 9. Results of different YOLO variants on facemask data.

Model Type	mAP50
YOLOv7	0.927
YOLOv6	0.6771
YOLOv5	0.791

YOLOv7 achieved the highest mAP50 (mean average precision at 50% Intersection over Union (IoU) threshold) score of 0.927, outperforming both YOLOv6 and YOLOv5. This higher score suggests that YOLOv7 is particularly well-suited for simple object detection tasks involving clear and distinguishable objects. YOLOv7's efficiency and architectural simplicity enabled it to outperform even newer models like YOLO-NAS in tasks with fewer complexities, where lighter architectures excel.

- YOLOv7's performance highlights its capability to handle real-time detection while balancing precision, making it suitable for applications such as facemask detection.
- On the other hand, YOLOv6 and YOLOv5 underperformed relative to YOLOv7, with mAP50 scores of 0.6771 and 0.791, respectively. YOLOv6 and YOLOv5, while capable of decent performance in general object detection, require further optimization, including additional epochs of training and fine-tuning of model parameters to improve their accuracy in specialized tasks like facemask detection.

The results show that older models like YOLOv5 and YOLOv6 could still be relevant with appropriate adjustments, but for tasks that prioritize high speed and accuracy on relatively simple datasets, YOLOv7 stands out as the optimal choice.

These results underscore the importance of selecting models based on the complexity of the dataset and task. While newer models may offer advanced features for handling complex image detection, older, simpler architectures can still perform optimally when the task at hand involves more straightforward detection.

5.3. Discussions

5.3.1. Limitations, Challenges, and Integration of YOLO with Emerging Technologies

Despite its broad applicability and success, YOLO faces several significant limitations that constrain its performance in certain scenarios. A major challenge is its difficulty in detecting small objects, particularly in cluttered or complex environments. Small objects often lack sufficient feature representation in YOLO's grid-based framework, as the resolution of feature maps tends to diminish with increasing model depth [143]. This limitation becomes critical in applications such as traffic monitoring, where distinguishing between distant vehicles and pedestrians is essential, or in medical imaging, where small anomalies like microcalcifications in mammograms can go undetected. Overlapping or occluded objects exacerbate this issue, as YOLO relies on anchor boxes and non-maximum suppression for object localization, which can lead to false negatives and overlooked detections.

Another limitation is YOLO's computational demands, which hinder its deployment on resource-constrained devices like IoT sensors, mobile platforms, and drones [144]. While lightweight variants such as YOLOv5s address this issue to some extent, they often sacrifice accuracy for efficiency, making them unsuitable for tasks that require high precision. The high computational cost also limits YOLO's usability in real-time applications where latency is a critical factor, such as autonomous vehicles and emergency response systems. Additionally, YOLO's fixed input size requirement may necessitate resizing images, potentially leading to loss of important details or distortions in object shapes, further degrading performance in scenarios where fine-grained detail is crucial.

Domain adaptability is another pressing challenge for YOLO. The model's performance tends to degrade significantly in domains with irregular or noisy data, such as low-light environments, underwater imaging, or thermal imagery [145]. These domains often present unique challenges that YOLO's conventional architecture is not optimized to address, resulting in reduced detection accuracy and robustness. For example, in underwater exploration, YOLO may struggle to distinguish objects due to variable lighting conditions, reflections, and distortions caused by water. Similarly, in medical imaging, variations in resolution, contrast, and texture can negatively impact YOLO's ability to generalize across datasets, necessitating extensive domain-specific tuning and pre-processing.

A further challenge is YOLO's vulnerability to adversarial attacks, which can manipulate the model by introducing imperceptible perturbations to input images [146]. These attacks can cause YOLO to misclassify objects, leading to potentially disastrous consequences in high-stakes applications such as security, defense, or healthcare. For instance, an adversarial attack on a surveillance system powered by YOLO might result in failing to detect a weapon or misidentifying a harmless object as a threat. This vulnerability underscores the need for robust defenses, such as adversarial training, input filtering, and enhanced feature extraction mechanisms. Additionally, ethical concerns related to privacy and dataset biases present another layer of challenges. YOLO's deployment in surveillance and facial recognition systems often raises privacy issues, while biases in training datasets can result in unfair or inaccurate detections, especially in diverse populations or underrepresented environments. These challenges highlight the importance of not only technical advancements but also ethical considerations in YOLO's design and application.

5.3.2. Advancing YOLO Through Integration with AI Tools and Emerging Technologies

To address the challenges faced by YOLO, researchers are exploring innovative trends to enhance its adaptability and performance. Few-shot learning has emerged as a promising approach, enabling YOLO to operate effectively even with limited labeled data by leveraging transfer learning and meta-learning techniques [147]. This reduces the dependency on large-scale datasets, making YOLO more accessible for specialized applications where data scarcity is common. Another advancement is the development of dynamic detection models, which allow YOLO to adapt to evolving criteria in real-time scenarios [148]. Applications such as robotics, where conditions change rapidly, or personalized retail systems, which require tailored recommendations, greatly benefit from this adaptability. Additionally, extending YOLO to handle 3D object detection has become a critical focus area [149,150]. By incorporating technologies like LiDAR, depth maps, and volumetric analysis, YOLO is now applied in advanced fields such as autonomous vehicles and AR/VR systems [151], where spatial precision and contextual understanding are paramount [152]. These innovations not only address existing limitations but also open new opportunities for YOLO in emerging technologies and complex real-world environments.

The integration of YOLO with advanced AI tools, particularly Edge AI, has transformed the landscape of real-time object detection by significantly enhancing efficiency and functionality [153]. Leveraging hardware accelerators such as FPGAs and TPUs enables YOLO to achieve faster inference with reduced power consumption, making it ideal for deployment on resource-constrained devices such as IoT systems, drones, and mobile platforms. Lightweight YOLO models handle initial detection on edge devices, while more complex computations are offloaded to cloud infrastructure, creating a hybrid system that optimizes resource usage and minimizes latency. This architecture is particularly valuable for large-scale, real-time applications, including smart homes, wearable technologies, and industrial monitoring systems, where speed and efficiency are critical.

Integration with contextual AI frameworks, such as Vision Transformers, further enhances YOLO's ability to operate in dynamic environments [154]. This combination allows YOLO to incorporate spatial and temporal context into its predictions, improving accuracy and reliability in scenarios such as crowded public spaces or rapidly changing industrial sites. Such advancements streamline real-time analytics, making it possible to process large volumes of data for applications like traffic management, crowd monitoring, and safety systems in smart cities. By providing actionable insights derived from real-time data, this integration empowers informed decision-making and enhances operational efficiency across various sectors.

These synergistic advancements have unlocked transformational applications across numerous domains. In autonomous vehicles, YOLO integrated with Edge AI ensures reliable, real-time object detection even under resource constraints, improving safety and navigation. In agriculture, UAVs equipped with YOLO and Edge AI enable large-scale crop monitoring, identifying pests, nutrient deficiencies, and other yield-impacting factors, reducing manual interventions and optimizing efficiency. In industrial automation, these systems perform real-time defect detection on production lines, maintaining consistent quality control. Additionally, YOLO's integration with multimodal AI, such as combining visual and auditory data, has expanded its utility to innovative areas like assistive technologies and advanced surveillance systems. Together, these advancements redefine the boundaries of intelligent detection and decision-making across diverse, real-world applications.

6. Ethical Considerations in the Deployment of YOLO: A Deeper Examination

The YOLO (You Only Look Once) framework, with its transformative real-time object detection capabilities, has significantly reshaped a broad range of industries. Its efficiency and speed have enabled breakthroughs in fields such as healthcare, autonomous driving, agriculture, and industrial automation. However, as with any disruptive technology, the widespread use of YOLO raises profound ethical questions. These issues extend beyond basic concerns of privacy or fairness and tap into deeper societal, philosophical, and environmental considerations. To responsibly harness YOLO's potential, we must delve into these ethical challenges with a nuanced understanding.

6.1. The Erosion of Privacy and the Threat of Surveillance Dystopias

As YOLO continues to enhance surveillance capabilities, we face the risk of creating a society where individuals are constantly monitored without their consent. Beyond the simple argument of privacy violations, YOLO-enabled systems threaten to embed a culture of surveillance into the fabric of daily life. The rapid pace of technological innovation is outpacing legislative and ethical frameworks, leading to a world where the omnipresent eye of cameras, drones, and smart devices can track and analyze human behavior in granular detail.

The ethical challenge here is not just about balancing security and privacy; it is about safeguarding the very concept of autonomy and freedom. In an environment where every action is logged and analyzed by real-time object detection systems, individuals may begin to self-censor or alter their behavior to avoid suspicion. This normalization of constant surveillance can lead to a dystopian future where free expression and individuality are compromised, and dissenting voices are stifled.

6.2. Bias and the Reinforcement of Social Inequalities

YOLO models, like many AI technologies, are only as fair as the data on which they are trained. However, the bias problem runs deeper than simple data misrepresentation. The use of YOLO in critical systems such as predictive policing, healthcare diagnostics, or hiring processes can reinforce systemic inequalities. By automating decision-making processes, we risk entrenching the biases present in historical data and perpetuating discriminatory practices.

In healthcare, for example, biased YOLO models could lead to unequal diagnostic outcomes across different racial or socioeconomic groups, where misdiagnosis or delayed detection could be life-threatening. In law enforcement, biased models might disproportionately target certain communities, leading to over-policing and further marginalization. The ethical dilemma lies in how we reconcile the tension between technological advancement and social justice. It is not enough to train YOLO on more diverse datasets; we must rigorously interrogate how the algorithms themselves make decisions, ensuring that they do not replicate or amplify existing biases.

6.3. Accountability in an Age of Automated Decision-Making

One of the most complex ethical issues surrounding YOLO's deployment is accountability. As these systems become increasingly autonomous, the line between human and machine responsibility blurs. When a YOLO-powered system makes a wrong decision whether in diagnosing a disease, misidentifying a pedestrian, or flagging an innocent person as a security threat who is accountable for the consequences?

The issue of accountability goes beyond merely ensuring transparency in the development of YOLO models. It extends into legal and moral territory, where developers, deployers, and users must navigate an intricate web of responsibility. If a YOLO-powered autonomous vehicle is involved in an accident, who should be held responsible the developer who designed the model, the organization that deployed it, or the user who trusted it? As we integrate YOLO into critical decision-making systems, we must establish clear ethical and legal frameworks for accountability, ensuring that responsibility is distributed appropriately across all stakeholders.

6.4. The Ethical Dilemmas in Medical and Life-Critical Applications

YOLO's application in healthcare particularly in diagnostics, surgery, and patient monitoring holds immense promise, but it also raises high-stakes ethical questions. Errors in object detection in these domains can have life-or-death consequences. A misdiagnosis caused by an incorrect detection of a tumor or a missed abnormality in a critical scan can lead to delayed treatments or improper medical interventions.

This challenges the trust between healthcare professionals and AI systems. While YOLO can assist in increasing the accuracy of medical assessments, it should not undermine the authority and expertise of healthcare professionals. Ensuring that YOLO remains a tool that complements human judgment, rather than replaces it, is vital. The ethical debate extends to questions about the humanization of care how much reliance on automated systems is acceptable before the personal touch of medical practitioners is lost?

6.5. Environmental Sustainability and the Hidden Cost of Automation

One of the overlooked ethical issues with YOLO is its environmental impact. The growing demand for AI and machine learning models has led to significant increases in energy consumption, particularly in training and deploying large-scale YOLO models. While the technology itself is seen as cutting-edge, the infrastructure required to support its deployment is resource-intensive, contributing to the carbon footprint of AI technologies.

This ethical concern goes beyond efficiency in training and into the realm of sustainability. As YOLO models are integrated into a broader range of industries, the need for high-performance computing resources grows. Data centers, GPUs, and cloud computing infrastructures essential for training large-scale models consume vast amounts of energy. Therefore, it is essential that we focus on developing greener AI technologies and optimizing YOLO variants for energy efficiency. This includes prioritizing lightweight models that maintain performance while minimizing environmental harm, as well as exploring renewable energy sources for data centers.

6.6. The Social Impact of YOLO and the Displacement of Human Labor

The automation potential of YOLO extends beyond its technical capabilities and into societal concerns. As industries adopt YOLO for object detection and automation, particularly in manufacturing, agriculture, and logistics, the displacement of human labor becomes a significant ethical concern. The technology that drives efficiency in industrial settings often comes at the cost of jobs, particularly in sectors reliant on manual labor for tasks such as quality control and monitoring.

The ethical challenge here is twofold. First, there is a need to address the potential economic disruption caused by widespread automation. Policymakers, businesses, and technology developers must collaborate to create strategies for retraining and upskilling displaced workers. Second, there is the broader philosophical question about the value of human labor in an automated society. As machines take over more tasks, how do we ensure that humans are not rendered obsolete? A society that over-automates without regard for the social consequences risks creating deep divides between those who benefit from automation and those who are left behind.

6.7. Ethical Frameworks for Responsible YOLO Deployment

The rapid pace of YOLO's evolution demands the parallel development of ethical frameworks that guide its responsible use. These frameworks should prioritize human dignity, fairness, privacy, and sustainability. At the core of this endeavor is the commitment to responsible AI development, where transparency, accountability, and inclusivity are foundational principles.

Developers and organizations must adopt stringent ethical guidelines for training, deploying, and monitoring YOLO-powered systems. These guidelines should include considerations of data fairness, model interpretability, privacy protections, and energy efficiency. By embedding ethical principles into the development lifecycle, we can ensure that YOLO is deployed in ways that benefit society without compromising fundamental rights or causing harm.

7. Conclusions

This paper has examined the remarkable evolution of the YOLO (You Only Look Once) family of object detection models, from earlier versions like YOLOv6, YOLOv7, and YOLOv8, through to groundbreaking innovations such as YOLO-NAS, YOLOv9, and the most recent releases, YOLOv10 and YOLOv11. Each iteration has brought advancements in speed, accuracy, and computational efficiency, solidifying YOLO's role as a dominant framework in real-time object detection. YOLO's single-stage detection architecture has enabled rapid, efficient object identification across diverse and time-sensitive fields, such as healthcare, autonomous driving, agriculture, and industrial automation.

YOLO-NAS introduced a key innovation with Post-Training Quantization (PTQ), optimizing the model for resource-constrained environments without compromising accuracy. YOLOv9 further enhanced performance by introducing features like Programmable Gradient Information (PGI) and Generalized Efficient Layer Aggregation Networks (GELAN), allowing the model to tackle more complex detection tasks, including those with occlusions and intricate patterns.

The recent developments in YOLOv10 and YOLOv11 have further pushed the boundaries of performance. YOLOv10's C3k2 blocks and YOLOv11's Cross-Stage Partial with Spatial Attention (C2PSA) blocks significantly improved the models' ability to detect small and occluded objects while maintaining computational efficiency. In particular, YOLOv11 emerged as the most accurate and efficient model in benchmark tests, outperforming previous versions in tasks such as facemask detection, blood cell analysis, and autonomous vehicle applications.

Comprehensive benchmarks across datasets like Roboflow 100, Object365, and COCO have demonstrated the distinct advantages of YOLOv9, YOLOv10, and YOLOv11, particularly in complex object detection scenarios. Among these, YOLOv11 consistently achieved the highest performance, confirming its status as the current gold standard for real-time detection tasks in applications that require high precision, such as healthcare, environmental monitoring, and autonomous systems.

However, with these technological advancements come important ethical considerations. YOLO's ability to enable real-time object tracking and identification raises concerns about privacy and the potential for intrusive surveillance, which could threaten individual freedoms and civil liberties. Additionally, the automation of tasks previously performed by humans, especially in industries such as manufacturing and agriculture, could lead to job displacement. Therefore, the need for stringent ethical frameworks and guidelines becomes crucial to ensure that YOLO's powerful capabilities are used responsibly and for the benefit of society.

Therefore, YOLO has demonstrated itself as a highly adaptable and powerful tool for real-time object detection across multiple domains. As research continues to refine its performance, particularly through the development of lightweight and energy-efficient models, YOLO will undoubtedly remain at the forefront of object detection technology. However, ensuring its responsible and ethical deployment will be essential in maximizing its potential while safeguarding societal values.

This research provides a comprehensive review of the YOLO framework, emphasizing its evolution and transformative applications across diverse domains. By analyzing performance benchmarks for YOLO versions from YOLOv8 to YOLOv11, the study sheds light on key technical advancements, such as improved feature aggregation and attention mechanisms, and their implications for real-time object detection. It offers domain-specific insights into YOLO's effectiveness in areas such as precision farming, healthcare diagnostics, and autonomous systems, demonstrating its adaptability and utility. Furthermore, the discussion of ethical considerations addresses critical issues like privacy, bias, and societal impact, offering a holistic perspective on the responsible deployment of YOLO models. This work serves as a resource for researchers and practitioners by synthesizing innovations and applications in the YOLO framework while pointing toward future research directions.

Despite its breadth, this review has certain limitations. The performance benchmarks rely heavily on open-source datasets, limiting validation with real-world samples. The analysis focuses primarily on YOLO's internal evolution rather than comparing it extensively with other object detection frameworks. Additionally, models were evaluated using a fixed number of training epochs, which might not fully capture their optimal performance potential. Finally, dataset biases inherent to publicly available data may influence the reported outcomes and generalizability of the results. These limitations highlight areas for further research, including extended training and validation with practical, real-life scenarios.

Funding: This research received no external funding.

Conflicts of Interest: The authors declare no conflict of interest.

References

1. Diwan, T.; Anirudh, G.; Tembhurne, J.V. Object detection using YOLO: Challenges, architectural successors, datasets and applications. *Multimed. Tools Appl.* **2023**, *82*, 9243–9275. [CrossRef] [PubMed]
2. Vijayakumar, A.; Vairavasundaram, S. YOLO-based Object Detection Models: A Review and its Applications. *Multimed. Tools Appl.* **2024**, *83*, 83535–83574. [CrossRef]
3. Wang, X.; Li, H.; Yue, X.; Meng, L. A comprehensive survey on object detection YOLO. In Proceedings of the 5th International Symposium on Advanced Technologies and Applications in the Inter of Things (ATAIT), Kusatsu, Japan, 28–29 August 2023.
4. Soviany, P.; Ionescu, R.T. Optimizing the trade-off between single-stage and two-stage object detectors using image difficulty prediction. *arXiv* **2018**, arXiv:1803.08707.
5. Chandana, R.; Ramachandra, A. Real time object detection system with YOLO and CNN models: A review. *arXiv* **2022**, arXiv:2208.00773.
6. Kaur, R.; Singh, S. A comprehensive review of object detection with deep learning. *Digit. Signal Process.* **2023**, *132*, 103812. [CrossRef]
7. Zhao, X.; Ni, Y.; Jia, H. Modified object detection method based on YOLO. In Proceedings of the CCF Chinese Conference on Computer Vision, Singapore, 11–14 October 2017; pp. 233–244.
8. Zhao, Z.-Q.; Zheng, P.; Xu, S.-T.; Wu, X. Object detection with deep learning: A review. *IEEE Trans. Neural Netw. Learn. Syst.* **2019**, *30*, 3212–3232. [CrossRef] [PubMed]
9. Ragab, M.G.; Abdulkader, S.J.; Muneer, A.; Alqushaibi, A.; Sumiea, E.H.; Qureshi, R.; Al-Selwi, S.M.; Alhussian, H. A Comprehensive Systematic Review of YOLO for Medical Object Detection (2018 to 2023). *IEEE Access* **2024**, *12*, 57815–57836. [CrossRef]
10. Shetty, A.K.; Saha, I.; Sanghvi, R.M.; Save, S.A.; Patel, Y.J. A review: Object detection models. In Proceedings of the 2021 6th International Conference for Convergence in Technology (I2CT), Maharashtra, India, 2–4 April 2021; pp. 1–8.
11. Du, J. Understanding of object detection based on CNN family and YOLO. *J. Phys. Conf. Ser.* **2018**, *1004*, 012029. [CrossRef]
12. Zou, X. A review of object detection techniques. In Proceedings of the 2019 International Conference on Smart Grid and Electrical Automation (ICSGEA), Xiangtan, China, 10–11 August 2019; pp. 251–254.
13. Sanchez, S.; Romero, H.; Morales, A. A review: Comparison of performance metrics of pretrained models for object detection using the TensorFlow framework. *IOP Conf. Ser. Mater. Sci. Eng.* **2020**, *844*, 012024. [CrossRef]
14. Ashraf, I.; Hur, S.; Kim, G.; Park, Y. Analyzing performance of YOLOx for detecting vehicles in bad weather conditions. *Sensors* **2024**, *24*, 522. [CrossRef]
15. Wu, S.; Li, X.; Wang, X. IoU-aware single-stage object detector for accurate localization. *Image Vis. Comput.* **2020**, *97*, 103911. [CrossRef]
16. Carranza-García, M.; Torres-Mateo, J.; Lara-Benítez, P.; García-Gutiérrez, J. On the performance of one-stage and two-stage object detectors in autonomous vehicles using camera data. *Remote Sens.* **2020**, *13*, 89. [CrossRef]
17. Yasmine, G.; Maha, G.; Hicham, M. Overview of single-stage object detection models: From YOLOV1 to Yolov7. In Proceedings of the 2023 International Wireless Communications and Mobile Computing (IWCMC), Marrakesh, Morocco, 19–23 June 2023; pp. 1579–1584.
18. Ren, S.; He, K.; Girshick, R.; Sun, J. Faster R-CNN: Towards real-time object detection with region proposal networks. *IEEE Trans. Pattern Anal. Mach. Intell.* **2016**, *39*, 1137–1149. [CrossRef] [PubMed]

19. Deng, J.; Xuan, X.; Wang, W.; Li, Z.; Yao, H.; Wang, Z. A review of research on object detection based on deep learning. *J. Phys. Conf. Ser.* **2020**, *1684*, 012028. [CrossRef]
20. Zhong, Y.; Wang, J.; Peng, J.; Zhang, L. Anchor box optimization for object detection. In Proceedings of the IEEE/CVF Winter Conference on Applications of Computer Vision, Snowmass, CO, USA, 1–5 March 2020; pp. 1286–1294.
21. Luo, S.; Dai, H.; Shao, L.; Ding, Y. M3dssd: Monocular 3D single stage object detector. In Proceedings of the IEEE/CVF Conference on Computer Vision and Pattern Recognition, Nashville, TN, USA, 20–25 June 2021; pp. 6145–6154.
22. Devi, S.; Thopalli, K.; Malarvezhi, P.; Thiagarajan, J.J. Improving single-stage object detectors for nighttime pedestrian detection. *Int. J. Pattern Recognit. Artif. Intell.* **2022**, *36*, 2250034. [CrossRef]
23. Hosang, J.; Benenson, R.; Schiele, B. Learning non-maximum suppression. In Proceedings of the IEEE Conference on Computer Vision and Pattern Recognition, Honolulu, HI, USA, 21–26 July 2017; pp. 4507–4515.
24. Yang, Z.; Sun, Y.; Liu, S.; Jia, J. 3DSSD: Point-based 3d single stage object detector. In Proceedings of the IEEE/CVF Conference on Computer Vision and Pattern Recognition, Seattle, WA, USA, 13–19 June 2020; pp. 11040–11048.
25. Wang, L.; Hua, S.; Zhang, C.; Yang, G.; Ren, J.; Li, J. YOLOdrive: A Lightweight Autonomous Driving Single-Stage Target Detection Approach. *IEEE Internet Things J.* **2024**, *11*, 36099–36113. [CrossRef]
26. Dai, X. HybridNet: A fast vehicle detection system for autonomous driving. *Signal Process. Image Commun.* **2019**, *70*, 79–88. [CrossRef]
27. Ortiz Castello, V.; del Tejo Catalá, O.; Salvador Igual, I.; Perez-Cortes, J.-C. Real-time on-board pedestrian detection using generic single-stage algorithms and on-road databases. *Int. J. Adv. Robot. Syst.* **2020**, *17*, 1729881420929175. [CrossRef]
28. Ren, J.; Chen, X.; Liu, J.; Sun, W.; Pang, J.; Yan, Q.; Tai, Y.-W.; Xu, L. Accurate single stage detector using recurrent rolling convolution. In Proceedings of the IEEE Conference on Computer Vision and Pattern Recognition, Honolulu, HI, USA, 21–26 July 2017; pp. 5420–5428.
29. Zhang, H.; Li, P.; Du, Z.; Dou, W. Risk entropy modeling of surveillance camera for public security application. *IEEE Access* **2020**, *8*, 45343–45355. [CrossRef]
30. Lu, Z.; Rathod, V.; Votel, R.; Huang, J. Retinatrack: Online single stage joint detection and tracking. In Proceedings of the IEEE/CVF Conference on Computer Vision and Pattern Recognition, Seattle, WA, USA, 13–19 June 2020; pp. 14668–14678.
31. Liu, W.; Anguelov, D.; Erhan, D.; Szegedy, C.; Reed, S.; Fu, C.-Y.; Berg, A.C. Ssd: Single shot multibox detector. In Proceedings of the Computer Vision–ECCV 2016: 14th European Conference, Amsterdam, The Netherlands, 11–14 October 2016; Proceedings, Part I 14. pp. 21–37.
32. Huang, L.; Yang, Y.; Deng, Y.; Yu, Y. Densebox: Unifying landmark localization with end to end object detection. *arXiv* **2015**, arXiv:1509.04874.
33. Lin, T.-Y.; Goyal, P.; Girshick, R.; He, K.; Dollár, P. Focal loss for dense object detection. *arXiv* **2017**, arXiv:1708.02002.
34. Liu, S.; Huang, D. Receptive field block net for accurate and fast object detection. In Proceedings of the European Conference on Computer Vision (ECCV), Munich, Germany, 8–14 September 2018; pp. 385–400.
35. Tan, M.; Pang, R.; Le, Q.V. Efficientdet: Scalable and efficient object detection. In Proceedings of the IEEE/CVF Conference on Computer Vision and Pattern Recognition, Seattle, WA, USA, 13–19 June 2020; pp. 10781–10790.
36. Jiang, Z.; Zhao, L.; Li, S.; Jia, Y. Real-time object detection method based on improved YOLOv4-tiny. *arXiv* **2020**, arXiv:2011.04244.
37. Kumar, C.; Punitha, R. Yolov3 and yolov4: Multiple object detection for surveillance applications. In Proceedings of the 2020 Third International Conference on Smart Systems and Inventive Technology (ICSSIT), Tirunelveli, India, 20–22 August 2020; pp. 1316–1321.
38. Das, A.; Nandi, A.; Deb, I. Recent Advances in Object Detection Based on YOLO-V4 and Faster RCNN: A Review. In *Mathematical Modeling for Computer Applications*; Wiley Online Library: Hoboken, NJ, USA, 2024; pp. 405–417.
39. Redmon, J. You only look once: Unified, real-time object detection. In Proceedings of the IEEE Conference on Computer Vision and Pattern Recognition, Las Vegas, NV, USA, 27–30 June 2016.
40. Mahasin, M.; Dewi, I.A. Comparison of CSPDarkNet53, CSPResNeXt-50, and EfficientNet-B0 backbones on YOLO v4 as object detector. *Int. J. Eng. Sci. Inf. Technol.* **2022**, *2*, 64–72. [CrossRef]
41. Chen, H.; Chen, Z.; Yu, H. Enhanced YOLOv5: An Efficient Road Object Detection Method. *Sensors* **2023**, *23*, 8355. [CrossRef] [PubMed]
42. Li, R.; Zeng, X.; Yang, S.; Li, Q.; Yan, A.; Li, D. ABYOLOv4: Improved YOLOv4 human object detection based on enhanced multi-scale feature fusion. *EURASIP J. Adv. Signal Process.* **2024**, *2024*, 6. [CrossRef]
43. Gao, C.; Zhang, Q.; Tan, Z.; Zhao, G.; Gao, S.; Kim, E.; Shen, T. Applying optimized YOLOv8 for heritage conservation: Enhanced object detection in Jiangnan traditional private gardens. *Herit. Sci.* **2024**, *12*, 31. [CrossRef]
44. Fu, X.; Angkawisittpan, N. Detecting surface defects of heritage buildings based on deep learning. *J. Intell. Syst.* **2024**, *33*, 20230048. [CrossRef]
45. Su, X.; Zhang, J.; Ma, Z.; Dong, Y.; Zi, J.; Xu, N.; Zhang, H.; Xu, F.; Chen, F. Identification of Rare Wildlife in the Field Environment Based on the Improved YOLOv5 Model. *Remote Sens.* **2024**, *16*, 1535. [CrossRef]
46. Byeon, H. YOLO v10-Based Brain Tumor Detection: An Innovative Approach in CT Imaging. *Nanotechnol. Percept.* **2024**, *20*, 113–125.
47. Li, T.; Zhang, L.; Lin, J. Precision agriculture with YOLO-Leaf: Advanced methods for detecting apple leaf diseases. *Front. Plant Sci.* **2024**, *15*, 1452502. [CrossRef]

48. Xiao, G.; Hou, S.; Zhou, H. PCB defect detection algorithm based on CDI-YOLO. *Sci. Rep.* **2024**, *14*, 7351. [CrossRef]
49. Nguyen, H.H.; Ta, T.N.; Nguyen, N.C.; Pham, H.M.; Nguyen, D.M. Yolo based real-time human detection for smart video surveillance at the edge. In Proceedings of the 2020 IEEE Eighth International Conference on Communications and Electronics (ICCE), Phu Quoc Island, Vietnam, 13–15 January 2021; pp. 439–444.
50. Kaur, A.; Singh, Y.; Neeru, N.; Kaur, L.; Singh, A. A Survey on Deep Learning Approaches to Medical Images and a Systematic Look up into Real-Time Object Detection. *Arch. Comput. Methods Eng.* **2022**, *29*, 2071–2111. [CrossRef]
51. Coşkun, D.; Karaboğa, D.; Baştürk, A.; Akay, B.; Nalbantoğlu, Ö.U.; Doğan, S.; Paçal, İ.; Karagöz, M.A. A comparative study of YOLO models and a transformer-based YOLOv5 model for mass detection in mammograms. *Turk. J. Electr. Eng. Comput. Sci.* **2023**, *31*, 1294–1313. [CrossRef]
52. Han, Z.; Huang, H.; Fan, Q.; Li, Y.; Li, Y.; Chen, X. SMD-YOLO: An efficient and lightweight detection method for mask wearing status during the COVID-19 pandemic. *Comput. Methods Programs Biomed.* **2022**, *221*, 106888. [CrossRef]
53. Vibhuti; Jindal, N.; Singh, H.; Rana, P.S. Face mask detection in COVID-19: A strategic review. *Multimed. Tools Appl.* **2022**, *81*, 40013–40042. [CrossRef] [PubMed]
54. Yu, C.J.; Yeh, H.J.; Chang, C.C.; Tang, J.H.; Kao, W.Y.; Chen, W.C.; Huang, Y.J.; Li, C.H.; Chang, W.H.; Lin, Y.T.; et al. Lightweight deep neural networks for cholelithiasis and cholecystitis detection by point-of-care ultrasound. *Comput. Methods Programs Biomed.* **2021**, *211*, 106382. [CrossRef] [PubMed]
55. Monemian, M.; Rabbani, H. Detecting red-lesions from retinal fundus images using unique morphological features. *Sci. Rep.* **2023**, *13*, 3487. [CrossRef] [PubMed]
56. Alyoubi, W.L.; Abulkhair, M.F.; Shalash, W.M. Diabetic Retinopathy Fundus Image Classification and Lesions Localization System Using Deep Learning. *Sensors* **2021**, *21*, 3704. [CrossRef] [PubMed]
57. Farahat, Z.; Zrira, N.; Souissi, N.; Benamar, S.; Belmekki, M.; Ngote, M.N.; Megdiche, K. Application of Deep Learning Methods in a Moroccan Ophthalmic Center: Analysis and Discussion. *Diagnostics* **2023**, *13*, 1694. [CrossRef] [PubMed]
58. Sobek, J.; Medina Inojosa, J.R.; Medina Inojosa, B.J.; Rassoulinejad-Mousavi, S.M.; Conte, G.M.; Lopez-Jimenez, F.; Erickson, B.J. MedYOLO: A Medical Image Object Detection Framework. *J. Imaging Inform. Med.* **2024**, *37*, 3208–3216. [CrossRef] [PubMed]
59. Vasker, N.; Sowrov, A.R.A.; Hasan, M.; Ali, M.S.; Rashid, M.R.A.; Islam, M.M. Unmasking Ovary Tumors: Real-Time Detection with YOLOv5. In Proceedings of the 2023 4th International Conference on Big Data Analytics and Practices (IBDAP), Bangkok, Thailand, 25–27 August 2023; pp. 1–6.
60. Sadeghi, M.H.; Sina, S.; Omidi, H.; Farshchitabrizi, A.H.; Alavi, M. Deep learning in ovarian cancer diagnosis: A comprehensive review of various imaging modalities. *Pol. J. Radiol.* **2024**, *89*, e30–e48. [CrossRef] [PubMed]
61. Zhang, S.; Wang, K.; Zhang, H.; Wang, T.; Gao, X.; Song, Y.; Wang, F. An improved YOLOv8 for fiber bundle segmentation in X-ray computed tomography images of 2.5D composites to build the finite element model. *Compos. Part A Appl. Sci. Manuf.* **2024**, *185*, 108337. [CrossRef]
62. Hossain, A.; Islam, M.T.; Islam, M.S.; Chowdhury, M.E.H.; Almutairi, A.F.; Razouqi, Q.A.; Misran, N. A YOLOv3 Deep Neural Network Model to Detect Brain Tumor in Portable Electromagnetic Imaging System. *IEEE Access* **2021**, *9*, 82647–82660. [CrossRef]
63. Chen, A.; Lin, D.; Gao, Q. Enhancing brain tumor detection in MRI images using YOLO-NeuroBoost model. *Front. Neurol.* **2024**, *15*, 1445882. [CrossRef] [PubMed]
64. Sara, U.; Akter, M.; Uddin, M.S. Image Quality Assessment through FSIM, SSIM, MSE and PSNR—A Comparative Study. *J. Comput. Commun.* **2019**, *7*, 8–18. [CrossRef]
65. Amin, J.; Anjum, M.A.; Sharif, M.; Kadry, S.; Nadeem, A.; Ahmad, S.F. Liver Tumor Localization Based on YOLOv3 and 3D-Semantic Segmentation Using Deep Neural Networks. *Diagnostics* **2022**, *12*, 823. [CrossRef]
66. Iriani Sapitri, A.; Nurmaini, S.; Naufal Rachmatullah, M.; Tutuko, B.; Darmawahyuni, A.; Firdaus, F.; Rini, D.P.; Islami, A. Deep learning-based real time detection for cardiac objects with fetal ultrasound video. *Inform. Med. Unlocked* **2023**, *36*, 101150. [CrossRef]
67. Baccouche, A.; Garcia-Zapirain, B.; Zheng, Y.; Elmaghraby, A.S. Early detection and classification of abnormality in prior mammograms using image-to-image translation and YOLO techniques. *Comput. Methods Programs Biomed.* **2022**, *221*, 106884. [CrossRef]
68. Loey, M.; Manogaran, G.; Taha, M.H.N.; Khalifa, N.E.M. Fighting against COVID-19: A novel deep learning model based on YOLO-v2 with ResNet-50 for medical face mask detection. *Sustain. Cities Soc.* **2021**, *65*, 102600. [CrossRef]
69. Pang, S.; Ding, T.; Qiao, S.; Meng, F.; Wang, S.; Li, P.; Wang, X. A novel YOLOv3-arch model for identifying cholelithiasis and classifying gallstones on CT images. *PLoS ONE* **2019**, *14*, e0217647. [CrossRef] [PubMed]
70. Pham, T.-L.; Le, V.-H. Ovarian Tumors Detection and Classification from Ultrasound Images Based on YOLOv8. *J. Adv. Inf. Technol.* **2024**, *15*, 264–275. [CrossRef]
71. Safdar, M.F.; Alkobaisi, S.S.; Zahra, F.T. A Comparative Analysis of Data Augmentation Approaches for Magnetic Resonance Imaging (MRI) Scan Images of Brain Tumor. *Acta Inf. Med.* **2020**, *28*, 29–36. [CrossRef]
72. Li, S.; Li, Y.; Yao, J.; Chen, B.; Song, J.; Xue, Q.; Yang, X. Label-free classification of dead and live colonic adenocarcinoma cells based on 2D light scattering and deep learning analysis. *Cytom. Part A* **2021**, *99*, 1134–1142. [CrossRef]
73. Pandey, S.; Chen, K.-F.; Dam, E.B. Comprehensive Multimodal Segmentation in Medical Imaging: Combining YOLOv8 with SAM and HQ-SAM Models. *arXiv* **2023**, arXiv:2310.12995.

74. Priyanka; Baranwal, N.; Singh, K.N.; Singh, A.K. YOLO-based ROI selection for joint encryption and compression of medical images with reconstruction through super-resolution network. *Future Gener. Comput. Syst.* **2024**, *150*, 1–9. [CrossRef]
75. Haimer, Z.; Mateur, K.; Farhan, Y.; Madi, A.A. YOLO Algorithms Performance Comparison for Object Detection in Adverse Weather Conditions. In Proceedings of the 2023 3rd International Conference on Innovative Research in Applied Science, Engineering and Technology (IRASET), Casablanca, Morocco, 18–19 May 2023; pp. 1–7.
76. Ding, Q.; Li, P.; Yan, X.; Shi, D.; Liang, L.; Wang, W.; Xie, H.; Li, J.; Wei, M. Cf-yolo: Cross fusion yolo for object detection in adverse weather with a high-quality real snow dataset. *IEEE Trans. Intell. Transp. Syst.* **2023**, *24*, 10749–10759. [CrossRef]
77. Lv, Z.; Wang, R.; Wang, Y.; Zhou, F.; Guo, N. Road Scene Multi-Object Detection Algorithm Based on CMS-YOLO. *IEEE Access* **2023**, *11*, 121190–121201. [CrossRef]
78. Rothmeier, T.; Wachtel, D.; von Dem Bussche-Hünnefeld, T.; Huber, W. I had a bad day: Challenges of object detection in bad visibility conditions. In Proceedings of the 2023 IEEE Intelligent Vehicles Symposium (IV), Anchorage, AK, USA, 4–7 June 2023; pp. 1–6.
79. Guo, X. A novel Multi to Single Module for small object detection. *arXiv* **2023**, arXiv:2303.14977.
80. Zhang, Y.; Sun, Y.; Wang, Z.; Jiang, Y. YOLOv7-RAR for Urban Vehicle Detection. *Sensors* **2023**, *23*, 1801. [CrossRef] [PubMed]
81. Elesawy, A.; Mohammed Abdelkader, E.; Osman, H. A Detailed Comparative Analysis of You Only Look Once-Based Architectures for the Detection of Personal Protective Equipment on Construction Sites. *Eng* **2024**, *5*, 347–366. [CrossRef]
82. Jia, X.; Tong, Y.; Qiao, H.; Li, M.; Tong, J.; Liang, B. Fast and accurate object detector for autonomous driving based on improved YOLOv5. *Sci. Rep.* **2023**, *13*, 9711. [CrossRef] [PubMed]
83. Dazlee, N.M.A.A.; Khalil, S.A.; Abdul-Rahman, S.; Mutalib, S. Object Detection for Autonomous Vehicles with Sensor-based Technology Using YOLO. *Int. J. Intell. Syst. Appl. Eng.* **2022**, *10*, 129–134. [CrossRef]
84. Xu, L.; Yan, W.; Ji, J. The research of a novel WOG-YOLO algorithm for autonomous driving object detection. *Sci. Rep.* **2023**, *13*, 3699. [CrossRef] [PubMed]
85. Aloufi, N.; Alnori, A.; Thayananthan, V.; Basuhail, A. Object Detection Performance Evaluation for Autonomous Vehicles in Sandy Weather Environments. *Appl. Sci.* **2023**, *13*, 10249. [CrossRef]
86. Li, Y.; Wang, J.; Huang, J.; Li, Y. Research on Deep Learning Automatic Vehicle Recognition Algorithm Based on RES-YOLO Model. *Sensors* **2022**, *22*, 3783. [CrossRef]
87. Kumar, D.; Muhammad, N. Object Detection in Adverse Weather for Autonomous Driving through Data Merging and YOLOv8. *Sensors* **2023**, *23*, 8471. [CrossRef] [PubMed]
88. Afdhal, A.; Saddami, K.; Sugiarto, S.; Fuadi, Z.; Nasaruddin, N. Real-Time Object Detection Performance of YOLOv8 Models for Self-Driving Cars in a Mixed Traffic Environment. In Proceedings of the 2023 2nd International Conference on Computer System, Information Technology, and Electrical Engineering (COSITE), Banda Aceh, Indonesia, 2–3 August 2023; pp. 260–265.
89. Al Mudawi, N.; Qureshi, A.M.; Abdelhaq, M.; Alshahrani, A.; Alazeb, A.; Alonazi, M.; Algarni, A. Vehicle Detection and Classification via YOLOv8 and Deep Belief Network over Aerial Image Sequences. *Sustainability* **2023**, *15*, 14597. [CrossRef]
90. Azevedo, P.; Santos, V. Comparative analysis of multiple YOLO-based target detectors and trackers for ADAS in edge devices. *Robot. Auton. Syst.* **2024**, *171*, 104558. [CrossRef]
91. He, Q.; Xu, A.; Ye, Z.; Zhou, W.; Cai, T. Object Detection Based on Lightweight YOLOX for Autonomous Driving. *Sensors* **2023**, *23*, 7596. [CrossRef] [PubMed]
92. Sarda, A.; Dixit, S.; Bhan, A. Object Detection for Autonomous Driving using YOLO [You Only Look Once] algorithm. In Proceedings of the 2021 Third International Conference on Intelligent Communication Technologies and Virtual Mobile Networks (ICICV), Tirunelveli, India, 4–6 February 2021; pp. 1370–1374.
93. Puliti, S.; Astrup, R. Automatic detection of snow breakage at single tree level using YOLOv5 applied to UAV imagery. *Int. J. Appl. Earth Obs. Geoinf.* **2022**, *112*, 102946. [CrossRef]
94. Jemaa, H.; Bouachir, W.; Leblon, B.; Bouguila, N. Computer vision system for detecting orchard trees from UAV images. *Int. Arch. Photogramm. Remote Sens. Spat. Inf. Sci.* **2022**, *XLIII-B4-2022*, 661–668. [CrossRef]
95. Idrissi, M.; Hussain, A.; Barua, B.; Osman, A.; Abozariba, R.; Aneiba, A.; Asyhari, T. Evaluating the Forest Ecosystem through a Semi-Autonomous Quadruped Robot and a Hexacopter UAV. *Sensors* **2022**, *22*, 5497. [CrossRef] [PubMed]
96. Tian, Y.; Yang, G.; Wang, Z.; Wang, H.; Li, E.; Liang, Z. Apple detection during different growth stages in orchards using the improved YOLO-V3 model. *Comput. Electron. Agric.* **2019**, *157*, 417–426. [CrossRef]
97. Bahhar, C.; Ksibi, A.; Ayadi, M.; Jamjoom, M.M.; Ullah, Z.; Soufiene, B.O.; Sakli, H. Wildfire and Smoke Detection Using Staged YOLO Model and Ensemble CNN. *Electronics* **2023**, *12*, 228. [CrossRef]
98. Hong, S.-J.; Han, Y.; Kim, S.-Y.; Lee, A.-Y.; Kim, G. Application of Deep-Learning Methods to Bird Detection Using Unmanned Aerial Vehicle Imagery. *Sensors* **2019**, *19*, 1651. [CrossRef] [PubMed]
99. Gai, R.; Chen, N.; Yuan, H. A detection algorithm for cherry fruits based on the improved YOLO-v4 model. *Neural Comput. Appl.* **2021**, *35*, 13895–13906. [CrossRef]
100. Yang, G.; Wang, J.; Nie, Z.; Yang, H.; Yu, S. A Lightweight YOLOv8 Tomato Detection Algorithm Combining Feature Enhancement and Attention. *Agronomy* **2023**, *13*, 1824. [CrossRef]
101. Qin, Z.; Wang, W.; Dammer, K.-H.; Guo, L.; Cao, Z. Ag-YOLO: A Real-Time Low-Cost Detector for Precise Spraying with Case Study of Palms. *Front. Plant Sci.* **2021**, *12*, 753603. [CrossRef] [PubMed]

102. Zhang, W.; Huang, H.; Sun, Y.; Wu, X. AgriPest-YOLO: A rapid light-trap agricultural pest detection method based on deep learning. *Front. Plant Sci.* **2022**, *13*, 1079384. [CrossRef] [PubMed]
103. Liu, D.; Lv, F.; Guo, J.; Zhang, H.; Zhu, L. Detection of Forestry Pests Based on Improved YOLOv5 and Transfer Learning. *Forests* **2023**, *14*, 1484. [CrossRef]
104. Jayagopal, P.; Purushothaman Janaki, K.; Mohan, P.; Kondapaneni, U.B.; Periyasamy, J.; Mathivanan, S.K.; Dalu, G.T. A modified generative adversarial networks with Yolov5 for automated forest health diagnosis from aerial imagery and Tabu search algorithm. *Sci. Rep.* **2024**, *14*, 4814. [CrossRef]
105. Dandekar, Y.; Shinde, K.; Gangan, J.; Firdausi, S.; Bharne, S. Weed Plant Detection from Agricultural Field Images using YOLOv3 Algorithm. In Proceedings of the 2022 6th International Conference On Computing, Communication, Control and Automation (ICCUBEA), Pune, India, 26–27 August 2022; pp. 1–4.
106. Dang, F.; Chen, D.; Lu, Y.; Li, Z. YOLOWeeds: A novel benchmark of YOLO object detectors for multi-class weed detection in cotton production systems. *Comput. Electron. Agric.* **2023**, *205*, 107655. [CrossRef]
107. MacEachern, C.B.; Esau, T.J.; Schumann, A.W.; Hennessy, P.J.; Zaman, Q.U. Detection of fruit maturity stage and yield estimation in wild blueberry using deep learning convolutional neural networks. *Smart Agric. Technol.* **2023**, *3*, 100099. [CrossRef]
108. Rai, N.; Zhang, Y.; Ram, B.G.; Schumacher, L.; Yellavajjala, R.K.; Bajwa, S.; Sun, X. Applications of deep learning in precision weed management: A review. *Comput. Electron. Agric.* **2023**, *206*, 107698. [CrossRef]
109. Han, Y.; Duan, B.; Guan, R.; Yang, G.; Zhen, Z. LUFFD-YOLO: A Lightweight Model for UAV Remote Sensing Forest Fire Detection Based on Attention Mechanism and Multi-Level Feature Fusion. *Remote Sens.* **2024**, *16*, 2177. [CrossRef]
110. Wu, Z.; Xue, R.; Li, H. Real-Time Video Fire Detection via Modified YOLOv5 Network Model. *Fire Technol.* **2022**, *58*, 2377–2403. [CrossRef]
111. Badgujar, C.M.; Poulose, A.; Gan, H. Agricultural object detection with You Only Look Once (YOLO) Algorithm: A bibliometric and systematic literature review. *Comput. Electron. Agric.* **2024**, *223*, 109090. [CrossRef]
112. Qiao, Y.; Guo, Y.; He, D. Cattle body detection based on YOLOv5-ASFF for precision livestock farming. *Comput. Electron. Agric.* **2023**, *204*, 107579. [CrossRef]
113. Kaiyu, T.; Lei, N.; Bozedan, G.; Congsheng, J.; Yuanmeng, F.; Liang, T.; Zhongling, H.; Xiang, J.; Kun, J. Application of Yolo Algorithm in Livestock Counting and Identificatiom System. In Proceedings of the 2023 20th International Computer Conference on Wavelet Active Media Technology and Information Processing (ICCWAMTIP), Chengdu, China, 15–17 December 2023; pp. 1–6.
114. Zhu, L.; Zhang, J.; Jia, C. An Improved YOLOv5-based Method for Surface Defect Detection of Steel Plate. In Proceedings of the 2022 China Automation Congress (CAC), Xiamen, China, 25–27 November 2022; pp. 2233–2238.
115. Wang, B.; Wang, M.; Yang, J.; Luo, H. YOLOv5-CD: Strip steel surface defect detection method based on coordinate attention and a decoupled head. *Meas. Sens.* **2023**, *30*, 100909. [CrossRef]
116. Guo, Z.; Wang, C.; Yang, G.; Huang, Z.; Li, G. MSFT-YOLO: Improved YOLOv5 Based on Transformer for Detecting Defects of Steel Surface. *Sensors* **2022**, *22*, 3467. [CrossRef] [PubMed]
117. Dong, C.; Pang, C.; Li, Z.; Zeng, X.; Hu, X. PG-YOLO: A Novel Lightweight Object Detection Method for Edge Devices in Industrial Internet of Things. *IEEE Access* **2022**, *10*, 123736–123745. [CrossRef]
118. Tianjiao, L.; Hong, B. A optimized YOLO method for object detection. In Proceedings of the 2020 16th International Conference on Computational Intelligence and Security (CIS), Nanning, China, 27–30 November 2020; pp. 30–34.
119. Wang, J.; Dai, H.; Chen, T.; Liu, H.; Zhang, X.; Zhong, Q.; Lu, R. Toward surface defect detection in electronics manufacturing by an accurate and lightweight YOLO-style object detector. *Sci. Rep.* **2023**, *13*, 7062. [CrossRef]
120. Schneidereit, S.; Yarahmadi, A.M.; Schneidereit, T.; Breuß, M.; Gebauer, M. YOLO-Based Object Detection in Industry 4.0 Fischertechnik Model Environment. In *Intelligent Systems and Applications*; Arai, C.K., Ed.; Springer: Cham, Switzerland, 2024; pp. 1–20.
121. Vu, T.-T.-H.; Pham, D.-L.; Chang, T.-W. A YOLO-based Real-time Packaging Defect Detection System. *Procedia Comput. Sci.* **2023**, *217*, 886–894. [CrossRef]
122. Yu, M.; Wan, Q.; Tian, S.; Hou, Y.; Wang, Y.; Zhao, J. Equipment Identification and Localization Method Based on Improved YOLOv5s Model for Production Line. *Sensors* **2022**, *22*, 10011. [CrossRef] [PubMed]
123. Liu, Z.; Lv, H. YOLO_Bolt: A lightweight network model for bolt detection. *Sci. Rep.* **2024**, *14*, 656. [CrossRef] [PubMed]
124. Dai, Z. Uncertainty-aware accurate insulator fault detection based on an improved YOLOX model. *Energy Rep.* **2022**, *8*, 12809–12821. [CrossRef]
125. Zendehdel, N.; Chen, H.; Leu, M.C. Real-time tool detection in smart manufacturing using You-Only-Look-Once (YOLO)v5. *Manuf. Lett.* **2023**, *35*, 1052–1059. [CrossRef]
126. Le, H.F.; Zhang, L.J.; Liu, Y.X. Surface Defect Detection of Industrial Parts Based on YOLOv5. *IEEE Access* **2022**, *10*, 130784–130794. [CrossRef]
127. Cong, P.; Lv, K.; Feng, H.; Zhou, J. Improved YOLOv3 Model for Workpiece Stud Leakage Detection. *Electronics* **2022**, *11*, 3430. [CrossRef]
128. Xu, X.; Zhang, X.; Zhang, T. Lite-YOLOv5: A Lightweight Deep Learning Detector for On-Board Ship Detection in Large-Scene Sentinel-1 SAR Images. *Remote Sens.* **2022**, *14*, 1018. [CrossRef]

129. Nishant, B.; Gill, S.S.; Raj, B. Improving Quality Assurance: Automated Defect Detection in Soap Bar Packaging Using YOLO-V5. In Proceedings of the 2023 International Conference on Electrical, Electronics, Communication and Computers (ELEXCOM), Roorkee, India, 26–27 August 2023; pp. 1–6.
130. Tran, V.T.; To, T.S.; Nguyen, T.-N.; Tran, T.D. Safety Helmet Detection at Construction Sites Using YOLOv5 and YOLOR. In *Intelligence of Things: Technologies and Applications*; Nguyen, N.-T., Dao, N.-N., Pham, Q.-D., Le, H.A., Eds.; Springer International Publishing: Cham, Switzerland, 2022; pp. 339–347.
131. Chen, Y.; Liu, H.; Chen, J.; Hu, J.; Zheng, E. Insu-YOLO: An Insulator Defect Detection Algorithm Based on Multiscale Feature Fusion. *Electronics* **2023**, *12*, 3210. [CrossRef]
132. Wang, C.-Y.; Yeh, I.H.; Hong, Y. YOLOv9: Learning What You Want to Learn Using Programmable Gradient Information. *arXiv* **2024**, arXiv:2402.13616.
133. Ultralytics. YOLO-NAS. 2023. Available online: https://docs.ultralytics.com/models/yolo-nas/#which-tasks-and-modes-are-supported-by-yolo-nas-models (accessed on 15 October 2024).
134. Liu, Z.; Wang, Y.; Han, K.; Zhang, W.; Ma, S.; Gao, W. Post-training quantization for vision transformer. *Adv. Neural Inf. Process. Syst.* **2021**, *34*, 28092–28103.
135. Chu, X.; Li, L.; Zhang, B. Make RepVGG Greater Again: A Quantization-aware Approach. *arXiv* **2022**, arXiv:2212.01593. [CrossRef]
136. Wang, C.-Y.; Hong, Y.; Yeh, I.H.; Wu, Y.-H.; Chen, P.-Y.; Hsieh, J.-W. CSPNet: A New Backbone that can Enhance Learning Capability of CNN. *arXiv* **2019**, arXiv:1911.11929.
137. Zhang, X.; Zeng, H.; Guo, S.; Zhang, L. Efficient Long-Range Attention Network for Image Super-resolution. *arXiv* **2022**, arXiv:2203.06697.
138. Wang, A.; Chen, H.; Liu, L.; Chen, K.; Lin, Z.; Han, J.; Ding, G. YOLOv10: Real-Time End-to-End Object Detection. *arXiv* **2024**, arXiv:2405.14458.
139. Khanam, R.; Hussain, M. YOLOv11: An Overview of the Key Architectural Enhancements. *arXiv* **2024**, arXiv:2410.17725.
140. Ciaglia, F.; Zuppichini, F.S.; Guerrie, P.; McQuade, M.; Solawetz, J. Roboflow 100: A rich, multi-domain object detection benchmark. *arXiv* **2022**, arXiv:2211.13523.
141. Shao, S.; Li, Z.; Zhang, T.; Peng, C.; Yu, G.; Zhang, X.; Li, J.; Sun, J. Objects365: A large-scale, high-quality dataset for object detection. In Proceedings of the IEEE/CVF International Conference on Computer Vision, Seoul, Republic of Korea, 27 October–2 November 2019; pp. 8430–8439.
142. Lin, T.-Y.; Maire, M.; Belongie, S.; Hays, J.; Perona, P.; Ramanan, D.; Dollár, P.; Zitnick, C.L. Microsoft coco: Common objects in context. In Proceedings of the Computer Vision–ECCV 2014: 13th European Conference, Zurich, Switzerland, 6–12 September 2014; Proceedings, Part V 13. pp. 740–755.
143. Mittal, P. A comprehensive survey of deep learning-based lightweight object detection models for edge devices. *Artif. Intell. Rev.* **2024**, *57*, 242. [CrossRef]
144. Hussain, M. Yolov1 to v8: Unveiling each variant–a comprehensive review of yolo. *IEEE Access* **2024**, *12*, 42816–42833. [CrossRef]
145. Wang, J.; Yang, P.; Liu, Y.; Shang, D.; Hui, X.; Song, J.; Chen, X. Research on improved yolov5 for low-light environment object detection. *Electronics* **2023**, *12*, 3089. [CrossRef]
146. Kazmi, S.M.K.A.; Aafaq, N.; Khan, M.A.; Khalil, M.; Saleem, A. From Pixel to Peril: Investigating Adversarial Attacks on Aerial Imagery Through Comprehensive Review and Prospective Trajectories. *IEEE Access* **2023**, *11*, 81256–81278. [CrossRef]
147. Wen, Y.; Wang, L. Yolo-sd: Simulated feature fusion for few-shot industrial defect detection based on YOLOv8 and stable diffusion. *Int. J. Mach. Learn. Cybern.* **2024**, *15*, 4589–4601. [CrossRef]
148. Chen, J.; Er, M.J. Dynamic YOLO for small underwater object detection. *Artif. Intell. Rev.* **2024**, *57*, 165. [CrossRef]
149. Liu, L.; Song, X.; Song, H.; Sun, S.; Han, X.-F.; Akhtar, N.; Mian, A. Yolo-3DMM for Simultaneous Multiple Object Detection and Tracking in Traffic Scenarios. *IEEE Trans. Intell. Transp. Syst.* **2024**, *25*, 9467–9481. [CrossRef]
150. El Ghazouali, S.; Mhirit, Y.; Oukhrid, A.; Michelucci, U.; Nouira, H. FusionVision: A comprehensive approach of 3D object reconstruction and segmentation from RGB-D cameras using YOLO and fast segment anything. *Sensors* **2024**, *24*, 2889. [CrossRef] [PubMed]
151. Ali, M.L.; Zhang, Z. Natural Human-Computer Interface Based on Gesture Recognition with YOLO to Enhance Virtual Lab Users' Immersive Feeling. In Proceedings of the 2024 ASEE Annual Conference & Exposition, Portland, OR, USA, 23–26 June 2024.
152. Talha, S.A.; Manasreh, D.; Nazzal, M.D. The Use of Lidar and Artificial Intelligence Algorithms for Detection and Size Estimation of Potholes. *Buildings* **2024**, *14*, 1078. [CrossRef]
153. Al Amin, R.; Hasan, M.; Wiese, V.; Obermaisser, R. FPGA-based Real-Time Object Detection and Classification System using YOLO for Edge Computing. *IEEE Access* **2024**, *12*, 73268–73278. [CrossRef]
154. Xue, C.; Xia, Y.; Wu, M.; Chen, Z.; Cheng, F.; Yun, L. EL-YOLO: An efficient and lightweight low-altitude aerial objects detector for onboard applications. *Expert Syst. Appl.* **2024**, *256*, 124848. [CrossRef]

computers

MDPI

Review

Object Tracking Using Computer Vision: A Review

Pushkar Kadam *,†, Gu Fang *,† and Ju Jia Zou †

School of Engineering, Design and Built Environment, Western Sydney University, Locked Bag 1797, Penrith, NSW 2751, Australia; j.zou@westernsydney.edu.au
* Correspondence: 18745753@student.westernsydney.edu.au (P.K.); g.fang@westernsydney.edu.au (G.F.)
† These authors contributed equally to this work.

Abstract: Object tracking is one of the most important problems in computer vision applications such as robotics, autonomous driving, and pedestrian movement. There has been a significant development in camera hardware where researchers are experimenting with the fusion of different sensors and developing image processing algorithms to track objects. Image processing and deep learning methods have significantly progressed in the last few decades. Different data association methods accompanied by image processing and deep learning are becoming crucial in object tracking tasks. The data requirement for deep learning methods has led to different public datasets that allow researchers to benchmark their methods. While there has been an improvement in object tracking methods, technology, and the availability of annotated object tracking datasets, there is still scope for improvement. This review contributes by systemically identifying different sensor equipment, datasets, methods, and applications, providing a taxonomy about the literature and the strengths and limitations of different approaches, thereby providing guidelines for selecting equipment, methods, and applications. Research questions and future scope to address the unresolved issues in the object tracking field are also presented with research direction guidelines.

Keywords: object tracking; computer vision; image processing; data association; deep learning

1. Introduction

Object tracking using computer vision is one of the most important functions of machines that interact with the dynamics of the real world, such as autonomous ground vehicles [1], autonomous aerial drones [2], robotics [3], and missile tracking systems [4]. For machines to operate and adapt according to real-world dynamics, it is essential to monitor changes. These changes are usually the motions that must be sensed through different sensors, followed by the machines responding according to these changes [4]. Computer vision mimics the human ability to observe these changes. Humans intuitively understand the change in their environment due to different senses, which helps them navigate their world. Vision is one of the primary senses that allow humans to navigate their environment. To design autonomous machines that perform human tasks such as driving [1,3,5–10], fishing [11], agricultural activities [2], and medical diagnoses [12–16], computer vision can help increase productivity. The inclusion of computer vision in human–computer interaction, robotics, and medical diagnoses provides humans with better tools for completing tasks efficiently and making decisions with better insights. Therefore, it is essential to investigate different methods, tools, and potential applications to evaluate their limitations and future scope for object tracking problems in computer vision to improve work efficiency and develop an autonomous system that works well with humans.

Different insights can be gained by looking at a holistic view of object tracking in computer vision that complements various aspects of the problem. Therefore, this review synthesises and categorises information regarding different aspects, such as sensors, datasets, approaches, and applications of object tracking problems in computer vision. The main contributions of this review are as follows:

- A systemic literature review in object tracking based on hardware usage, datasets, image processing and deep learning methods, and application areas.
- Recommendations and guidelines for selecting sensors, datasets, and application methodologies based on their advantages and limitations.
- A taxonomy for sensor equipment and methodologies.
- Research questions and future scope to address unresolved issues in the object tracking field.

This review highlights the development of object tracking methods in computer vision over the last ten years. The review takes major journal articles published since 2013 in object tracking in computer vision and aims to outline the progress made in this field. This review highlights the different approaches, methods, equipment, datasets, and object tracking applications. By highlighting current development, the review consolidates the data on methods, applications, and types of vision sensors, enabling engineers and software developers to make informed choices while developing their systems for different applications. Furthermore, this review identifies different limitations in current methods and proposes future developments to help push the boundaries of object tracking.

In this paper, Section 2 outlines different reviews performed in object tracking and distinguishes this review from these previous reviews. Section 3 discusses the types of equipment for different vision sensors and how they impact development. Section 4 provides the overview of available datasets for benchmarking object tracking results. Section 5 lays out the different approaches and methods used in object tracking. Section 6 lists the different areas where object tracking in computer vision is deployed. Section 7 provides a discussion of object tracking methods and datasets. Section 8 provides limitations and future work along with the research questions and recommendations to address them. Section 9 outlines the conclusion of this study. Figure 1 shows the structure of the review.

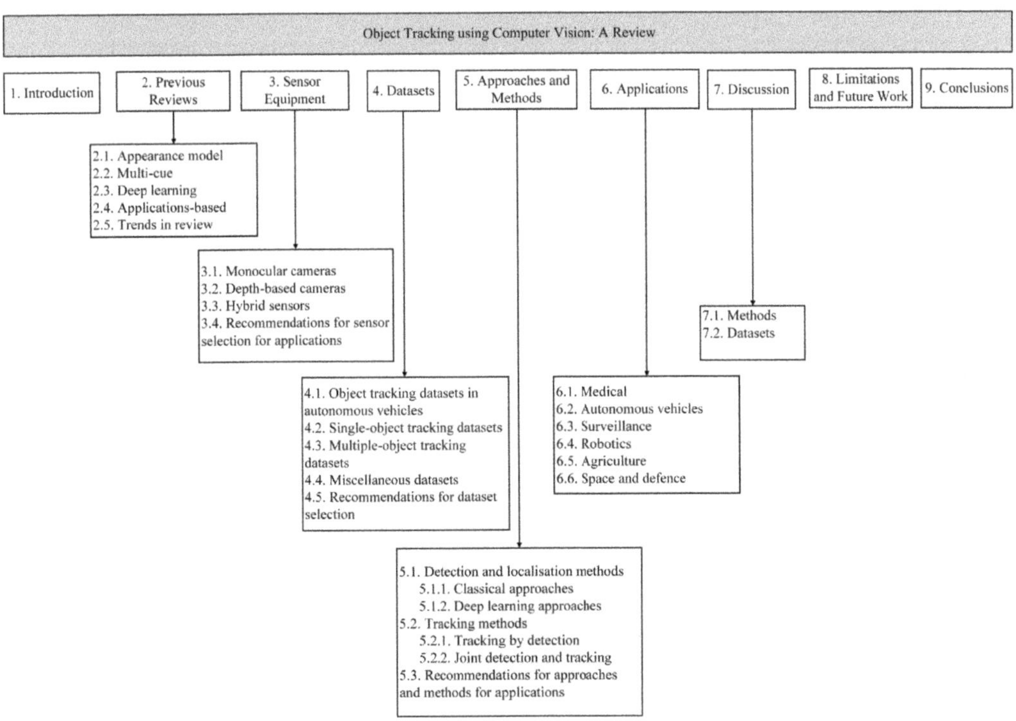

Figure 1. Structure of the review.

2. Previous Reviews

There has been a considerable development in object tracking using computer vision. Previous review articles and surveys focus on a niche area of the object tracking problem. A review focusing exclusively on a subarea of the research field is often beneficial in investigating specific gaps in the literature. However, widening the scope of the literature review helps to identify whether a particular approach has an advantage over the others. Furthermore, a review of the field of research provides a roadmap for researchers and engineers to investigate the problem further according to the needs of the application. This section identifies different reviews covering different aspects of the object tracking problem and distinguishes this review from these previous reviews. This section also outlines the main contribution of each review, which acts as a roadmap for different research niches in the object tracking literature.

2.1. *Appearance Model*

Any object, such as circles, squares, cylinders, and triangles, can be deconstructed to its basic geometry. Identifying these geometric features can assist in detecting the objects in an image frame. These types of visual appearance form object descriptors, which use different features of the object, such as edges and corners, to construct a mathematical model for object identification.

In their survey of appearance models, Li et al. [17] reviewed the literature on visual representation as per their feature-construction mechanism. Since object tracking methods have problems handling complex object appearance changes due to illumination, occlusion, shape deformation, and camera motion, Li et al. [17] concluded that it was essential to effectively model the 2D appearance of tracked objects for successful visual tracking. Their survey focused on the detection methods as a precursor to the tracking-by-detection approach. While appearance models are advantageous in object detection, they are still handcrafted to particular object detection. Handcrafted feature models for face detection will differ from human body detection. While that survey proposed learning techniques such as support vector machines and particle filtering, their learning is dependent upon the training sample selection.

2.2. *Multi-Cue*

Since the publication of the review by Li et al. [17] in 2013, there have been significant improvements in deep learning methods, which have proven effective in object detection [18,19]. In their survey, Kumar et al. [19] identified the research in multi-cue object tracking that used appearance models in traditional and deep learning approaches. Multi-cue methods rely on multiple cues in the image, such as colour, texture, contour, and object features, to develop descriptors to identify the object. They surveyed methods that used handcrafted features integrated with deep learning-based models to provide robust tracking algorithms.

2.3. *Deep Learning*

There was a surge in the review of deep learning methods for object tracking, with two reviews in 2021 and three reviews in 2022. Park et al. [20] reviewed the evolution of multiple-object tracking in deep learning by categorising the previous multiple object tracking algorithm in 12 approaches. They also reviewed the benchmark datasets and standard evaluation methods. Kalake et al. [21] reviewed deep learning-based online multiple-object tracking and ranked the networks on different public benchmark datasets. Mandal et al. [22] provided an empirical review of the state-of-the-art deep learning methods for change detection by categorising the existing approaches into different deep learning methods. Furthermore, they provided an empirical analysis of the evaluation settings adopted by existing deep learning methods. Guo et al. [23] reviewed deep learning methods for multiple-object tracking in autonomous driving. Their review categorised the algorithms based on tracking by detection, joint detection and tracking, and transformer-based tracking.

They identified multiple-object tracking datasets and provided an experimental analysis and future research direction in deep learning. While it is important to examine deep learning methods in isolation to identify the best methods according to the solution, it is also important to consider traditional appearance-based and statistical models for certain types of applications. Therefore, studying and reviewing traditional and deep learning methods can provide insights into method selection based on hardware and applications.

2.4. Applications-Based

Recent reviews have looked into detection-based multiple-object tracking [24], data association methods [25], long-term visual tracking [26], and methods used in ship tracking [27]. Dai et al. [24] introduced a taxonomy of multiple-object tracking and provided a detailed summary of the results of algorithms on popular datasets. Liu et al. [26] reviewed long-term tracking algorithms while describing existing benchmarks and evaluation protocols. Rocha et al. [27] reviewed datasets and state-of-the-art algorithms for single and multiple-object tracking with the view of applying them to ship tracking. Furthermore, they provided insights into developing novel datasets, benchmarking metrics, and novel ship-tracking algorithms. These reviews are focused on specific applications, such as single- or multiple-object tracking, and provide direction for research in their respective fields.

2.5. Trend in Reviews

Different approaches, such as appearance models, data association, and long-term tracking, were reviewed from previous reviews over the last ten years. A summary of reviews works on object tracking is provided in Table 1. Figure 2 shows the number of reviews covering different areas of object tracking from 2013 to 2023. A trend is noticed in Figure 2 where there is a peak of interest in object tracking in 2022, with five papers, out of which three focus exclusively on deep learning methods. The exclusive nature of the literature surveyed in recent reviews necessitates a comparative evaluation of the different approaches. Also, hardware equipment and hardware constraints in the application require investigating different types of sensors and their corresponding methods, applications, and scopes. Furthermore, based on an overview of the object tracking field, guidelines, and recommendations for the methods will contribute to the decision-making process for specific applications. Therefore, this survey aims to investigate different sensor equipment, datasets, approaches and methods, and object tracking applications in computer vision.

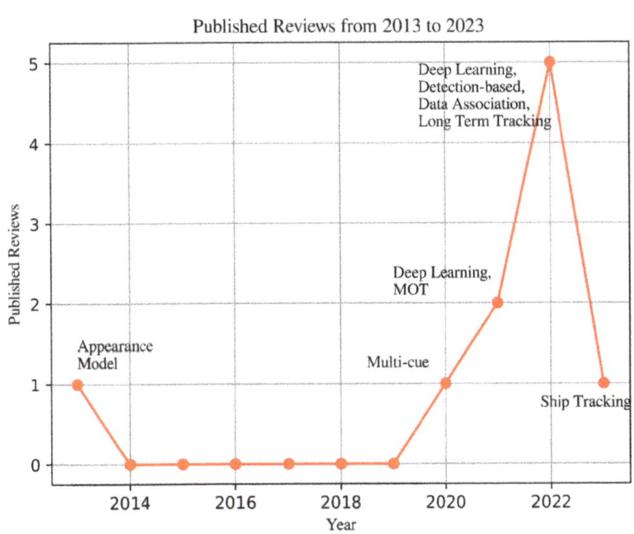

Figure 2. Trend in reviews from 2013 to 2023.

Table 1. Summary of the review works on object tracking.

Paper	Year	Topic	Main Contributions
[17]	2013	Appearance models in visual object tracking	• Review of visual representation according to their feature-construction mechanism. • Existing statistical modelling schemes for tracking by detection.
[19]	2020	Multi-cue-based visual tracking	• Categorisation of multi-cue object tracking based on the exploited appearance model into traditional architecture and deep learning-based tracker.
[20]	2021	Multiple object tracking in deep learning approach.	• Categorisation of previous MOT algorithms into 12 approaches and discussion of the main procedures for each category. • A review of the benchmark datasets and standard evaluation methods for evaluating MOT.
[21]	2021	Deep learning approaches in real-time multiple-object tracking	• Review of deep learning-based online MOT methods and networks that rank highest in the public benchmark.
[22]	2022	Deep learning frameworks for change detection	• Model design-based categorisation of the existing approaches. • Presentation of empirical analysis of evaluation settings for deep learning. • Future directions for change detection.
[23]	2022	Deep learning-based visual multiple-object tracking algorithm for autonomous driving	• Detailed review of object tracking methods: tracking by detection (TBD), joint detection and tracking (JDT), and transformer-based tracking.
[24]	2022	Detection-based video multiple-object tracking	• Taxonomy based on the MOT problem. • Summary of the results of 40 algorithms on popular datasets.
[25]	2022	Data association in multiple-object tracking	• Review of data association techniques via uniquely defined similarity functions and filters for multiple-object tracking. • Taxonomy of data association methods.
[26]	2022	Long term visual tracking	• Thorough review of long-term tracking, summarising the long-term tracking algorithms from framework architectures, and utilisation of intermediate tracking results' perspective.
[27]	2023	Ship tracking	• Review of datasets and state-of-the-art tracking algorithms for single- and multiple-object tracking. • Provides insights for developing novel datasets, benchmarking metrics, and novel ship-tracking algorithms.
Ours	2024	Object tracking in computer vision	• Systemic literature review on hardware usage, datasets, image processing and deep learning methods, and application areas. • Recommendations and guidelines for selecting sensors, datasets, and application methodologies based on their advantages and limitations. • Taxonomy for the sensor equipment and methodologies. • Research questions and future scope to address unresolved issues in the object tracking field.

3. Sensor Equipment

The development and implementation of object tracking methods begin with the sensor input. The choice of sensor equipment depends upon different constraints of the problem, such as depth requirement [10,28,29], tracking objects from multiple viewpoints [30], or intercepting the object following a certain trajectory [4]. Based upon the different problem constraints, different types of vision sensors such as monocular, stereo, depth-based camera, and hybrid vision sensors are used. Figure 3 shows the taxonomy of sensor equipment studied in the literature. The following sections categorise the research based on the types of vision sensors.

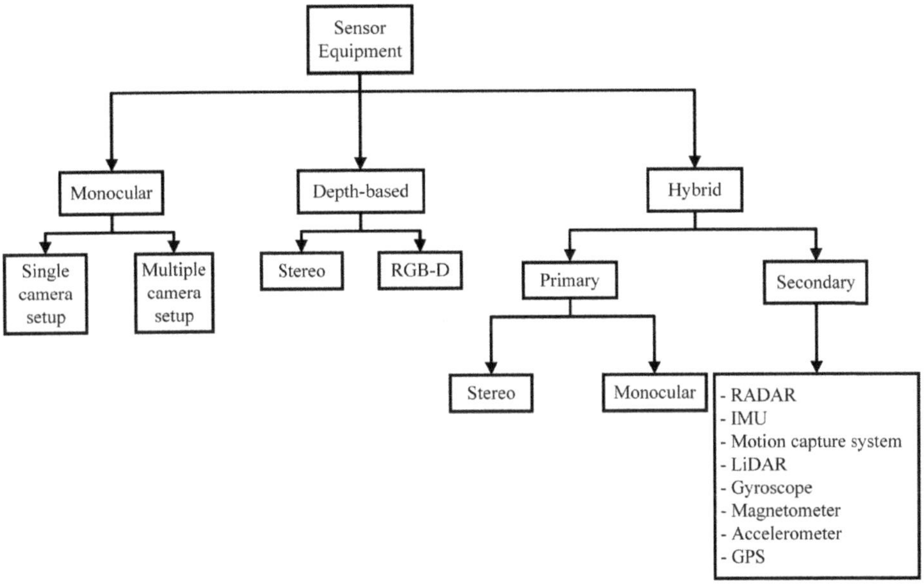

Figure 3. Taxonomy of sensor equipment.

3.1. Monocular Cameras

Monocular cameras are widely used in object tracking. A monocular camera refers to a single camera in a computer vision system, where the system relies on extracting information from a single image form the camera. While it is difficult to estimate the depth from a single image, some researchers incorporate multiple monocular cameras with the principles of stereoscopy that give the 3D position of the target object [30]. Considering the advantages and limitations of monocular vision, different methods are developed based on the information available from the single image or a modified system that incorporates multiple monocular cameras [30], eventually becoming uncalibrated stereo vision [31]. Since the cost and availability of cameras are important considerations in some applications, monocular cameras become a suitable option.

The camera setup is important for developing application-specific datasets. Kwon et al. [4] used a monocular camera to acquire images from a moving camera. Their approach for using a monocular camera was to derive homography matrices in estimating the pose of a target in six DOFs. Their proposed methods were to be used in a missile application, where the camera of the missile tracks a target missile as a moving object for interception. Their approach for overcoming depth and size information was to use the image sequences from the moving camera on the missile. The motion estimator used these images to estimate the rotational and translation motion of the free-moving target. Their research focused on deriving homography matrices for estimating the motion of a moving target using a monocular camera, and a practical simulation was designed. However, the performance of their methods depended upon accurate feature matching. Thus, any high-resolution monocular camera could be used to apply their methods.

Zarrabeitia et al. [16] used a single and two monocular cameras to detect the trajectories of a water droplet. Two monocular cameras allowed them to construct a stereo system for 3D trajectories. Yan et al. [32] used four fixed monocular cameras for handover problems in computer vision to track a skater as the skater escapes the field of view (FOV) of one camera to another. Gionfrida et al. [13] used a single monocular camera to capture the participant's images to develop a markerless hand motion capture system. They developed the ground truth for the hand movement with a marker-based approach using an eight-camera Qualisys motion capture system. They compared the motion obtained from a markerless monocular camera system with the ground truth. Huang et al. [33] developed a setup consisting of an overhead crane trolley, a camera, a spherical marker, a computer with a GUI connected to a motion control system, and a vision computer to process images and track the motion of a payload. The setup was designed in the lab, but it had the potential to be applied on outdoor overhead handling cranes.

The monocular camera setups have a unique application that solves a particular problem; however, the methods developed using these setups often require some modifications if the constraints of the problems change. The advantage of constructing a monocular camera setup is that multiple camera views can be used, which helps detect depth and address occlusion. Furthermore, multiple cues become accessible in the image by using different types of monocular cameras, such as infrared and RGB, on a setup. However, the disadvantage of such a system could be that a thorough calibration must be performed. Also, the delay in sequentially triggering multiple monocular cameras must be addressed since the data could be lost due to a delay in image capture in a dynamic environment. Knowing the capability and application is essential before selecting the appropriate camera system. Table 2 summarises the different types of camera systems used in literature with their depth estimation capability provided by the methods in the paper and their respective applications. Therefore, monocular camera setups are often developed when the problem has a unique requirement.

Table 2. Summary of monocular camera systems.

Paper	Camera System	Depth Estimation	Depth Estimation Method	Application
[4]	Moving camera	✓	Homography matrices	Missile interception
[16]	One or two cameras	✓	Stereo reconstruction	Bloodletting events (medical)
[32]	Four cameras	x	-	Tracking skaters (sports)
[13]	Single camera	x	-	Biomechanical assessment (Medical)
[33]	Single camera	x	-	Overhead crane

3.2. Depth-Based Cameras

Depth-based cameras provide images of the scene along with depth information. Stereo and RGB-D (RGB-Depth) cameras are the two types of depth-based cameras used in the object tracking literature. A stereo camera system comprises two or more monocular cameras, often as a single unit such as Bumblebee2 [10,28,29] or built from multiple monocular cameras [30]. RGB-D cameras such as Microsoft's Kinect sensor collect RGB images and depth information using an infrared (IR) projector and camera based on the principle of structured light [34]. Object tracking methods are developed by setting up the depth-based camera [12,28] or by using a public dataset [35] as in the case of monocular camera data. Since depth information is vital for machines to interact with their environment and know the location of the object in the real world, it is important to consider different depth-based camera setups for object tracking.

Stereo cameras are widely used in applications where depth measurement is required. Garcia et al. [36] developed a prototype of a stereo camera by using two static low-cost cameras. That stereo camera could be overhead in different urban environments with constant lighting. With the constraint of constant lighting conditions, the system was designed to track the movement, size, and height of the people passing under the camera. The system could be adjusted to operate at different heights depending on the urban environment by adjusting the system parameters to comply with the average height of the people and the camera location from the ground. Chuang et al. [11] used a stereo camera with six LED strobes, batteries, and computer housing for underwater operation. Their camera could have 4-megapixel images, and the data transfer rate was five frames per second using an Ethernet cable. Hu et al. [37] used two AVT F-504B cameras to construct a binocular stereo camera mounted on a tripod. They calibrated the camera using the calibration toolbox [38] in MATLAB. Yang et al. [15] used a binocular stereo placed in front of a person to collect data for hand gestures. Sinisterra et al. [29] mounted a Bumblebee2 stereo camera on top of an unmanned surface vehicle that was used for chasing a moving marine vehicle. Busch et al. [2] mounted their stereo camera on a manipulator arm attached to a drone for tracking tree branch movement. During the experimental procedures, they placed the stereo camera in front of the tree branch on an actuation system capable of performing sway action. Wu et al. [39] also developed a stereo camera mounted on a quadcopter with an NUC computer to detect and track a target. Richey et al. [12] used a stereo camera to track breast surface deformation for medical applications. Their setup consisted of an optical tracker, ultrasound, guidance display, and pen-marked fiducial points on the skin whose ground truth was collected by an optically tracked stylus. The depth information measured with the help of the stereo-matching process helps in the respective applications. Czajkowska et al. [14] used a stereo camera setup and a stereoscopic navigation system called Polaris Vicra to evaluate ground truth. Since a binocular stereo camera can be constructed by aligning two cameras or purchased as a single unit, the stereo setup is becoming popular when depth information is required.

RGB-D is another depth-based camera with an infrared projector and collector system to measure depth along with the RGB channels of the image [34]. The depth value relative to the position of the camera is collected for every pixel in the RGB-D camera. Kriechbaumer et al. [28] used RGB-D data for developing their methods; however, their methods were adapted to stereo later. Similarly, Rasoulidanesh et al. [40] used the RGB-D Princeton pedestrian dataset [41]. The use of RGB-D for tracking in the literature has been limited to public datasets developed using RGB-D cameras and in the indoor environment, as outlined by Kriechbaumer et al. [28]. An RGB-D camera has certain limitations when the object is far away, making it difficult for applications to track objects using drones [42]. Therefore, while RGB-D cameras have advantages in the indoor environment, they may not be suitable for outdoor applications due to their limited sensor range, which misses faraway objects.

Depth-based cameras are useful for localising the tracking object in a 3D space relative to the depth camera. Table 3 summarises the different types of depth-based vision sensors used in the surveyed literature. The table categorises cameras based on "Off the shelf" and "Constructed". As the name suggests, off-the-shelf cameras are purchased as a single unit, while constructed cameras use different components, such as two monocular cameras, to construct a stereo camera. The advantage of using off-the-shelf products is that they often come with a software development kit that allows the user to use pre-built tools such as calibration, depth detection, disparity map, and point cloud map generation. The constructed camera would have an advantage where the problem constraint requires a custom baseline or camera lens, which may not be part of the off-the-shelf product. Furthermore, other aspects such as depth calculation methods, frames per second (FPS), and resolution play an important role in depth measurement accuracy and are often constraints on applications. Therefore, a depth-based camera has an advantage over a monocular camera as it provides all the information obtained from monocular (RGB image) and depth estimation capability.

Table 3. Summary of depth-based cameras.

Paper	Type	Off the Shelf	Constructed	Camera	Depth Calculation Method	Application	FPS	Resolution
[36]	Stereo	x	✓	Two static cameras	Epipolar geometry	Pedestrian tracking	30	320 × 240
[11]	Stereo	✓	x	Cam-trawl	Stereo triangulation	Tracking fish	5	2048 × 2048
[37]	Stereo	x	✓	AVT F-504B	Epipolar geometry	Pedestrian tracking	25.6	1360 × 1024
[29]	Stereo	✓	x	Bumblebee2	Stereo matching using SAD	Tracking ship	15	320 × 240
[2]	Stereo	✓	x	ZED	3D point cloud	Tree branch tracking	30	1920 × 1080
[39]	Stereo	✓	x	Mynteye	Stereo matching	Air and ground target tracking	25	752 × 480
[12]	Stereo	✓	x	Grasshopper	Stereo matching	Fiducial tracking for surgical guidance	5	1200 × 1600
[28]	Stereo	✓	x	Bumblebee2	Stereo triangulation	Autonomous ship localisation	8.2	1024 × 768
[40]	RGB-D	✓	x	KinectV2	Time of flight	Pedestrian tracking	30	1920 × 1080

3.3. *Hybrid Sensors*

In applications with uncertainties in vision data collection, additional sensors whose data can complement that of the vision data are used. These sensor setups are classified as hybrid sensors as they incorporate multiple sensors, which is important in the development of the method. Cesic et al. [10] mounted a stereo camera and radar on a moving vehicle in urban scenarios. Similarly, Ram et al. [43] also used radar and a monocular camera for autonomous cars, while Feng et al. [5] used a combination of monocular camera with an inertial measurement unit (IMU). Persic et al. [3] used a combination of stereo, monocular, and motion capture systems, monocular and radar, and monocular and LiDAR systems mounted on a car for autonomous driving. Kriechbaumer et al. [28] based their system on a platform on a survey vessel consisting of a Bumblebee2 stereo camera, an inertial measurement unit (IMU) fused with tri-axial MEMS gyroscope, accelerometer and magnetometers, a GPS receiver, a 360-degree prism, and a total station, which is an equipment used for land surveying. Contrary to detecting targets using drones, Zheng et al. [42] developed a panoramic stereo camera system on the ground to detect flying drones. Their platform comprised four stereo cameras mounted on a stand with a computer, IMU, router, and GPS module. The IMU and GPS were located on the ground node and used to measure the attitude and position of each sensing node in a global coordinate frame. Since the KITTI [35] dataset consists of different types of sensors, the research in [1,5,8,9,44] using this dataset also fit under hybrid sensors with the primary goal of localising a vehicle. Table 4 summarises the sensors based on primary sensors and a vision sensor along with the secondary sensor that complements the primary sensor. From the applications of different methods, hybrid sensors are used where the risk and uncertainties are high, such as in autonomous vehicles and drones. Therefore, for outdoor applications, combining vision sensor data with other sensor data to create a hybrid system is beneficial for high-risk applications.

Table 4. Summary of hybrid camera systems.

Paper	Primary Sensor	Secondary Sensors	Application
[10]	Stereo camera	• RADAR	Autonomous driving
[43]	Monocular camera	• RADAR	Autonomous driving
[5]	Monocular camera	• IMU	Autonomous driving
[3]	Stereo camera	• Motion capture systems • RADAR • LiDAR	Moving target tracking
[28]	Stereo camera	• IMU • Gyroscope • Accelerometer • Magnetometer • GPS	Autonomous ship tracking
[42]	Stereo camera	• IMU • GPS	Drone tracking

3.4. Recommendations for Sensor Selection for Applications

The sensor equipment is the first step to consider based on the type of object tracking application. The correct selection process for the sensor equipment is essential as it relies upon the capabilities of the sensor. Table 5 summarises the category of papers reviewed in the literature in this section. While application plays an important role in selecting a sensor type, other constraints, such as computing and hardware cost, must also be considered. This subsection aims to summarise, compare, and suggest guidelines for selecting sensors.

Monocular cameras, such as webcams, are accessible and less expensive than depth-based cameras. A high-resolution webcam can provide more details in terms of pixel density. However, the higher the resolution, the higher the computation cost to process the images. Furthermore, monocular cameras cannot provide depth information in the scene, but the depth information can be obtained using multiple monocular cameras [16] or a moving camera [4] along with the principles of stereography.

From the insights derived from the literature review, the following guidelines can be used to determine when monocular cameras are sufficient:

- If the tracking application does not require depth information.
- If the system does interact with its environment, such as tracking in sports [32], a biomechanical assessment [13], or observing pedestrian movements, a monocular camera is sufficient.
- If depth information is required, uncalibrated stereo methods can be used with either a moving camera [4] or multiple monocular cameras [16].

Depth-based cameras are more expensive compared to monocular cameras. The advantage of using depth-based cameras such as stereo cameras or RGB-D is that they provide depth information about objects relative to the position of the camera. This is beneficial information for localising a target object in the 3D space. Off-the-shelf depth-based cameras often have the advantage of proprietary software or a software development kit (SDK) provided by the manufacturer. The software provides functionality such as camera calibration, disparity map generation, and point cloud generation. An SDK often comes with the option of multiple programming languages, which provides pre-built code packages. These camera code packages, with features such as depth detection and point cloud generation, can be integrated within projects without the need to develop code from scratch for the camera input processing. Some of the functionalities of the SDK, such as real-time point cloud generation, often require high computer hardware specifications such as a GPU [2]. However, alternative software libraries such as OpenCV can be used to develop methods that do not require GPUs for image processing.

The following guidelines are recommended for selecting depth-based cameras for applications:

- Depth-based cameras are ideal if the depth information of the target object is needed.
- Stereo cameras are better than RGB-D ones in outdoor settings since an RGB-D camera relies on structured light, which may not be suitable for outdoor environments.
- RGB-D cameras are a better option than stereo cameras for indoor applications as the depth accuracy will be higher due to the structured light.
- A constructed stereo setup is a better option for a custom baseline, and the focal length of the lens is required for applications such as in panoramic stereo systems [42].

Hybrid sensors provide additional data for the overall application. For highly critical applications, such as autonomous vehicles, more data that can benefit the dynamic system, such as a moving vehicle in a dynamic environment, are essential. Sensors like IMUs, gyroscopes, and accelerometers can help maintain the stability of the dynamic system, while GPS helps localise it in 3D space. It is important to consider the stability of autonomous vehicles, their localisation in the environment, and other moving objects such as pedestrians and other vehicles.

The following are the recommendations for deciding on a hybrid system:

- Hybrid sensors are the best choice for a dynamic system interacting with a dynamic environment such as an autonomous vehicle [5,10,28,43].
- GPS as an additional sensor with the camera helps localise the camera system in the real world, thereby allowing the localisation of target objects.
- An IMU, accelerometer, and gyroscope provide additional data that can help the control system of the dynamic system for stability while tracking objects.

Table 5. Categorisation of papers based on the vision sensors.

Vision Sensor	Papers
Monocular	[4,13,16,32,33]
Depth-based	[2,6,11,12,14,15,29,36,37,39]
Hybrid	[3,5,10,28,42,43]

4. Datasets

Datasets are essential for evaluating methods and setting standards which cover a wide variety of scenarios. A diverse dataset is helpful to develop methods that can be evaluated before they are deployed in real-world systems. Some public datasets such as HumanEVA [45] and KITTI [35] cover various data catering to specific applications. In contrast, some others [7,42,43,46] develop their datasets for general tracking applications. Researchers who create an in-house dataset are looking for specific scenarios for their applications. The dataset is used for machine learning and deep learning methods to train a classifier for detection and tracking. Therefore, the availability of a dataset is essential for benchmarking the methods and training a machine learning or deep learning model to accomplish the tasks.

4.1. Object Tracking Datasets in Autonomous Vehicles

Research on autonomous driving has significantly increased in the past few years [47]. The KITTI dataset [35] is widely used for benchmarking the methods in autonomous driving applications. The KITTI dataset consists of high-resolution colour and greyscale stereo images, laser scans, GPS, and IMU data. Several researchers [1,5,8,9,44] developed their object tracking methods using the KITTI dataset in the application of autonomous driving. Deepambika and Rahman [9] also used the DAIMLER dataset [48], a pedestrian dataset, to evaluate their methods for autonomous driving. The DAIMLER dataset consists of stereo images captured from a calibrated stereo camera mounted on a vehicle in an urban environment. The pedestrian cutout is comprised of 24-bit PNG format images, float disparity maps, and ground truth shapes.

The Multivehicle Stereo Event Camera (MVSEC) dataset [49] is another stereo image dataset for event-based cameras developed for autonomous driving cars. The MVSEC dataset consists of greyscale images along with IMU data. The stereo camera was constructed from two Dynamic Vision and Active Pixel Sensors (DAVIS) cameras. A Visual Inertial (VI) sensor [50] was mounted on top of the stereo camera. This setup was mounted on a motorcycle handlebar along with GPS. A Velodyne LiDAR system was used to get the ground-truth depth information.

HCI [51] is a synthetic dataset comprising 24 designed scenes with the ground truth of a light field. The dataset comprises four images for three scenes: stratified, test, and training. These scenes consist of patterns and household images with their ground truth. They provide an additional 12 scenes with their ground truth in the dataset, which is not used for official benchmarking. Shen et al. [7] created their dataset for developing their methods by building on the HCI dataset for a potential application in autonomous driving. An autonomous driving dataset is often accompanied by additional sensor data such as GPS, IMU, and stereo camera images. Autonomous navigation is treated as an object tracking problem, and the dataset's availability can help benchmark the methods before deploying them for autonomous cars to avoid dynamic obstacles by tracking them in real time.

4.2. Single-Object Tracking Datasets

Single-object tracking (SOT) is the research area where a single object, as opposed to multiple objects, is the subject of the tracking. There have been different versions of Visual Object Tracking (VOT) datasets from its inception in 2013, with the latest being VOT2022 [52] as a part of the VOT Challenge. The VOT dataset consists of monocular images and is used to benchmark the methods for visual object tracking. Unlike MOT datasets, VOT datasets are for single object tracking.

In VOT2022 [52], the following evaluation protocols were used:

- **Short-term tracker** :
  - Target is localised and reported in each frame.
  - For the target that goes out of frame or gets occluded, there is no target re-detection from these trackers.
  - The information on the target object is not retained when the object is occluded.
- **Short-term tracking with conservative updating**:
  - Similar to the short-term tracker, the target is localised in each frame, and there is no re-detection of the target.
  - Tracking robustness is increased by a selective updating of the visual model based on the estimation confidence.
  - The tracking reliability relies on the confidence estimation, which is based on the object detection confidence, thereby performing a detection operation when the tracking estimation confidence is low.
- **Pseudo-long-term tracker**:
  - When the target position is predicted to be "not visible" due to occlusion or when the target is out of the image frame, it is not reported.
  - There is no explicit tracking re-detection, which means that when the object is occluded, the detection failure is reported, and there are no further efforts to search the object in the image frame.
  - There is an internal mechanism to identify tracking failure where the failure could be due to low confidence in the estimation, object detection, or both.
- **Re-detecting long-term tracker**:
  - Target position is not reported when the target prediction is "not visible".

- Unlike a pseudo-long-term tracker, there is an explicit search over the image frame when the object is lost during tracking.
- Object detection techniques can be employed to detect the object in the entire image frame.
- Upon re-detection, the tracking is continued from the new location.

Object Tracking Benchmark (OTB) [53] is another single-object tracking dataset. OTB-50, consisting of 50 difficult target objects out of 100 targets from OTB [53], was used by Yan et al. [32] to evaluate their trackers. OTB has annotations consisting of 11 attributes: illumination variation, scale variation, occlusion, deformation, motion blur, fast motion, in-plane rotation, out-of-plane rotation, out-of-view, background clutters, and low resolution [53]. The Rigid Pose dataset [54] is a single-object tracking dataset created synthetically. Along with tracking, the dataset can also be used to evaluate methods for occlusion. The dataset consists of four objects from public KIT object model data [55]. These object models are placed on the image and manually manipulated to record the trace, which is used as ground truth.

Zhong et al. [56] used the Rigid Pose dataset for their evaluation. Furthermore, the ACCV14 dataset [57], an RGB-D dataset, was used for their evaluation. The Princeton [41] dataset is an RGB-D dataset used by Rasoulidanesh et al. [40] for evaluating their method for tracking the object along with depth. The Princeton dataset comprises 100 video clips with RGB and depth information and manually annotated bounding boxes as ground truth. Microsoft's Kinect 1.0 sensor was used for data collection with a depth range between 0.5 and 10 m. The Princeton dataset consists of three types of targets, with each scene having a different level of clutter in the background and occlusion.

HumanEva [45] is a multi-view synchronised motion capture dataset consisting of 40,000 frames for each camera. The HumanEva dataset is a pose estimation dataset of four human subjects performing six predefined actions. The ground truth for the motion was captured with ViconPeak, a commercial motion capture system.

Web crawling to download publicly available images on different websites has become more relevant [58]. The Stanford Cars Dataset [59] uses 16,185 images of 196 classes of cars. This dataset was used by Mdfaa et al. [46] to train a classifier for the moving-object class such as a car, and the Describable Textures Dataset (DTD) [60] was used for the non-moving class, such as buildings, in their application of tracking using a drone in a simulated urban environment. Stanford's car images dataset [59] was collected by web crawling popular websites. Then, a deduplication process was applied using perceptual hashing [61] to ensure distinct images belonged to a class. Then, Amazon Mechanical Turk was used to crowdsource the annotations. The DTD [60] consists of 5640 texture images annotated with 47 describable attributes. Like the Stanford dataset, DTD was also downloaded online instead of collecting images in the lab. Although both the Stanford and describable texture datasets are not developed for object tracking, they were used by Mdfaa et al. [46] for training a classifier that would be used for tracking by a detection approach. To evaluate their tracking methods, they used Visual Object Tracker (VOT) benchmarks [62–65]. Thus, a large dataset was available for training.

4.3. Multiple-Object Tracking Datasets

Multiple-object tracking (MOT) is a method in which multiple objects are tracked simultaneously in a given scene. Several datasets have been developed to benchmark the methods where multiple objects are present in a crowded environment. Pedestrian tracking is one such example where the video from a CCTV can be tracked over time. However, any problem in detecting and tracking multiple objects can be classified as an MOT-based problem. MOT [66] is a widely used dataset for evaluating multiple object problems. The MOT dataset, a part of MOTChallenge, has had several versions (MOT15 [67], MOT16 [68], MOT17 [68], and MOT20 [69]) over the years. The images in these datasets are a collection of images from publicly available datasets with standardised annotations. Luo et al. [70] reviewed the MOT tracking methods that outlined the collection of different MOT datasets.

The evaluation metrics are different for multiple object tracking. MOT20 [66] provided the following evaluation metrics:

- **Tracker to target assignment**:
  - No target re-identification.
  - Target object ID is not maintained when the object is not visible.
  - Matching is not performed independently but by a temporal correspondence in each consecutive video frame.
- **Distance measure**:
  - The Intersection over Union (IoU) is used to detect similarity between target and ground truth.
  - The IOU threshold is set to 0.5.
- **Target-like annotations**:
  - Static objects such as pedestrians sitting on a bench or humans in a vehicle are not annotated for tracking; however, the detector is not penalised for tracking these objects.
- **Multiple-Object Tracking Accuracy (MOTA)**:
  MOTA combines three sources of error: false negatives, false positives, and mismatch error.
  $$MOTA = 1 - \frac{\sum_t (FN_t + FP_t + IDSW_t)}{\sum_t GT_t} \quad (1)$$
  - t is the video frame index.
  - GT is the number of ground-truth objects.
  - FN and FP are false negatives and false positives, respectively.
  - $IDSW$ is the mismatch error or identity switch.
- **Multiple-Object Tracking Precision (MOTP)**:
  MOTP is the measure of localisation precision, and it quantifies the localisation accuracy of the detection, thereby providing the actual performance of the tracker.
  $$MOTP = \frac{\sum_{t,i} d_{t,i}}{\sum_t c_t} \quad (2)$$
  - c_t is the number of matches in frame t
  - $d_{t,i}$ is the bounding box's overlap of target i with the ground truth object
- **Tracking quality measures**:
  Tracking quality measures how well the object is tracked over its lifetime.
  - The target is mostly tracked for successful tracking for at least 80% of its lifetime.
  - The target is mostly lost for successful tracking of less than 20% of its lifetime.
  - The target is partially tracked for the rest of the tracks.

Caltech's Pedestrian [71] dataset consists of a video recorded from a car comprising low-resolution images and occluded pedestrians. Wang et al. [72] used the first 1000 frames of the Caltech dataset for their Centretown sequence. Caltech's dataset consists of 10 h of video in traffic in an urban area taken from a vehicle. The dataset consists of 250,000 images along with 350,000 bounding boxes with labels and 2300 unique pedestrian annotations. Caltech's dataset also considered occlusion in their annotation, where they annotated the image frame with a bounding box even when the object was occluded. Three sequences were included in the data. MOT challenges keep improving upon their datasets by including different conditions in the image dataset for future development of MOT methods.

Different datasets were used to evaluate the object tracking methods over different applications. A diverse dataset helps evaluate the methods in different scenarios, improving their potential for adaptability to different real-world circumstances. For the pedestrian tracking problem, the PETS2009 sequence [73] was used. The PETS2009 sequence consists of an image sequence and its ground truth from the footage recorded outdoors in different weather conditions of people performing different behaviours [73]. The PETS2009 dataset was used by Gennaro et al. [30] and Wang et al. [72] for pedestrian tracking application. The region-based object tracking (RBOT) [74] dataset is a monocular RGB dataset developed to determine the pose, such as translation and rotation, of the objects. These are known objects, and their pose is relative to the camera.

4.4. Miscellaneous Datasets

Different from the public datasets, some researchers create their in-house datasets. The reason for creating a dataset is either the unavailability of the data for an application or the application of their methods in a niche case where public datasets are insufficient.

Several datasets were developed using stereo or multiple cameras to detect the 3D location of an object. Zheng et al. [42] developed a stereo vision dataset for tracking unknown MAVs. Yan et al. [32] built a dataset of skaters where the movements of the skaters were tracked over four different monocular cameras as a part of the handover problem in computer vision. Busch et al. [2] collected a dataset using a stereo ZED camera of a pine tree branch. The pine tree branch was mounted on an actuator system to simulate the movement of the branch when capturing the images. Hu et al. [37] build a fully labelled dataset of seven sequence pairs and 20 objects using a calibrated binocular camera. They annotated their dataset with similar attributes to that of OTB [53]. Cesic et al. [10] developed a radar and stereo vision-based dataset for an application in autonomous driving and MOT. The data were collected by mounting the sensors on a car driving in the centre of a three-way street. Kriechbaumer et al. [28] collected more than 15,000 images on a 50 m long reach of the river for the application of tracking surface vehicles. Most of these datasets are either private or available upon request. The use of multiple cameras helps in the localisation and tracking of an object in 3D space.

Datasets developed on monocular cameras are also helpful in 2D tracking. These types of datasets are often accompanied by additional sensor data such as radar or IMU data. Ram et al. [43] created a dataset using a monocular camera and radar equipment for automotive target tracking. Gionfrida et al. [13] developed a labelled dataset for monocular 2D tracking. Garcia and Younes [75] developed a dataset with 8746 images of a mock drogue for the automatic refuelling application of unmanned aircraft. Monocular camera-based datasets are useful when the object's 3D information is not required. However, they are often accompanied by additional sensor data for 3D tracking.

The data collection process is not feasible for some applications, such as aerospace and different illumination conditions. Therefore, researchers create synthetic datasets generated using mathematical models or computer-generated designs. Kwon et al. [4] developed a simulated dataset based on a mathematical model for the applications of missile interception. Biondi et al. [76] developed simulated data by exploiting mathematical models of a smooth Keplerian motion of the target. The Keplerian motion of the target was assumed to describe the equation that provides the position of the centre of mass of the target object and chaser vehicle in the earth-centred inertial frame of reference. They also included the occlusion period in their dataset. While synthetic datasets are readily available to test different methods, they must be evaluated to ensure their authenticity for application.

4.5. Recommendations for Dataset Selection

There are several public datasets available for evaluating methods. The public datasets used for developing and testing object tracking methods are mentioned in Table 6. Developing more datasets by addressing the lack of diversity in current datasets is helpful for the research community in developing better methods.

While the two main categorisations of datasets are single-object tracking and multiple-object tracking, they are further categorised based on their applications. Different uncertainties must be taken into account for autonomous driving, such as self-localisation, safe navigation, obstacle avoidance, and pedestrian detection. Therefore, while autonomous vehicles can be classified as a multiple-object detection problem, they deserve their own category due to their complexity and the research area dedicated to the application of autonomous navigation. Since autonomous vehicles include a range of vehicles, such as automobiles, ships, and aerial vehicles, different datasets cater to each type of application. This dataset is often developed with the help of hybrid sensors because they can provide multiple types of data for high-risk operations.

Single- and multiple-object detection datasets are similar with one exception: their names suggest that they track single or multiple objects. The approach to developing the datasets for single and multiple objects differs from its application and evaluation metrics. Miscellaneous datasets do not fit in either the SOT or MOT categories and were developed by researchers to solve particular problems. The trackers developed for these datasets are limited to the application for which the datasets were developed.

The following are the recommendations for selecting the datasets:

- SOT datasets are sufficient for indoor environments where the tracker is focused on one object.
- MOT datasets are ideal for any outdoor applications where multiple objects are tracked, and their trajectories need to be remembered by the tracker.
- A dataset can be developed and annotated manually or crowd-sourced using platforms like Mechanical Turk [59].
- A simulated or synthetic tracking dataset such as Kwon et al.'s [4] can be developed for applications where the data collection process is not feasible.

Table 6. Datasets used for developing and evaluating object tracking methods.

Dataset	Description	Sensor Type	Data Type	Used by	Links +
KITTI [35]	High-resolution colour and greyscale stereo images, laser scans, GPS, IMU	Stereo + hybrid	MOT	[1,5,8,9,44]	https://www.cvlibs.net/datasets/kitti/
PETS2009 [73]	RGB images from the real world with multiple synchronised cameras	Monocular	MOT	[30,72]	ftp://ftp.cs.rdg.ac.uk/pub/PETS2009/Crowd_PETS09_dataset/a_data/
RBOT [74]	Semi-synthetic dataset with 6-DOF pose tracking	Monocular	SOT	[77]	https://github.com/henningtjaden/RBOT
MVSEC [49]	Event-based stereo images with IMU and GPS data	Stereo + hybrid + event-based	MOT	[6]	https://daniilidis-group.github.io/mvsec/
VOT [62–65]	Visual object tracking dataset	Monocular	SOT	[46]	https://www.votchallenge.net/
MOT (MOT15 [67], MOT16 [68], MOT17 [68], and MOT20 [69])	Collection of publicly available dataset	Monocular	MOT	[78–80]	https://motchallenge.net/
Rigid Pose [54]	Synthetic dataset with varying objects, background motion, occlusions, and noise.	Stereo	SOT	[56]	http://www.karlpauwels.com/datasets/rigid-pose/
Princeton [41]	Video clips along with depth information with manually annotated bounding boxes.	RGB-D	SOT	[40]	http://tracking.cs.princeton.edu
DAIMLER [48]	Pedestrian dataset with a single object class	Stereo	MOT	[9]	http://www.gavrila.net/Datasets/Daimler_Pedestrian_Benchmark_D/daimler_pedestrian_benchmark_d.html
Caltech pedestrian [71]	Pedestrian dataset with ten hours of footage	Monocular	MOT	[72]	https://data.caltech.edu/records/f6rph-90m20
HumanEva [45]	Human subjects performing predefined actions	Monocular + motion sensor	SOT	[81]	https://github.com/mhd-medfa/Single-Object-Tracker

+ The links to the datasets were accessed on 27 February 2024.

5. Approaches and Methods

Computer vision problems are being addressed with two main approaches: classical image processing and deep learning. Since object tracking is also a computer vision problem, these two approaches address this problem. Object tracking problems in computer vision are often divided into two steps: first, the object of interest is detected and then tracked over a sequence of images. The tracking is further divided into different approaches, such as tracking by detection, where the target object is detected in each image frame, and joint tracking, where the detection and tracking happen simultaneously. The tracking can be performed only when the input is a sequence where the object is within the image frame. There are instances where the object disappears because it goes out of the field of view of the camera or is obstructed by other objects. Keeping track of these objects in the middle of the video when they partially disappear has created a class of problems called occlusion. Different filtering and morphological operations are performed in the image processing methods to develop a model for detection and tracking [11,15].

Deep learning models use training data to develop a classifier that detects and locates the object [82–84]. After detecting the objects, both approaches involve using statistical or data association methods to track them. Some researchers aim to develop an end-to-end deep learning model using attention mechanisms to learn a classifier that can track the objects [40].

Apart from tracking by detection, joint detection methods detect the object in a frame and connect the location of the object for every subsequent frame in the video sequence. Another approach is detection by tracking where the objects are located in the first frame of the video. Then, statistical methods predict the future location, and the confidence score is increased further by detection [8,15,44].

Figure 4 gives the taxonomy of the approaches and methods used for object tracking that classifies the approach and categorises the methods in each approach. The following subsections also highlight the strengths and limitations of each approach. This section categorises the methods that rely solely on image processing and deep learning detection methods. Each of the tracking procedures and type of problem, such as MOT and SOT, are outlined in each category.

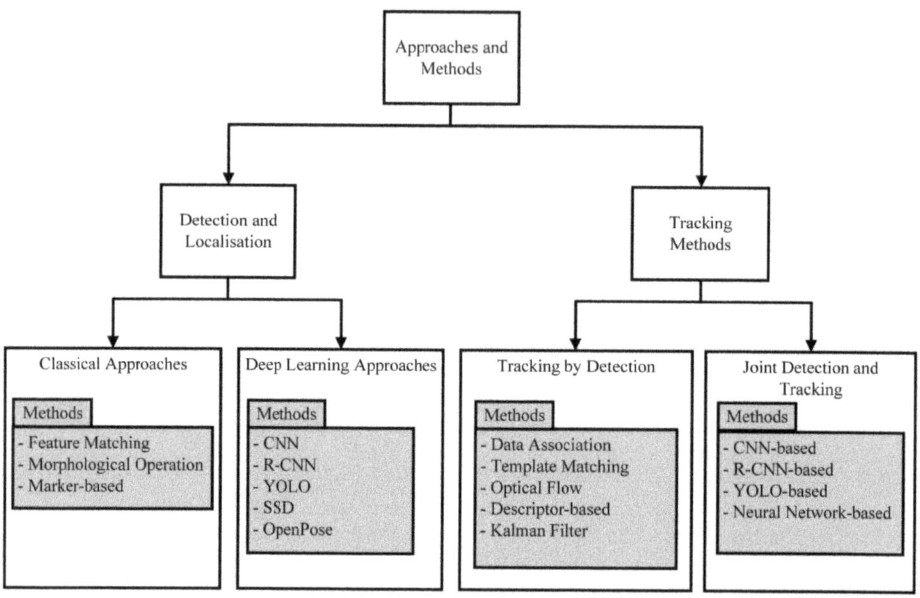

Figure 4. Taxonomy of approaches and methods for object tracking.

5.1. Detection and Localisation Methods

The first step in most tracking problems is detecting and localising the object. Detecting features and tracking those features using image processing has been an approach in many research studies for a long time. However, deep learning methods are becoming more prominent due to their higher accuracy and the use of end-to-end networks for localising and classifying objects. This section categorises and reviews the detection and localisation problems into image processing and deep learning approaches.

5.1.1. Classical Approaches

The classical approach encompasses the methods built using different image processing operations and algorithms. Since the operations and algorithms are tailored to fit the applications and datasets, no standard sets of operations are generalised for all the use cases. Furthermore, kernel size and threshold values are often empirically selected for different filtering and morphological operations in image processing [85]. Despite the tailored approach to solving the detection and tracking problem, some generalised steps are often used in many research approaches. However, researchers tweak the parameters to fit into their applications to find the optimal values that work with different operations and algorithms. The classical approach can be grouped by the methods that dominate these approaches. This paper further categorises the classical detection approaches into feature matching, morphological operation-based, and marker-based detection.

A. *Using feature matching*

Image matching deals with identifying features in the image and then matching them with the corresponding features on other images [86]. Kriechbaumer et al. [28] developed two algorithms for visual odometry for aquatic surface vehicles in a GPS-denied location. The first algorithm was based on image matching of sparse features [87] from the left and right input of the stereo camera along with consecutive stereo image frames where the input was a rectified greyscale image from a calibrated stereo camera. Additionally, a Kalman filter [88] was used for smoothing the estimated trajectory. The second algorithm was an appearance-based algorithm modified from the methods [89] developed for RGB-D cameras where the input of depth information was provided. Their experimental results were evaluated using ground-truth data collected using an electronic theodolite integrated with an electronic distance meter (EDM) and a total station, which is the equipment used in land surveying. Visual odometry enhances navigational accuracy on different types of surfaces. The position error with the feature-based technique was smaller than the appearance-based algorithm with a mean of ± 0.067 m, under the permitted limit of 1 m considered accurate. They performed a linear regression analysis that revealed that the error depended on the movement of the ship and the image features of the scene. Thus, the methods for environment surveying required further modifications depending on the type of application for river monitoring.

Jenkins et al. [90] developed methods for fast motion tracking by developing a fast compressive tracking method. They implemented a template matching technique using weighted multi-frame template matching and similarity metrics to detect the objects in consecutive video frames. They aimed to address problems such as occlusion, motion blur, and tracker offset. A bounding box with a confidence score was incorporated over the object detected with template matching over the image sequences. Overall, they developed a robust method to identify and keep track of the object in real time at an operating speed upwards of 120 FPS with minimal computation time. This was still dependent on the frame-by-frame template matching, and there was a potential of missed object detection in an image frame in case of occlusion.

Busch et al. [2] developed a method for detecting the branch of a pine tree by using the depth information from the stereo camera. They mounted the camera on a drone, and after calculating the depth of the features of the pine tree, they set a threshold of 0.6 metres to identify the ROI. The 0.6-metre threshold was arbitrarily selected as it would be the closest distance between the branch and the drone during the application. The distance threshold was used to generate a mask to isolate the ROI. They used a brute-force feature matching for the stereo matching operation from the

OpenCV [91] software library to calculate a 3D map of the tree branch to generate a point cloud of the branch. This detection approach was only limited to the pine tree branch detection.

B. *Morphological operation*

Morphological operations are a set of image processing operations that apply a structuring element that changes the structure of the features in the image. Two common types of morphological operations are erosion, where an object is reduced in size, and dilation, where the object is increased in size. A generalised way of approaching object tracking problems is tracking by detection. In tracking by detection, the focus is on detection operation in every image frame of a video sequence. Figure 5 shows a generalised diagram of tracking by detection, where the target object is detected, and the location information is stored and tracked for each video frame. The location of the object detected in each image frame of the video sequence is the tracking location of the object. Using stereo images, Chuang et al. [11] tracked underwater fish as an MOT problem. Their method included image processing steps such as double local thresholding, which includes Otsu's method [92] for object segmentation, histogram back-projection to address unstable lighting conditions underwater, the area of the object, and the variance of the pixel values within the object region. They developed a block-matching algorithm that broke the fish object down into four equal blocks and matched them using a minimum sum of the absolute difference (SAD) criterion. This detection process had too many morphological operations with varied parameters, such as kernel sizes and threshold values. Furthermore, the block-sized stereo-matching approach was innovative in reducing computation. However, it may not be a generalised solution to detect other aquatic life for applications in the fishing industry.

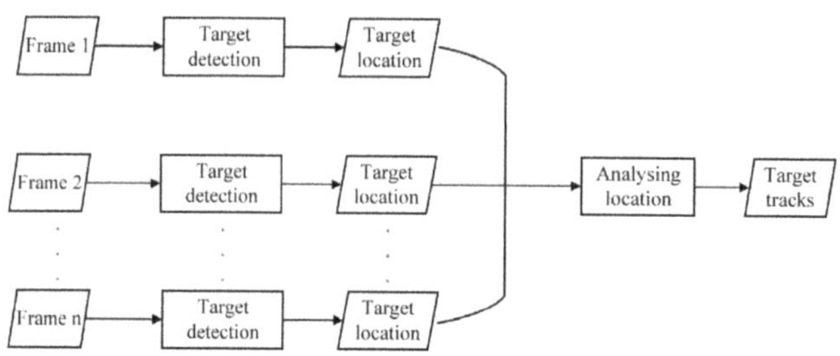

Figure 5. A generalised diagram of tracking by detection.

Yang et al. [15] developed a process for 3D character recognition with a potential for medical applications such as sign language communication or human–computer interaction in medical care by using binocular cameras. Their hand detection process involved converting the image from the RGB to YCbCr colour space and then applying morphological operations such as erosion [85] to eliminate small blobs not part of the hand. Then, they used Canny edge detection [93] to calculate the minimum and maximum distance of the edges in the image frame to determine the centre of the hand and then calculate the finger position, which would be the maximum distance from the centre. The tracking process relied on detecting the hand in each video sequence frame. The validity of hand gestures was determined by calculating the distance between the centre and the outermost feature. The distance value helped to know if the hand was not in a fist position and therefore, ready to be tracked. They further used stereo distance computing methods to track the feature in 3D space. Their method had several limitations, such as the hand needing to be the only skin exposed during the recording because if the face was visible, it would have been difficult to eliminate it during morphological operation, and it would have led to confusion regarding the location of the hand. Since the tracking relied upon detection, object location data were lost for any false negatives. The morphological operations could cause a loss of the exact location of the fingertip. Also, multiple processing stages in detection and tracking meant that the overall robustness of the system relied upon each stage working efficiently. Due to these reasons, there is a need for improvement in these methods for a robust implementation.

Deepambika and Rahman [9] developed methods for detecting and tracking vehicles in different illumination settings. They addressed motion detection using a symmetric mask-based discrete wavelet transform (SMDWT). Their system combined background subtraction, frame differencing, SMDWT, and object tracking with dense stereo disparity-variance. They used the SMDWT instead of the convolution or finite impulse response (FIR) filter method, as these lifting-based [94] methods are good in terms of computation cost. They used background subtraction and frame differencing, binarization and logical OR operations, and morphological operations for motion detection. Background subtraction allows the detection of moving objects from the present frame based on a reference frame. The output from the background subtraction and frame differencing was binarized for the thresholding operation to eliminate the noise in the image. Morphological operations could eliminate other undesired pixels. The next step was to obtain a motion-based disparity mask to extract the ROI for the object. Furthermore, the disparity map was constructed using SAD [95], a useful component for depth detection and stereo matching.

Czajkowska et al. [14] used a set of image processing steps to detect a biopsy needle and estimate its trajectory. They began by performing needle puncture detection. The detection algorithm applied a weighted fuzzy c-means clustering [96] technique to identify ultrasonic elastography recording before the needle touched the tissue. The needle detection was performed using the Histogram of Oriented Gradients (HoG) [97] detector.

C. *Marker-based*

Some detection methods use predefined markers. Markers are physically known objects the vision system has prior knowledge about. These markers are relatively easier to detect than markerless detection, which relies on feature extraction and comparison with the features of the target object. Huang et al. [33] developed a detection method for tracking the payload swing attached to an overhead crane. The payload detection was performed using the spherical marker attached to the payload. Similarly, Richey et al. [12] used a marker-based approach to detect breast surface deformations. Their marker-based detection approach used alphabets with specific ink colour and KAZE feature [98] detection for stereo matching. Using a marker-based approach reduces the computation cost in detection because the features to be detected in the image are known beforehand. However, the marker-based approach has certain problems, as object tracking only works for known objects in a controlled indoor environment. These methods are not ideal for tracking objects in the outdoor environment where the markers may be compromised due to external environmental factors such as wind or rain.

5.1.2. Deep Learning Approaches

Object detection uses a Convolutional Neural Network (CNN), a deep learning method. The primary use of CNNs in object tracking methods is to extract features for further template matching. Any deep learning methods capable of localisation and classifying the object in the image frame can be deployed in the object detection stage. This section investigates the different deep learning methods used to detect objects within the context of object tracking.

A. *R-CNN*

R-CNN [99] is an object localisation and classification method. R-CNN performs localisation and classification in two steps. First, different regions of the images are extracted and passed through a CNN for classification. If the object is detected in these extracted regions, it is localised in the image. Fast R-CNN [84] and its variants, such as Mask R-CNN [100] and Faster R-CNN [101] are other prominent object detection methods used within the context of object tracking for the detection stage. Meneses et al. [79] used R-CNN [99] to extract the detection features. Garcia and Younes [75] used Faster R-CNN [101] for object detection, where they trained the network on 8746 images of a mock drogue for its application to detecting a beacon. Li et al. [1] used Mask R-CNN [100] for object segmentation for segmenting vehicles in the application of autonomous driving. They developed the DyStSLAM method, which modified SLAM [102] to work in dynamic environments.

R-CNN [99] is beneficial for the localisation and classification of objects in an image. Detection windows of different sizes scan the image to extract small regions that are passed through the CNN for classification. This process ensures that different scales of objects are detected. However, the problem with this approach is that scanning multiple times over the images with different window sizes and passing each extracted region to classify the object is time-consuming. For the tracking-by-detection approach, the object detection process will be time-consuming for each image frame of a video sequence. Therefore, using R-CNN may not be ideal for real-time applications.

B. *Single-shot detection methods*

Single-shot detection methods such as Single-Shot Multibox Detector (SSD) [103] and You Only Look Once (YOLO) [82] can perform localisation and classification. These methods use default bounding boxes with different aspect ratios within the image to classify objects. The bounding boxes with higher confidence scores are responsible for object detection. YOLO [82] and its subsequent versions identified in the review by Terven et al. [104] have significantly improved object localisation, classification, pose estimation, and segmentation.

In the object detection for tracking, Aladem and Rawashdeh [8], Zhang et al. [80], Ngoc et al. [44], Wu et al. [39] used YOLOv3 [83], while Zheng et al. [42] used YOLOv5 [105]. Xiao et al. [78] used a Fast YOLO [106] network to localise a pedestrian object in each video frame and at the same time, they used the MegaDepth [107] CNN for the depth estimation.

The advantage of SSD [103] or YOLO [82] over R-CNN [99] is that both the localisation and classification process happen in a single pass through the CNN. Due to the single-pass detection, these methods are better than R-CNN for real-time applications. SSD and YOLO require a large dataset and computational power to train. Also, the detection is limited to the training images used to train the network. Therefore, it is important to consider if the target object class is present in the training dataset for these networks before deploying these methods for tracking.

C. *Other CNN methods*

Yan et al. [32] used CNN as a feature extractor and used these features in the template matching approach. Mdfaa et al. [46] used a CNN whose architecture was designed with the augmentation of SiamMask [108] and MiDaS [109] architectures where each of them was trained separately. ResNet18 [110] was used for binary classification, and two datasets, the Stanford Cars Dataset and Describable Textures Dataset (DTD) [60], were used for training. Gionfrida et al. [13] used OpenPose [111] to detect the hand pose for further tracking. DyStSLAM helps localise an autonomous vehicle by extracting dynamic information from the scene. The deep learning methods incorporated in detection are used or developed based on the applications. Faster detection methods are helpful when the applications are on a real-time system like autonomous driving. Thus, deep learning methods should be evaluated on these datasets with the development of new datasets. If the results are not accurate enough, they will motivate the development of new methods.

5.2. Tracking Methods

The tracking process takes place after object detection. The tracking method keeps track of the movement of the object over multiple video sequence frames. This subsection highlights the tracking methods based on the image processing framework, while identifying their strengths and weaknesses. Approaches towards tracking methods use the multi-step image processing approach or end-to-end deep learning methods. In image matching, the standard procedure is to identify the features of the object and match them in consecutive video frames. The image matching technique is often accompanied by data association methods that help to keep track of the object. The deep learning methods often use end-to-end networks trained on image sequences. Deep learning can also be a two-step approach where detection occurs before tracking, and the network tracks the features in the subsequent frames. The literature outlines the two approaches used for object tracking.

5.2.1. Tracking by Detection

Tracking-by-detection (TBD) methods involve detecting objects in each image frame without prior knowledge or estimation of their future state. The object is associated with the previous detection [23].

A. *Data association*
Data association is the process of using previously known information about the object pose, movement, and change in appearance and comparing it with the newly identified objects and tracking movements of the object [25]. Data association is one of the most used methods for tracking and it is often modified as per the specifications of the applications. Chuang et al. [11] developed tracking for low-frame-rate video to track live fish. Their method used stereo matching by dividing the fish object into four blocks of equal size. The four blocks were formed by taking four equal column widths of the object's bounding box. These blocks in each of the left and right images of the stereo were matched using the sum of absolute difference (SAD). The stereo-matching process was followed by feature-based temporal matching, where four cues, such as vicinity, area, motion direction, and histogram distance, were considered. They further modified the Viterbi data association used in single-target tracking to multiple tracking, using the Viterbi algorithm [112] for tracking. Since the video had low contrast and a low frame rate, the Viterbi data association process helped track the object in multiple frames.
Feng et al. [5] used 3D bounding boxes generated by an object detector [113]. These bounding boxes were the basis for a multilevel data association method and a geometry-based dynamic object classification method, enabling robust object tracking. The system also introduced a sliding window-based tightly coupled estimator that optimised the poses of the ego vehicle with the sensors mounted on it, IMU biases, and object-related factors that formed different features of the dynamic objects. This approach allowed for the optimisation of both the vehicle and object states. These tracking methods used visual odometry data for self-localisation and object detection to know the position of the object relative to the vehicle. Their approach required further development for tracking non-rigid objects and testing their methods in real-world applications.
Zhang et al. [80] proposed a Multiplex Label Graph based on graph theory. This graph was developed so that each node stored information about multiple detectors. A CNN generated these detectors from the Part-Based Convolution Baseline (PCB) [114] network that was trained on the Market-1501 dataset [115]. They treated the object tracking in the frame as a graph optimisation problem where the goal is to find the path of a detector in multiple image frames of a video sequence. To achieve this, they broke down the video frames into a group of images called "window" and detected the object within each successive frame in the window. They tested different window sizes on MOT16 and MOT17 [68] datasets and determined that a window size of 20 was the optimal value that increased tracking accuracy. Then,

a data association was performed with certain threshold functions that identified whether the nodes in the successive frames were associated. The distance between the nodes in the successive frames checked that association.

B. *Template matching*

Template matching is a process of identifying small parts of the target image that match the features using cross-correlation methods to a template image of the object by scanning the target image [116]. Jenkins et al. [90] developed their methods to track different types of objects available in the tracking dataset [117]. For this purpose, they implemented a template matching technique using weighted multi-frame template matching to detect the objects in consecutive video frames. The weighted multi-frame template approach was tested using similarity metrics such as normalised cross-correlation and cosine similarity. The results of the similarity metrics showed a significant increase in accuracy on their chosen evaluation dataset. Overall, they developed a robust method to identify and keep track of the object in real time with minimal computation time. Tracking robustness depended upon frame-by-frame template matching, which may pose problems during the detection of any false negatives during the tracking stage.

Yang et al. [15] developed tracking methods for tracking the movement of hands in medical applications. The tracking process was performed by detection. They used hand gestures to automate the decision-making process regarding the beginning and end of the tracking process. They further used stereo-matching methods to compute the distance between the camera and the hand, allowing them to track the hand in 3D space. Their method relied on detection, which means that tracking information would be lost for any false negative detection.

Richey et al. [12] developed tracking methods for breast deformation while the patient was supine, and the video frames were collected using stereo cameras during the hand movement of the patient. The labelled fiducial points, with the alphabet written in blue ink on the breasts, were tracked over the video frame. The labels were propagated through a camera stream by matching the key points to previous key points. The features obtained from these fiducial points leveraged the ink colours and adaptive thresholding, which were tracked using KAZE [98] feature matching. The features were stored in order to be tracked over the sequences of images. This method relied upon detecting all 26 English alphabets written on the breast; therefore, a detection failure may disrupt the tracking process.

Zheng et al. [42] tracked drones from a ground camera setup. They proposed a trajectory-based Micro Aerial Vehicle (MAV) tracking algorithm that operated in two parts: individual multi-target trajectory tracking within each sensing node based on its local measurements and the fusion of these trajectory segments at a central node using the Kuhn–Mumkres [118] matching matrix algorithm. This research introduced an MAV monitoring system that effectively detected, localised, and tracked aerial targets by combining panoramic stereo cameras and advanced algorithms.

C. *Optical flow*

Optical flow deals with the analysis of the moving patterns in the image due to the relative motion of the objects or the viewer [119]. Czajkowska et al. [14] developed a tracking method for needle tracking. The detection step provided information about the position of the needle. The tracking of needle tips focused on the single-point tracking technique. Methods like Canny edge detection [93] and Hough transform [120] were used for the trajectory detection. To implement the tracking process in real time with low computation resources, they considered using the Lucas–Kanade [121] approach that helped solve the optical flow equation using the least square method. Finally, they used the Kanade–Lucas–Tomasi (KLT) [122] algorithm that introduces the Harris corner [123] features. Furthermore, the pyramid representation of the KLT algorithm was combined with minimum eigenvalue-based feature extraction to avoid missing the tracking point of the needle. The two paths used for tracking were helpful in addressing both cases of fully and partially visible needles with ultrasonic images. Their method had a low computational cost in tracking, so it could be used in real time.

Wu et al. [39] designed and implemented a target tracking system for quadcopters for steady and accurate tracking of ground and air targets without prior information. Their research was motivated by the limitations of existing unmanned aerial vehicle (UAV) systems that failed to track targets accurately in the long term and could not relocate targets after they were lost. Therefore, they developed a vision detection algorithm that used a correlation filter, support vector machines, Lucas–Kanade [121] optical flow tracking, and the Extended Kalman Filter (EKF) [124] with stereo vision on a quadcopter to solve the existing detection problems in UAVs. Their visual tracking algorithm consisted of translation and scale tracking, tracking quality evaluation and drift correction, tracking loss detection, and target relocation. The target position was inferred from the correlation response map of the translation filter. Based on the target position, the target scale was predicted by a scale filter [125]. Then, the drift of the target position was corrected with an appearance filter that detected if the target was lost and allowed the tracking quality evaluation, which had a similar structure to that of the translation filter. Furthermore, the tracking quality was evaluated by the confidence score, composed of the average peak-to-correlation energy (APCE) and the maximum response of the appearance filter. If the confidence score exceeded the re-detection threshold, the target was tracked successfully, and the translation and scale filters were updated. Otherwise, the SVM classifier was activated for target re-detection. They made improvements on the Lucas–Kanade [121] optical flow and Extended Kalman filter algorithms to estimate the local and global states of the target. Their simulation and real-world experiments showed that the tracking system they developed was stable.

D. *Descriptor-based*

Descriptors are the feature vectors of the object that capture unique features that help to classify a particular object [126]. Aladem and Rawashdeh [8] used the YOLOv3 detector as a tool to create an elliptical mask by using a bounding box to extract the features for a feature detector such as Shi–Tomasi's [127] for feature matching. The feature matching process was followed by Binary Robust and Oriented Features (BRIEF) [128] for matching between the consecutive frames. Their method was for the odometry data evaluated on the KITTI [35] dataset. There were certain limitations, such as losing the objects and being unable to detect them. When the same objects reappeared, they were classified as new objects. They suggested that using a Kalman filter [88] in the future would help to deal with the missing object problem during detection.

Ngoc et al. [44] used the features from YOLOv3 [83] for tracking. The features extracted within the bounding box of this object detector were used in the particle filter algorithm [129]. These particles were tracked in the subsequent frames of the KITTI dataset [35]. While solving this problem, they also focused on identifying multiple objects when the camera was in motion. They took a hybrid approach, using stereo and IMU data for target tracking. Their method also took into account the camera movement. Their method had a future scope of application in mobile robotics.

E. *Kalman Filter*

Kalman filtering is an algorithm that uses prior measurements or states and produces estimates for future states over a time period [88]. The Kalman filter has a wide range of applications where the future state estimate of the object of interest is required , such as guidance, navigation, and control of autonomous vehicles. Since the target object in a video sequence shows the same property of moving states where state estimates are required, the Kalman filter is applied in object tracking problems.

Busch et al. [2] tracked the movement of a pine tree branch. They tested different types of feature descriptors such as SIFT [130], SURF [131], ORB [132], FAST [133], and Shi–Tomasi [127]. Their results showed that FAST-SIFT and Shi–Tomasi combinations performed best at 1 m and a camera perspective of 0 degrees. These numbers indicated the optimal position and orientation of the camera on the drone for collecting the pine tree branch data. These features were further filtered and mapped to 3D space to create a point cloud. The principal component analysis method was used to detect the direction of the branch. A developed Kalman filter [88] was derived that improved the intercept point estimation of the pine tree branch, which was the point at 75 mm from the tip of the branch. This developed Kalman filter reduced the intercept point error, which was helpful when determining the intercept point as the sway parameter.

Huang et al. [33] developed a method where a Kalman filter initially predicted the target position [88]. The tracking ball area was obtained through mean shift iteration and target model matching. Since mean shift has problems with tracking fast objects, combining it with a Kalman filter offers stability in detection since a Kalman filter is useful in estimating the minimum mean square error in the dynamic system. Then, the minimum area circular method was integrated to identify the position of the tracking ball correctly and quickly. The recognition part was more robust when an auxiliary module that pre-processed the area determined by the mean shift iteration was proposed. Geometric methods obtained the swing angle for the ball mounted on the crane payload. Their method was tested on an experimental overhead crane with a swing payload setup. Therefore, the methods may need further modification when the vision tracking system is applied to an outdoor overhead traveling crane with background disturbances and unexpected outdoor environmental factors such as wind and illumination.

5.2.2. Joint Detection and Tracking

Different from tracking by detecting, joint tracking methods are end-to-end trainable networks where tracking and detection are performed in a single network [23]. Different research groups have experimented with available CNN architectures, with more research literature being added. With the development of more methods, the deep learning approach can be further classified based on their methods. In this section, deep learning approaches for tracking are categorised based on CNN-based, R-CNN-based, YOLO, and other neural network-based methods. Deep learning methods for tracking are investigated by different reviews [21–23] that focus on MOT methods and their application for autonomous driving. In this subsection, the deep learning approach is classified based on the primary methods used for localisation for tracking by detection and joint tracking.

A. *CNN-based approaches*

Convolutional Neural Network-based approaches involve using deep learning methods for feature extraction to track these features in consecutive video frames. Rasoulidanesh et al. [40] developed a tracking method with an RGB and depth frame input. The spatial attention network extracted a glimpse from these data as the part of the frame where the object of interest was probably located. Then, the features of the object were extracted from the glimpse using a CNN with the first three layers of AlexNet [18]. The glimpse could extract two types of features: ventral and dorsal. The former extracted appearance-based features, while the latter aimed to compute the foreground and background segmentation. These features were then fed to an LSTM [134] network and fully connected neural networks to give a bounding-box correction. The bounding-box correction was fed back to the spatial attention section to compute the new glimpse and appearance for the next frame to improve object detection and foreground segmentation. They showed that adding depth increased accuracy, especially in more challenging environments. Their results showed that the depth-based models could perform accurate tracking with only depth information, without RGB.

Zhong et al. [56] used an encoder–decoder network. They proposed to combine a learning-based video object segmentation module with an optimisation-based pose estimation module in a closed loop. After solving the current object pose, they rendered the 3D object model generated on a computer to obtain a refined, model-constrained mask of the current frame. It was then fed back to the segmentation network for processing the next frame, closing the whole loop. To detect the occluded object, they designed a novel six-DOF object tracking pipeline based on a mutual guidance loop of video object segmentation along with six-DOF object pose estimation and combining learning and optimisation methods. They presented a robust six-DOF object pose tracker that could handle heavy occlusions. The experiments showed that their method could achieve competitive performance on non-occluded sequences and significantly better robustness on occluded sequences.

Yan et al. [32] developed a tracking method for the handover problem. They proposed a tracking algorithm that improved the tracking accuracy based on the MDNET [135], which is a multi-domain network. The target state in the initial frame of the video sequence was given, and the tracking was started. Then, the target handover began when the target crossed the field of view (FOV) line of the camera. The target feature extracted by a CNN was used for template matching. When the target handover was completed, the target was tracked in the next camera. In their research, they mainly improved the accuracy of target tracking and target handover. In terms of tracking, they improved on the original MDNET algorithm. In addition, they combined perspective transformation with features extracted by a CNN to realise the target handover.

B. *R-CNN-based approaches*

Meneses et al. [79] used R-CNN to extract features. The data association method used these features to track the object. They developed SmartSORT, which modelled the frame-by-frame association between new detections and existing targets as an assignment problem. They considered neural networks trained with the backpropagation algorithm as the regression model. Thus, given that the feature vector from R-CNN was related to the detection and the target, the regression model calculated their association cost. Once the regression model had computed every association cost, it optimally solved the assignment problem via the Hungarian method [136], which is an optimisation method that selects the best possible cost for a combination of activities, in this case, the tracking path over the frame of images.

Garcia and Younes [75] developed a tracking system that worked by capturing an image with a Kinect camera sensor, which acted as an input to a deep learning object detector using Faster R-CNN [101], which output the bounding box around each of the eight beacons on a drogue used to refuel an aircraft. Then, the navigation algorithms that used non-linear least squares and collinearity equations were used to find the position and orientation of the drogue, thereby allowing the aircraft to align with the beacon for refuelling. They performed their experiments on a mock drogue and verified their solution using the VICON motion tracking system. There were issues with the trained detectors with the inference time being too large. Also, they made several assumptions regarding using a mock drogue, and their image dataset was too small for training with limited augmentation.

C. *YOLO and other neural network-based approaches*

Mdfaa et al. [46] developed methods that used depth information and training data to train a Siamese network [137] to track an object. Since their application involved tracking a moving object using an aerial drone, they developed a system in which the drone kept following the object until it reached its location or the moving object stopped. In this type of tracking, there are two sub-tasks: identifying the tracked object and estimating its state, which is its position and orientation. The objective of the tracking mission is to automatically predict the state of the moving object in consecutive frames given its initial state. Their proposed framework combined

2D SOT with monocular depth estimation (RGB-D) to track moving objects in 3D space. Using this information, the Siamese network tracked the target object, which produced a mask, a bounding box, an object class, and an RPN score for the object. Xiao et al. [78] used Fast YOLO [106] and MegaDepth [107] for detection and depth estimation. The results from these two networks were used as features for object detection and tracking using a Kalman Filter [88]. They proposed an algorithm that helped them track the pedestrian object in the video frame and developed data association rules regarding remembering the objects in case of occlusion. They developed a method that tracked the movement of multiple objects in 3D space on a video. However, their real-time tracking needed improvement for a dynamic system that interacts with the environment.

Yang et al. [6] developed the Self-Attention Optical Flow Estimation Network (SA-FlowNet) for applications on event-based cameras. SA-FlowNet independently uses crisscross and temporal self-attention mechanisms that help capture long-range dependencies and efficiently extract the temporal and spatial features from the event stream. Their proposed network used an end-to-end learning method to adopt a spiking-analogue neural network architecture. It gained significant computational energy benefits, especially for Spiking Neural Networks (SNNs) [138]. Their network architecture was based on a deep spike-analogue neural network architecture that combined event cameras for energy-efficient optical flow estimation. Their network could achieve higher performance and save energy consumption. It could also be used for object detection, motion segmentation, and challenging scenery tasks in dim light, occlusions, and high-speed conditions.

5.3. Recommendations for Approaches and Methods for Applications

The methods for object tracking in computer vision rely on object detection followed by tracking the detected object. The reliance on object detection before tracking ensures that object detection methods are studied and improved. This review outlines a detailed study of the detection methods incorporated into the object tracking literature over the last ten years.

Based on the insights gained from the literature survey and the identification of advantages and limitations of different methods as presented in Tables 7 and 8, the following recommendations are made for the selection of object detection methods:

- The classical approach is helpful when the target object can be identified by its geometry and where the computation resources and annotated datasets are limited to train a deep learning model.
- Deep learning approach in detection for tracking applications is helpful for objects with no standard geometry where the annotated dataset and computational resources are available.

The object tracking process involves keeping track of the detected objects over different video frames. Some methods detect objects in each video frame and then use association techniques to match the detection. This process of detecting objects in each image frame and later connecting the tracks is called tracking by detection (TBD). A different approach to tracking involves joint detection and tracking (JDT), where an end-to-end framework is used with estimation techniques to predict the objects in the next frame by using object features from the previous frame. Figure 6 shows a generalised diagram of end-to-end tracking using prior knowledge.

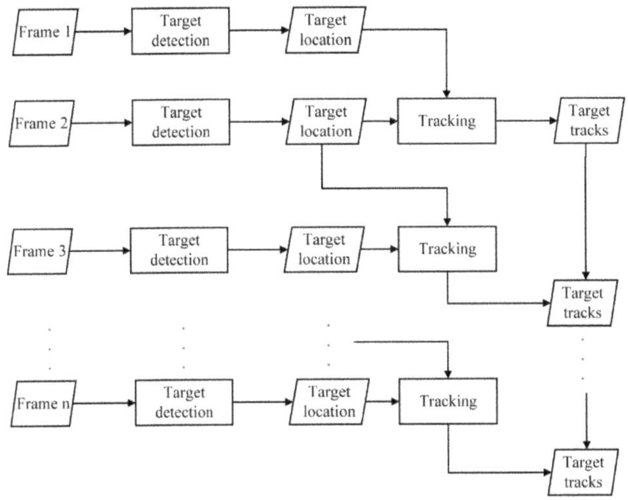

Figure 6. A generalised diagram of end-to-end tracking using prior knowledge.

Table 7. Summary of classical approaches for detection.

Paper	Key Methods	Advantages	Limitations
[28]	Sparse feature image matching, Kalman filter	Enhances navigational accuracy using visual odometry techniques, particularly useful in GPS-denied environments.	Relies on accurate feature matching and may not be ideal for objects without known feature geometries.
[90]	Template matching, weighted multi-frame template, confidence scoring	Provides a fast and robust method for object tracking in real-time video streams.	Template matching methods may not be suitable for different environmental conditions.
[2]	Depth-based feature matching, thresholding, point cloud generation	Effective for detecting specific objects in complex environments using depth information.	Limited to applications where depth information is available and may not generalise well to scenarios with different types of objects or backgrounds.
[9]	Morphological operations, wavelet transform, object tracking	Robust approach for vehicle detection and tracking in varying illumination conditions.	Accurate motion detection and further tests are required to address fast-moving uncertain objects.
[14]	Fuzzy clustering, HoG feature detection	Effective for detecting and tracking biopsy needles in medical applications.	Requires accurate needle puncture detection and feature extraction. Further tests are needed to ensure higher performance in scenarios with complex tissue structures or noisy ultrasound images.
[33]	Marker-based detection, geometric methods	Provides a reliable method for tracking payload swing in overhead cranes.	The methods were tested on a prototype in the laboratory setting, and the results of real-world data would confirm the robustness of the methods.
[12]	Marker-based detection, KAZE feature matching	Effective for detecting breast surface deformations using markers and stereo matching.	Using alphabets as markers sets the marker limits to 26 markers based on the English alphabet. A different marker identification system is required to overcome this limitation. Also, the method is suitable for detecting markers with a particular ink colour.
[11]	Stereo matching, block matching, Otsu's thresholding	Enables tracking of underwater fish using stereo image processing techniques.	The block stereo matching helps detect the fish. Morphological operations with arbitrary threshold values are used. The block-matching approach is not general enough to detect a variety of aquatic life.
[15]	Morphological operations, feature detection, stereo tracking	Provides a method for 3D character recognition and tracking using stereo vision.	The hand must be the only skin exposed during the recording because if the face is visible, it would be difficult to eliminate it during morphological operation, and it would lead to confusion regarding the location of the hand.

From the insights in terms of advantages and limitations of different methods and approaches presented in Tables 9 and 10, the following are the recommendations for the selection of tracking approaches:

- The tracking-by-detection method is useful to track multiple objects when the objects are not often occluded.
- Using data association methods is useful to track the trajectories of the target objects.
- Joint detection and tracking is useful when a dataset for tracking for a specific application and the computational resources are available to develop an end-to-end framework.

Table 8. Summary of deep learning approaches for detection.

Paper	Key Methods	Advantages	Limitations
[1,75,79]	R-CNN, Faster R-CNN for object detection, Mask R-CNN for object segmentation	Effective for object localisation, classification, and segmentation. Widely used in various applications like beacon detection and autonomous driving.	Time-consuming due to scanning multiple regions with different window sizes for each image frame and may not be suitable for real-time applications. Requires extensive training on target-specific datasets.
[8,39,42,44,78,80]	YOLOv3, YOLOv5, Fast YOLO for object detection	Performs localisation and classification in a single pass through a CNN; suitable for real-time applications. Efficient object detection for tracking without prior information.	Requires large datasets and computational power for training. Detection limited to classes present in the training dataset and may misclassify untrained class of object.
[32,46]	Custom CNN architecture for feature extraction, object detection	Combines deep learning features with traditional approaches. Incorporates multiple architectures for improved object detection performance.	Resource-intensive training process. Requires large datasets and computational power.
[13]	OpenPose for hand pose detection	Provides accurate hand pose detection for further tracking applications.	Dependent on the quality of the input data and the performance of the OpenPose model.

Table 9. Summary of tracking-by-detection methods.

Paper	Key Methods	Advantages	Limitations
[11]	Stereo matching, feature-based temporal matching, Viterbi data association	Effective for low-frame-rate video tracking, integrates stereo matching and feature-based matching for robust tracking.	Viterbi data association may introduce computational cost and may not perform optimally in scenarios with high object occlusions.
[5]	Multilevel data association, geometry-based dynamic object classification	Robust tracking based on 3D bounding boxes and dynamic object classification.	Further development is needed for tracking non-rigid objects and testing in real-world applications.
[80]	Multiplex Label Graph based on graph theory, CNN-based object detectors	Offers a novel approach to object tracking using graph optimisation techniques.	Computational complexity may be high, and optimisation parameters may require tuning for different scenarios.
[90]	Weighted multi-frame template matching	Robust template matching technique for real-time object tracking.	Relies on accurate template matching in consecutive frames, and it may suffer from computational complexity in scenarios with high frame rates.
[15]	Stereo matching, 3D tracking	Enables 3D tracking of hands in medical applications using stereo matching.	Tracking relies on accurate detection, may lose tracking information for false negative detections.
[12]	Feature extraction, fiducial tracking, KAZE feature matching	Tracks fiducial points on the breast for deformation analysis using stereo cameras.	Relies on accurate fiducial detection and may face challenges with detection in scenarios with complex backgrounds or lighting conditions.
[42]	Trajectory-based tracking, Kuhn–Mumkres matching matrix algorithm	Effective for tracking MAVs using panoramic stereo cameras and trajectory optimisation algorithms.	The method may face challenges with fast-moving objects or environments with limited visual cues.
[14]	Lucas–Kanade optical flow, KLT algorithm	Provides real-time needle tracking using optical flow and feature matching techniques.	Requires robust feature extraction and matching algorithms, and the accuracy may be affected in scenarios with rapid motion or complex backgrounds.
[39]	Correlation filter, SVM classifier, Lucas–Kanade optical flow, EKF	Stable and accurate target tracking system for UAVs using a combination of visual detection algorithms.	Complex algorithmic pipelines may introduce computational overhead and require fine-tuning for different UAV platforms or tracking scenarios.
[8]	YOLOv3 object detection, Shi–Tomasi feature matching, BRIEF descriptor	Efficient tracking using YOLOv3 features and robust feature matching techniques.	Relies on accurate object detection and feature matching, and robustness may be affected in scenarios with object occlusions or cluttered backgrounds.
[44]	YOLOv3 object detection, particle filter	Hybrid approach for object tracking using YOLOv3 features and particle filtering.	Parameter tuning may be required, and computational cost will increase in scenarios with large numbers of objects.

Table 9. *Cont.*

Paper	Key Methods	Advantages	Limitations
[2]	SIFT, SURF, ORB, FAST, Shi–Tomasi feature descriptors, Kalman filter	Provides accurate tracking of pine tree branches using a combination of feature descriptors and Kalman filtering.	Requires careful selection and tuning of feature descriptors and may face challenges in complex branch motion or occlusion scenarios.
[33]	Mean shift, Kalman filter, geometric methods	Effective for tracking crane-mounted objects using mean shift and Kalman filtering.	There is a possibility of reduced robustness in outdoor environments with unpredictable factors such as wind or lighting changes.

Table 10. Summary of joint detection and tracking methods.

Paper	Key Methods	Advantages	Limitations
[40]	Use of depth information for tracking accuracy enhancement	Improved accuracy, especially in challenging environments	Depth-based models may require additional hardware or sensors, increasing complexity and cost
[56]	Combination of video object segmentation and pose estimation in a closed loop	Robust tracking performance, particularly in handling occlusions	Complexity of closed-loop system may increase computational overhead
[32]	Integration of CNN features for template matching and perspective transformation	Improved accuracy for handover tracking tasks	The method is specific to handover tracking tasks and may not generalise well to other tracking scenarios
[79]	R-CNN features for frame-by-frame association	Accurate frame-by-frame association for tracking objects	Computational complexity may increase with the use of R-CNN features, potentially limiting real-time performance
[75]	Implementation of Faster R-CNN for object detection and navigation algorithms	Accurate object detection and navigation for aircraft refuelling	Issues with large inference time and limited training data may hinder real-world applicability
[46]	Integration of Siamese networks with depth information for 3D object tracking	Capability to track objects in 3D space, useful for applications like drone surveillance	Depth information may not always be available or reliable, limiting the applicability of the method
[78]	Usage of Fast YOLO and MegaDepth for pedestrian tracking	Efficient pedestrian tracking with consideration of occlusions	Real-time performance may be impacted by the computational demands of YOLO and MegaDepth networks
[6]	Introduction of SA-FlowNet for energy-efficient optical flow estimation	Reduced energy consumption and improved performance for object detection and motion segmentation	Specific to event-based cameras, may not be directly applicable to conventional camera systems

6. Applications

The main reason for developing different methods and datasets is to ensure they are applied to solve real-world problems. Each real-world scenario and problem is different, and each has its constraints. In object tracking using computer vision, each problem, depending upon the environmental conditions such as indoor or outdoor applications, available computational resources, and the cost of the system, can become a constraint. This section outlines the different domains in which the object tracking methods are applied. Table 11 categorises different papers based on their applications studied in this review. Some of the papers in Table 11 overlap the application domains, such as multiple-object tracking (MOT) application methods that can be applied to detect multiple pedestrians for surveillance applications. The following subsections are grouped by their primary applications, and Figure 7 shows the structure of the categorisation of the application.

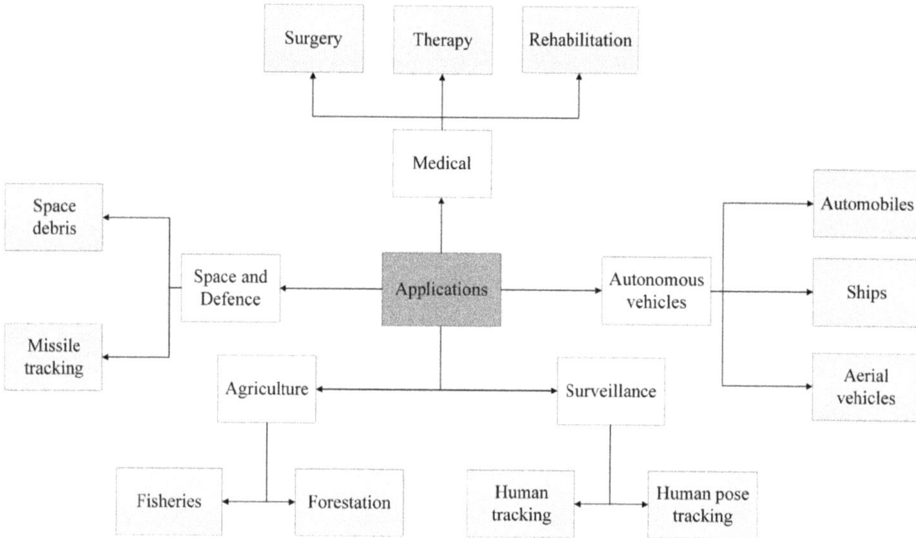

Figure 7. Structure of primary applications of object tracking.

6.1. Medical

Computer vision is preferred in medical applications where non-intrusive diagnoses are required. Non-intrusive diagnoses involve imaging and computational methods that elaborate results to help medical practitioners better diagnose patients. Richey et al. [12] used object tracking to track marked fiducial points for breast conservation surgery. Gionfrida et al. [13] used hand-pose tracking in the clinical setting to study hand kinematics using pose with a potential application in rehabilitation. Czajkowska et al. [14] developed processes for tracking a biopsy needle. Zarrabeitia et al. [16] applied their method for tracking 3D trajectories of droplets, which has a potential application in medicine for bloodletting events. Yang et al. [15] developed the 3D character recognition methods by tracking hand movement, which has an application in physical health examination and communicating using sign language. The results from object tracking provide insights into the operation procedure, providing greater details to the practitioners to make informed decisions. Thus, object tracking has a wider scope of application in numerous medical fields.

6.2. Autonomous Vehicles

An accurate object tracking solution is required in fields with a lot of dynamic movement, and autonomous driving is a primary example. Several types of research focus on detecting objects that could be observed in potential driving scenarios, thereby creating evaluation datasets of cars [35] and pedestrians [48] in the autonomous driving context. Different methods [1,3,5–10] have been proposed for applications in autonomous driving for detecting objects. Object tracking in autonomous driving involves detecting all moving objects, such as cars and pedestrians, from the sensor systems of the car. The datasets [35,49] collected for autonomous driving come with different attributes such as GPS, IMU, radar, and images. Yet, the scope of object detection for autonomous driving applications is limited to the few attributes in the dataset, such as radar, IMU, and images.

Similar to autonomous driving, water surface vehicle applications [28,29] face similar problem constraints. These attributes help detect objects and compute their trajectories in 3D space from the relative position of the vision system mounted on the vehicle. Knowing the movement of different objects around the autonomous vehicle, a future aim is to use this information for cruise control.

Autonomous aerial vehicles need to be aware of the dynamic environment around them. There are multiple applications in the field of aerial vehicles. Some applications track objects using sensors mounted on the aerial vehicle, while others track the flying aerial vehicle from the ground. Regarding tracking flying drones, Zheng et al. [42] applied their methods to develop a panoramic stereo to track rogue drones. Mdfaa et al. [46] developed a single-object tracker to be mounted on an aerial vehicle. Garcia and Younes [75] applied their method in automatically refuelling unmanned aerial vehicles using a drogue. Busch et al. [2] developed object tracking for the application of drones in agriculture. Wu et al. [39] applied target tracking on a quadcopter. The wide range of applications of unmanned aerial vehicles indicates that there are different niche cases to consider in aerial applications, which demand more datasets and methods. Figure 8 provides an overview of object tracking methods and their application to autonomous vehicles.

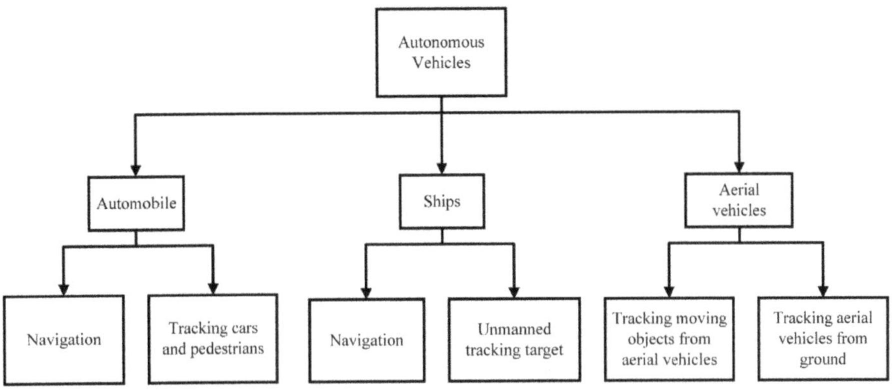

Figure 8. Overview of object tracking in autonomous vehicles.

6.3. Surveillance

Human movement tracking is one of the methods that is used in surveillance and sports. It is important to track the path of human movement in the scene and detect and track it over a longer period using multiple cameras. The application of human movement tracking also has to consider the problem of occlusion [56]. Yan et al. [32] tracked human skaters over multiple cameras to solve the object handover problem. Multiple methods [30,36,37,72,78,80,139,140] were developed for their applications in human pedestrian tracking. Along with human movement, pose estimation is another problem that fits well with action tracking. Different methods [13,77,81] were developed for pose estimation, which has applications in human action tracking and robotics [3,8]. The action tracking methods have different applications in surveillance, pose estimation, and robotics. Further development in these methods will have a wider scope for human–computer interaction problems.

6.4. Robotics

In robotic applications, a robot is an example of a dynamic system that interacts and manoeuvres itself autonomously within its environment. A robot needs to localise itself and the objects around it. Different sensors provide environmental input data to the robot, helping it accomplish its goals and operate safely without breaking itself, damaging nearby objects, or harming humans. Vision sensors on robots provide fine-grained data of the objects of interest, enabling the robots to perceive their surroundings. Busch et al. [2] used an object tracking method on aerial robots to investigate the movement of tree branches. Similarly, Wu et al. [39] also deployed a vision-based target-tracking method on aerial robots to track both ground and aerial objects. Therefore, using robots in object tracking applications is essential when the environment is too hostile or fast-paced for humans to operate, such as examining tree tops [2] or tracking aerial vehicles [39].

Persic et al.'s [3] method has an application in autonomous vehicles and robotics. Since their method focused on moving target tracking, it has a potential application in mobile or industrial robotics where there are different moving objects with higher uncertainty of object collisions. Similarly, Aladem and Rawashdeh [8] also developed their methods for safe navigation for mobile robots.

The field of robotics can benefit from object tracking as it allows the robots to perceive their environment while ensuring safe operation and preventing harm to humans. There is further potential for the application of object tracking methods in human–robot interaction, where the robots track human actions to work together to achieve a common goal.

6.5. Agriculture

Object tracking has potential in agriculture applications. Collecting information about plants and trees constantly swaying due to environmental factors such as wind and rain is important in agriculture. Busch et al. [2] applied object tracking to identify the swaying motion of a pine tree branch. Their motivation for developing tracking methods for tree branches was to allow researchers in the forestry industry to select trees for breeding, analyse genetics, and monitor plant diseases. The use of aerial vehicles with computer vision to examine tree branches outdates the use of ladders or manually climbing trees with a rope. In their application, they mounted their camera on an unmanned aerial vehicle with a manipulator arm to collect data on pine tree branches. Their proposed application has the potential to be used in the forestry industry to improve the efficiency of collecting tree data and thus maintain healthy forests.

Using an autonomous system in fishing is an important application in the fishing industry. Chuang et al. [11] developed methods for tracking live fish underwater. Tracking the movement of fish underwater is beneficial as it improves the efficiency of fishing operations. Knowing the positions of the fish, an autonomous system can deploy a trawl to catch fish. Furthermore, a computer vision system with object detection and tracking algorithms can lead to sustainable fishing techniques without damaging the ecosystem. Drawing inspiration from these applications, many more potential applications can be developed in agriculture using object tracking and computer vision.

6.6. Space and Defence

Object tracking has been applied to space and defence applications. Tracking space debris is an important application in the space industry. The damage caused by space debris could lead to the loss of space shuttles and human lives. Tracking space debris is essential for safer space flight, and thus, the space debris must be removed. Biondi et al. [76] developed their method to estimate the dynamic rotational state of space debris. Using computer vision to track space debris could lead to potential unmanned space missions to clear the space debris for safer space flights.

Defence applications are also using computer vision for object tracking tasks. Kwon et al. [4] developed a method for tracking and intercepting missiles with applications in defence technology. Their method aimed to solve the problem where both the target and the camera are moving. Thus, the method had potential applications in mobile robotics and unmanned aerial vehicles.

Garcia and Younes [75] developed methods for applications in autonomous aerial refuelling of aircraft. In the aerial refuelling task, a tanker aerial vehicle provides a refuelling probe to the drogue of the receiving aircraft and the refuelling is performed mid-air. In their research, their vision system, comprising a monocular camera on an unmanned aerial vehicle, used object detection to track the refuelling drogue in mid-flight and automatically refuel without human intervention. The refuelling task accounted for turbulence, and both the camera system and refuelling drogue were in motion.

The above-mentioned applications are reported based on computer simulation or experimental tests only. Further development will need to be conducted before they can be reliably deployed to real-world and critical applications.

Table 11. Categorisation of papers based on applications.

Application	Papers
Medical	[12–16]
Aerial vehicles	[2,39,42,46,75]
SOT	[33,40,46]
MOT	[11,44,76,79]
Human action tracking	[30,32,36,37,56,72,78,80,139,140]
Pose estimation	[13,77,81]
Autonomous driving	[1,3,5–10]
Aquatic surface vehicle	[28,29]
Robotics	[3,8]
Agriculture	[2,11]
Space/Defence	[4,76]

7. Discussion

Despite extensive research, object tracking using computer vision is still an active research area. The different solutions proposed to solve the tracking problem emerge from the constraints of the problem regarding resources and applications. The application of object tracking in different domains drives the development of the datasets, methods, and evaluation processes. Object tracking methods have several potential applications in different industries and research domains. The development of methods to address the problem constraints has evolved the approach from a set of image processing steps to using end-to-end deep learning models. While significant progress has been made in the last ten years in object tracking using computer vision, there is still room for improvement in addressing issues such as developing generalised procedures or frameworks, addressing lighting conditions, tracking fast-moving objects, and occlusion.

7.1. Methods

Despite the lack of a formal generalised procedure or framework for object tracking, the closest generalisation of procedure in the literature is first object detection and then object tracking. While this generalised tracking procedure is becoming more common, the dependency on multiple processing steps during the detection affects the overall robustness of the method. These image processing steps are developed iteratively, adjusting their parameters empirically or using statistical methods based on the results. When the algorithm receives the least error, it is ready for deployment. However, the method's accuracy is set based on the dataset upon which it was evaluated. Therefore, the two-step detection and tracking process can be combined into a single end-to-end deep learning framework.

Deep learning detection methods also incorporate an iterative process; however, since different architectures are already evaluated on a large and varied detection dataset with multiple classes, they become useful out of the box for detection. The object detection community is incrementally improving the detection method to be faster in real time [83]. Yet, these efficiency improvements come at higher computation costs. Classification and localisation can be performed simultaneously in real time with the detection architectures, such as YOLO [82] and subsequent versions. This dual functionality of deep learning methods to localise and classify in real time has led to a considerable leap in multiple-object tracking problems. However, in unique applications where the network was not trained to include a class of objects, the network needs to be trained either from scratch or using transfer learning [141] methods. Training a deep network requires computational resources; the image processing steps are preferred where such resources are unavailable. However, image processing methods in recent years have declined due to the availability of computational resources and pre-trained deep network architectures for detection. Apart from detection, very few methods use deep learning architecture for tracking. Tracking objects is still performed using estimation methods such as data association and Kalman filter. Using methods such as LSTM has helped create an end-to-end detection process in deep learning.

One of the important reasons for developing object tracking methods is for the machines to interact with their dynamic environment. This problem falls under the domain of ego-based problems where the sensors are mounted on machines such as robots or autonomous vehicles [5]. For ego-based problems, the objects are localised and tracked from the point of view of the machines. At the same time, the machines must also be able to localise themselves in the dynamic environment to function in a complex environment such as traffic or manufacturing. Therefore, there is a future scope for developing methods and procedures to adapt these vision systems on robots or autonomous vehicles to make an adaptive system in a dynamic environment.

Autonomous aerial vehicles such as unmanned drones are being used to track vehicles [39,46] and in the agricultural sector [2]. Since the range of vision sensors is limited, these drones often have to fly closer to the target, which can interfere with the object's natural state, such as vegetation, or distract humans in a crowded environment. Also, tracking drones from the ground station is an important application, and the distance from the ground station to the drone impacts the localisation and tracking of the drones [42]. Furthermore, in space applications for tracking debris, it is essential to track a fast-moving object at a faraway distance [76]. The range of measuring distance using a stereo camera depends upon the stereo camera parameters, such as the baseline between the two cameras. Zheng et al. [42] calculated the effective sensing range of the entire system of panoramic stereo reached 80 metres. Therefore, progress in increasing the current range of a state-of-the-art system will be significant progress in detecting faraway objects. Therefore, there is further scope for developing vision sensors and methods to track faraway objects.

7.2. Datasets

The applications of object tracking in diverse domains, from medical applications to autonomous navigation, have led to the creation of datasets catering to specific domains. The availability of the dataset ensures that all possible conditions of applications are considered. Since consistently testing on real-world applications can be expensive, the datasets can often simulate the real world to test the applications. In this case, the data can be manually collected from the real world or generated synthetically. However, if the methods are only evaluated on the dataset, it leaves further questions about their applicability in real-world dynamic situations.

In the iterative development process, real-world scenarios may often not be considered, and the method may be more accurate than the dataset. Still, it may not perform well in real-world applications. The most widely used odometry dataset, KITTI [35], consists of different sensor data types that help localise autonomous driving. Researchers combine different object detection datasets and develop methods to cater to real-world applications in a dynamic driving environment. The methods are developed on simulated datasets since some applications are particular, such as space applications [4,76]. For such applications, it is difficult to obtain real datasets and to experiment on such systems, which is an expensive process. While the ground truths often consist of object location, it will be helpful to have additional ground truths about tracking in different situations, such as variations in illumination, at high speed, and with occlusions.

While it is important to develop vision sensors and methods for detecting and tracking faraway objects, developing the dataset for training a deep learning network and evaluating methods is equally important. For applications such as missile tracking or missile intercepting systems [4], collecting data can be a cumbersome process. An alternative in this situation is to generate a synthetic dataset that imitates the real-world application. However, this synthetic dataset needs to be validated before the methods and equipment are developed for the applications. Therefore, researching approaches to create synthetic datasets and evaluating their validity for complex applications such as faraway object detection can be an important research focus.

Several problems in object tracking incorporate the use of multiple cameras [30,32]. A class of problem that uses multiple cameras is the handover problem [32] in object tracking, where the object disappears from the field of view of a camera and appears in the field of view of the next camera. A large-scale dataset can be generated using multiple cameras with ground truths that track objects over multiple cameras.

8. Limitations and Future Work

As computer vision systems are being incorporated into different engineering domains, these systems' ability to interact with the dynamic world relies on tracking objects in real time. New problems are encountered in object tracking as new applications are investigated. While developing a generalised method is often the researchers' goal, addressing all the issues encountered in object tracking in one method is challenging. Therefore, the scope for developing methods in object tracking using computer vision is wide, and several areas can be further investigated to address each problem.

The literature review in this paper raised significant questions about the future scope of research. The research questions, along with recommendations, are outlined as follows:

Q1 Could an end-to-end deep learning approach be developed to detect, classify, estimate the pose, and track the object in a 3D space?
Recommendation: There is significant development in object detection and classification methods such as YOLO [82], R-CNN [99], and Fast R-CNN [84]. Since methods such as YOLO [105] can localise, classify, segment objects, and estimate object pose, it will be worth investigating if the additional feature of tracking can be incorporated in this deep learning framework over video frame sequence. A sequence of video frames could act as an input to these networks, and post-processing steps such as estimating the tracks and stereo matching can be incorporated to detect and track objects. Methods such as SA-FlowNet [6] use a sequence of images for event-based cameras to track objects over time. Spatial attention networks [40] address the tracking using a sequence of video frames for depth estimation using RGB-D sensors. These methods can be further investigated for both calibrated and uncalibrated stereo cameras for depth estimation using a deep CNN.

Q2 Could the range of 3D tracking for faraway objects be extended?
Recommendation: Object tracking is being incorporated in applications of aerial vehicles where the long-range for depth estimation is important. The current state-of-the-art system uses a DS-2CD6984F-IHS/NFC HIKVISION camera and achieves a tracking range of 80 metres using panoramic stereo on a ground station for drone detection [42]. The range may be enhanced by using cameras with a higher zoom factor to construct a similar panoramic system. However, it will be worth investigating whether changing the camera parameters will significantly impact the results using the same methods or if the current state-of-the-art method will require modifications to track faraway objects.

Q3 How can object tracking be implemented on adaptive systems in a dynamic environment?
Recommendation: Robotics is an example of an adaptive system where the robots are subjected to a dynamic environment with moving objects. In this environment, robots need to know the position of the moving objects relative to their position and estimate their location with respect to their trajectory to avoid a collision. This problem may be addressed by developing methods in robots that monitor their environment in real time. The tracking process used in the present methods is performed as a post-processing method where the entire video sequence is available. This creates a limitation in a real-time system, where future information about the environment is unavailable. A predictive tracking algorithm will be helpful for the robot to avoid collision with moving objects. Therefore, for applications in adaptive systems, object tracking accompanied with tracking prediction will have a wider scope for robotics application.

Q4 What improvements are required in the current datasets for object tracking?

Recommendation: The datasets currently used for object tracking, as highlighted in Section 4, were developed for their respective applications. Datasets such as KITTI [35] are specific for autonomous driving, which consist of not only stereo camera video data but also IMU, GPS, and laser scan data. Other datasets such as pedestrian tracking [48,71] were developed for surveillance applications. These datasets are specific to their applications, and their limitation is that they are not generalised enough for a wider application in multiple scenarios.
To develop a dataset for 3D object tracking, stereo camera data of diverse objects similar to ImageNet [142] or MS COCO [143] with their ground truth will provide a common ground to evaluate the performance of object tracking methods. Along with a wider range of object classes, this dataset should also consider the 3D position of the object with respect to the camera. Therefore, an object-tracking dataset may consist of the following attributes:

- Stereo camera video sequence;
- Object classes in each video frame;
- Object location with its bounding-box coordinates in each video frame;
- Ground truth for object tracks for each video sequence;
- Ground truth for object's 3D position relative to the camera.

Generating such a dataset may require extensive effort. However, some data collection processes could be automated, such as using ultrasonic sensors and structured light sensors such as RGB-D [34] to collect ground truth for distance where possible, and the annotation for the dataset could be crowd-sourced using Amazon Mechanical Turk as used by Stanford's dataset [59]. Therefore, there is a scope for developing methods and processes for data collection and benchmarking the dataset for object tracking in computer vision.

Q5 Should hybrid sensors be used for object tracking, or should object tracking completely rely on computer vision?
Recommendation: Having more sensor data when possible is always beneficial. In the case of the KITTI [35] dataset, multiple sensor data are available to the user. Since the application is focused on autonomous driving, using a variety of sensors helps this type of adaptive system make better decisions based on its dynamic environment.
There are systems where having more sensors could create an additional payload on the mechanical system. Aerial drones and industrial robots are examples of adaptive systems where the additional payload can create functional problems. Having a single vision sensor on these devices, such as a stereo or RGB-D camera, could reduce their weight, thereby reducing the additional power requirement for operation. In these situations, relying on computer vision is beneficial. Thus, there is a requirement for better methods that address the diverse scenarios where these systems are deployed.

9. Conclusions

Object tracking is still an ongoing research area, and there is no standardised approach to solving it. Many approaches are developed using different hardware, datasets, and application methodologies. This paper conducted a synthesised review to group these methods according to the hardware and datasets used, the methodologies adopted, and the application areas for object tracking.

In particular, we divided the literature according to the type of cameras used, such as monocular, stereo, depth, and hybrid sensors. The datasets were grouped according to their focused research applications, such as autonomous driving, single-object tracking, multiple-object tracking, and other miscellaneous applications. We also classified the existing literature according to the methodologies used. The application of object tracking is also grouped based on their area of focus, such as medical, autonomous vehicles, single-object tracking, multiple-object tracking, surveillance, robotics, agriculture, space, and defence.

The contribution of this review is the systemic categorisation of different aspects of the object tracking problem. This review highlighted the trends and interest in object tracking research over the last ten years, thereby contributing to the detailed literature review on hardware, datasets, approaches, and applications. Furthermore, tabulated information summarised different tools and methods to develop an object tracking system. A taxonomy was provided for the methods, while identifying the advantages and limitations of different approaches and methods. The review also recommended when the equipment, datasets, and methods can be used. Also, from the review of the literature, different research questions were identified with a recommended approach to address these questions.

Author Contributions: Conceptualisation, P.K. and G.F.; investigation, P.K.; data curation, P.K.; writing—original draft preparation, P.K.; writing—review and editing, P.K., G.F. and J.J.Z.; supervision, G.F. and J.J.Z. All authors have read and agreed to the published version of the manuscript.

Funding: This research received no external funding.

Institutional Review Board Statement: Not applicable.

Informed Consent Statement: Not applicable.

Data Availability Statement: No new data were created or analysed in this study. Data sharing is not applicable to this article.

Conflicts of Interest: The authors declare no conflicts of interest.

Abbreviations

The following abbreviations are used in this manuscript:

APCE	Average peak-to-correlation energy
CNN	Convolutional Neural Networks
DTD	Describable Textures Dataset
EDM	Electronic distance meter
FIR	Finite impulse response
FOV	Field of view
GUI	Graphical User Interface
HCI	Heidelberg Collaboratory for Image Processing
HoG	Histogram of Oriented Gradients
IMU	Inertial measurement unit
JDT	Joint detection and tracking
KITTI	Karlsruhe Institute of Technology and Toyota Technological Institute
LiDAR	Light Detection and Ranging
MEMS	Micro-Electromechanical System
MOT	Multiple-object tracking
MVSEC	Multivehicle Stereo Event Camera
NUC	Next Unit Computing
R-CNN	Regions with CNN features
RBOT	Region-based object tracking
RPN	Risk Priority Number
SAD	Sum of absolute difference
SMDWT	Symmetric mask-based discrete wavelet transform
SNN	Spiking Neural Networks
SOT	Single-object tracking
SSD	Single-Shot Multibox Detector
TBD	Tracking by detection
VI	Visual Inertial
VOT	Visual object tracking
YOLO	You Only Look Once

References

1. Li, X.; Shen, Y.; Lu, J.; Jiang, Q.; Xie, O.; Yang, Y.; Zhu, Q. DyStSLAM: An efficient stereo vision SLAM system in dynamic environment. *Meas. Sci. Technol.* **2023**, *34*, 205105. [CrossRef]
2. Busch, C.; Stol, K.; van der Mark, W. Dynamic tree branch tracking for aerial canopy sampling using stereo vision. *Comput. Electron. Agric.* **2021**, *182*, 106007. [CrossRef]
3. Persic, J.; Petrovic, L.; Markovic, I.; Petrovic, I. Spatiotemporal Multisensor Calibration via Gaussian Processes Moving Target Tracking. *IEEE Trans. Robot.* **2021**, *37*, 1401–1415. [CrossRef]
4. Kwon, J.H.; Song, E.H.; Ha, I.J. 6 Degree-of-Freedom Motion Estimation of a Moving Target using Monocular Image Sequences. *IEEE Trans. Aerosp. Electron. Syst.* **2013**, *49*, 2818–2827. [CrossRef]
5. Feng, S.; Li, X.; Xia, C.; Liao, J.; Zhou, Y.; Li, S.; Hua, X. VIMOT: A Tightly Coupled Estimator for Stereo Visual-Inertial Navigation and Multiobject Tracking. *IEEE Trans. Instrum. Meas.* **2023**, *72*, 3291011. [CrossRef]
6. Yang, F.; Su, L.; Zhao, J.; Chen, X.; Wang, X.; Jiang, N.; Hu, Q. SA-FlowNet: Event-based self-attention optical flow estimation with spiking-analogue neural networks. *IET Comput. Vision* **2023**, *17*, 925–935. [CrossRef]
7. Shen, Y.; Liu, Y.; Tian, Y.; Liu, Z.; Wang, F. A New Parallel Intelligence Based Light Field Dataset for Depth Refinement and Scene Flow Estimation. *Sensors* **2022**, *22*, 9483. [CrossRef] [PubMed]
8. Aladem, M.; Rawashdeh, S. A Combined Vision-Based Multiple Object Tracking and Visual Odometry System. *IEEE Sens. J.* **2019**, *19*, 11714–11720. [CrossRef]
9. Deepambika, V.; Rahman, M.A. Illumination invariant motion detection and tracking using SMDWT and a dense disparity-variance method. *J. Sens.* **2018**, *2018*, 1354316. [CrossRef]
10. Ćesić, J.; Marković, I.; Cvišić, I.; Petrović, I. Radar and stereo vision fusion for multitarget tracking on the special Euclidean group. *Robot. Auton. Syst.* **2016**, *83*, 338–348. [CrossRef]
11. Chuang, M.C.; Hwang, J.N.; Williams, K.; Towler, R. Tracking live fish from low-contrast and low-frame-rate stereo videos. *IEEE Trans. Circuits Syst. Video Technol.* **2015**, *25*, 167–179. [CrossRef]
12. Richey, W.; Heiselman, J.; Ringel, M.; Meszoely, I.; Miga, M. Soft Tissue Monitoring of the Surgical Field: Detection and Tracking of Breast Surface Deformations. *IEEE Trans. Biomed. Eng.* **2023**, *70*, 2002–2012. [CrossRef]
13. Gionfrida, L.; Rusli, W.; Bharath, A.; Kedgley, A. Validation of two-dimensional video-based inference of finger kinematics with pose estimation. *PLoS ONE* **2022**, *17*, e0276799. [CrossRef]
14. Czajkowska, J.; Pyciński, B.; Juszczyk, J.; Pietka, E. Biopsy needle tracking technique in US images. *Comput. Med. Imaging Graph.* **2018**, *65*, 93–101. [CrossRef]
15. Yang, J.; Xu, R.; Ding, Z.; Lv, H. 3D character recognition using binocular camera for medical assist. *Neurocomputing* **2017**, *220*, 17–22. [CrossRef]
16. Zarrabeitia, L.; Qureshi, F.; Aruliah, D. Stereo reconstruction of droplet flight trajectories. *IEEE Trans. Pattern Anal. Mach. Intell.* **2015**, *37*, 847–861. [CrossRef] [PubMed]
17. Li, X.; Hu, W.; Shen, C.; Zhang, Z.; Dick, A.; Van Den Hengel, A. A survey of appearance models in visual object tracking. *ACM Trans. Intell. Syst. Technol.* **2013**, *4*, 1–48 [CrossRef]
18. Krizhevsky, A.; Sutskever, I.; Hinton, G.E. ImageNet Classification with Deep Convolutional Neural Networks. *Commun. ACM* **2017**, *60*, 84–90. [CrossRef]
19. Kumar, A.; Walia, G.S.; Sharma, K. Recent trends in multicue based visual tracking: A review. *Expert Syst. Appl.* **2020**, *162*, 113711. [CrossRef]
20. Park, Y.; Dang, L.M.; Lee, S.; Han, D.; Moon, H. Multiple object tracking in deep learning approaches: A survey. *Electronics* **2021**, *10*, 2406. [CrossRef]
21. Kalake, L.; Wan, W.; Hou, L. Analysis Based on Recent Deep Learning Approaches Applied in Real-Time Multi-Object Tracking: A Review. *IEEE Access* **2021**, *9*, 32650–32671. [CrossRef]
22. Mandal, M.; Vipparthi, S.K. An Empirical Review of Deep Learning Frameworks for Change Detection: Model Design, Experimental Frameworks, Challenges and Research Needs. *IEEE Trans. Intell. Transp. Syst.* **2022**, *23*, 6101–6122. [CrossRef]
23. Guo, S.; Wang, S.; Yang, Z.; Wang, L.; Zhang, H.; Guo, P.; Gao, Y.; Guo, J. A Review of Deep Learning-Based Visual Multi-Object Tracking Algorithms for Autonomous Driving. *Appl. Sci.* **2022**, *12*, 10741. [CrossRef]
24. Dai, Y.; Hu, Z.; Zhang, S.; Liu, L. A survey of detection-based video multi-object tracking. *Displays* **2022**, *75*, 102317. [CrossRef]
25. Rakai, L.; Song, H.; Sun, S.; Zhang, W.; Yang, Y. Data association in multiple object tracking: A survey of recent techniques. *Expert Syst. Appl.* **2022**, *192*, 116300. [CrossRef]
26. Liu, C.; Chen, X.F.; Bo, C.J.; Wang, D. Long-term Visual Tracking: Review and Experimental Comparison. *Mach. Intell. Res.* **2022**, *19*, 512–530. [CrossRef]
27. Rocha, R.d.L.; de Figueiredo, F.A.P. Beyond Land: A Review of Benchmarking Datasets, Algorithms, and Metrics for Visual-Based Ship Tracking. *Electronics* **2023**, *12*, 2789. [CrossRef]
28. Kriechbaumer, T.; Blackburn, K.; Breckon, T.; Hamilton, O.; Casado, M. Quantitative evaluation of stereo visual odometry for autonomous vessel localisation in inland waterway sensing applications. *Sensors* **2015**, *15*, 31869–31887. [CrossRef] [PubMed]
29. Sinisterra, A.; Dhanak, M.; Ellenrieder, K.V. Stereovision-based target tracking system for USV operations. *Ocean Eng.* **2017**, *133*, 197–214. [CrossRef]

30. Gennaro, T.D.; Waldmann, J. Sensor Fusion with Asynchronous Decentralized Processing for 3D Target Tracking with a Wireless Camera Network. *Sensors* **2023**, *23*, 1194. [CrossRef]
31. Hartley, R.; Zisserman, A. *Multiple View Geometry in Computer Vision*, 2nd ed.; Cambridge University Press: Cambridge, UK, 2004.
32. Yan, M.; Zhao, Y.; Liu, M.; Kong, L.; Dong, L. High-speed moving target tracking of multi-camera system with overlapped field of view. *Signal Image Video Process* **2021**, *15*, 1369–1377. [CrossRef]
33. Huang, J.; Xu, W.; Zhao, W.; Yuan, H. An improved method for swing measurement based on monocular vision to the payload of overhead crane. *Trans. Inst. Meas. Control* **2022**, *44*, 50–59. [CrossRef]
34. Zhang, Z. Microsoft Kinect Sensor and Its Effect. *IEEE MultiMedia* **2012**, *19*, 4–10. [CrossRef]
35. Geiger, A.; Lenz, P.; Stiller, C.; Urtasun, R. Vision meets robotics: The KITTI dataset. *Int. J. Robot. Res.* **2013**, *32*, 1231–1237. [CrossRef]
36. García, J.; Gardel, A.; Bravo, I.; Lázaro, J.; Martínez, M. Tracking people motion based on extended condensation algorithm. *IEEE Trans. Syst. Man Cybern. Part A Syst. Hum.* **2013**, *43*, 606–618. [CrossRef]
37. Hu, M.; Liu, Z.; Zhang, J.; Zhang, G. Robust object tracking via multi-cue fusion. *Signal Process* **2017**, *139*, 1339–1351. [CrossRef]
38. Bouguet, J.Y. Camera Calibration Toolbox for Matlab. 2022. Available online: https://data.caltech.edu/records/jx9cx-fdh55 (27 February 2024).
39. Wu, S.; Li, R.; Shi, Y.; Liu, Q. Vision-Based Target Detection and Tracking System for a Quadcopter. *IEEE Access* **2021**, *9*, 62043–62054. [CrossRef]
40. Rasoulidanesh, M.; Yadav, S.; Herath, S.; Vaghei, Y.; Payandeh, S. Deep attention models for human tracking using RGBD. *Sensors* **2019**, *19*, 750. [CrossRef] [PubMed]
41. Song, S.; Xiao, J. Tracking Revisited using RGBD Camera: Unified Benchmark and Baselines. In Proceedings of the IEEE International Conference on Computer Vision, Sydney, Australia, 1–8 December 2013. [CrossRef]
42. Zheng, Y.; Zheng, C.; Zhang, X.; Chen, F.; Chen, Z.; Zhao, S. Detection, Localization, and Tracking of Multiple MAVs with Panoramic Stereo Camera Networks. *IEEE Trans. Autom. Sci. Eng.* **2023**, *20*, 1226–1243. [CrossRef]
43. Ram, S. Fusion of Inverse Synthetic Aperture Radar and Camera Images for Automotive Target Tracking. *IEEE J. Sel. Top. Signal Process* **2023**, *17*, 431–444. [CrossRef]
44. Ngoc, L.; Tin, N.; Tuan, L. A New framework of moving object tracking based on object detection-tracking with removal of moving features. *Int. J. Adv. Comput. Sci. Appl.* **2020**, *11*, 35–46. [CrossRef]
45. Sigal, L.; Balan, A.O.; Black, M.J.; Balan, A.O.; Black, M.J.; Black, M.J. HUMANEVA: Synchronized Video and Motion Capture Dataset and Baseline Algorithm for Evaluation of Articulated Human Motion. *Int. J. Comput. Vis.* **2010**, *87*, 4–27. [CrossRef]
46. Mdfaa, M.A.; Kulathunga, G.; Klimchik, A. 3D-SiamMask: Vision-Based Multi-Rotor Aerial-Vehicle Tracking for a Moving Object. *Remote Sens.* **2022**, *14*, 5756. [CrossRef]
47. Karangwa, J.; Liu, J.; Zeng, Z. Vehicle Detection for Autonomous Driving: A Review of Algorithms and Datasets. *IEEE Trans. Intell. Transp. Syst.* **2023**, *24*, 11568–11594. [CrossRef]
48. Flohr, F.; Gavrila, D. PedCut: An iterative framework for pedestrian segmentation combining shape models and multiple data cues. In Proceedings of the British Machine Vision Conference (BMVC), Bristol, UK, 9–13 September 2013.
49. Zhu, A.Z.; Thakur, D.; Ozaslan, T.; Pfrommer, B.; Kumar, V.; Daniilidis, K. The Multi Vehicle Stereo Event Camera Dataset: An Event Camera Dataset for 3D Perception. *IEEE Robot. Autom. Lett.* **2018**, *3*, 2800793. [CrossRef]
50. Nikolic, J.; Rehder, J.; Burri, M.; Gohl, P.; Leutenegger, S.; Furgale, P.T.; Siegwart, R. A synchronized visual-inertial sensor system with FPGA pre-processing for accurate real-time SLAM. In Proceedings of the 2014 IEEE International Conference on Robotics and Automation (ICRA), Hong Kong, China, 31 May–7 June 2014; pp. 431–437. [CrossRef]
51. Honauer, K.; Johannsen, O.; Kondermann, D.; Goldluecke, B. A dataset and evaluation methodology for depth estimation on 4D light fields. In *Computer Vision–ACCV 2016, Proceedings of the 13th Asian Conference on Computer Vision, Taipei, Taiwan, 20–24 November 2016*; Revised Selected Papers, Part III 13; Lecture Notes in Computer Science; Springer: Cham, Switzerland, 2017; Volume 10113, pp. 19–34. [CrossRef]
52. Kristan, M.; Leonardis, A.; Matas, J.; Felsberg, M.; Pflugfelder, R.; Kämäräinen, J.K.; Chang, H.J.; Danelljan, M.; Čehovin Zajc, L.; Lukežič, A.; et al. The Tenth Visual Object Tracking VOT2022 Challenge Results. In Proceedings of the European Conference on Computer Vision, Tel Aviv, Israel, 23–27 October 2022; Lecture Notes in Computer Science; Springer: Cham, Switzerland, 2023; Volume 13808, pp. 431–460. [CrossRef]
53. Wu, Y.; Lim, J.; Yang, M.H. Object tracking benchmark. *IEEE Trans. Pattern Anal. Mach. Intell.* **2015**, *37*, 1834–1848. [CrossRef] [PubMed]
54. Pauwels, K.; Rubio, L.; Díaz, J.; Ros, E. Real-time Model-based Rigid Object Pose Estimation and Tracking Combining Dense and Sparse Visual Cues. In Proceedings of the IEEE Conference on Computer Vision and Pattern Recognition, Portland, OR, USA, 23–28 June 2013. [CrossRef]
55. Kasper, A.; Xue, Z.; Dillmann, R. The KIT object models database: An object model database for object recognition, localization and manipulation in service robotics. *Int. J. Robot. Res.* **2012**, *31*, 927–934. [CrossRef]
56. Zhong, L.; Zhang, Y.; Zhao, H.; Chang, A.; Xiang, W.; Zhang, S.; Zhang, L. Seeing through the Occluders: Robust Monocular 6-DOF Object Pose Tracking via Model-Guided Video Object Segmentation. *IEEE Robot. Autom. Lett.* **2020**, *5*, 5159–5166. [CrossRef]

57. Krull, A.; Michel, F.; Brachmann, E.; Gumhold, S.; Ihrke, S.; Rother, C. 6-DOF Model Based Tracking via Object Coordinate Regression. In Proceedings of the Computer Vision—ACCV, Singapore, 1–5 November 2014; Springer International Publishing: Berlin/Heidelberg, Germany, 2015. [CrossRef]
58. Hwang, J.; Kim, J.; Chi, S.; Seo, J. Development of training image database using web crawling for vision-based site monitoring. *Autom. Constr.* **2022**, *135*, 104141. [CrossRef]
59. Krause, J.; Stark, M.; Deng, J.; Li, F.-F. 3D Object Representations for Fine-Grained Categorization. In Proceedings of the IEEE International Conference on Computer Vision Workshops, Sydney, Australia, 2–8 December 2013. [CrossRef]
60. Cimpoi, M.; Maji, S.; Kokkinosécole, I.; Mohamed, S.; Vedaldi, A. Describing Textures in the Wild. In Proceedings of the IEEE Conference on Computer Vision and Pattern Recognition, Columbus, OH, USA, 23–28 June 2014. [CrossRef]
61. Zauner, C. Implementation and Benchmarking of Perceptual Image Hash Functions. 2010. Available online: http://www.phash.org/docs/pubs/thesis_zauner.pdf (accessed on 27 February 2024).
62. Kristan, M.; Matas, J.; Leonardis, A.; Felsberg, M.; Fernández, G.; Vojí, T.; Häger, G.; Nebehay, G.; Pflugfelder, R.; Gupta, A.; et al. The Visual Object Tracking VOT2015 challenge results 2015 IEEE International Conference on Computer Vision Workshop 2015 IEEE International Conference on Computer Vision Workshop. *Chin. Acad. Sci.* **2015**, *32*, 79. [CrossRef]
63. Kristan, M.; Leonardis, A.; Matas, J.; Felsberg, M.; Pflugfelder, R.; Čehovin, L.; Vojír, T.; Häger, G.; Lukežič, A.; Fernández, G.; et al. The visual object tracking VOT2016 challenge results. In *Computer Vision–ECCV 2016 Workshops: Amsterdam, The Netherlands, October 8–10 and 15–16, 2016, Proceedings, Part II*; Lecture Notes in Computer Science (Including Subseries Lecture Notes in Artificial Intelligence and Lecture Notes in Bioinformatics); Springer: Cham, Switzerland, 2016; Volume 9914, pp. 777–823. [CrossRef]
64. Kristan, M.; Leonardis, A.; Matas, J.; Felsberg, M.; Pflugfelder, R.; Čehovin Zajc, L.; Vojír, T.; Bhat, G.; Lukežič, A.; Eldesokey, A.; et al. The sixth visual object tracking VOT2018 challenge results. In Proceedings of the Computer Vision—ECCV 2018 Workshops, Munich, Germany, 8–14 September 2018; Lecture Notes in Computer Science; Volume 11129, pp. 3–53. [CrossRef]
65. Kristan, M.; Matas, J.; Leonardis, A.; Felsberg, M.; Pflugfelder, R.; Kämäräinen, J.K.; Zajc, L.C.; Drbohlav, O.; Lukezic, A.; Berg, A.; et al. The seventh visual object tracking VOT2019 challenge results. In Proceedings of the 2019 International Conference on Computer Vision Workshop, ICCVW 2019, Seoul, Republic of Korea, 27–28 October 2019; pp. 2206–2241. [CrossRef]
66. Dendorfer, P.; Rezatofighi, H.; Milan, A.; Shi, J.; Cremers, D.; Reid, I.; Roth, S.; Schindler, K.; Leal-Taixé, L.; Taixé, T. MOT20: A Benchmark for Multi Object Tracking in Crowded Scenes. *arXiv* **2020**, arXiv:2003.09003.
67. Leal-Taixé, L.; Taixé, T.; Milan, A.; Reid, I.; Roth, S.; Schindler, K. MOTChallenge 2015: Towards a Benchmark for Multi-Target Tracking. *arXiv* **2015**, arXiv:1504.01942.
68. Milan, A.; Leal-Taixé, L.; Taixé, T.; Reid, I.; Roth, S.; Schindler, K. MOT16: A Benchmark for Multi-Object Tracking. *arXiv* **2016**, arXiv:1603.00831.
69. Dendorfer, P.; Rezatofighi, H.; Milan, A.; Shi, J.; Cremers, D.; Reid, I.; Roth, S.; Schindler, K.; Leal-Taixé, L.; Taixé, T. CVPR19 Tracking and Detection Challenge: How crowded can it get? *arXiv* **2019**, arXiv:1906.04567.
70. Luo, W.; Xing, J.; Milan, A.; Zhang, X.; Liu, W.; Kim, T.K. Multiple object tracking: A literature review. *Artif. Intell.* **2021**, *293*, 103448. [CrossRef]
71. Dollar, P.; Wojek, C.; Schiele, B.; Perona, P. Pedestrian detection: A benchmark. In Proceedings of the 2009 IEEE Conference on Computer Vision and Pattern Recognition, Miami, FL, USA, 20–25 June 2009; pp. 304–311. [CrossRef]
72. Wang, Z.; Yoon, S.; Park, D. Online adaptive multiple pedestrian tracking in monocular surveillance video. *Neural Comput. Appl.* **2017**, *28*, 127–141. [CrossRef]
73. Ferryman, J.; Ellis, A.L. Performance evaluation of crowd image analysis using the PETS2009 dataset. *Pattern Recognit. Lett.* **2014**, *44*, 3–15 [CrossRef]
74. Tjaden, H.; Schwanecke, U.; Schömer, E.; Cremers, D. A Region-Based Gauss-Newton Approach to Real-Time Monocular Multiple Object Tracking. *IEEE Trans. Pattern Anal. Mach. Intell.* **2019**, *41*, 1797–1812. [CrossRef]
75. Garcia, J.; Younes, A. Real-Time Navigation for Drogue-Type Autonomous Aerial Refueling Using Vision-Based Deep Learning Detection. *IEEE Trans. Aerosp. Electron. Syst.* **2021**, *57*, 2225–2246. [CrossRef]
76. Biondi, G.; Mauro, S.; Pastorelli, S.; Sorli, M. Fault-tolerant feature-based estimation of space debris rotational motion during active removal missions. *Acta Astronaut.* **2018**, *146*, 332–338. [CrossRef]
77. Wang, Q.; Zhou, J.; Li, Z.; Sun, X.; Yu, Q. Robust and Accurate Monocular Pose Tracking for Large Pose Shift. *IEEE Trans. Ind. Electron.* **2023**, *70*, 8163–8173. [CrossRef]
78. Xiao, P.; Yan, F.; Chi, J.; Wang, Z. Real-Time 3D Pedestrian Tracking with Monocular Camera. *Wirel. Commun. Mob. Comput.* **2022**, *2022*, 7437289. [CrossRef]
79. Meneses, M.; Matos, L.; Prado, B.; Carvalho, A.; Macedo, H. SmartSORT: An MLP-based method for tracking multiple objects in real-time. *J. Real-Time Image Process.* **2021**, *18*, 913–921. [CrossRef]
80. Zhang, Y.; Sheng, H.; Wu, Y.; Wang, S.; Ke, W.; Xiong, Z. Multiplex Labeling Graph for Near-Online Tracking in Crowded Scenes. *IEEE Internet Things J.* **2020**, *7*, 7892–7902. [CrossRef]
81. Du, M.; Nan, X.; Guan, L. Monocular human motion tracking by using de-mc particle filter. *IEEE Trans. Image Process.* **2013**, *22*, 3852–3865. [CrossRef]

82. Redmon, J.; Divvala, S.; Girshick, R.; Farhadi, A. You Only Look Once: Unified, Real-Time Object Detection. In Proceedings of the 2016 IEEE Conference on Computer Vision and Pattern Recognition (CVPR), Las Vegas, NV, USA, 27–30 June 2016; pp. 779–788. [CrossRef]
83. Redmon, J.; Farhadi, A. YOLOv3: An Incremental Improvement. *arXiv* **2018**, arXiv:1804.02767. [CrossRef]
84. Girshick, R. Fast R-CNN. In Proceedings of the 2015 IEEE International Conference on Computer Vision (ICCV), Santiago, Chile, 7–13 December 2015; pp. 1440–1448. [CrossRef]
85. Soille, P. Erosion and Dilation. *Morphol. Image Anal.* **2004**, *2*, 63–103. [CrossRef]
86. Ma, J.; Jiang, X.; Fan, A.; Jiang, J.; Yan, J.; Lepetit, V.; Yan, J.; Jiang, X. Image Matching from Handcrafted to Deep Features: A Survey. *Int. J. Comput. Vis.* **2021**, *129*, 23–79. [CrossRef]
87. Geiger, A.; Ziegler, J.; Stiller, C. StereoScan: Dense 3d reconstruction in real-time. In Proceedings of the 2011 IEEE Intelligent Vehicles Symposium (IV), Baden, Germany, 5–9 June 2011; pp. 963–968. [CrossRef]
88. Kalman, R.E. A new approach to linear filtering and prediction problems. *J. Fluids Eng. Trans. ASME* **1960**, *82*, 35–45. [CrossRef]
89. Steinbrücker, F.; Sturm, J.; Cremers, D. Real-time visual odometry from dense RGB-D images. In Proceedings of the IEEE International Conference on Computer Vision, Barcelona, Spain, 6–13 November 2011; pp. 719–722. [CrossRef]
90. Jenkins, M.; Barrie, P.; Buggy, T.; Morison, G. Extended fast compressive tracking with weighted multi-frame template matching for fast motion tracking. *Pattern Recognit. Lett.* **2016**, *69*, 82–87. [CrossRef]
91. Itseez. Open Source Computer Vision Library. 2015. Available online: https://github.com/itseez/opencv (accessed on 27 February 2024).
92. Otsu, N. A Threshold Selection Method from Gray-Level Histograms. *IEEE Trans. Syst. Man Cybern* **1979**, *9*, 62–66. [CrossRef]
93. Canny, J. A Computational Approach to Edge Detection. *IEEE Trans. Pattern Anal. Mach. Intell.* **1986**, *PAMI-8*, 679–698. [CrossRef]
94. Hsia, C.H.; Guo, J.M.; Chiang, J.S. Improved Low-Complexity Algorithm for 2-D Integer Lifting-Based Discrete Wavelet Transform Using Symmetric Mask-Based Scheme. *IEEE Trans. Circuits Syst. Video Technol.* **2009**, *19*, 1202–1208. [CrossRef]
95. Kanade, T.; Kano, H.; Kimura, S.; Yoshida, A.; Oda, K. Development of a video-rate stereo machine. In Proceedings of the 1995 IEEE/RSJ International Conference on Intelligent Robots and Systems. Human Robot Interaction and Cooperative Robots, Pittsburgh, PA, USA, 5–9 August 1995; Volume 3, pp. 95–100. [CrossRef]
96. Szwarc, P.; Kawa, J.; Pietka, E. White matter segmentation from MR images in subjects with brain tumours. In *Information Technologies in Biomedicine, Proceedings of the Third International Conference, ITIB 2012, Gliwice, Poland, 11–13 June 2012*; Lecture Notes in Computer Science; Springer: Berlin/Heidelberg, Germany, 2012; Volume 7339 LNBI, pp. 36–46. [CrossRef]
97. Dalal, N.; Triggs, B. Histograms of oriented gradients for human detection. In Proceedings of the 2005 IEEE Computer Society Conference on Computer Vision and Pattern Recognition (CVPR'05), San Diego, CA, USA, 20–25 June 2005; Volume 1, pp. 886–893. [CrossRef]
98. Alcantarilla, P.F.; Bartoli, A.; Davison, A.J. KAZE features. In Proceedings of the Computer Vision–ECCV 2012: 12th European Conference on Computer Vision, Florence, Italy, 7–13 October 2012; Part VI 12; Springer: Berlin/Heidelberg, Germany, 2012; pp. 214–227. [CrossRef]
99. Girshick, R.; Donahue, J.; Darrell, T.; Malik, J. Rich Feature Hierarchies for Accurate Object Detection and Semantic Segmentation. In Proceedings of the 2014 IEEE Conference on Computer Vision and Pattern Recognition, Columbus, OH, USA, 23–28 June 2014; pp. 580–587. [CrossRef]
100. He, K.; Gkioxari, G.; Dollár, P.; Girshick, R. Mask R-CNN. In Proceedings of the 2017 IEEE International Conference on Computer Vision (ICCV), Venice, Italy, 22–29 October 2017; pp. 2980–2988. [CrossRef]
101. Ren, S.; He, K.; Girshick, R.; Sun, J. Faster R-CNN: Towards Real-Time Object Detection with Region Proposal Networks. *IEEE Trans. Pattern Anal. Mach. Intell.* **2017**, *39*, 1137–1149. [CrossRef] [PubMed]
102. Leonard, J.; Durrant-Whyte, H. Mobile robot localization by tracking geometric beacons. *IEEE Trans. Robot. Autom.* **1991**, *7*, 376–382. [CrossRef]
103. Liu, W.; Anguelov, D.; Erhan, D.; Szegedy, C.; Reed, S.; Fu, C.Y.; Berg, A.C. SSD: Single shot multibox detector. In *Computer Vision–ECCV 2016, Proceedings of the 14th European Conference, Amsterdam, The Netherlands, 11–14 October 2016*; Proceedings, Part I 14; Lecture Notes in Computer Science; Springer: Cham, Switzerland, 2016; Volume 9905, pp. 21–37. [CrossRef]
104. Terven, J.; Córdova-Esparza, D.M.; Romero-González, J.A. A Comprehensive Review of YOLO Architectures in Computer Vision: From YOLOv1 to YOLOv8 and YOLO-NAS. *Mach. Learn. Knowl. Extr.* **2023**, *5*, 1680–1716. [CrossRef]
105. Jocher, G. YOLOv5 by Ultralytics. 2020. Available online: https://doi.org/10.5281/zenodo.3908559 (accessed on 1 October 2023).
106. Shafiee, M.J.; Chywl, B.; Li, F.; Wong, A. Fast YOLO: A Fast You Only Look Once System for Real-time Embedded Object Detection in Video. *arXiv* **2017**, arXiv:1709.05943. [CrossRef]
107. Li, Z.; Snavely, N. MegaDepth: Learning Single-View Depth Prediction from Internet Photos. In Proceedings of the IEEE Conference on Computer Vision and Pattern Recognition, Salt Lake City, UT, USA, 18–23 June 2018. [CrossRef]
108. Wang, Q.; Zhang, L.; Bertinetto, L.; Hu, W.; Torr, P.H. Fast Online Object Tracking and Segmentation: A Unifying Approach. In Proceedings of the IEEE/CVF Conference on Computer Vision and Pattern Recognition, Long Beach, CA, USA, 15–20 June 2019. [CrossRef]
109. Ranftl, R.; Lasinger, K.; Hafner, D.; Schindler, K.; Koltun, V. Towards Robust Monocular Depth Estimation: Mixing Datasets for Zero-Shot Cross-Dataset Transfer. *IEEE Trans. Pattern Anal. Mach. Intell.* **2022**, *44*, 1623–1637. [CrossRef] [PubMed]

110. He, K.; Zhang, X.; Ren, S.; Sun, J. Deep Residual Learning for Image Recognition. In Proceedings of the 2016 IEEE Conference on Computer Vision and Pattern Recognition (CVPR), Las Vegas, NV, USA, 27–30 June 2016; pp. 770–778. [CrossRef]
111. Cao, Z.; Hidalgo, G.; Simon, T.; Wei, S.E.; Sheikh, Y. OpenPose: Realtime Multi-Person 2D Pose Estimation Using Part Affinity Fields. *IEEE Trans. Pattern Anal. Mach. Intell.* **2021**, *43*, 172–186. [CrossRef]
112. Forney, G. The viterbi algorithm. *Proc. IEEE* **1973**, *61*, 268–278. [CrossRef]
113. Li, P.; Zhao, H.; Liu, P.; Cao, F. RTM3D: Real-Time Monocular 3D Detection from Object Keypoints for Autonomous Driving. In Proceedings of the European Conference on Computer Vision, Glasgow, UK, 23–28 August 2020; Lecture Notes in Computer Science; Springer: Cham, Switzerland, 2020; Volume 12348, pp. 644–660. [CrossRef]
114. Sun, Y.; Zheng, L.; Yang, Y.; Tian, Q.; Wang, S. Beyond Part Models: Person Retrieval with Refined Part Pooling (and A Strong Convolutional Baseline). In Proceedings of the European Conference on Computer Vision, Munich, Germany, 8–14 September 2018; Lecture Notes in Computer Science; Springer: Cham, Switzerland, 2018; Volume 11208, pp. 501–518. [CrossRef]
115. Zheng, L.; Shen, L.; Tian, L.; Wang, S.; Wang, J.; Tian, Q. Scalable Person Re-identification: A Benchmark. In Proceedings of the 2015 IEEE International Conference on Computer Vision (ICCV), Santiago, Chile, 7–13 December 2015; pp. 1116–1124. [CrossRef]
116. Brunelli, R.; Poggiot, T. Template matching: Matched spatial filters and beyond. *Pattern Recognit.* **1997**, *30*, 751–768. [CrossRef]
117. Wu, Y.; Lim, J.; Yang, M.H. Online Object Tracking: A Benchmark. In Proceedings of the IEEE Conference on Computer Vision and Pattern Recognition, Portland, OR, USA, 23–28 June 2013. [CrossRef]
118. Munkres, J. Algorithms for the Assignment and Transportation Problems. *J. Soc. Ind. Appl. Math.* **1957**, *5*, 32–38. [CrossRef]
119. Horn, B.K.; Schunck, B.G. Determining optical flow. *Artif. Intell.* **1981** , *17* 185–203. [CrossRef]
120. Hough, P.V. Method and Means for Recognizing Complex Patterns. U.S. Patent 3,069,654, 18 December 1962.
121. Lucas, B.D.; Kanade, T. An Iterative Image Registration Technique with an Application to Stereo Vision. In Proceedings of the 7th International Joint Conference on Artificial Intelligence—Volume 2, San Francisco, CA, USA, 24–28 August 1981; IJCAI'81, pp. 674–679.
122. Tomasi, C.; Kanade, T. Detection and tracking of point. *Int. J. Comput. Vis.* **1991**, *9*, 3.
123. Harris, C.; Stephens, M. A combined corner and edge detector. In Proceedings of the Alvey Vision Conference, Manchester, UK, 15–17 September 1988; Volume 15, pp. 10–5244.
124. Li, Q.; Li, R.; Ji, K.; Dai, W. Kalman Filter and Its Application. In Proceedings of the 2015 8th International Conference on Intelligent Networks and Intelligent Systems (ICINIS), Tianjin, China, 1–3 November 2015; pp. 74–77. [CrossRef]
125. Witkin, A.P. Scale-Space Filtering. In *Readings in Computer Vision*; Morgan Kaufmann: Burlington, MA, USA, 1987; Volume 2, pp. 329–332. [CrossRef]
126. Persoon, E.; Fu, K.S. Shape Discrimination Using Fourier Descriptors. *IEEE Trans. Syst. Man Cybern.* **1977**, *7*, 170–179. [CrossRef]
127. Shi, J.; Tomasi. Good features to track. In Proceedings of the 1994 IEEE Conference on Computer Vision and Pattern Recognition, Seattle, WA, USA, 21–23 June 1994; pp. 593–600. [CrossRef]
128. Calonder, M.; Lepetit, V.; Strecha, C.; Fua, P. BRIEF: Binary Robust Independent Elementary Features. In *Computer Vision—ECCV 2010, Proceedings of the 11th European Conference on Computer Vision, Heraklion, Crete, Greece, 5–11 September* 2010; Lecture Notes in Computer Science; Springer: Berlin/Heidelberg, Germany, 2010; pp. 778–792. [CrossRef]
129. Mozhdehi, R.J.; Medeiros, H. Deep convolutional particle filter for visual tracking. In Proceedings of the 2017 IEEE International Conference on Image Processing (ICIP), Beijing, China, 17–20 September 2017; pp. 3650–3654. [CrossRef]
130. Lowe, D.G. Distinctive Image Features from Scale-Invariant Keypoints. *Int. J. Comput. Vis.* **2004**, *60*, 91–110. [CrossRef]
131. Bay, H.; Tuytelaars, T.; Van Gool, L. SURF: Speeded Up Robust Features. In Computer Vision–ECCV 2006, Proceedings of the 9th European Conference on Computer Vision, Graz, Austria, 7–13 May 2006; Lecture Notes in Computer Science; Springer: Berlin/Heidelberg, Germany, 2006; Volume 3951, pp. 404–417. [CrossRef]
132. Rublee, E.; Rabaud, V.; Konolige, K.; Bradski, G. ORB: An efficient alternative to SIFT or SURF. In Proceedings of the 2011 International Conference on Computer Vision, Barcelona, Spain, 6–13 November 2011; pp. 2564–2571. [CrossRef]
133. Rosten, E.; Porter, R.; Drummond, T. Faster and Better: A Machine Learning Approach to Corner Detection. *IEEE Trans. Pattern Anal. Mach. Intell.* **2010**, *32*, 105–119. [CrossRef]
134. Hochreiter, S.; Schmidhuber, J. Long Short-Term Memory. *Neural Comput.* **1997**, *9*, 1735–1780. [CrossRef] [PubMed]
135. Nam, H.; Han, B. Learning Multi-domain Convolutional Neural Networks for Visual Tracking. In Proceedings of the IEEE Computer Society Conference on Computer Vision and Pattern Recognition, Las Vegas, NV, USA, 27–30 June 2016; pp. 4293–4302. [CrossRef]
136. Kuhn, H.W. The Hungarian method for the assignment problem. *Nav. Res. Logist.* **2005**, *52*, 7–21. [CrossRef]
137. Koch, G.; Zemel, R.; Salakhutdinov, R. Siamese neural networks for one-shot image recognition. In Proceedings of the ICML Deep Learning Workshop, Lille, France, 6–11 July 2015; Volume 2.
138. Gerstner, W.; Kistler, W.M. *Spiking Neuron Models: Single Neurons, Populations, Plasticity*; Cambridge University Press: Cambridge, UK, 2002. [CrossRef]
139. Varga, D.; Szirányi, T.; Kiss, A.; Spórás, L.; Havasi, L. A Multi-View Pedestrian Tracking Method in an Uncalibrated Camera Network. In Proceedings of the IEEE International Conference on Computer Vision, Santiago, Chile, 7–13 December 2015; pp. 184–191. [CrossRef]
140. Koppanyi, Z.; Toth, C.; Soltesz, T. Deriving Pedestrian Positions from Uncalibrated Videos. In Proceedings of the ASPRS Imaging & Geospatial Technology Forum (IGTF), Tampa, FL, USA, 12–16 March 2017; pp. 4–8.

141. Hosna, A.; Merry, E.; Gyalmo, J.; Alom, Z.; Aung, Z.; Azim, M.A. Transfer learning: A friendly introduction. *J. Big Data* **2022**, *9*, 102. [CrossRef]
142. Russakovsky, O.; Deng, J.; Su, H.; Krause, J.; Satheesh, S.; Ma, S.; Huang, Z.; Karpathy, A.; Khosla, A.; Bernstein, M.; et al. ImageNet Large Scale Visual Recognition Challenge. *Int. J. Comput. Vis.* **2015**, *115*, 211–252. [CrossRef]
143. Lin, T.Y.; Maire, M.; Belongie, S.; Hays, J.; Perona, P.; Ramanan, D.; Dollár, P.; Zitnick, C.L. Microsoft coco: Common objects in context. In *Computer Vision–ECCV 2014, Proceedings of the 13th European Conference, Zurich, Switzerland, 6–12 September 2014;* Part V 13; Springer: Berlin/Heidelberg, Germany, 2014; pp. 740–755. [CrossRef]

computers

MDPI

Review

Quantum Image Compression: Fundamentals, Algorithms, and Advances

Sowmik Kanti Deb and W. David Pan *

Department of Electrical and Computer Engineering, University of Alabama in Huntsville, Huntsville, AL 35899, USA; sd0129@uah.edu
* Correspondence: pand@uah.edu

Abstract: Quantum computing has emerged as a transformative paradigm, with revolutionary potential in numerous fields, including quantum image processing and compression. Applications that depend on large scale image data could benefit greatly from parallelism and quantum entanglement, which would allow images to be encoded and decoded with unprecedented efficiency and data reduction capability. This paper provides a comprehensive overview of the rapidly evolving field of quantum image compression, including its foundational principles, methods, challenges, and potential uses. The paper will also feature a thorough exploration of the fundamental concepts of quantum qubits as image pixels, quantum gates as image transformation tools, quantum image representation, as well as basic quantum compression operations. Our survey shows that work is still sparse on the practical implementation of quantum image compression algorithms on physical quantum computers. Thus, further research is needed in order to attain the full advantage and potential of quantum image compression algorithms on large-scale fault-tolerant quantum computers.

Keywords: quantum computing; quantum image compression; quantum image processing

1. Introduction

In recent years, in accordance with Moore's law [1], the computing ability of electronic computers has exponentially increased. However, the growth in power of CPUs has plateaued in over the last few years due to various constraints, prompting the search for alternative methods to boost computational performance. In 1982, Richard Feynman, an American theoretical physicist, introduced the concept of quantum computing. This innovative model leverages quantum mechanics principles like superposition and entanglement to enhance data storage, processing, and transmission capabilities far beyond those of traditional computers [2]. The potential of quantum computing was further underscored by Peter Shor's introduction of a quantum algorithm for prime number factorization in 1994 [3], and by Lov Grover's quantum search algorithm in 1996 [4].

As the field of digital image processing evolves, it faces the challenge of handling an ever-growing volume and complexity of images, propelled by advances in pattern recognition, image understanding, and the development of sophisticated image sensors. Traditional image processing algorithms, foundational to numerous applications within information science, are inherently parallel in nature, demanding extensive computational resources for execution. The surge in image quantity and resolution has rendered these classical algorithms increasingly time-consuming and hardware-intensive. In response to these challenges, the integration of quantum computing into image processing emerges as a promising solution. Quantum computing utilizes qubits for data storage and leverages the properties of quantum physics, such as superposition and entanglement, to offer unparalleled parallel processing capabilities. This shift in paradigm provides a significant improvement in efficiency for tasks related to image processing.

The quantum approach to image processing significantly reduces the computational complexity associated with storing and manipulating large sets of image data. While a classical computer requires exponential resources $O(n \times 2^n)$ to store sequences of n-bit length, a quantum computer can achieve this with linear complexity O(n) [5]. Moreover, operations that are inherently sequential and resource-intensive on classical computers, such as bitwise inversion, can be executed more efficiently on quantum computers. This is due to the quantum computer's ability to perform operations on entangled qubits in parallel, dramatically reducing the time and resources needed for complex image processing tasks. This innovative method of leveraging quantum computing for image processing not only accelerates classical algorithms but also paves the way for the development of novel quantum image processing algorithms. These improvements have the potential to completely transform the field by greatly decreasing time it requires to analyze data and the amount of hardware needed. This will allow for the development of more advanced image processing applications that need a lot of resources. Hence, how can we use the quantum computing technique for image processing is crucial for surpassing the constraints of conventional computational techniques. This advancement presents a novel opportunity to efficiently and effectively process digital images.

To process images in quantum state, we need to follow three steps as Figure 1, (i) prepare the image and store it into quantum state, (ii) process quantum image, (iii) processed digital image from quantum state. The quantum image compression and encryption techniques lie in the preparation of the image into quantum state. Similar to the traditional digital image compression, the quantum image compression methods have lossy and lossless compression.

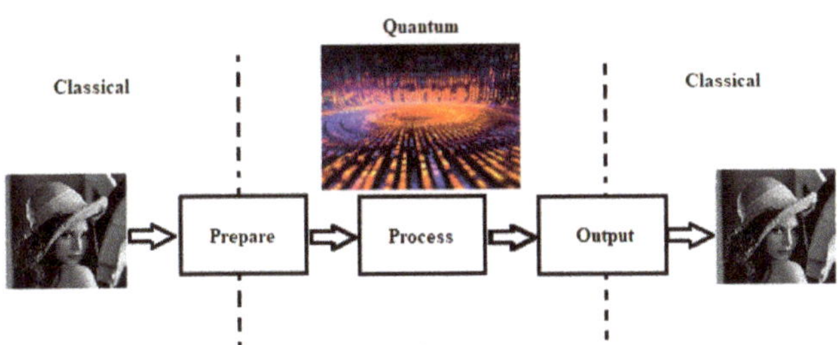

Figure 1. The processing steps of quantum image processing, converting the image from classical state to quantum state, then processing in quantum state, next convert the processed image from quantum to classical state as output.

The early 21st century witnessed several pivotal advancements aimed at enhancing the efficiency and quality of image compression techniques. In 2002, Lewis et al. introduced a method that utilized a two-dimensional orthogonal wavelet transform for compressing digital images. This innovative approach enabled the decomposition of images into coefficients that are localized both spatially and spectrally, offering a nuanced balance between preserving image quality and achieving substantial compression [6]. Another noteworthy development came in the form of an advanced bit plane coding strategy specifically designed for quantizing discrete cosine transform (DCT) coefficients [7]. This technique was lauded for its ability to deliver superior decoding quality compared to the JPEG2000 standard [8], which was the benchmark at the time. Kouda et al. introduced a hierarchical quantum neural network-based image compression scheme, assessing the utility of large quantum neural networks in tackling complex image compression scenarios [9]. This approach underscored the potential of quantum computing to revolutionize traditional practices by offering novel solutions that could outperform conventional algorithms in both efficiency and effectiveness. A significant challenge in image compression has always been the time-consuming nature of traditional image coding methods. To address this issue, Yang R. introduced a cutting-edge algorithm that employed a quantum BP (back-propagation) network for image compression [10]. This method not only accelerated the encoding process but also enhanced the quality of the reconstructed images, showcasing the synergy between quantum computing and neural network methodologies in improving computational processes. In 2016, Yuen et al. unveiled an algorithm that combined discrete cosine transform (DCT) with the Secure Hashing Algorithm (SHA-1) for both compressing and encrypting images [11]. This dual-purpose algorithm highlighted the growing need for secure and efficient image processing techniques in an increasingly digital and interconnected world. In the same year, based on hyper-chaotic system Zhou et al. proposed an image encryption-compression scheme [12]. The same authors also published image encryption and compression scheme based on Mellin transform and compressive sensing [13]. In 2018, an image compression–encryption algorithms by combining hyper-chaotic system with discrete fractional random transform was introduced by Gong et al. [14].

While the above work is on the traditional images, as the field of quantum computing is advancing rapidly many of these classical techniques have been expanded to encompass the quantum realm. In this paper, we will focus on the quantum image processing and will discuss about the recent advancements in the field of quantum image compression. We start in Section 2 with a brief introduction to quantum computing. Readers already familiar with these fundamental concepts can skip Section 2 and proceed directly to Section 3.

2. Brief Introduction to Quantum Computing

2.1. Vector

Quantum states are mathematically expressed as vectors in a complex vector space called Hilbert space. Hilbert space is a fundamental framework in quantum mechanics because it can effectively capture the probabilistic and superpositional characteristics of quantum systems. The nomenclature used to represent vectors in Hilbert space is a distinctive and sophisticated formalism, generally known as Dirac notation, or more informally, the "bra-ket" notation [15].

$$|\psi\rangle = \begin{bmatrix} a_1 \\ a_2 \\ \vdots \\ a_n \end{bmatrix}, \tag{1}$$

In Dirac notation, a vector (representing a quantum state) in Hilbert space is symbolized by a ket, denoted as $|\psi\rangle$, where $|\cdot\rangle$ signifies the ket and ψ is a label that identifies the specific quantum state. The ket is a column vector that encompasses all the essential information required to completely explain the quantum state within the mathematical framework of quantum mechanics. Complementary to the ket is the bra, denoted as $\langle\phi|$, where $\langle\cdot|$ represents the bra, and ϕ is a label for the vector. The bra is essentially the conjugate transpose of the ket. In more concrete terms, if the ket represents a column vector, then the bra represents a row vector, with its complex elements conjugated. The usage of this bra vector is essential in the construction of quantum mechanical algorithms, particularly in the computation of probabilities and expectation values, which are key aspects of quantum mechanics.

The implementation of bra-ket notation brought about a significant transformation in the mathematical handling of quantum mechanics, providing a potent and intuitive mechanism for managing the abstract concepts essential to the theory. It simplifies the depiction of quantum processes, such as measurements and transformations, and offers a standardized framework for discussing and evaluating quantum states. It also enables the succinct definition of quantum mechanical processes, such as unitary transformations and observables. In summary, the bra-ket notation encapsulates the abstract and counterintuitive nature of quantum mechanics in a mathematically rigorous yet accessible language, enabling the exploration and exploitation of quantum phenomena for computational purposes.

2.2. Tensor Products

The tensor product is a mathematical operation that combines vector spaces to create a bigger vector space.

1. Assume, we have a scaler α. $|v\rangle$ is an element in V space and $|w\rangle$ is an element in W space. Then we can write:

$$\alpha(|v\rangle \otimes |w\rangle) = (\alpha|v\rangle \otimes |w\rangle) = |v\rangle \otimes \alpha(|w\rangle), \tag{2}$$

2. Now if we have two elements, $|v_1\rangle$, $|v_2\rangle$ in V space and an element $|w\rangle$ in W space

$$(|v_1\rangle + |v_2\rangle) \otimes |w\rangle = |v_1\rangle \otimes |w\rangle + |v_2\rangle \otimes |w\rangle \tag{3}$$

3. Similarly, $|v\rangle$ in V space and $|w_1\rangle$ and $|w_2\rangle$ in W space

$$|v\rangle \otimes (|w_1\rangle + |w_2\rangle) = |v\rangle \otimes |w_1\rangle + |v\rangle \otimes |w_2\rangle \tag{4}$$

We can find the tensor product of two matrices X (dimension $m \times n$) and Y (dimension $i \times j$) as

$$X \otimes Y = \begin{bmatrix} x_{11}Y & x_{12}Y & \cdots & X_{1n}Y \\ x_{21}Y & x_{22}Y & \cdots & x_{2n}Y \\ \vdots & \vdots & \ddots & \vdots \\ x_{m1}Y & x_{m2}Y & \cdots & x_{mn}Y \end{bmatrix} \tag{5}$$

2.3. Quantum Bit

In a classical computer bit is the core component, which functions inside a binary system, alternating between two distinct states: 0 and 1. The binary system serves as the foundation for classical computing architectures, allowing for the representation, manipulation, and retention of data. Quantum computing, in contrast, presents a sophisticated and intricate alternative to the classical bit, known as the quantum bit or qubit. Qubits are fundamental units that encapsulate the laws of quantum physics, forming the essential foundation for both the theoretical and practical aspects of quantum computing. Qubits, unlike traditional bits, exist inside a mathematical domain that is more flexible and abstract, rather than being limited to the binary certainties of 0 and 1. This abstraction enables the conceptualization and advancement of quantum computing theory without being limited by the physical implementation in specific hardware platforms. Qubits, being very versatile mathematical entities, allow for extensive study of the potential of quantum computing, without being restricted by the limits of physical systems.

A qubit is characterized by its capacity to exist in states that extend beyond the binary values of 0 and 1. The ability to simultaneously exist in several states is demonstrated by the phenomenon called quantum superposition, in which a qubit occupies a state that is a combination of $|0\rangle$ and $|1\rangle$. Mathematically, the superposed state can be represented as:

$$|\psi\rangle = \alpha|0\rangle + \beta|1\rangle \tag{6}$$

where α and β denote the probability amplitudes. The amplitudes represent the probability of the qubit collapsing into either the $|0\rangle$ or $|1\rangle$ state when measured. A qubit's state is represented as a vector in a two-dimensional complex vector space, with $|0\rangle$ and $|1\rangle$ being the basis states used for computation. The basis states constitute an orthonormal basis set, serving as a structured framework for the definition and manipulation of qubits.

The superposition principle grants qubits the ability to exist in several states simultaneously, which is in striking contrast to the binary restriction of conventional bits. Quantum computers have the ability to process and interpret data in ways that are fundamentally distinct from traditional computing methods due to their multi-state nature. When a measurement is performed on a superposed qubit state $|\psi\rangle$, it collapses into one of its component states, either $|0\rangle$ or $|1\rangle$. The probability of each event is defined by the square of the associated probability amplitude ($|\alpha|^2$ for $|0\rangle$ and $|\beta|^2$ for $|1\rangle$). The stochastic character of qubit measurement forms the basis for the quantum mechanical phenomena that quantum algorithms utilize for purposes such as encryption, search optimization, and simulation of quantum systems. Also,

$$|\alpha|^2 + |\beta|^2 = 1 \tag{7}$$

In quantum computing, $|0\rangle$ is expressed as:

$$|0\rangle = \begin{bmatrix} 1 \\ 0 \end{bmatrix} \tag{8}$$

In quantum computing, $|1\rangle$ is expressed as:

$$|1\rangle = \begin{bmatrix} 0 \\ 1 \end{bmatrix} \tag{9}$$

$$|\psi\rangle = \alpha|0\rangle + \beta|1\rangle = \begin{bmatrix} \alpha \\ \beta \end{bmatrix} \tag{10}$$

Let us consider a pair of qubits. From a classical perspective, a pair of bits has the capability to represent four unique values (00, 01, 10, 11) simultaneously. However, within a quantum system, two qubits have the ability to simultaneously exist in a superposition of all four of these states. Consequently, the two-qubit system can be characterized by a state vector that encompasses this superposition, denoting a quantum state that is a linear combination of its four fundamental states: $|00\rangle$, $|01\rangle$, $|10\rangle$, and $|11\rangle$. So, the quantum state for two qubit system can be written as:

$$|\psi\rangle = \alpha_{00}|00\rangle + \alpha_{01}|01\rangle + \alpha_{10}|10\rangle + \alpha_{11}|11\rangle \tag{11}$$

where

$$|\alpha_{00}|^2 + |\alpha_{01}|^2 + |\alpha_{10}|^2 + |\alpha_{11}|^2 = 1 \tag{12}$$

These four states can be represented as:

$$|00\rangle = |0\rangle \otimes |0\rangle = \begin{bmatrix} 1 \\ 0 \\ 0 \\ 0 \end{bmatrix} \tag{13}$$

$$|01\rangle = |0\rangle \otimes |1\rangle = \begin{bmatrix} 0 \\ 1 \\ 0 \\ 0 \end{bmatrix} \tag{14}$$

$$|10\rangle = |1\rangle \otimes |0\rangle = \begin{bmatrix} 0 \\ 0 \\ 1 \\ 0 \end{bmatrix} \tag{15}$$

$$|11\rangle = |1\rangle \otimes |1\rangle = \begin{bmatrix} 0 \\ 0 \\ 0 \\ 1 \end{bmatrix} \tag{16}$$

2.3.1. Qubit Measurements and Unit Circle Theory

The basic states of a qubit in quantum computing are represented by the states $|0\rangle$ and $|1\rangle$ in quantum physics. In a two-dimensional coordinate system, where the state $|0\rangle$ aligns with the X-axis and the state $|1\rangle$ aligns with the Y-axis, these states can be visually depicted. Every state has a basis vector: the vector for $|0\rangle$ is $[1\ 0]^T$, indicating that it is a unit vector along the X-axis; the vector for $|1\rangle$ is $[0\ 1]^T$, indicating that it is a unit vector along the Y-axis.

We can take into consideration additional vectors that create different angles with the X-axis in order to investigate the idea of superposition. For example, the vector $[1/\sqrt{2}\ 1/\sqrt{2}]^T$ can be used to represent a vector that forms a 45-degree angle with the X-axis. According to this vector, there is an equal chance that this qubit will be measured and found in the states of $|0\rangle$ or $|1\rangle$. This indicates that the quantum state is an equal superposition of $|0\rangle$ and $|1\rangle$. In addition, another vector that forms a 60-degree angle with the X-axis can be represented by the column vector $[1/2\ \sqrt{(3/2)}]$. This vector represents a quantum state that is not an equal superposition of $|0\rangle$ and $|1\rangle$. Instead, it has distinct probabilities for being observed in each state, with a greater likelihood for the state $|1\rangle$ due to the larger coefficient in the vector representation.

Thus, a qubit can be mathematically described as a unit vector within a two-dimensional complex vector space (Figure 2). When we apply this principle to the geometric model known as the "Bloch sphere", the state $|0\rangle$ correlates to the X-axis, whereas the state $|1\rangle$ aligns with the Y-axis on this sphere. It is crucial to emphasize that any point on the surface of the Bloch sphere represents a qubit in a state of superposition, which is a weighted combination of the states $|0\rangle$ and $|1\rangle$. In the practice of quantum measurement, two primary approaches are utilized. The first is the measurement in the standard basis, also known as the computational basis, which corresponds precisely to the previously mentioned states $|0\rangle$ and $|1\rangle$. The second methodology incorporates measurements taken on an arbitrary basis, enabling the evaluation of the qubit's state across various Bloch sphere orientations. The selection of these arbitrary bases is not obligatory and can be chosen to accommodate particular quantum computing tasks or algorithms, thereby offering a versatile structure for the assessment and application of quantum states.

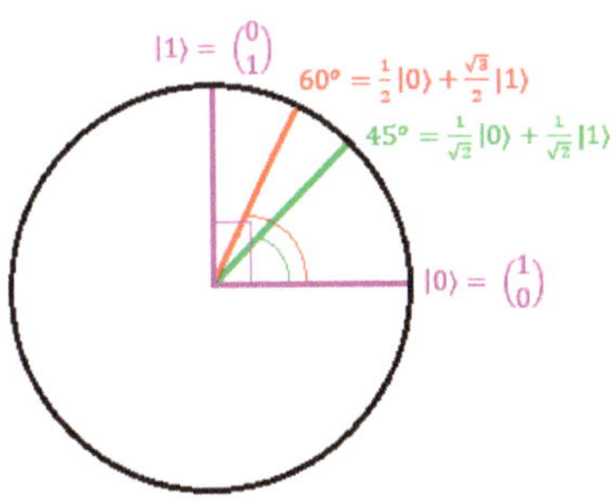

Figure 2. Unit circle representation on various angles. The vector $[1/\sqrt{2}\ 1/\sqrt{2}]^T$ can be used to represent a vector that forms a 45-degree angle with the X-axis and there is an equal chance that qubit will be measured and found in the states of $|0\rangle$ or $|1\rangle$. Another vector that forms a 60-degree angle with the X-axis can be represented by the column vector $[1/2\ \sqrt{(3/2)}]$. This vector represents a quantum state that is not an equal superposition of $|0\rangle$ and $|1\rangle$.

2.3.2. Measuring on Standard Basis

Let us assume, state $|S\rangle$ has an angle θ with $|0\rangle$ state in X axis. The figure is drawn in a 2D real space (Figure 3), and all of its amplitudes are real.

$$|S\rangle = a|0\rangle + b|1\rangle = \begin{pmatrix} \cos\theta \\ \sin\theta \end{pmatrix} \tag{17}$$

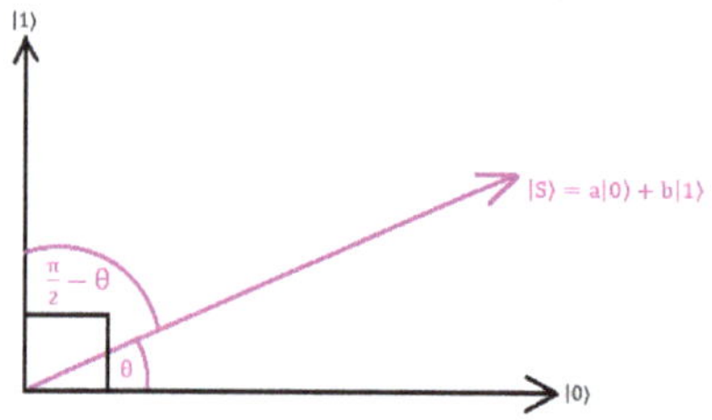

Figure 3. Projection on standard basis states. State |S⟩ has an angle θ with |0⟩ state in X-axis. Then the angle of |S⟩ with |1⟩ state would be (π/2 − θ).

From the figure, the state |0⟩ has the probability $\cos^2\theta$ and state |1⟩ has the probability $\sin^2\theta$, which can be written as $\cos^2(\pi/2-\theta)$. Thus, depending on the stated above probabilities, the state S is projected onto either the |0⟩ state or |1⟩ state.

2.3.3. Measuring on Arbitrary Basis

In this case, measurement is completed on any orthogonal basis rather than onto |0⟩ and |1⟩ basis. From Figure 4, state |S⟩ is measure using $|u\rangle$ and $|u'\rangle$ basis. Here $|u\rangle$ has the probability $\cos^2\theta$ and $|u'\rangle$ has the probability $\sin^2\theta$. The amplitude of $|u\rangle$ and $|u'\rangle$ given by:

$$|u\rangle = \frac{1}{\sqrt{2}}|0\rangle + \frac{1}{\sqrt{2}}|1\rangle \tag{18}$$

$$|u\prime\rangle = -\frac{1}{\sqrt{2}}|0\rangle + \frac{1}{\sqrt{2}}|1\rangle \tag{19}$$

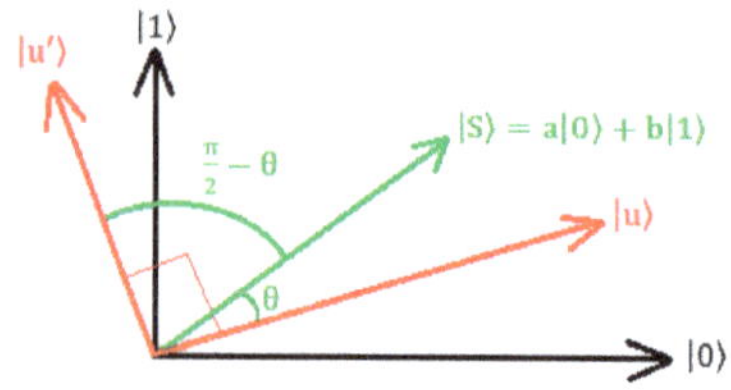

Figure 4. Projection onto arbitrary orthogonal basis states. State |S⟩ is measured with respect to |u⟩ and |u′⟩. |u⟩ and |u′⟩ is measured with probability of $\cos^2\theta$ and $\sin^2\theta$, respectively.

These concepts will come in handy when we will talk about the FRQI (flexible representation of quantum images) representation of quantum images where rotation operation will be required.

2.4. Circuit and Gates

Logic gates are essential components in traditional digital circuits, responsible for manipulating and transforming information. They serve as the fundamental building blocks for complicated computing functions. Similarly, quantum circuits utilize a distinct set of logic gates that are specifically intended to function based on the principles of quantum mechanics. Quantum logic gates enable the manipulation of quantum information by applying unitary transformations to quantum states, allowing for the execution of logical operations. The mathematical description of these changes is commonly conveyed by matrices, which accurately capture the specific operation being applied to the quantum state.

One significant category of quantum logic gates is the single quantum gate (Figure 5). As the name implies, it only requires the participation of one qubit to perform its action. In contrast, multi-qubit gates are capable of performing quantum operations and interactions that are more intricate, as they involve two or more qubits. Quantum circuits employ horizontal lines to represent qubits in their graphical depiction. The lines depicted in the schematic of a quantum circuit, commonly known as wires, represent the pathway through which quantum information travels. The symbol "U" is used to represent a single quantum gate on these wires. This symbol indicates the unitary operation that the gate performs on the qubit it interacts with. When $|\psi\rangle$ state is used as an input to this gate it gives $U|\psi\rangle$ as an output. Unitary transformations play a crucial role in the functioning of quantum gates. These transformations are invertible and maintain the norm of the quantum state, a necessity for quantum operations based on the principles of quantum physics. The utilization of a matrix representation for a quantum gate offers a potent means of comprehending and formulating quantum algorithms, as it enables the accurate computation of the gate's impact on a certain quantum state.

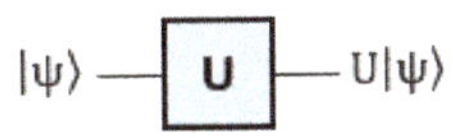

Figure 5. Single quantum gate.

The single quantum gate can be expressed in a matrix form:

$$|\psi\rangle = \begin{bmatrix} \alpha \\ \beta \end{bmatrix}, U = \begin{bmatrix} a & b \\ c & d \end{bmatrix} \tag{20}$$

$$U|\psi\rangle = \begin{bmatrix} a & b \\ c & d \end{bmatrix} \begin{bmatrix} \alpha \\ \beta \end{bmatrix} = \begin{bmatrix} a\alpha + b\beta \\ c\alpha + d\beta \end{bmatrix} \tag{21}$$

It is impossible to overstate the significance of single quantum gates in quantum computation. Although they are the most basic form of quantum gates, single quantum gate executes critical operations that are indispensable for quantum computation, including the initialization, manipulation, and preparation of measurements of qubits. The Pauli gates (X, Y, Z), which alter the state of a qubit in multiple dimensions, and the Hadamard gate, which generates superposition states, are both instances of single quantum gates. These gates function as the quantum equivalents of classical logic gates such as NOT and XOR, albeit within a domain where quantum states can be superimposed and entangled.

Hadamard gate:

$$H = \begin{bmatrix} \frac{1}{\sqrt{2}} & \frac{1}{\sqrt{2}} \\ \frac{1}{\sqrt{2}} & -\frac{1}{\sqrt{2}} \end{bmatrix} = \frac{1}{\sqrt{2}} \begin{bmatrix} 1 & 1 \\ 1 & -1 \end{bmatrix} \tag{22}$$

Applying the Hadamard gate to $|0\rangle$ state or $|1\rangle$ state:

$$H|0\rangle = \frac{1}{\sqrt{2}} \begin{bmatrix} 1 & 1 \\ 1 & -1 \end{bmatrix} \begin{bmatrix} 1 \\ 0 \end{bmatrix} = \frac{1}{\sqrt{2}}|0\rangle + \frac{1}{\sqrt{2}}|1\rangle = |+\rangle \tag{23}$$

$$H|1\rangle = \frac{1}{\sqrt{2}} \begin{bmatrix} 1 & 1 \\ 1 & -1 \end{bmatrix} \begin{bmatrix} 0 \\ 1 \end{bmatrix} = \frac{1}{\sqrt{2}}|0\rangle - \frac{1}{\sqrt{2}}|1\rangle = |-\rangle \tag{24}$$

So, by using the Hadamard H gate, the state $|0\rangle$ and $|1\rangle$ can be convert into a superposition state. The new state is known as $|+\rangle$ state and $|-\rangle$ state, respectively.

Pauli-X:

$$X = \begin{bmatrix} 0 & 1 \\ 1 & 0 \end{bmatrix} \tag{25}$$

The Pauli-X gate has the ability to change the state of a single qubit. That is why this gate is also called bit-flip or Not gate.

Table 1 shows some common single quantum gates.

Table 1. Example of some single quantum gates.

Gate Name/Operator	Circuit Diagram	Matrix Representation
Hadamard	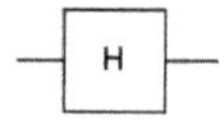	$H = \frac{1}{\sqrt{2}}\begin{bmatrix} 1 & 1 \\ 1 & -1 \end{bmatrix}$
Pauli-X	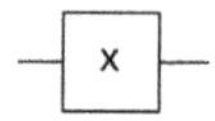	$X = \begin{bmatrix} 0 & 1 \\ 1 & 0 \end{bmatrix}$
Identity	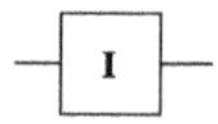	$I = \begin{bmatrix} 1 & 0 \\ 0 & 1 \end{bmatrix}$

Within the sophisticated realm of quantum computing, in addition to the simplicity and grace of individual quantum gates, there exists a more intricate category of quantum gates that require the participation of several qubits for their functioning. Multi-qubit quantum gates enhance the complexity and functionality of quantum circuits, allowing for a wider range of computational operations that exploit the distinct characteristics of quantum mechanics, such as entanglement and superposition, to perform tasks that are beyond the capabilities of single-qubit gates.

One prominent example of multi-qubit gates is the Controlled-NOT (CNOT) gate, which represents the idea of quantum control dynamics. The CNOT gate functions by manipulating two qubits, with one qubit acting as the control and the other as the target.

$$\text{CNOT} = \begin{bmatrix} 1 & 0 & 0 & 0 \\ 0 & 1 & 0 & 0 \\ 0 & 0 & 0 & 1 \\ 0 & 0 & 1 & 0 \end{bmatrix} \tag{26}$$

The CNOT gate operates by flipping the state of the target qubit, changing it from $|0\rangle$ to $|1\rangle$ or vice versa, only when the control qubit is in the state $|1\rangle$ as shown in the Equations (27)–(30). The conditional operation described here is the quantum equivalent of the conventional XOR gate. It showcases how quantum computing may imitate and expand upon traditional logic operations within a quantum context.

$$\text{CNOT}|00\rangle = \begin{bmatrix} 1 & 0 & 0 & 0 \\ 0 & 1 & 0 & 0 \\ 0 & 0 & 0 & 1 \\ 0 & 0 & 1 & 0 \end{bmatrix} \begin{bmatrix} 1 \\ 0 \\ 0 \\ 0 \end{bmatrix} = \begin{bmatrix} 1 \\ 0 \\ 0 \\ 0 \end{bmatrix} = |00\rangle \tag{27}$$

$$\text{CNOT}|01\rangle = \begin{bmatrix} 1 & 0 & 0 & 0 \\ 0 & 1 & 0 & 0 \\ 0 & 0 & 0 & 1 \\ 0 & 0 & 1 & 0 \end{bmatrix} \begin{bmatrix} 0 \\ 1 \\ 0 \\ 0 \end{bmatrix} = \begin{bmatrix} 0 \\ 1 \\ 0 \\ 0 \end{bmatrix} = |01\rangle \tag{28}$$

$$\text{CNOT}|10\rangle = \begin{bmatrix} 1 & 0 & 0 & 0 \\ 0 & 1 & 0 & 0 \\ 0 & 0 & 0 & 1 \\ 0 & 0 & 1 & 0 \end{bmatrix} \begin{bmatrix} 0 \\ 0 \\ 1 \\ 0 \end{bmatrix} = \begin{bmatrix} 0 \\ 0 \\ 0 \\ 1 \end{bmatrix} = |11\rangle \tag{29}$$

$$\text{CNOT}|11\rangle = \begin{bmatrix} 1 & 0 & 0 & 0 \\ 0 & 1 & 0 & 0 \\ 0 & 0 & 0 & 1 \\ 0 & 0 & 1 & 0 \end{bmatrix} \begin{bmatrix} 0 \\ 0 \\ 0 \\ 1 \end{bmatrix} = \begin{bmatrix} 0 \\ 0 \\ 1 \\ 0 \end{bmatrix} = |10\rangle \tag{30}$$

Expanding on the concept of conditional operations, the quantum computing also has the 0-Controlled-NOT (0CNOT) gate. This gate inverts the target qubit only when the control qubit is in the state $|0\rangle$. This gate expands the spectrum of quantum logic operations.

The Toffoli gate, also referred to as the CCNOT gate, is a significant expansion of the CNOT gate. It involves the use of two control qubits and one target qubit. The Toffoli gate performs a bit-flip operation on the target qubit exclusively when both control qubits are in the state $|1\rangle$. The significance of this gate in quantum computing lies in its ability to facilitate reversible computation, which is essential for the development of universal quantum computers. Also, as we explore farther into the domain of multi-qubit operations, the idea of scalability becomes apparent with the introduction of the n-CNOT gate. The gate expands the concept of conditional operation to n control qubits, providing a flexible method for coordinating intricate quantum processes that may be customized to meet the specific needs of advanced quantum algorithms.

Another important example of multi-qubit gate is the Swap gate. It facilitates the exchange of states between two qubits. The function of this gate is crucial in quantum algorithms as it allows for the reorganization of qubit states without impacting the overall quantum state of the system. This facilitates operations that necessitate particular qubit configurations.

Table 2 shows some common multiple quantum gates.

Table 2. Example of multiple quantum gates and their matrix representation.

Gate Name/Operator	Circuit Diagram	Matrix Representation
CNOT or CX	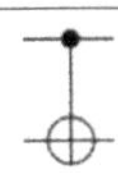	$\text{CNOT} = \begin{bmatrix} 1 & 0 & 0 & 0 \\ 0 & 1 & 0 & 0 \\ 0 & 0 & 0 & 1 \\ 0 & 0 & 1 & 0 \end{bmatrix}$
0CNOT	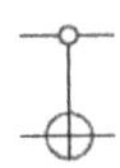	$\text{0CNOT} = \begin{bmatrix} 0 & 1 & 0 & 0 \\ 1 & 0 & 0 & 0 \\ 0 & 0 & 1 & 0 \\ 0 & 0 & 0 & 1 \end{bmatrix}$
Toffoli or CCX	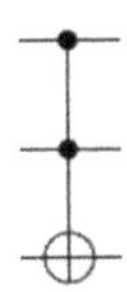	$\text{Toffoli} = \begin{bmatrix} 1 & 0 & 0 & 0 & 0 & 0 & 0 & 0 \\ 0 & 1 & 0 & 0 & 0 & 0 & 0 & 0 \\ 0 & 0 & 1 & 0 & 0 & 0 & 0 & 0 \\ 0 & 0 & 0 & 1 & 0 & 0 & 0 & 0 \\ 0 & 0 & 0 & 0 & 1 & 0 & 0 & 0 \\ 0 & 0 & 0 & 0 & 0 & 1 & 0 & 0 \\ 0 & 0 & 0 & 0 & 0 & 0 & 0 & 1 \\ 0 & 0 & 0 & 0 & 0 & 0 & 1 & 0 \end{bmatrix}$
Swap	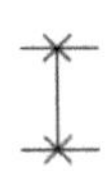	$\text{swap} = \begin{bmatrix} 1 & 0 & 0 & 0 \\ 0 & 0 & 1 & 0 \\ 0 & 1 & 0 & 0 \\ 0 & 0 & 0 & 1 \end{bmatrix}$

Having a basic understanding of these gates and how these work is very important because these gates are useful to build a quantum circuit. For instance, if we are working with the FRQI representation of quantum images, we need to understand the use of the Hadamard gate, Identity gate, Pauli-X gate, CNOT gate [16], etc. Another popular quantum image representation technique is NEQR (short for Novel Enhanced Quantum Representation) in which an image can be defined as:

$$|I\rangle = \frac{1}{2^n} \sum_{y=0}^{2^n-1} \sum_{x=0}^{2^n-1} \prod_{i=0}^{q-1} \left| c_{yx}^{i} \right\rangle |yx\rangle \tag{31}$$

To implement this, we need to use Hadamard gate, Toffoli gate, Swap gate [17], etc. We discuss this technique in detail in the next section. So, before jumping into the image processing part, knowing the basic concept of these gates are important because these will be required to represent the images in quantum state.

3. Quantum Image Representations

Before we delve into quantum image compression, we need to understand how an image can be represented in quantum state, since a number of quantum image representations have been proposed. The first attempt to represent an image in quantum system was proposed after introducing Qubit Lattice in 2003 [18]. Then in 2005 quantum superposition was introduced in Real Ket [19] to represent image. In 2010, Venegas et al. proposed entangled image which used quantum entanglement [20]. Le et al. also published their work FRQI or flexible representation of quantum images [16] in the same year. Here, they utilized an n-qubit sequence to represent the coordinate information. To store the color information of the image they used angle. An image in FRQI model can be represented as follows [16]:

$$|I(\theta)\rangle = \frac{1}{2^n}\sum_{i=0}^{2^{2n}-1}(\cos\theta_i|0\rangle + \sin\theta_i|1\rangle)\otimes|i\rangle \tag{32}$$

$$\theta_i \in \left[0, \frac{\pi}{2}\right], i = 0, 1, \ldots, 2^{2n} - 1 \tag{33}$$

Here, $|i\rangle$ (=0, 1, . . ., $2^{2n} - 1$) are 2^{2n} computational basis quantum states and $\theta = (\theta_0, \theta_1, \ldots, \theta_2{}^{2n} - 1)$ is the vector of angles encoding colors. Here the coordinate information is represented with $|i\rangle$ and the grey scale information is represented using $\cos\theta_i\ |0\rangle + \sin\theta_i\ |1\rangle$. This model can represent the greyscale information as well as the coordinate system of an image in quantum state properly.

This FRQI model was extended further in the following year and a new model called Multi-Channel Representation for Quantum Image (MCRQI) [21] was proposed, which also consider the RGB space. This model represents images as follows:

$$|I(\theta)\rangle = \frac{1}{2^{n+1}}\sum_{i=0}^{2^{2n}-1}\left|c^i_{RGB\alpha}\right\rangle\otimes|i\rangle \tag{34}$$

$$\begin{aligned}\left|c^i_{RGB\alpha}\right\rangle = {} & \cos\theta_{Ri}|000\rangle + \cos\theta_{Gi}|001\rangle + \cos\theta_{Bi}|010\rangle + \cos\theta_{\alpha i}|011\rangle \\ & + \sin\theta_{Ri}|100\rangle + \sin\theta_{Gi}|101\rangle + \sin\theta_{Bi}|110\rangle + \sin\theta_{\alpha i}|111\rangle\end{aligned} \tag{35}$$

As we can see, in MCRQI to store RGB channels and opacity, three qubits are required. Here, θ_{Ri}, θ_{Gi}, θ_{Bi} vectors represent the RGB colors and $\theta_{\alpha i}$ represents the channels.

In FRQI scheme while encoding the image pixels, normalized superposition state is utilized, allowing simultaneous operations on all pixels, thereby addressing the need for real-time processing in image applications. A number of algorithms have been introduced based on this principle. However, FRQI's restriction to one qubit per pixel for grayscale information makes certain complex color operations challenging.

The NEQR model for digital images representation, was introduced in 2013 by Zhang et al. [17], uses entangled qubit sequences to encode an image's grayscale and spatial information in a quantum superposition. This method converts grayscale values into binary using q qubits, improving simplicity and accessibility. The binary-encoded grayscale data are stored in a q-qubit sequence, whereas the coordinates for a 2^n-by-2^n pixel image are retained in a 2n-qubit sequence. To better illustrate the algorithm, let us consider a 2-by-2 image as shown in Figure 6. In order to apply NEQR to an image, first q + 2n qubits needs to be initialized to the $|0\rangle$ state. This is followed by applying identity (I) gates and Hadamard (H) gates to this initial state. Subsequently, the grayscale values for all pixels are established using 2n-CNOT gates. So, in the figure, to store the coordinate information H-gate needs to be applied to two of the ten $|0\rangle$ qubits. Then, 2-CNOT gates need to be used to store the grayscale information. The quantum circuit for the NEQR preparation is shown in Figure 7.

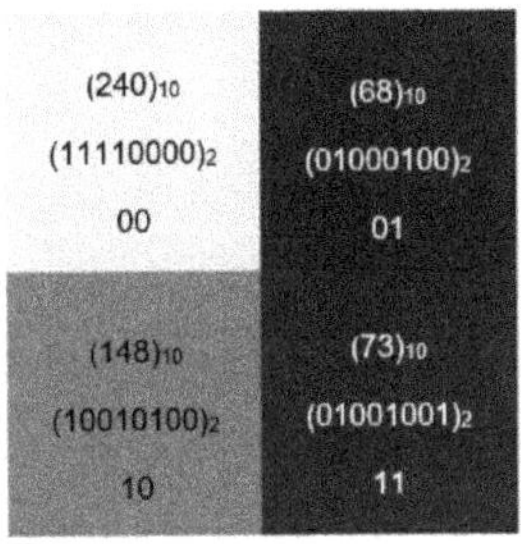

Figure 6. A 2-by-2 example image where $(240)_{10}$ and $(11110000)_2$ is the intensity of pixel in decimal and binary at position 00. Same goes for other three pixels.

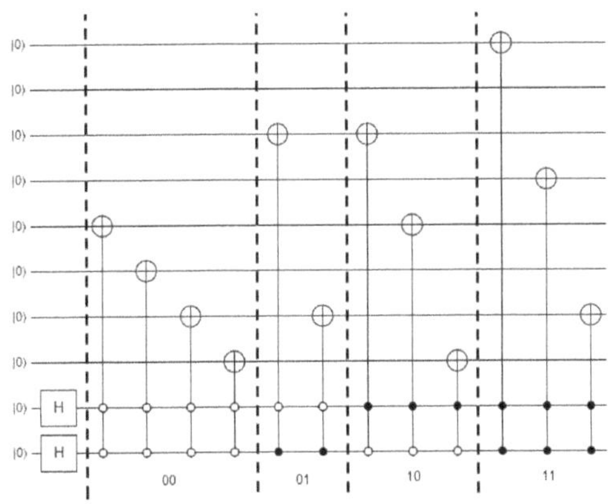

Figure 7. A 2-by-2 image represented in a quantum circuit by using the NEQR scheme.

The NEQR model is a substantial improvement over the FRQI model. NEQR requires more qubits than FRQI but solves the problem of reliably measuring grayscale information with a limited number of measurements. NEQR simplifies color operations, giving it a more practical and often useful framework in quantum image processing. However, both NEQR and FRQI have a constraint in that they are designed to store images that are strictly square because their horizontal and vertical coordinate lengths are equal. This limitation presents an issue for depicting images that are not square or rectangular, which are prevalent. To address this issue, the improved novel enhanced quantum representation (INEQR) [22] was introduced in 2015 by Jiang et al. INEQR allows for storing and processing rectangular images by supporting uneven horizontal and vertical coordinates. This improvement broadens the applicability of quantum image representations, making them more suitable for real-world scenarios where images may not have square dimensions.

GQIR or Generalized Quantum Image Representation was presented to represent non-square, rectangular images of arbitrary dimension by utilizing logarithmic coordinates [23]. Despite its versatility, GQIR adds redundancy to the representation process. The Novel Quantum Representation for Log-Polar Images (QUALPI) offers a framework for image representation in polar coordinates, diverging from conventional Cartesian-based methods [24]. In 2014, Li et al. introduced a new encoding approach for multi-dimensional color images called the n-qubit normal arbitrary superposition state (NASS). This method creatively encodes grayscale values using quantum states' angles and assigns certain states to represent different dimensions, enabling the compression of multi-dimensional color images on a quantum computer [25]. In 2016, the FRQI method was improved, and a new model called the FRQCI or Flexible Representation for Quantum Color Image, which improved the management of color in quantum image representations [26]. Sang et al. developed the Novel Quantum Representation of Color Digital Images (NCQI) by integrating enhancements from MCRQI and NEQR within a similar period [27]. The new model modifies the qubits in NEQR from q to 3q to symbolize the RGB color channels, making color operations, such as intricate color transformations, much simpler to perform. Yet, a downside of the NCQI paradigm is the heightened need for qubits.

In 2018, Liu et al. introduced an Optimized Quantum Representation for Color Digital Images (OCQR) to tackle this problem [28]. OCQR requires fewer qubits, about one-third of what NCQI uses, to hold pixel values, while having a similar time complexity for preparing quantum pictures. OCQR optimizes computational resources by minimizing qubit usage and improves the efficiency of specific color changes. In 2017, the NEQR model was expanded to include Red–Green–Blue (RGB) color schemes by creating the Quantum Multi-Channel RGB Representation (QMCR) [29]. Although this new method demands more qubits than the MCRQI model, it streamlines the picture preparation process and allows for accurate image retrieval. In the same year, Jiang et al. introduced a new framework for three-dimensional imaging in the quantum realm, called the quantum point cloud [30]. This novel approach expands quantum image processing to 3D visual data, providing new opportunities for manipulating and analyzing digital images in quantum computing.

In the following year, BRQI (Bitplane Representation of Quantum Images) was published by Li et al. [31], which allows for altering color complements, reversing, and translating bitplanes within the BRQI framework. This BRQI method divides the grayscale values into eight different binary bits, converting a grayscale image into eight distinct bit planes. It requires three qubits to express the bitplane index, while n qubits are assigned to encode the spatial coordinates of the image. Moreover, Wang et al. in 2019, published a model where a bitplane is used to represent color digital images. They named this model QRCI [32]. An improved FRQI model called FRQCI was proposed by Li et al. [33]. Interestingly, in this model they talked about some image processing operators for pixel coordinate information and color representation. Khan explored FRQI and NEQR model further and came up with an improved flexible representation of quantum images (IFRQI) [34]. In this model, every pair of bits was represented using angle, enabling single qubit to store information equivalent to 2-bit grayscale values. This method significantly enhances the precision in retrieving the original image data. In the following year Grigoryan et al. published a new algorithm to store the images in quantum state by using Fourier transform representation [35]. In the same year, Wang et al. came up with a method called DQRCI (double quantum color images encryption scheme) in which two color images are stored into quantum superposition state simultaneously [36].

4. Quantum Image Compression

In this section, we provide a review of the literature in quantum image compression. To make it understandable for the readers this section is divided into two subsections. In the first subsection we talk about the papers focusing on direct methods and algorithms for compressing images using quantum computing techniques. These typically involve novel quantum algorithms that enhance or replace classical compression methods. In the second one, we give an overview of the papers that explore not only the quantum image compression technique but also quantum image representation, storage and retrieval.

4.1. Quantum Image Compression Techniques

In 2006, Yang et al. proposed a quantum vector quantization encoding algorithm for image compression [37]. This study presents a hybrid quantum-classical vector quantization (VQ) encoding algorithm that is more efficient than the pure quantum version. It requires fewer than $\sqrt{N}$ (N = number of pixels) operations for most images and achieves close to a 100% success rate. The same group also published another work on image compression by using the quantum discrete cosine transform (QDCT) [38]. The proposed algorithms for 1-D and 2-D DCT decrease the time complexity to $O(\sqrt{N})$ for 1-D and O(N) for 2-D, in contrast to the classical complexities of $O(N \log_2 N)$ for 1-D and $O(N^2 \log_2 N)$ for 2-D. it also expands Grover's algorithm, known for its effectiveness in quantum searching, to tackle more complex unstructured search problems.

Nodehi et al. in 2009, proposed an image compression method for fractal images based on Functional Sized population Quantum Evolutionary Algorithm (FSQEA) [39]. The Quantum Evolutionary Algorithm (QEA) represents an emerging optimization technique that adopts probabilistic solution representation, proving to be especially effective for combinatorial challenges such as the Knapsack problem. Given that fractal image compression falls under the NP-Hard category, genetic algorithms (GAs) have traditionally been the go-to approach for such issues. However, the application of QEA to fractal image compression remains unexplored territory. In the paper, not only FSQEA for fractal image compression is proposed but also optimized by fine-tuning different parameters to enhance the performance, where it was shown that the PSNR of the proposed algorithm is better, i.e., 27.44 dB instead of 27.27 dB for GA. Notably, the time complexity of the FSQEA mirrors that of the original QEA, attributed to the fact that the average population size for the FSQEA is equivalent to that of the conventional QEA, and the number of function evaluations remains constant across both algorithms. Given the inherently time-intensive nature of fractal image compression, and the need for multiple iterations to ascertain optimal parameters, the study utilizes benchmark functions as a preliminary step. However, the temporal complexity of the FSQEA is similar to that of the original QEA because the average population size and the number of function evaluations are the same in both algorithms.

Qi et al. proposed an algorithm that uses Quantum Backpropagation (QBP) for image compression [40]. They showed a quantum neuron model that uses a combination of quantum gates, especially phase-shift and controlled-NOT gates as the basic building block for the operation. Incorporating the principles of traditional backpropagation (BP) they showed that the QBP network outperforms its classical BP counterpart. The work demonstrates a quicker learning rate ($\eta = 0.09$ compared to QNN with $\eta = 3.6$) as well as superior image compression capabilities (with a compression rate of $R = 0.16$ compared to QNN with 0.15).

Another work on fractal image compression (FIC) was presented by Du et al. in 2015 [41]. Grover's quantum search algorithm (QSA) was applied to accelerate the encoding process of FIC. Both theoretically and experimentally they showed that substantial amount of speedup was achieved by this method over the traditional FIC. Additionally, in terms of preserving the quality of retrieved images, the proposed QAFIC outperforms other contemporary FIC methods. A quantum image compression scheme based on JPEG was proposed by Jiang et al. in 2017 [42]. Figure 8 depicts the workflow of the JPEG based quantum image compression algorithm. As depicted in the workflow, first, the image is quantized, then the quantized JPEG coefficients are inputted into qubits and finally converted into pixel values. Compared with the Boolean expression compression (BEC) method, this scheme is less complicated and faster (with a running time of 0.164 s compared to 5.54 h in BEC), with high compression ratios (84.66% for the "cameraman" image compared to 69.07% in BEC).

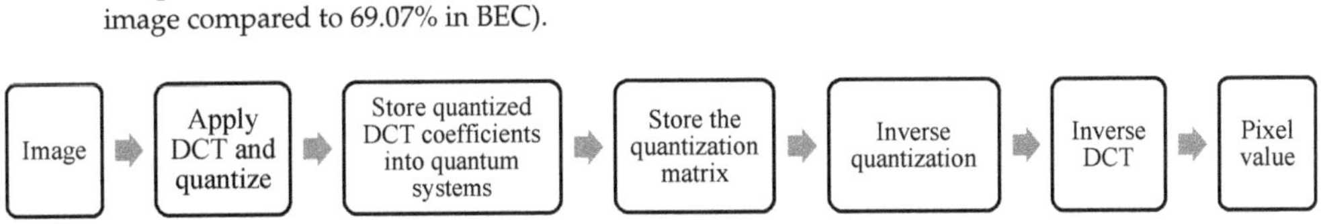

Figure 8. Workflow of JPEG based quantum image compression algorithm.

Pang et al. proposed a signal and image compression technique using the quantum discrete cosine transform (QDCT) [43]. In order to compress images and signals, this study introduces a quantum algorithm for the discrete cosine transform (DCT) that is specifically engineered to be computationally more efficient than its classical counterpart. This is accomplished by the algorithm calculating the DCT coefficients concurrently and identifying the most significant coefficients. The conventional Grover's iteration is improved through the incorporation of a novel iteration method called the quantum DCT iteration (G_{DCT}), which is specifically designed for DCT operations and compression tasks.

The construction of the 1D-DCT using this method demonstrates an $O(\sqrt{N})$ complexity for a vector of size N. Conversely, the 2D-DCT computation for an N-by-N matrix manifests an O(N) complexity. The quantum DCT algorithm was developed by taking advantage of two inherent properties of the DCT: its energy conservation capability and the fact that numerous DCT coefficients are insignificant and can therefore be excluded with minimal degradation to the quality of the reconstructed image. A study by Dai et al. introduces a quantum technique that utilizes the quantum DCT along with a 4-dimensional hyper chaotic Henon map to compress multiple images simultaneously [44]. Using QDCT, this method combines four grayscale images into a single quantum image, resulting in an efficient compression ratio that reduces the requirements for data transmission. Encryption involves using the 4D hyper-chaotic Henon map to manipulate the quantum image, uniformly spreading pixel values to create a large key space for increased security. A logistic map-guided quantum image cycle shift technique is used to scatter pixel data for improved encryption. The authors also showed by simulation that their model seems to be efficient with lower computational complexity (O(n)) than traditional picture encryption approaches ($O(n2^{3n})$ and $O(2^{6n})$).

In 2023, Ma er al. proposed a scheme to apply compression to quantum RGB images by using the quantum Haar wavelet transform (HQWT) and iterative quantum Fibonacci transform (IQFT) [45]. They converted multiple RGB images into a unified hybrid image. This hybrid image then undergoes compression at varying ratios using a measurement matrix built from Hadamard gates. The compressed image is then encrypted by using the Generalized Inverse Quantum Fourier Transform (IQFT), resulting in a compacted image form. The proposed scheme has total computation complexity of $O(n^3)$. In the following year, Wang et al. published a quantum version of autoencoder based on parameterized quantum circuits for image compression [46]. They combined quantum image processing with the machine learning, especially the autoencoder to apply image compression on the quantum images. Ji et al. proposed an image compression and reconstruction algorithm by leveraging the quantum network (QN) in 2024 [47]. QN is a network structure where the fundamentals of quantum mechanics are used to transmit and process information. In their approach, first the image is converted to a quantum state from classical state. Then this quantum state is used as an input for the quantum compression network. The measurements of the output state are converted into compressed image which are utilized to train the QN based on the gradient descent algorithm. Lastly, the simulation of compression of grayscale images is realized by this quantum algorithm. Haque et al. proposed a block-wise lossy SCMNEQR (state connection modification novel enhanced quantum representation) compression scheme for quantum gray-scale images [48]. Their algorithm was able to minimize the total computational time by 99.66% and 7.36% compared to JPEG and DCT-EFRQI (Direct Cosine Transform Efficient Flexible Representation of Quantum Image) approaches, respectively.

4.2. Quantum Image Storage, Representation, Compression, and Retrieval Techniques

In 2011, one of the pioneering works on quantum image processing was published by Le et al. [16]. A flexible representation of quantum images (FRQI) was proposed in this paper. Quantum image compression (QIC) aims to decrease the quantum resources necessary for preparing and reconstructing quantum images by lowering the number of simple quantum gates needed, which is crucial in both the theoretical and practical realms of quantum computing, as seen in the FRQI model, where simplifying basic gates such as controlled rotation gates is critical.

A way is suggested to combine these gates with identical rotation angles by leveraging the limited ability of the human visual system to differentiate between numerous colors, which enables a distinct range of color values for representation. Grouping controlled rotation operators with the same angles and combining their conditions can greatly decrease the required number of gates. We can consider an 8 × 8 pixel image as shown in Figure 9 with only two colors: blue and red. This image would need 64 $C^6(\cdot)$ controlled-rotation gates for its initial quantum state preparation. Here the dot $(\cdot)$ in these notations is a placeholder indicating that the gate can be applied to any arbitrary target gate. Categorizing these gates into two groups based on color can significantly decrease the total number. The 64 gates can be simplified to 4 as shown in Figure 10, resulting in a 93.75% reduction, by using simpler gates such as one $C^1(\cdot)$ and two $C^2(\cdot)$ gates for the red locations.

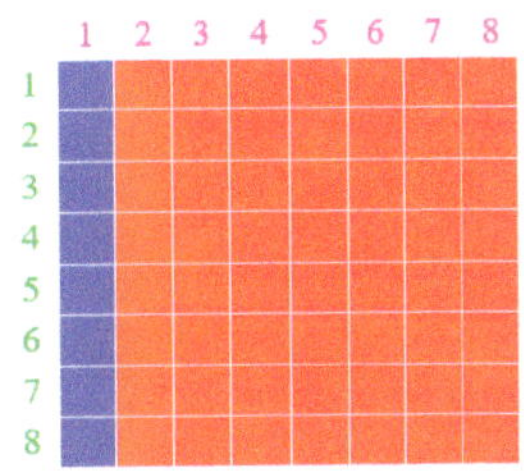

Figure 9. Two color 8 × 8 pixel image, 8 blue pixels and 56 red pixels.

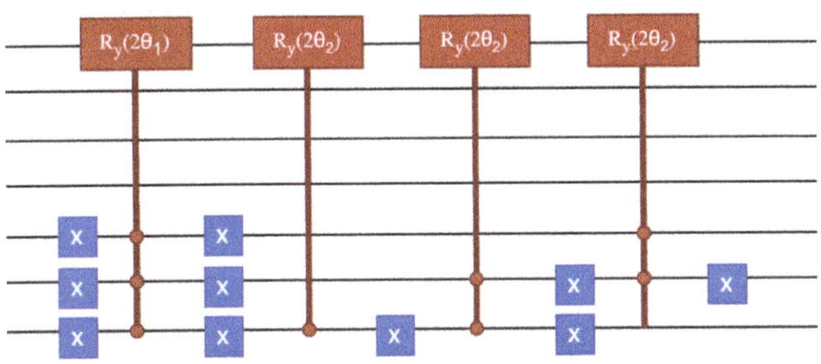

Figure 10. Minimized circuit for a two-color 8 × 8 pixel image. Here, X is the Pauli-X gates, θ is the vector of angles encoding colors (two in this case) and $R_y(2\theta_i)$ is the controlled-rotation gate.

The controlled-rotation gate is given by the following equation:

$$R_y(2\theta_i) = \begin{pmatrix} cos\ \theta_i & -sin\ \theta_i \\ sin\ \theta_i & cos\ \theta_i \end{pmatrix} \tag{36}$$

A key step in this process involves translating binary strings that represent pixel positions into Boolean minterms. Each binary digit is treated as a Boolean variable, with "1" represented by the variable (x) and "0" represented by its negation $(\overline{x})$. After organizing the gates by color, we can condense them by merging the binary strings of each color group into a unified Boolean expression. This phrase includes all the necessary conditions for the controlled-rotation gates of that group. An 8-position group in the blue color category as shown in Figure 11, which would have needed 8 individual gates, can be depicted by a single term in a simplified Boolean expression. This suggests that replacing the original eight gates with a single controlled-rotation gate can simplify the quantum circuit and decrease the quantum resources required for image representation.

The 8 position of blue pixels and their binary string and Boolean expression

$$
\begin{aligned}
|0\rangle &\longrightarrow |000000\rangle \longrightarrow \overline{x_5x_4x_3x_2x_1x_0}\\
|8\rangle &\longrightarrow |001000\rangle \longrightarrow \overline{x_5x_4}x_3\overline{x_2x_1x_0}\\
|16\rangle &\longrightarrow |010000\rangle \longrightarrow \overline{x_5}x_4\overline{x_3x_2x_1x_0}\\
|24\rangle &\longrightarrow |011000\rangle \longrightarrow \overline{x_5}x_4x_3\overline{x_2x_1x_0}\\
|32\rangle &\longrightarrow |100000\rangle \longrightarrow x_5\overline{x_4x_3x_2x_1x_0}\\
|40\rangle &\longrightarrow |101000\rangle \longrightarrow x_5\overline{x_4}x_3\overline{x_2x_1x_0}\\
|48\rangle &\longrightarrow |110000\rangle \longrightarrow x_5x_4\overline{x_3x_2x_1x_0}\\
|56\rangle &\longrightarrow |111000\rangle \longrightarrow x_5x_4x_3\overline{x_2x_1x_0}
\end{aligned}
$$

$$
\begin{aligned}
\text{Minimized Boolean expression} &= \overline{x_5x_4x_3x_2x_1x_0} + \overline{x_5x_4}x_3\overline{x_2x_1x_0} + \overline{x_5}x_4\overline{x_3x_2x_1x_0} + \overline{x_5}x_4x_3\overline{x_2x_1x_0} +\\
&\quad x_5\overline{x_4x_3x_2x_1x_0} + x_5\overline{x_4}x_3\overline{x_2x_1x_0} + x_5x_4\overline{x_3x_2x_1x_0} + x_5x_4x_3\overline{x_2x_1x_0}\\
&= \overline{x_2x_1x_0}
\end{aligned}
$$

Figure 11. Boolean expression and its minimized expression for an 8-position group.

The QIC algorithm aims to decrease the number of controlled rotation gates within color groups by minimizing their Boolean expression, as depicted in Figure 12. The process begins with identifying places within the group of similar color and concludes with simplified Boolean expression.

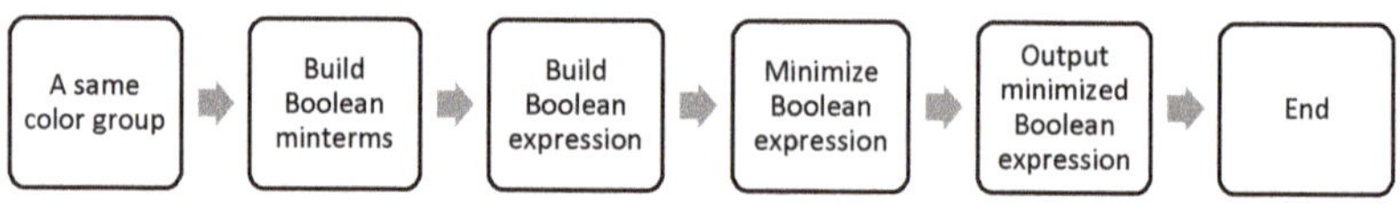

Figure 12. Quantum image compression flow chart.

In 2013, Li et al. proposed a method to store, retrieve and compress images in a quantum system [49]. More specifically, the authors proposed a compression algorithm where they achieve a lossless compression ratio of 2.058. In this algorithm, to compress an image, termed "newImage", we first determine the number m of unique colors the image contains. Each color relates to a quantum state from the QSMC set, and these states are lined up in a quantum queue. The compression procedure involves scanning the "newImage" in a certain direction as shown in Figure 13, either row-wise starting from the second pixel of the first row (1,2) or column-wise starting from the second row's first pixel (2,1). We record only the initial pixel of each continuous sequence of pixels with identical colors as we scan. When the scan encounters a pixel of a different color, it stops to record the color and sequence length before continuing from the last pixel of the uniform sequence. s is the length of the longest sequence of pixels with matching color. n is the number of pixels in the compressed "newImage".

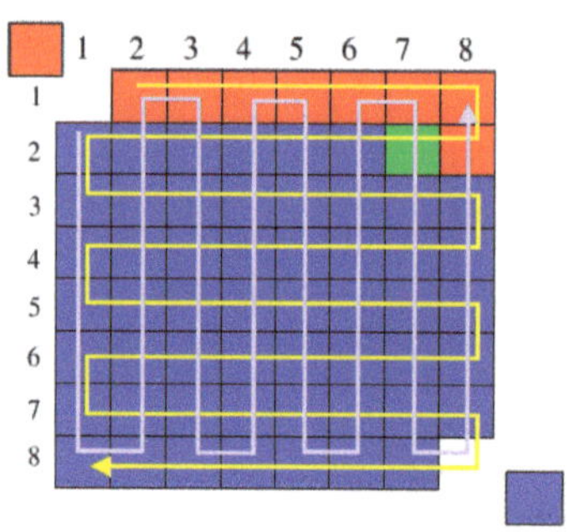

Figure 13. Scanning a 3-color 8 × 8 image by rows (indicated by the purple line) starting from the second pixel of the first row (1,2), and by columns (indicated by the yellow line) starting from the second row's first pixel (2,1).

Next, a bijective function is created as:

$$F_4 : posNum \leftrightarrows \gamma, \tag{37}$$

where $posNum = \{1, 2, \ldots, m, m+1, m+s\}$ and $\gamma = \{\gamma_1, \gamma_2, \ldots, \gamma_{m+s}\}(\gamma_i = \frac{\pi(i-1)}{2(m+s-1)}, i \in \{1, 2, \ldots, m+s\})$. $R_y(2\gamma_i)$, which is rotation operator given by Equation (38), converts state $|0\rangle$ to m+s states.

$$R_y(2\gamma_i) = \begin{bmatrix} \cos\gamma_i & -\sin\gamma_i \\ \sin\gamma_i & \cos\gamma_i \end{bmatrix}, (i = 1, 2, \ldots, m+s) \tag{38}$$

$$\begin{cases} |\overline{\omega}_i\rangle = \cos\gamma_i|0\rangle + \sin\gamma_i|1\rangle, \ i\epsilon\{1, 2, \ldots, m\} \\ |x_i\rangle = \cos\gamma_{m+i}|0\rangle + \sin\gamma_{m+i}|1\rangle, i\epsilon\{1, 2, \ldots, m\} \end{cases} \tag{39}$$

Here $|\overline{\omega}_j\rangle$ is the jth position of queue Q_1 and $|x_i\rangle$ represents an integer i. $|\overline{\psi}_i\rangle$ represents the ith pixel and can be defined as:

$$|\overline{\psi}_i\rangle = \begin{cases} |\overline{\omega}_j\rangle \otimes |u_x\rangle, i = 1, |u_x\rangle\epsilon\text{QSNC}, x\epsilon\{1, 2, \ldots, N\} \\ |\overline{\omega}_j\rangle \otimes |u_y\rangle, i = n, |u_y\rangle\epsilon\text{QSNC}, y\epsilon\{1, 2, \ldots, N\} \\ |\overline{\omega}_j\rangle \otimes |x_k\rangle, \quad i\epsilon\{2, 3, \ldots, n-1\}, k \geq 2 \\ |\overline{\omega}_j\rangle, \quad i\epsilon\{2, 3, \ldots, n-1\}, k = 1 \end{cases} \tag{40}$$

where u_x is the coordinate of the first pixel and u_y is the coordinate of the last pixel of the newImage, k represents consecutive pixels of same color depending on the direction of the scanning. After that $|\overline{\psi}_i\rangle$ is stored in another quantum queue Q_2 and the process is repeated. Suppose three colors in Figure 13 are represented, respectively, by $|\upsilon_r\rangle$, $|\upsilon_g\rangle$, $|\upsilon_b\rangle$ and saved in Q_1. Q_2 has five states as follows: $|\overline{\psi}_1\rangle = |\overline{\omega}_1\rangle \otimes |u_1\rangle$, $|\overline{\psi}_2\rangle = |\overline{\omega}_1\rangle \otimes |x_8\rangle$, $|\overline{\psi}_3\rangle = |\overline{\omega}_2\rangle$, $|\overline{\psi}_4\rangle = |\overline{\omega}_3\rangle \otimes |x_{53}\rangle$, $|\overline{\psi}_5\rangle = |\overline{\omega}_3\rangle \otimes |u_{120}\rangle$. The compressed image stored in Q_1 and Q_2 is shown in Figure 14.

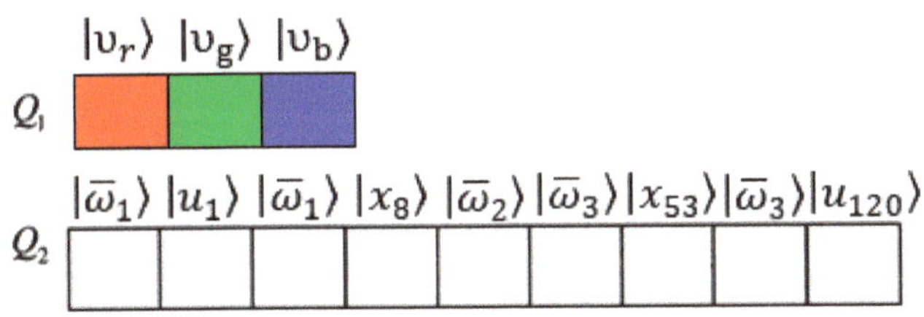

Figure 14. The compressed image stored in Q1 and Q2.

Another milestone in quantum image processing was the NEQR model [17] proposed in 2013 by Zhang et al., in which 15X compression ratio on quantum images was achieved. While FRQI relies on one qubit per pixel to store grayscale data, which restricts compression to areas with consistent grayscale values, NEQR stores grayscale data by distributing it among a series of qubits, enabling optimization of each qubit separately. By employing Boolean expression minimization, NEQR can obtain higher compression ratios for quantum images by simplifying the preparation of each qubit individually. An operation set Φ consists of all the quantum operations of quantum image preparation can be expressed as

$$\phi = \bigcup_{Y=0}^{2^n-1} \bigcup_{X=0}^{2^n-1} \bigcup_{i=0}^{q-1} \phi^i_{YX}, \ \phi^i_{YX} \in \{\text{I}, 2n-\text{CNOT}\} \tag{41}$$

where ϕ^{i}_{YX} represents the quantum operation for the ith qubit. These operations can be categorized into q groups as shown in the following equation:

$$\phi = \bigcup_{Y=0}^{2^n-1}\bigcup_{X=0}^{2^n-1}\bigcup_{i=0}^{q-1}\phi^{i}_{YX} = \bigcup_{i=0}^{q-1}\left(\bigcup_{Y=0}^{2^n-1}\bigcup_{X=0}^{2^n-1}\phi^{i}_{YX}\right) = \bigcup_{i=0}^{q-1}\phi_i \tag{42}$$

Depending on the value of $C^{i}{}_{YX}$, the style of the operation ϕ^{i}_{YX} will change such that, when $C^{i}{}_{YX} = 0$, ϕ^{i}_{YX} will be the identity gate I. Otherwise, it will be 2n − CNOT qubit gate. This will invert the ith qubits in the color qubit sequence when the pixel position is (Y, X). Thus ϕ can be written as:

$$\begin{aligned}\phi &= \bigcup_{Y=0}^{2^n-1}\bigcup_{X=0}^{2^n-1}\phi^{i}_{YX}\\ \phi &= \left(\bigcup_{Y=0}^{2^n-1}\ \bigcup_{X=0,\ C^{i}_{YX}=0}^{2^n-1} I\right)\cup\left(\bigcup_{Y=0}^{2^n-1}\ \bigcup_{X=0,\ C^{i}_{YX}=1}^{2^n-1}(2n-CNOT)_{YX}\right)\end{aligned} \tag{43}$$

The identity operation will not affect the quantum state; hence, the operation can be ignored from the first part in the ith group of quantum operation. The espresso algorithm [50] which is used in the second part of the operation, compresses the control information of controlled not gates. The espresso algorithm is a program use to reduce the complexity of digital logic gate circuits by using heuristic and specific algorithms.

$$\bigcup_{Y=0}^{2^n-1}\ \bigcup_{X=0,\ C^{i}_{YX}=1}^{2^n-1} YXEspresso\overrightarrow{\bigcup_{K_i}} K_i \tag{44}$$

The expression builds a new quantum controlled-not gates $\bigcup_{K_i} K_i - CNOT$ for the new ith group $\phi'{}_i$ by providing the equivalent and compact control information sets $\bigcup_{K_i} K_i$. So, the new circuit will be given by,

$$\phi' = \bigcup_{i=0}^{q-1}\phi'_i = \bigcup_{i=0}^{q-1}\bigcup_{K_i} K_i - CNOT \tag{45}$$

Figure 15 shows the workflow for image compression in the NEQR algorithm.

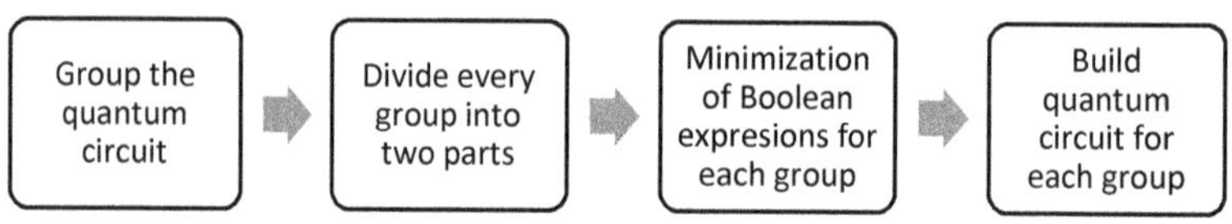

Figure 15. Workflow of image compression in the NEQR algorithm.

A study from 2014 shows the multidimensional color image compression based on quantum amplitudes and phases [25]. Both the lossless and lossy quantum image compression algorithms were developed. About 72.6 compression ratio was achieved by this algorithm. For lossless compression, the process is divided into two steps. The first step is dimensionality reduction and sorting algorithm for a k-dimensional color image (called DRS). In the second step, the lossless compression algorithm was applied for quantum images (LCQI). For lossy image compression Quantum Fourier Transform (QFT) was used to generate a NASS (n-qubit normal arbitrary superposition state) state $|\psi_A\rangle$. About 1.4 quantum compression ratio was achieved in this case. They also applied QWT (Quantum Wavelet Transform) instead of QFT and achieved 1.5 quantum compression ratio. In 2022, Amankwah et al. published a paper that introduced quantum compression for

N-dimensional images [51]. They applied their algorithm to prepare an FRQI state, which reduced the number of necessary gates by up to 90%, without lowering the image quality. Haque et al. published a peper on quantum image representation and compression technique using DCT-EFRQI (Direct Cosine Transform Efficient Flexible Representation of Quantum Image) in 2023 [52]. Both experimental and theoretical results showed that the proposed DCT-EFRQI had better compression ratio compared with EFRQI (Efficient Flexible Representation of Quantum Image). For example, for the "cameraman" image, the proposed algorithm had compression ratio of 8.4543:1 compared to 2.5864:1 for EFRQI. The work showed that DCT-EFRQI provided twice as much compression on medium-size images (512 × 512) than on large-size images (1024 × 1024).

5. Conclusions

Quantum image compression applies the laws of quantum mechanics to improve the effectiveness of image data reduction and compression. It utilizes qubits to encode image data by taking advantage of superposition and entanglement to process and compress images in a way that the classical algorithms cannot match. By leveraging quantum parallelism, these methods can theoretically achieve compression tasks at speeds unattainable by classical computers, with potentially higher compression ratios and lower losses of quality. Moreover, the inherent properties of quantum systems, like the ability to handle vast amounts of data simultaneously, make quantum image compression particularly suited for high-resolution and high-dimensional imaging applications, such as medical imaging, satellite imagery, and large-scale video data. However, the practical application of quantum image compression is still in its nascent stages. The field faces substantial challenges that stem primarily from the limitations of current quantum technology. These include the instability of quantum states (decoherence), the high error rates of quantum operations, the complexity of quantum circuit design, and the need for robust quantum error correction methods. We believe that rapid advances in quantum systems and hardware in the coming years will help address these constraints. Moreover, there are plenty of opportunities to conduct further research on quantum algorithms that mimic the classical transform coding methods like Fourier transforms or wavelet transforms, where we utilize the properties of quantum bits to perform quantum-specific transformations on quantum states representing images. This could lead to more efficient transformations, reducing the time and resources needed for encoding and decoding images. Moreover, if quantum entanglement can be utilized to compress correlated regions within an image by entangling qubits that represent similar or related image features (like colors or edges), it might be possible to reduce the overall number of qubits needed to represent an image, effectively compressing the image data. Furthermore, quantum machine learning models can be designed to learn optimal compression strategies based on the image content. These models could identify patterns and features in image data that classical algorithms might overlook and use these insights to compress images more effectively. Also, a hybrid algorithm can be developed where the initial stages of image processing and feature extraction are performed using classical techniques, and the heavy lifting of actual data compression is conducted on quantum hardware. This could make quantum image compression more practical and accessible with current technology. But it is needless to say, the development of scalable quantum computers that can handle real-world image compression tasks remains a significant hurdle. Work is still sparse on the practical feasibility in the implementation of quantum image compression algorithms on physical quantum computers, where a huge of amount of quantum gates will present challenges on achieving fidelity by dealing with noise and decoherence [53]. According to IBM's quantum road map "https://www.ibm.com/roadmaps/quantum/2024/ (accessed on 14 July 2024)", in about ten years or so, quantum computers will be able to support 2000 qubits working in a distributed 100,000-qubit machine, with distributed software tools that enable noise-free quantum computations working seamlessly with classical computations. While there seems to be a long way to go before we can attain the full advantage and potential of the many algorithms we have discussed above, the future of quantum image compression is bright as we are entering into the new age of quantum-centric computing.

Author Contributions: Conceptualization, W.D.P.; Methodology, S.K.D. and W.D.P.; Validation, S.K.D. and W.D.P.; Formal Analysis, S.K.D., W.D.P.; Investigation, S.K.D. and W.D.P.; Resources, S.K.D. and W.D.P.; Data Curation, S.K.D. and W.D.P.; Writing—Original Draft Preparation, S.K.D. and W.D.P.; Writing—Review & Editing, S.K.D. and W.D.P.; Visualization, S.K.D.; Supervision, W.D.P.; Project Administration, W.D.P. All authors have read and agreed to the published version of the manuscript.

Funding: This research received no external funding.

Conflicts of Interest: The authors declare no conflict of interest.

References

1. Moore, G. Cramming more components onto integrated circuits. *Proc. IEEE* **1998**, *86*, 82–85. [CrossRef]
2. Feynman, R.-P. Simulating physics with computers. *Int. J. Theor. Phys.* **1982**, *21*, 467–488. [CrossRef]
3. Shor, P.W. Algorithms for quantum computation: Discrete logarithms and factoring. In *Proceedings 35th Annual Symposium on Foundations of Computer Science*; IEEE: Piscataway, NJ, USA, 1994; pp. 124–134.
4. Grover, L.K. A fast quantum mechanical algorithm for database search. In Proceedings of the 28th Annual ACM Symposium on the Theory of Computing, ACM, Philadelphia, PA, USA, 22–24 May 1996; pp. 212–219.
5. Wang, Z.; Xu, M.; Zhang, Y. Review of Quantum Image Processing. *Arch. Comput. Methods Eng.* **2022**, *29*, 737–761. [CrossRef]
6. Lewis, A.S.; Knowles, G. Image compression using the 2-D wavelet transforms. *IEEE Trans. Image Process.* **2002**, *1*, 244–250. [CrossRef]
7. Ponomarenko, N.; Lukin, V.; Egiazarian, K.; Astola, J. DCT based high quality image compression. In Proceedings of the Image Analysis, Scandinavian Conference, SCIA 2005, Joensuu, Finland, 19–22 June 2005; Volume 3540, pp. 1177–1185.
8. Taubman, D.S.; Marcellin, M.W. JPEG2000: Standard for interactive imaging. *Proc. IEEE* **2002**, *90*, 1336–1357. [CrossRef]
9. Kouda, N.; Matsui, N.; Nishimura, H. Image compression by layered quantum neural networks. *Neural. Process. Lett.* **2002**, *16*, 67–80. [CrossRef]
10. Yang, R.; Zuo, Y.J.; Lei, W.J. Researching of image compression based on quantum BP network. *Telkomnika Indones. J. Elect. Eng.* **2013**, *11*, 6889–6896.
11. Yuen, C.H.; Wong, K.W. A chaos-based joint image compression and encryption scheme using DCT and SHA-1. *Appl. Soft Comput.* **2011**, *11*, 5092–5098. [CrossRef]
12. Zhou, N.R.; Pan, S.M.; Cheng, S. Image compression-encryption scheme based on hyper-chaotic system and 2D compressive sensing. *Opt. Laser Technol.* **2016**, *82*, 121–133. [CrossRef]
13. Zhou, N.R.; Li, H.L.; Wang, D.; Pan, S.M.; Zhou, Z.H. Image compression and encryption scheme based on 2D compressive sensing and fractional Mellin transform. *Opt. Commun.* **2015**, *343*, 10–21. [CrossRef]
14. Gong, L.; Deng, C.; Pan, S.; Zhou, N. Image compression-encryption algorithms by combining hyper-chaotic system with discrete fractional random transform. *Opt. Laser Technol.* **2018**, *103*, 48–58. [CrossRef]
15. Dirac, P.A.M. A new notation for quantum mechanics. *Math. Proc. Camb. Philos. Soc.* **1939**, *35*, 416–418. [CrossRef]
16. Le, P.Q.; Dong, F.; Hirota, K. A flexible representation of quantum images for polynomial preparation, image compression and processing operations. *Quant. Inf. Process* **2011**, *10*, 63–84. [CrossRef]
17. Zhang, Y.; Lu, K.; Gao, Y.; Wang, M. NEQR: A novel enhanced quantum representation of digital images. *Quant. Inf. Process* **2013**, *12*, 2833–2860. [CrossRef]
18. Venegas-Andraca, S.-E.; Bose, S. Storing processing and retrieving an image using quantum mechanics. *SPIE Conf. Quant. Inf. Comput.* **2003**, *5106*, 137–147.
19. Latorre, J.I. *Image Compression and Entanglement*; Tech. Rep. quant-ph/0510031; University of Barcelona: Barcelona, Spain, 2005.
20. Venegas-Andraca, S.E.; Ball, J.L. Processing images in entangled quantum system. *Quant. Inf. Process* **2010**, *9*, 1–11. [CrossRef]
21. Sun, B.; Iliyasu, A.M.; Le, P.; Dong, F.; Hirota, K. A multichannel representation for images on quantum computers using the RGB color space. In Proceedings of the IEEE 7th International Symposium on Intelligent, Signal Processing, Malta, Floriana, 19–21 September 2011; pp. 160–165.
22. Jiang, N.; Wang, L. Quantum image scaling using nearest neighbor interpolation. *Quant. Inf. Process* **2015**, *14*, 1559–1571. [CrossRef]
23. Jiang, N.; Wang, J.; Mu, Y. Quantum image scaling up based on nearest-neighbor interpolation with integer scaling ratio. *Quant. Inf. Process* **2015**, *14*, 4001–4026. [CrossRef]

24. Zhang, Y.; Lu, K.; Gao, Y.; Xu, K. A novel quantum representation for log-polar images. *Quant. Inf. Process* **2013**, *12*, 3103–3126. [CrossRef]
25. Li, H.S.; Zhu, Q.; Zhou, R.G.; Li, M.C.; Song, L.; Ian, H. Multidimensional color image storage, retrieval, and compression based on quantum amplitudes and phases. *Inf. Sci.* **2014**, *273*, 212–232. [CrossRef]
26. Li, P.; Xiao, H.; Li, B. Quantum representation and watermark strategy for color images based on the controlled rotation of qubits. *Quant. Inf. Process* **2016**, *15*, 4415–4440. [CrossRef]
27. Sang, J.; Wang, S.; Li, Q. A novel quantum representation of color digital images. *Quant. Inf. Process* **2017**, *16*, 42. [CrossRef]
28. Liu, K.; Zhang, Y.; Lu, K.; Wang, X.; Wang, X. An optimized quantum representation for color digital images. *Quant. Inf. Process* **2018**, *57*, 2938–2948. [CrossRef]
29. Abdolmaleky, M.; Naseri, M.; Batle, J.; Farouk, A.; Gong, L.H. Red-green-blue multi-channel quantum representation of digital images. *Opt. Int. J. Light. Electron. Opt.* **2017**, *128*, 121–132. [CrossRef]
30. Jiang, N.; Hu, H.; Dang, Y.; Zhang, W. Quantum point cloud and its compression. *Int. J. Theor. Phys.* **2017**, *56*, 3147–3163. [CrossRef]
31. Li, H.-S.; Chen, X.; Xia, H.-Y.; Liang, Y.; Zhou, Z. A quantum image representation based on bitplanes. *IEEE Access* **2018**, *6*, 62396–62404. [CrossRef]
32. Wang, L.; Ran, Q.; Ma, J.; Yu, S.; Tan, L. QRCI: A new quantum representation model of color digital images. *Opt. Commun.* **2019**, *438*, 147–158. [CrossRef]
33. Li, P.; Liu, X. Color image representation model and its application based on an improved frqi. *Int. J. Quant. Inf.* **2018**, *16*, 1850005. [CrossRef]
34. Khan, R.A. An improved flexible representation of quantum images. *Quant. Inf. Process.* **2019**, *18*, 1–9. [CrossRef]
35. Grigoryan, A.M.; Agaian, S.S. New look on quantum representation of images: Fourier transform representation. *Quant. Inf. Process.* **2020**, *19*, 148. [CrossRef]
36. Wang, L.; Ran, Q.; Ma, J. Double quantum color images encryption scheme based on DQRCI. *Multimed. Tools Appl.* **2020**, *79*, 6661–6687. [CrossRef]
37. Chao-Yang, P.; Zheng-Wei, Z.; Guang-Can, G. A hybrid quantum encoding algorithm of vector quantization for image compression. *Chin. Phys.* **2006**, *15*, 3039–3043. [CrossRef]
38. Chao-Yang, P.; Zheng-Wei, Z.; Guang-Can, G. Quantum Discrete Cosine Transform for Image Compression. *arXiv* **2006**, arXiv:quant-ph/0601043v2. [CrossRef]
39. Nodehi, A.; Tayarani, M.; Mahmoudi, F. A novel functional sized population quantum evolutionary algorithm for fractal image compression. In Proceedings of the 2009 14th International CSI Computer Conference, Tehran, Iran, 1–2 July 2009; pp. 564–569. [CrossRef]
40. Qi, F.; Zhou, H. Research of Image Compression Based on Quantum BP Network. *Indones. J. Electr. Eng. Comput. Sci.* **2014**, *12*, 197–205.
41. Du, S.; Yan, Y.; Ma, Y. Quantum-Accelerated Fractal Image Compression: An Interdisciplinary Approach. *IEEE Signal Process. Lett.* **2015**, *22*, 499–503. [CrossRef]
42. Jiang, N.; Lu, X.; Hu, H.; Dang, Y.; Cai, Y. A Novel Quantum Image Compression Method Based on JPEG. *Int. J. Theor. Phys.* **2018**, *57*, 611–636. [CrossRef]
43. Pang, C.Y.; Zhou, R.G.; Hu, B.Q.; Hu, W.; El-Rafei, A. Signal and image compression using quantum discrete cosine transform. *Inform. Sci.* **2019**, *473*, 121–141. [CrossRef]
44. Dai, J.Y.; Ma, Y.; Zhou, N.R. Quantum multi-image compression-encryption scheme based on quantum discrete cosine transform and 4D hyper-chaotic Henon map. *Quantum Inf. Process* **2021**, *20*, 246. [CrossRef]
45. Ma, Y.; Zhou, N.R. Quantum color image compression and encryption algorithm based on Fibonacci transform. *Quantum Inf. Process* **2023**, *22*, 39. [CrossRef]
46. Wang, H.; Tan, J.; Huang, Y.; Zheng, W. Quantum image compression with autoencoders based on parameterized quantum circuits. *Quantum Inf. Process* **2024**, *23*, 41. [CrossRef]
47. Ji, X.; Liu, Q.; Huang, S.; Chen, A.; Wu, S. Image Compression and Reconstruction Based on Quantum Network. *arXiv* **2024**, arXiv:2404.11994.
48. Haque, E.; Paul, M. BLOCK-WISE COMPRESSION OF THE QUANTUM GRAY-SCALE IMAGE USING LOSSY PREPARATION APPROACH. 2024. Available online: https://www.researchgate.net/profile/Md-Ershadul-Haque-3/publication/379894430_BLOCK-WISE_COMPRESSION_OF_THE_QUANTUM_GRAY-SCALE_IMAGE_USING_LOSSY_PREPARATION_APPROACH/links/66206bf243f8df018d163d27/BLOCK-WISE-COMPRESSION-OF-THE-QUANTUM-GRAY-SCALE-IMAGE-USING-LOSSY-PREPARATION-APPROACH.pdf (accessed on 12 July 2024).
49. Li, H.-S.; Qingxin, Z.; Lan, S.; Shen, C.-Y.; Zhou, R.; Mo, J. Image storage, retrieval, compression and segmentation in a quantum system. *Quantum Inf. Process* **2013**, *12*, 2269–2290. [CrossRef]
50. Brayton, R.K.; Sangiovanni-Vincentelli, A.; McMullen, C.; Hachtel, G. *Log Minimization Algorithms VLSI Synth*; Kluwer Academic Publishers: Dordrecht, The Netherlands, 1984.
51. Amankwah, M.G.; Camps, D.; Bethel, E.W.; Van Beeumen, R.; Perciano, T. Quantum pixel representations and compression for N-dimensional images. *Sci. Rep.* **2022**, *12*, 7712. [CrossRef] [PubMed]

52. Haque, M.E.; Paul, M.; Ulhaq, A.; Debnath, T. Advanced quantum image representation and compression using a DCT-EFRQI approach. *Sci. Rep.* **2023**, *13*, 4129. [CrossRef] [PubMed] [PubMed Central]
53. Mastriani, M. Quantum image processing: The pros and cons of the techniques for the internal representation of the image. A reply to: A comment on "Quantum image processing?". *Quantum Inf. Process.* **2020**, *19*, 156. [CrossRef]

MDPI AG
Grosspeteranlage 5
4052 Basel
Switzerland
Tel.: +41 61 683 77 34

Computers Editorial Office
E-mail: computers@mdpi.com
www.mdpi.com/journal/computers

www.ingramcontent.com/pod-product-compliance
Lightning Source LLC
Chambersburg PA
CBHW061612220926
51850CB00005B/489
9783725857838